& Graham's
UCTION TO
NEUROPATHOLOGY

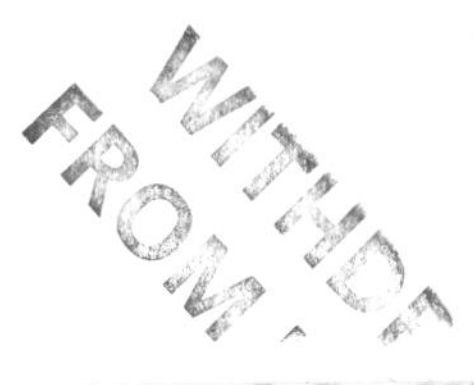

Adams & Graham's

INTRODUCTION TO NEUROPATHOLOGY

THIRD EDITION

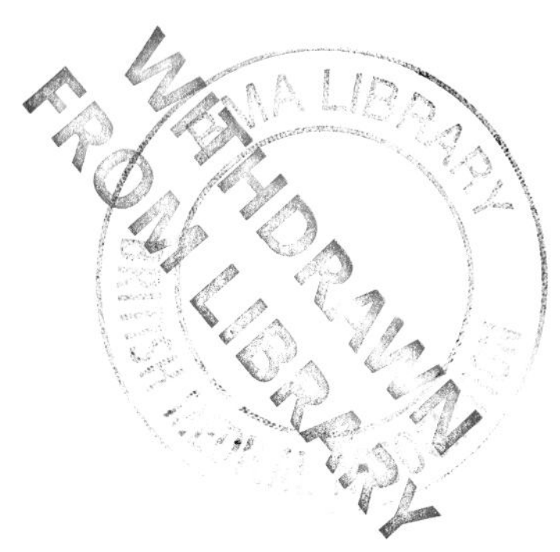

David I Graham
Professor of Neuropathology, Division of Clinical Neuroscience, University of Glasgow, Southern General Hospital, Glasgow, UK

James A R Nicoll
Professor of Neuropathology, Division of Clinical Neurosciences, University of Southampton, Southampton General Hospital, Southampton, UK

Ian Bone
Professor of Neurology, Division of Clinical Neuroscience, Institute of Neurological Sciences, Southern General Hospital, Glasgow, UK

Hodder Arnold

A MEMBER OF THE HODDER HEADLINE GROUP

First published in Great Britain in 1988 by Churchill Livingstone
Second edition 1994
This third edition published in 2006 by
Hodder Arnold, an imprint of Hodder Education, a member of the Hodder Headline Group,
338 Euston Road, London NW1 3BH

http://www.hoddereducation.com

Distributed in the United States of America by
Oxford University Press Inc.,
198 Madison Avenue, New York, NY10016
Oxford is a registered trademark of Oxford University Press

British Library Cataloguing in Publication Data
A catalogue record for this book is available from the British Library

Library of Congress Cataloging-in-Publication Data
A catalog record for this book is available from the Library of Congress

ISBN-10 0 340 81197 8
ISBN-13 978 0 340 81197 9

1 2 3 4 5 6 7 8 9 10

Commissioning Editor: Philip Shaw
Project Editor: Heather Fyfe
Production Controller: Karen Tate
Cover Designer: Laura de Grasse

Typeset in 9.5/12 Rotis serif by Charon Tec Ltd (A Macmillan Company), Chennai, India
www.charontec.com
Printed and bound in Great Britain by CPI Bath

CONTENTS

CONTRIBUTORS

Professor Jeanne E Bell
Department of Pathology (Neuropathology)
Western General Hospital
Edinburgh, UK

Dr Marjorie Black
Department of Forensic Medicine and Science
University of Glasgow
Glasgow, UK

Professor Ian Bone
Department of Neurology
Institute of Neurological Sciences
Southern General Hospital
Glasgow, UK

Professor David I Graham
Academic Unit of Neuropathology
Division of Clinical Neuroscience
Southern General Hospital
Glasgow, UK

Professor Donald M Hadley
Department of Neuroradiology
Institute of Neurological Sciences
Southern General Hospital
Glasgow, UK

Dr Tobias Hatter
Department of Forensic Medicine and Science
University of Glasgow
Glasgow, UK

Dr Jean W Keeling
Consultant Paediatric Pathologist
Royal Hospital for Sick Children
Edinburgh, UK

Professor James A R Nicoll
Department of Pathology
Division of Clinical Neurosciences
University of Southampton
Southampton General Hospital
Southampton, UK

Dr Robin Reid
Department of Pathology
Western Infirmary
Glasgow, UK

Dr Fiona Roberts
Department of Pathology
Western Infirmary
Glasgow, UK

Dr Susan Robinson
Department of Neuropathology
Institute of Neurological Sciences
Southern General Hospital
Glasgow, UK

Dr Colin Smith
School of Clinical and Molecular Medicine
Department of Pathology
Western General Hospital
Edinburgh, UK

FOREWORD

Previous editions of *Introduction to Neuropathology* have served as well-travelled portals of entry into neuropathology. Rather battered and much-thumbed copies still sit on the shelves of many clinical and basic neuroscience departments. It is a book that I have recommended to general histopathologists, neurologists, neurosurgeons in training and medical students with an inkling of interest in neuropathology: slim and light enough to carry around in a briefcase, readable and inexpensive. It is also very practical and can be used to guide the neophyte in cutting and interpreting the appearances of brain slices, and even more experienced pathologists in the differential diagnosis of neurological disease on microscopy.

Over the dozen or so years that have elapsed since the publication of the 2nd edition of this text there have been major advances in neuropathology. Our understanding and approach to the diagnosis of neurodegenerative diseases have undergone radical changes, the classification of brain neoplasms has been through several revisions (and the methods and criteria that we use for their diagnosis have been modified accordingly), and molecular genetic advances have had a substantial impact on almost all aspects of neuropathology.

The resurrection of *Introduction to Neuropathology* is therefore very welcome. Whilst the book has been renamed to reflect the major contributions of Hume Adams and David Graham to previous editions, the authorship of the current edition combines the experience of one of those founding editors with chapters from several new contributors, who have used their particular skills and expertise to strengthen the book still further. The chapters on diseases of the bony coverings of the central nervous system and on medicolegal aspects of neuropathology will be particularly welcomed by many readers. As noted in the preface to this edition, the book has also benefited from the feedback of many trainees, both past and present.

I have no doubt that this edition will be even more popular than its predecessors. The authors are to be congratulated on producing a well-focused, excellent neuropathology book that should still the appetite of some but will whet the appetite of the more inquiring and ambitious.

Professor Seth Love
Department of Neuropathology
Institute of Clinical Sciences
Frenchay Hospital
Bristol
UK

PREFACE

With the increasing use of information technology it might have been assumed that the traditional book format would become less often consulted due to the vast amount of information available on-line. Apparently, this is not so: rather, it would appear that both forms of information are complementary.

Perhaps, therefore, it was not too much of a surprise to be approached with a view to producing a third edition of *Introduction to Neuropathology* originally published in 1988 and subsequently in 1994. The lengthy interval between the second edition and now clearly indicated the need for a comprehensive rewrite of the book rather than simply editing it. However, in order to retain the spirit and purpose of the previous editions we have changed the title to honor the major contribution made by our Emeritus predecessor Professor J Hume Adams. We are grateful for his continuing support and encouragement.

The principal aims of the book have remained unchanged. They are to provide sufficient information about the more common and important disorders of the nervous system for doctors in training and basic scientists whose investigations require a human context and clinico-pathological correlation. We have endeavored to provide an account of fact which reflects recent advances in knowledge. As always the views and comments and criticisms of those trainees rotating through our departments have been noted and considered in compiling this new edition. We are thankful for these.

Careful consideration has been given to the scope of this book as there are already specialized reference texts on most, if not of all, of the topics covered in our various chapters, e.g. cerebrovascular disease, infections, tumors, trauma. The problem-based approach, modern in concept, initially seemed an attractive one but transpired to be a challenge too far. Thus we have opted for a more traditional style recognizing that the diagnostic needs of the clinician are different from those of the laboratory-based practitioner. By including more comparative imaging, we hope to have achieved a compromise thereby satisfying the needs of trainees in histopathology and the specialist sub-divisions of neuropathology, pediatric pathology and forensic medicine as well as those of our clinical colleagues in neurology, neurosurgery and psychiatry. Where there are close working relationships between clinical and basic neurosciences, we know from past experience that previous editions of *Introduction to Neuropathology* have been greatly appreciated by PhD students and research assistants.

The 18 chapters of both the second and third editions have been expanded to 21 in recognition of advances made and the need for a more comprehensive text which truly reflects the service normally provided by a regional neuropathology unit. Perhaps this is best illustrated by changes to the previous chapters on 'Metabolic and deficiency disorders' and 'Intoxications', with the creation of two new chapters encompassing peroxisomal and mitochondrial disorders and lysosomal diseases and the leukodystrophies. Similarly, there has been an adjustment of the titles and content of the previous chapters on 'System disorders' and 'Aging and the dementias'; the former now having been expanded into a new chapter on 'Neurodegenerative diseases, movement disorders and system degenerations'. Again, to reflect the practice in the west of

Scotland two new chapters have been commissioned. We are delighted that Dr Robin Reid has written on 'Disorders of the bony coverings of the brain and spine' and that Drs Marjorie Black and Tobias Hatter have provided a text on the 'The law and forensic neuropathology'.

We are also very grateful for the new authors who have been recruited to either co-author or rewrite existing chapters. Principal amongst these are Professor Donald Hadley on 'Structural and functional neuroanatomy', Professor Jeanne Bell and Dr Jean Keeling on 'Developmental and perinatal disorders', Dr Colin Smith on 'Tumors and paraneoplastic syndromes', Dr Susan Robinson on 'Skeletal muscle and peripheral nerve', and Dr Fiona Roberts on 'The orbit'. We are grateful to them all for their contributions. We are also grateful to Dr Will Maxwell, Senior Lecturer in Anatomy, Faculty of Biomedical Life Sciences, University of Glasgow and to Dr Willie Stewart, Department of Neuropathology, Southern General Hospital, Glasgow for providing illustrations and/or figures and advice on both the content and the style of the book.

We would emphasize that this text is an introduction to the discipline and hopefully will provide sufficient interest to foster a closer working relationship between basic and clinical neurosciences within the clinical disciplines and a better understanding of clinico-pathological correlations, and the difficulties encountered in daily practice.

It is certainly our experience that the development of closer working relationships between pathologist and clinician can greatly improve the need and consent rate for autopsy and maximize the potential of surgically derived specimens whether for diagnostic or research purposes.

Our sincere thanks are to those who have been invaluable in the planning, execution and completion of this book. In particular, to Mrs Marisa Hughes and Mrs Sandra Greenshields, secretaries; Mrs Janice Stewart and Mrs Mary Ann MacKinnon, research technicians; the enormous help over many years of Mr J Lynch, senior chief biomedical scientist in this department, and his staff; and the willing assistance of Mr A McIlroy, Head of the Department of Medical Illustration, Southern General Hospital and his staff, in particular Mrs Christine Prentice, medical photographer, and Mr John Main and Marian Littlejohn, medical artists. Last, but not least, we are indebted to the encouragement, support and patience of Dr Jo Koster, commissioning editor for medical and health sciences, Hodder Arnold Publishers and her staff; in particular, Miss Heather Fyfe, project editor, who has steered us to completion.

D I Graham
J A R Nicoll
I Bone
April 2006

ACKNOWLEDGEMENTS

We are indebted to Dr J Hume Adams, Emeritus Professor of Neuropathology at The University of Glasgow and to Hodder Arnold for permission to reproduce illustrations – modified or otherwise – used previously in the second edition of *An Introduction to Neuropathology* by J Hume Adams and D I Graham. These are Figures 1.12, 3.2, 3.4b, 3.6, 3.7, 3.8a and b, 3.9, 3.10, 3.12, 3.16a, 4.2, 4.7, 4.13a and b, 5.1, 5.2, 5.3, 5.4, 5.12, 5.17, 5.18, 5.19b, 5.25, 5.27, 5.30, 6.6, 6.7, 6.11, 8.27, 9.9a, 10.2, 10.11, 10.14, 11.6, 15.34, 15.45, and 16.35.

Professor Jeanne Bell and Dr Jean Keeling are grateful to Dr Roger Malcomson for assistance with some of the illustrations used in Chatper 14 and to Ms Angela Penman for having prepared the manuscript.

LIST OF ABBREVIATIONS

ABC	avidin–biotin complex
Ach	acetylcholine
ACTH	adrenocorticotrophic hormone
AD	Alzheimer's disease
ADEM	acute disseminated encephalomyelitis
ADH	antidiuretic hormone
ADP	adenosine diphosphate
AFP	alpha-fetoprotein
AHLE	acute hemorrhagic leukoencephalopathy
AIDP	acute inflammatory demyelinating polyradiculopathy
AIDS	acquired immunodeficiency syndrome
ALD	adrenoleukodystrophy
ALS	amyotrophic lateral sclerosis
AMAN	acute motor axonal neuropathy
AMN	adrenomyeloneuropathy
AMSAN	acute motor–sensory axonal neuropathy
ANA	anti-nuclear antibody
APOE	apolipoprotein E gene
APP	amyloid precursor protein (also named β-amyloid precursor protein)
ATP	adenosine triphosphate
ATR	atypical teratoid/rhabdoid tumor
BBB	blood–brain barrier
BDNF	brain-derived neurotrophic factor
BMAA	β-*N*-methylamino-L-alanine
BOAA	β-*N*-oxalylamino-L-alanine
BRI	protein of gene BRI which is related to the British familial form of Dementia
BSE	bovine spongiform encephalopathy
CAA	cerebral amyloid angiopathy
CADASIL	cerebral autosomal dominant arteriopathy with subcortical infarcts and leukoencephalopathy
c-ANCA	anti-neutrophil cytoplasmic antibody
CBD	corticobasal degeneration
CBF	cerebral blood flow
CEA	carcinoembryonic antigen
CGH	comparative genomic hybridizaition
CIDP	chronic inflammatory demyelinating neuropathy
CJD	Creutzfeldt–Jakob disease
CK	creatine kinase (same as CPK)
CMAP	compound motor action potential
CMV	cytomegalovirus
CPK	creatine phosphokinase (same as CK)
CPM	central pontine myelinolysis
CPP	cerebral perfusion pressure
CSF	cerebrospinal fluid
CT	computed tomography

DFP	di-isopropylfluorophosphonate
DIG	desmoplastic infantile ganglioglioma
DLB	dementia with Lewy bodies
DLBCL	diffuse large B-cell lymphoma
DMPK	dystrophy myotonic protein kinase gene
DNA	deoxyribonucleic acid
DNET	dysembryoplastic neuroepithelial tumor
DRPLA	dentatorubropallidoluysian atrophy
EAE	experimental allergic encephalitis
EBV	Epstein–Barr virus
EMG	electromyography
EMNL	extranodal marginal node lymphoma
EOM	external ocular muscle
ESR	erythrocyte sedimentation rate
FACS	fluorescence-activated cell sorter
FAE	fetal alcohol effect
FAI	fatal accident enquiry
FAS	fetal alcohol syndrome
FGF	fibroblast growth factor
FGFR3	fibroblast growth factor receptor 3
FISH	fluorescence *in situ* hybridization
fMRI	functional MRI
FSH	follicle-stimulating hormone
FTD	frontotemporal dementia
FTDP-17	frontotemporal dementia with parkinsonism linked to chromosome 17
GBS	Guillain–Barré syndrome
GFAP	glial fibrillary acidic protein
GH	growth hormone
GOM	granular osmiophilic material
GPI	general paralysis of the insane
HAART	highly active anti-retroviral therapy
HAM	HTLV-1-associated myleopathy
H&E	hematoxylin and eosin stain
HCl	hydrochloric acid
HIE	hypoxic/ischemic encephalopathy
HLA	human leukocyte antigen
HMPAO	hexamethyl-propyleneamine oxine
HTLV-1	human T-cell lymphotropic virus-1
H/VG	hematoxylin/van Gieson stain
ICH	intracranial hemorrhage
ICP	intracranial pressure
IHC	immunohistochemistry
IL	interleukin
ISH	*in situ* hybridization
JC	Jamestown Canyon (virus)
KSS	Kearns–Sayre syndrome
LCH	Langerhans cell histiocytosis
LFB	Luxol fast blue
LH	luteinizing hormone
MAG	myelin-associated glycoprotein
MCI	mild cognitive impairment
MELAS	mitochondrial encephalomyopathy lactic acidosis and stroke-like episodes
MEM	mini-chromosomal maintenance
MGMT	O^6-methylguanine methyltransferase
MHC	major histocompatibility complex
MND	motor neuron disease
MOG	myelin oligodendrocyte glycoprotein
MPTP	1-methyl-4-phenyl-1,2,3,6 – tetrahydropyridine
MRI	magnetic resonance imaging
MRS	magnetic resonance spectroscopy
MS	multiple sclerosis
MSA	multiple system atrophy
MSB	Martius scarlet blue
MtDNA	mitochondrial DNA
NADH-Tr	nicotinamide adenine dinucleotide–tetrazolium reductase
NAHI	non-accidental head injury
NALD	neonatal adrenoleukodystrophy
NCAM	nerve cell adhesion molecule
NCS	nerve conduction study
NDD	neurodegenerative disease

NDNA	nuclear DNA
NMDA	*N*-methyl-D-aspartate
NSE	neuron-specific enolase
NTD	neural tube defect
PABN	polyadenylate binding protein nuclear gene
PAS	periodic acid–Schiff stain
PCNSL	primary CNS lymphoma
PCR	polymerase chain reaction
PET	positron emission tomography
PKU	phenylketonuria
PLAP	placental alkaline phosphatase
PML	progressive multifocal leukoencephalopathy
PNET	primitive neuroectodermal tumor
PNS	peripheral nervous system
PRL	prolactin
PROMM	proximal myotonic myopathy
PrP	protease resistant peptide
PSP	progressive supranuclear palsy
PTAH	phosphotungstic acid hematoxylin
PTHrP	parathyroid hormone related protein
PXA	pleomorphic xanthroastrocytoma
RANK	receptor activator of the NFκB ligand
REAL	Revised European–American Classification of Lymphoid Neoplasms
SAH	subarachnoid hemorrhage
SCA	spinocerebellar ataxia
SFT	solitary fibrous tumor
SIDS	sudden infant death syndrome
SLE	systemic lupus erythematosus
SMN1	survival motor neuron 1 gene
SMON	subacute myelo-optic neuropathy
SNAP	sensory nerve action potential
SOD	superoxide dismutase
SOD1	superoxide dismutase-1 gene
SPECT	single photon emission computed tomography
SSPE	subacute sclerosing panencephalitis
SUDEP	sudden unexpected death in epilepsy
SUDI	sudden infant death in infancy
TAI	traumatic axonal injury
TB	tuberculosis
TBI	traumatic brain injury
TGF	transforming growth factor
TIA	transient ischemic attack
TNF-α	tumor necrosis factor alpha
TOCP	tri-orthocresyl phosphate
TSE	transmissible spongiform encephalopathy
TSH	thyroid-stimulating hormone
TTF1	thyroid transcription factor 1
VGCCA	voltage-gated calcium channel antibodies
VHL	von Hippel–Lindau disease
VLCFA	very long chain fatty acid
VZV	varicella zoster virus

CHAPTER 1

INTRODUCTION

David I Graham

BACKGROUND

The central nervous system (CNS) is complex, and its proper study requires special investigations, including the use of various staining methods, electron microscopy, and the application of immunohistochemistry and molecular techniques. Nonetheless, many of the principles of general pathology are relevant, so that a training in general pathology is advantageous to a proper appreciation of neuropathology.

Disease of the CNS is often manifest by the signs and symptoms of focal neurological deficit. It is for this reason that some knowledge of structure, function and metabolism is important. The ability to localize and better characterize lesions *in vivo* has improved enormously in the last decade with high resolution computed tomographic scanning (CT), magnetic resonance imaging (MRI), single photon emission computed tomography (SPECT) and positron emission tomography (PET). In spite of these advances, however, there remains a need for traditional methods such as examination of cerebrospinal fluid (CSF), the microscopic examination of biopsy specimens, and autopsies in order to achieve accurate clinico-pathological correlation. These mainstays of clinical neuropathology are now run, however, in parallel with techniques that include tissue culture and sampling of specimens for neurochemical analysis. As the fundamental nature of disease becomes better understood, so the importance of genetics and molecular pathology become increasingly apparent. This might suggest that the role of the neuropathologist is limited, but on the contrary he/she is in a singular position to make full use of the material and to help realize its full potential.

In this introductory chapter brief comment will be made on certain technical points, some of which have been dealt with in greater detail elsewhere, and a 'Further reading' section is given near the end of this book.

TECHNIQUES IN NEUROPATHOLOGY

The pathologist should see the clinical records so that the type of neurological illness can be determined and, if necessary, further advice sought from a neuropathologist. It can then be decided in advance if some brain tissue has to be retained unfixed for microbiological or neurochemical studies, the spinal cord and posterior ganglia require to be removed, and which, if any, muscles and peripheral nerves have to be taken for histological examination.

Health and Safety in the practice of autopsies has achieved considerable awareness during the last two decades in part due to the advent of the acquired immunodeficiency syndrome (AIDS) and more recently because of the transmissible spongiform encephalopathies (TSEs). The potential hazards of serum positivity for HBsAg and tuberculous meningitis have long been recognized but to these must now be added the extra risks associated with multiple drug resistance, infectious complications of chemotherapy and transplantation and intravenous drug abuse. Therefore, before starting an autopsy the pathologist must assess the potential hazard and in the context determine if the autopsy would in fact be high-risk and equally important if the mortuary is accredited with up to date codes of practice for the prevention of infections in clinical laboratories, aspects of which include the facilities, protective equipment and procedures.

The most common human TSE is the sporadic form of Creutzfeldt–Jakob disease (CJD) with a frequency of about 1 per million of the worldwide population per year. This would suggest that a department of neuropathology in a regional neuroscience center serving a population of about 3 million is likely to either undertake such a high-risk autopsy or to perform brain cut about three times each year. Special techniques have been developed for both procedures for which codes of practice are available in approved facilities. In addition to CJD there has been considerable awareness of the various iatrogenic forms of CJD (growth hormone treated, dural and corneal implants) and most recently of new variant CJD and its association with bovine spongiform encephalopathy.

Essential components of the risk assessment as to whether or not to undertake an autopsy on high-risk patients are the decontamination procedures and the codes of practice for injury (sharps) and unexpected exposure (meningitis).

Depending upon the clinical information and the radiological and laboratory investigations, the pathologist should be prepared to take samples of brain and other tissues for neurochemical studies, samples of CSF or other cystic fluids for microbiological study and samples for electron microscopy. The smooth conduct of these complex autopsies therefore requires a range of facilities that include the requisite specimen container methods for rapid freezing and storage at −80°C and a range of fixatives to optimize immunohistochemistry, molecular biological techniques and ultrastructure.

REMOVAL OF THE BRAIN AND SPINAL CORD

The pathologist should remove the brain – or at least witness the procedure – so that the tightness of the dura, the presence and volume of blood in either the extradural or subdural spaces can be ascertained. A saw cut through the calvaria should be made immediately above the supraorbital ridge and continued horizontally round the skull to the occiput. The dura should not be breached, although this may be difficult when it is tightly adherent to the skull as is common in infants and the elderly. The skull cap can be prised loose by twisting a T-shaped chisel along the saw cut and if necessary, this can be tapped gently with a mallet if the skull has not been completely cut through. Force, however, must be avoided as this may produce damage to the bone that might be misinterpreted as a fracture. If the dura is tightly adherent to the skull, a malleable retractor is a useful means of separating the two. The superior sagittal sinus is now opened and inspected to establish whether or not it contains thrombus. The dura is then incised along the line of the saw cut, preferably with curved scissors, taking care not to damage the underlying cortex. The tenseness of the dura is established at this stage. The falx is freed from the cribriform plate and the dura retracted to allow inspection of the bridging veins draining into the sagittal sinus. The frontal poles are then retracted gently and the rostral cranial nerves, the pituitary stalk and the internal carotid arteries cut. The attachment of the tentorium cerebelli to the skull is then incised to expose the structures of the posterior fossa. The next stage is to divide the remaining cranial nerves and the vertebral arteries as they enter the skull. The upper end of the spinal cord is transected and the brain gently removed from the skull taking care not to damage the brainstem.

If an abnormality in the lower brainstem or upper cervical cord is suspected, a central wedge of occipital bone should be removed along with the spines and the laminae of the upper cervical vertebrae, so that the brain and the upper segments of the spinal cord can be removed in one block – the Greenfield procedure.

The spinal cord may be removed by either an anterior or posterior approach. Advantages of the anterior approach are that the autopsy can be carried out through a single midline ventral incision, and the dorsal root ganglia and the vertebral arteries in the transverse processes of the cervical vertebrae are more easily identifiable. After the cord has been exposed fully, it should be removed within its dural sheaf. Angulation of the cord during its removal must be avoided since this can cause remarkable distortion of its intrinsic architecture (the so-called toothpaste effect). In some situations it is desirable to remove the vertebral column en bloc and to fix the cord *in situ*.

NEONATAL AUTOPSY

Because of the nature of the disease processes presenting in the neonatal period, as well as the physical characteristics of the brain and skull at this stage of development, the procedure for removal and handling of the brain requires a separate comment. Basically, the aim is to allow *in situ* inspection of the brain, dura and great blood vessels, to establish the sites of any traumatic tearing or hemorrhage, and to allow assessment of any developmental abnormalities in the relationship of brain, skull and meninges.

The calvaria is opened with scissors along the sutures. The sagittal suture is opened on each side of the midline and the cuts are extended laterally into the lambdoid and coronal sutures. Towards the base of the skull these cuts are then curved towards each other so that the flaps of skull and dura can be sprung out, petal-like. Gentle manipulation of the head and brain can then disclose the great blood vessels and the dura and its reflection. The frontal bones can be sprung out by scissors cuts made in the midline and base, and greater exposure obtained. The brain is then removed in the sequence described for the adult after dividing and freeing the falx. In suspected abnormalities of the posterior fossa, the foramen magnum and of the cervical spine, and in hydrocephalus, the posterior fossa and cervical spine require to be opened first.

The neonatal brain is very soft to touch and so great care is required in its handing and removal. This can be accomplished by an assistant positioning the head upright during removal, care being taken to support the brain at all times. Removal of the brain under water has some support. After removal, handling must be kept to a minimum, and the brain should be weighed after immersion in a previously weighed container of fixative. As suspension by the basilar artery is inappropriate for neonatal brains, several flotation methods have been devised to overcome distortion. These include fixation in formalin using a mattress of cotton wool, flotation in 20% formalin, and fixation in 10% formalin to which glacial acidic acid has been added until the brain begins to float. This last method has the advantage of providing a firmer brain for dissection and does not jeopardize routine staining procedures.

EXAMINATION OF RELATED STRUCTURES

Blood vessels

In cases of cerebrovascular disease the major extracranial arteries of the neck have to be examined. These should be dissected in one block rather than opened *in situ*. This is most easily done by exposing the arch of the aorta after opening the pericardium and then dissecting along its major branches. The block that is finally removed, therefore, consists of the arch of the aorta, the inominate artery, the common carotid arteries, the proximal parts of the external carotid arteries, the internal carotid arteries up to the base of the skull, the proximal parts of the subclavian arteries and the proximal parts of the vertebral artery to the point where they enter the foramina of the 6th cervical vertebra. After fixation the presence or absence of atheroma and/or occlusion can be assessed by serial transverse section. The cavernous portions of the carotid arteries should also be examined.

Base of the skull including the pituitary gland and the middle ear

Examination of the base of the skull depends on the type of lesion being sought. The dura, however, has to be stripped from the bone to identify fractures and to allow examination of the various air and venous sinuses and the middle ear. It may be necessary in certain cases to explore the contents of the orbits through the floor of the anterior cranial fossa.

The pituitary gland lies in the sella turcica (pituitary fossa) of the sphenoid bone bordered laterally by the thin-walled cavernous sinus, the siphon of the internal carotid artery, the III, IV and VI cranial nerves and ophthalmic–maxillary branches of the V nerve. Anteriorly, the fossa is formed by the anterior clinoid processes and posteriorly by a plate of bone called the dorsum sellae with superior bony projections called the posterior clinoid processes. The sellae turcica and pituitary gland are covered by a sheet of dura the diaphragma sella through which passes the pituitary stalk.

The gland may be approached posteriorly after the removal of the posterior clinoid processes and the dorsum sella by dissection of the diaphragma sella the gland then being free to be removed from the fossa or it may be removed en bloc by coronal cuts anterior and posterior to the clinoid processes and cuts in the lateral plane lateral to each cavernous sinus.

Examination of the middle ear

The middle ear lies within the petrous part of the temporal bone situated between the middle and posterior fossae. The lateral wall is formed mainly from the tympanic membrane and the roof is a thin plate of petrous temporal bone that separates it from the middle cranial fossa. The middle ear may be approached by de-roofing the middle ear cavity or by the en bloc removal of the petrous temporal bone after the dura has been stripped from the base of the skull.

Brain banks

It is increasingly recognized that advances in aspects of neurology, neurosurgery and psychiatry are dependent at least in part on the availability of samples of human brain. With the active support of various research councils and charities it has been possible to establish a network of UK, European and worldwide brain banks in which have been accrued portions of the nervous system of patients who have donated through living wills. Such facilities, among others, are available for patients with CJD, AIDS, Alzheimer's disease, Parkinson's disease, motor neuron disease, multiple sclerosis and muscle diseases. The death of a patient enrolling in such a scheme is usually notified to the regional neuropathologist who facilitates autopsy and the onward transport of appropriate materials to the brain bank usually on the same day as death.

Fixation

It is difficult to obtain precise information about the distribution of any lesion of the brain if it is cut in the unfixed state. Furthermore, some lesions, such as small foci of demyelination or a recent infarct, may not be identifiable in the unfixed brain, even by an experienced neuropathologist. Portions of the unfixed brain may of course have to be removed for bacteriological studies or neurochemical analysis. In cases of massive subarachnoid hemorrhage, it is advisable to dissect the arteries at the base of the brain prior to fixation and to wash away the blood clot with normal saline in an attempt to identify any saccular aneurysm or other vascular malformation.

After preliminary observations have been made, the brain should be fixed intact as soon as possible after removal from the skull. If it is allowed to lie on the dissecting table, even for a short time, it will become permanently deformed. The brain should be placed in a 10-L polythene bucket containing neutral 4% (10% of 40%) formaldehyde in normal saline. After the brain has been immersed, a paperclip attached to a piece of string tied across the top of the bucket can be slipped under the basilar artery and the brain allowed to hang freely, care being taken to ensure that no surface of the brain is in contact with the bottom or sides of the bucket. Fixative should be changed after 3 days and then at weekly intervals. The spinal cord still within the dura is best fixed vertically in a large measuring cylinder.

Increasingly, consent is being given for head-only autopsies or for the retention of sufficient samples of the brain to achieve a diagnosis, the remainder of the specimen being returned to the body for the funeral. Although still desirable practice, it is not always possible to retain the entire specimen and even if permission is given for this it is often the request to cut and examine it after only a few days fixation, again in order that the tissue not used for diagnostic purposes be returned to the body. Therefore, new working practices have had to be developed within neuropathology, each laboratory having to tailor its operating procedures to meet the requests of the consenting relatives and referring colleagues in pathology. Given this flexible approach and willingness to adapt to the changing circumstances together with protocols that ensure the proper sampling of the brain, it is still possible to achieve a high quality diagnostic service.

Dissection

If permitted the brain should be normally fixed for 3–4 weeks and then washed in running water for an hour or so prior to dissection. The plane in which the dissection is carried out depends to some extent on how best to correlate the morbid anatomy with the neuroradiological findings. In general, however, our standard procedure is to cut the cerebral hemispheres in the coronal plane, since we find this to be the most informative technique. Brain slices or blocks require to be fixed for a lesser time.

Prior to dissection the intact brain is examined for external abnormalities such as flattening of the convolutions, selective or generalized atrophy, thickening or other abnormalities of the meninges, vascular malformations, and tentorial or tonsillar herniations. Any focal abnormalities, such as areas of 'softening' are noted. Our initial procedure is to detach the hind brain from the cerebrum by transecting the upper pons. A further transverse section is made through the cerebral peduncles, to obtain a block of the midbrain including the aqueduct. A coronal cut is then made through the cerebral hemispheres at the level of the mamillary bodies, and the hemispheres cut into slices 1 cm thick with the aid of two angles made of brass. The brain knife should be sharp and of sufficient width and pulled smoothly across the brain. Sometimes a lesion in the cerebellum can best be displayed by a transverse cut, but it is usually more informative to separate the cerebellum from the brainstem by cutting through the cerebellar peduncles on each side. The hemispheres can then be cut at right angles to the folia and slightly nearer the vermis than the lateral border: this is the best method for demonstrating the folial pattern of the dentate nuclei. A further 1-cm thick slice of the lateral part of each hemisphere is then obtained by using the angle referred to above. A further cut is then made through the vermis. A series of transverse cuts is then made through the pons and medulla. Slices are laid out in a standard fashion so that any abnormalities, the size and shape of the ventricles, and the presence of any distortion and/or displacement of the midline structures can be identified easily (Fig. 1.1a–h).

The first step in examining the spinal cord is to open the dura in the midline along its dorsal and ventral aspects. Any external abnormalities are noted, including atrophy of nerve roots. A series of transverse cuts through the full thickness of the cord is then made and any intrinsic abnormalities noted. The ventral surface of the cord is easily identified by the single anterior spinal artery. Even if the cord has been damaged at post mortem, it is usually possible to identify the segments approximately by identifying the lowest large ventral root of the cervical plexus: this is usually T1.

There are occasions where the brain should be cut in the midline sagittal plane to demonstrate the third ventricle, the aqueduct and the pineal region and, increasingly, there is a need to cut the cerebral hemispheres in the horizontal plane in order to correlate appearances with CT scanning and magnetic resonance imaging (Fig. 1.2).

Block taking

Unless consented for research purposes the number of blocks and their location should be determined by the disease/disorder under study and whether the whole brain or only a part of it has been retained. In general, fewer samples are required if the disease is focal rather then multifocal or diffuse and the extent to which clinico-radiological-pathological correlations can be achieved from the available material. It is recommended that if there is uncertainty then the regional neuropathology center be contacted and the case discussed or arrangements

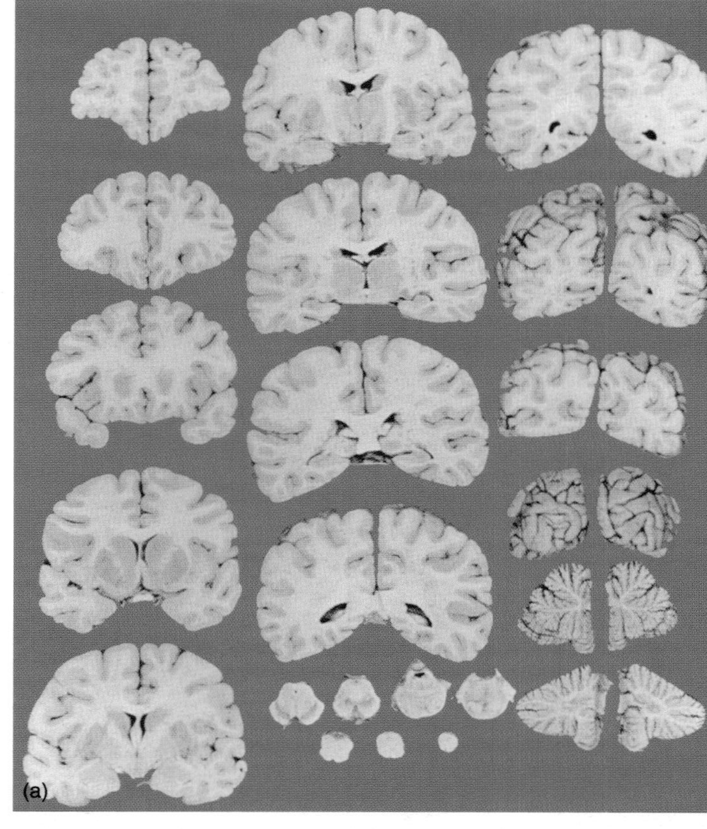
(a)

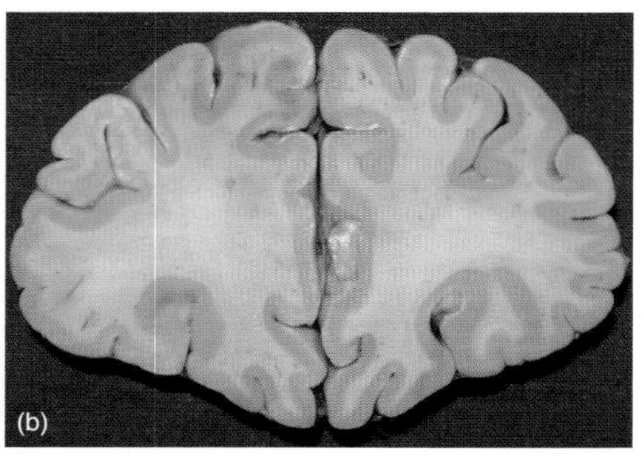
(b)

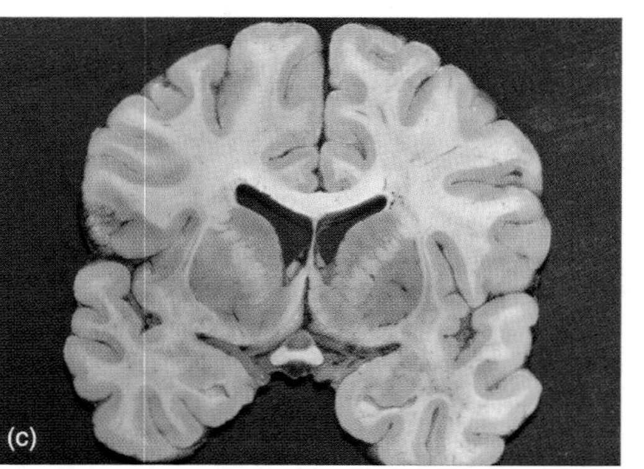
(c)

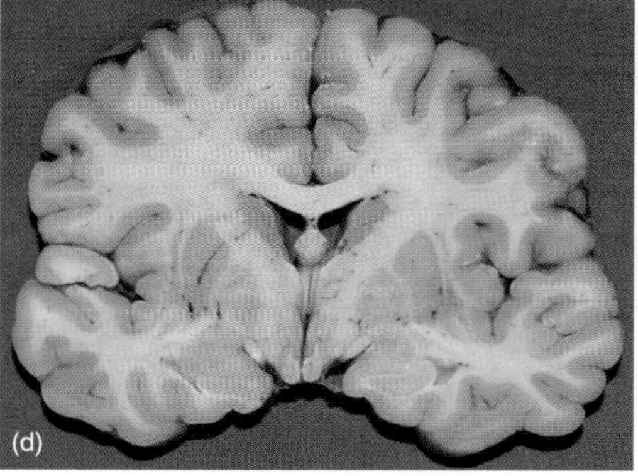
(d)

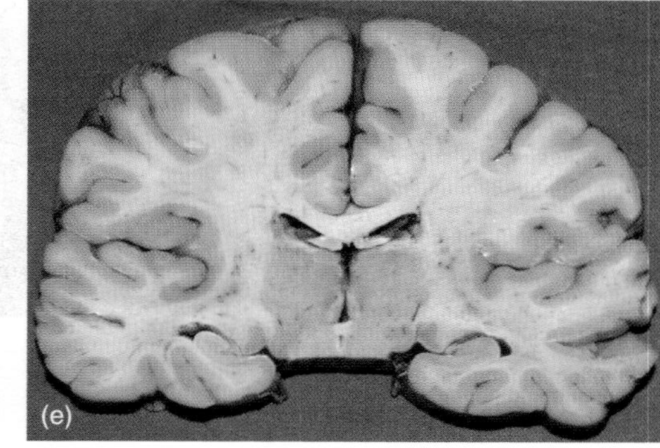
(e)

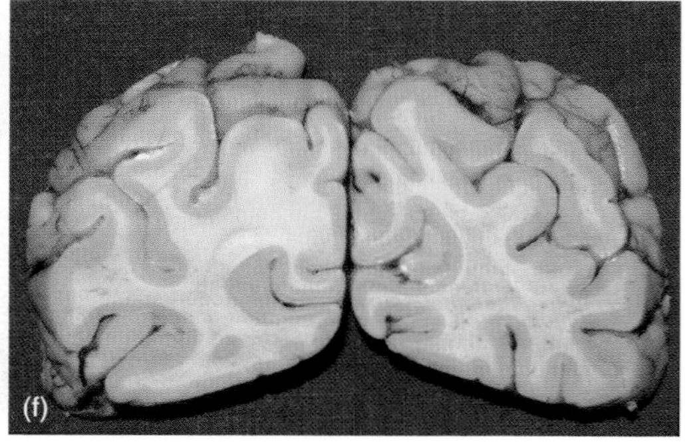
(f)

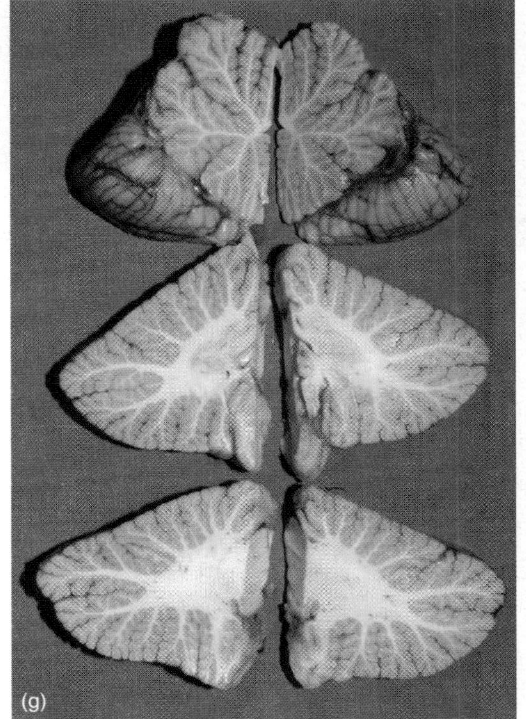

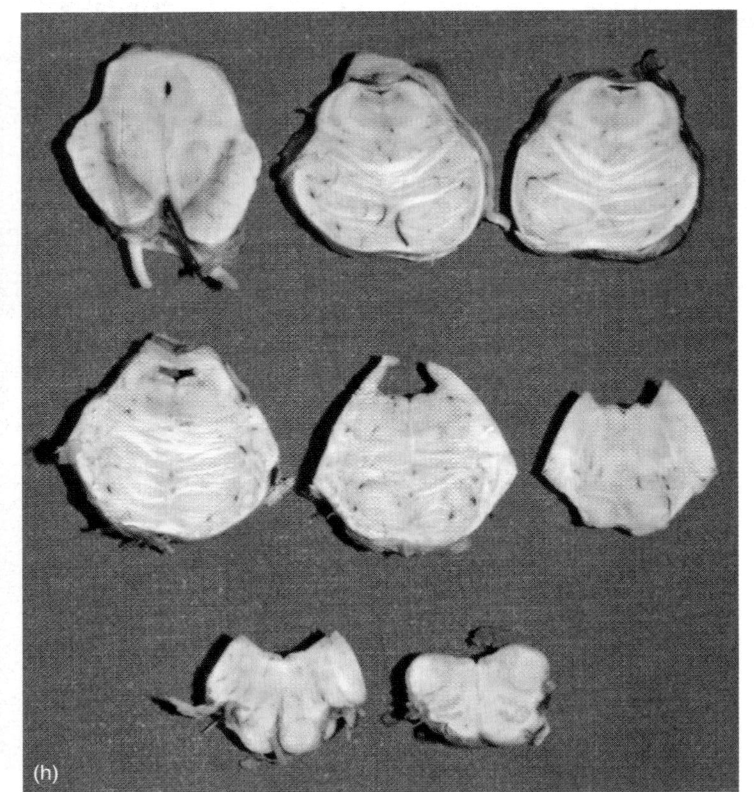

Figure 1.1 (a) Dissection of the brain. The brain laid out ready for inspection. (b) Coronal slice of normal brain at the level of the frontal lobes. (c) Coronal slice of normal brain at the level of the basal ganglia. (d) Coronal slice of normal brain at the level of the mamillary bodies. (e) Coronal slice of normal brain at the level of the lateral geniculate bodies. (f) Coronal slice of normal brain at the level of the occipital lobes. (g) Normal cerebellum. After bisection in the midline the hemispheres have been cut at right angles to the folial pattern on the upper surface of the specimen. (h) Normal brainstem. Horizontal slices have been cut at the levels of the midbrain, pons and medulla oblongata.

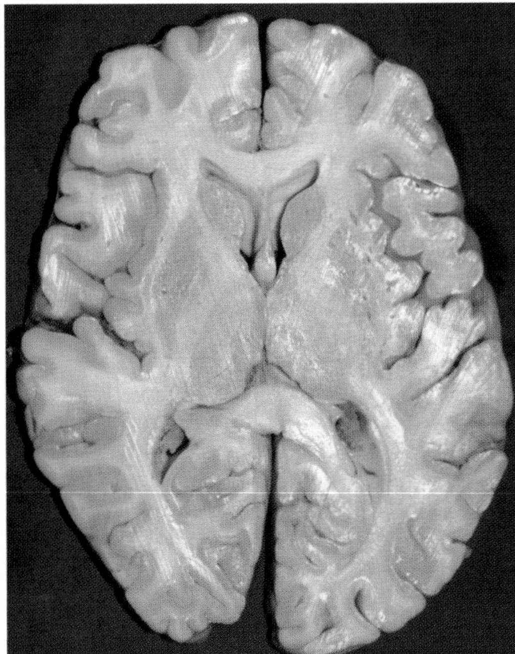

Figure 1.2 Horizontal slice of normal brain. This plane of sectioning allows good correlation with neuroimaging.

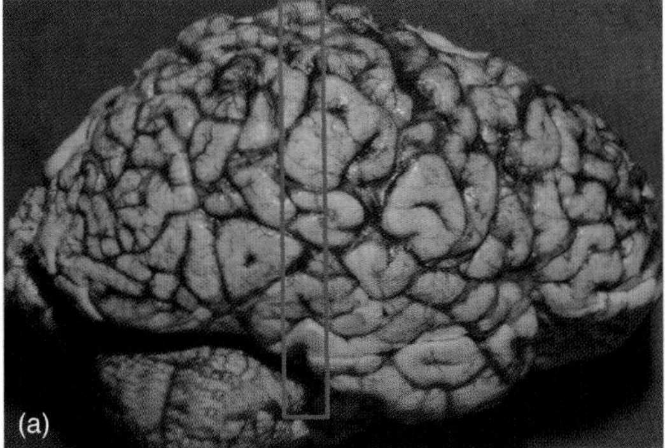

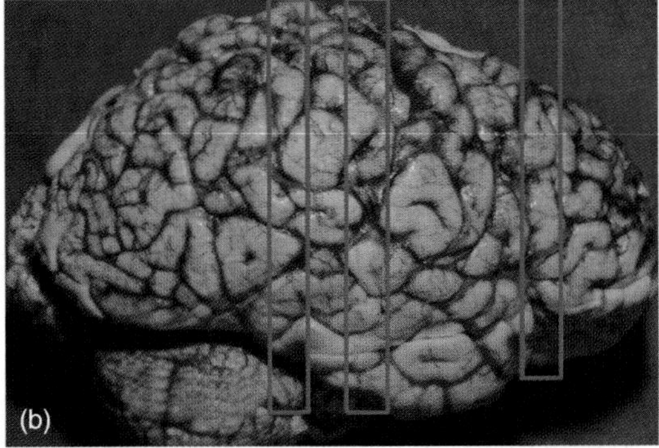

Figure 1.3 Surface markings of cerebral hemisphere for (a) minimal sampling (see Fig. 1.4) and (b) more extensive sampling (see Fig. 1.5) depending upon the nature of the presumed diffuse pathology.

be made for the neuropathologist to be in attendance at the time of autopsy. In any event it is helpful to know where to cut the unfixed brain from its surface markings in order to take blocks for minimal or more extensive sampling (Fig. 1.3a and b).

Focal pathologies include cerebrovascular disease, tumors and many infections and under these circumstances it might be appropriate to limit the sampling to only a few blocks for general screening (Fig. 1.4). On the other hand, a widely distributed multifocal pathology will require a larger number of blocks from more brain areas, in order to determine the full extent of the pathology, its nature and time course. In those cases in which the lesions are diffuse – metabolic encephalopathy, after certain types of head injury and the various neurodegenerative diseases including cases of dementia, movement disorder, sudden unexplained death in infancy or sudden unexpected death in epilepsy (Fig. 1.5).

The size, anatomical location and number of blocks which have been taken for microscopic examination should be recorded. It is often helpful to adopt some standard method for identifying from which side of the brain the blocks have been taken, e.g. by making in it a small hole or nick or a colored ink on all blocks taken from one or other hemisphere.

Examination of the autonomic nervous system

Detailed dissection of the entire system is seldom required, as usually an adequate sample for study can be obtained from the cervical sympathetic trunk together with the superior cervical ganglia, stellate ganglion and a portion of the vagus nerve including its inferior ganglion. The cervical sympathetic trunk lies beneath the prevertebral fascia and muscles

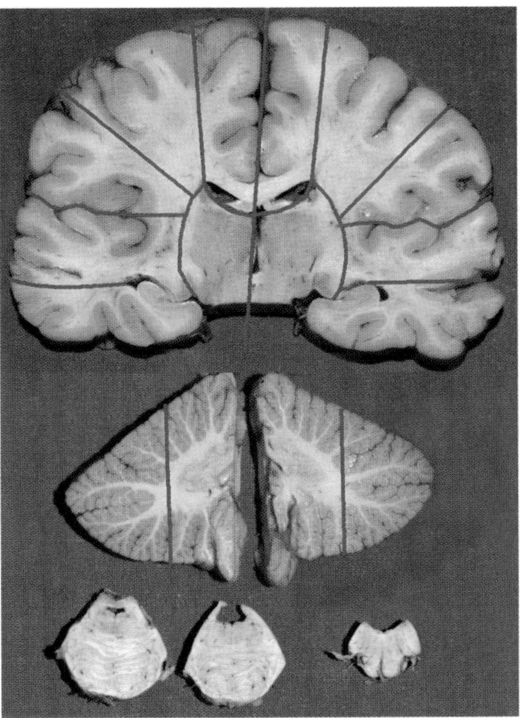

Figure 1.4 Minimum blocks taken for presumed diffuse pathology. Routine screening from coronal slice of both cerebral hemispheres at level of thalami (see Fig. 1.1e), to include the parasagittal cortex and corpus callosum, the boundary zone between the anterior and middle cerebral arteries in relation to the sides and depths of the intraparietal sulcus, the insula, hippocampus, and the thalamus including the internal capsule, the dentate nuclei of the cerebellum, and the brainstem at the levels of the midbrain, pons and medulla.

either side of the vertebral column immediately anterior to the neck of the ribs. Often difficult to identify, the best approach is an en-bloc removal so that each sample includes the cervical sympathetic trunk and the three ganglia although the inferior ganglion is often amalgamated with the first thoracic ganglion. The superior cervical ganglion is the largest and can be located ensheathed in loose connective tissue just below the point at which the vagus emerges from the skull, behind the glossopharyngeal and accessory nerves. The vagus nerve is easily recognized within the carotid sheath during the exploration of the common carotid artery.

Cranial and spinal nerves

There are 12 paired cranial nerves some of which have a mixed sensory and motor function others being purely motor or sensory. All, except the olfactory and the optic nerves, join the CNS at points within the brainstem.

Of the 31 pairs of spinal nerves, eight are cervical from C1 to C8, 12 are thoracic from T1 to T12, five are lumbar from L1 to L5, five are sacral from S1 to S5 and there is a single coccygeal nerve. Because of the differential growth rate between the spinal cord and the vertebral canal in the adult, the end of the spinal cord lies opposite the disc between the first and second lumbar vertebrae. As a result, the cord segments gradually move out of synchrony with their corresponding vertebral bodies and below C8 the roots have to make an increasingly longer caudal journey to transverse their appropriate intervertebral foramen. The mass of roots that form below the level of the cord in the lumbar region is called the cauda equina.

The dorsal root ganglia lie in the intervertebral canal just proximal to the union of the dorsal and ventral spinal roots.

Skeletal muscle and the peripheral nervous system

From which muscles the samples should be taken is best determined by the clinical picture supplemented by electrophysiology. In many instances a previous biopsy may have been undertaken which may well have provided a diagnosis and therefore guide the need for further samples. However, not all disorders are symmetrical and, increasingly, CT and MRI scanning are being used to map the distribution of muscle disease. In general, a severely wasted muscle is unlikely to provide a diagnosis.

Sampling of peripheral nerve and/or muscle will depend on the nature and distribution of the disorders under study and, on occasion, dissection of the small muscles of the hand or foot can be justified. Samples may be taken for neurochemistry and histochemistry, other samples being laid out on labeled cardboard and air dried to achieve adhesion between the sample and the cardboard prior to immersion fixation.

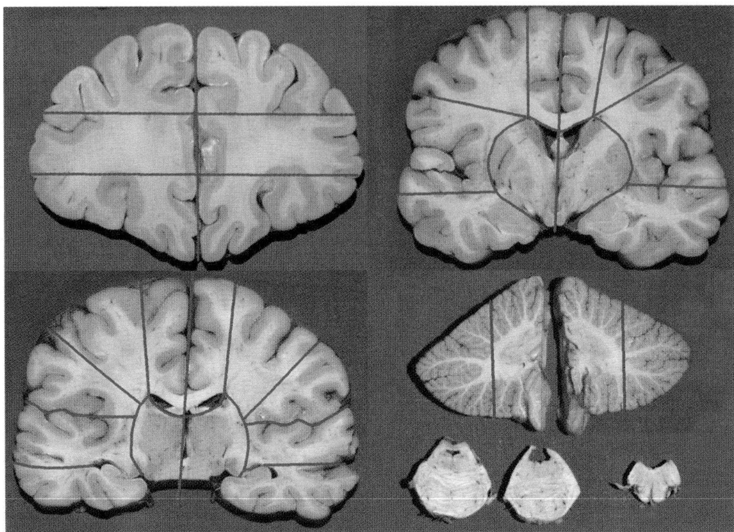

Figure 1.5 Block taking for cases of dementia, diffuse traumatic brain injury, movement disorders, sudden unexpected death in infancy and epilepsy. Routine screening from three coronal slices of the cerebral hemisphere at levels of the frontal lobes, the basal ganglia, the thalami, the cerebellum, and the brainstem.

Whereas the afferent and efferent components may vary from nerve to nerve the overall structure remains the same. However, in order to sample appropriately, in some cases detailed knowledge of the various plexuses and the peripheral nervous system is required.

HISTOLOGICAL TECHNIQUES

The principal histological techniques used in neuropathology are listed in Table 1.1, from which it can be seen that much information can be gained from a limited number of techniques that are also often used routinely in departments of pathology.

Brain biopsy is a standard procedure in most neurosurgical units. Two principal techniques are available when a rapid diagnosis is required: smears or frozen sections, both of which are simple and rapid. After fixation in alcohol the smears can be stained with 1% toluidine blue, polychrome methylene blue, hematoxylin and eosin (H&E), for example. If the biopsy is too tough to smear, frozen sections are indicated.

In paraffin-embedded material abnormalities in cells and myelin can be identified in sections stained with H&E, provided fairly thick sections (7–8 μm) are examined. It is easy to recognize the differences between gray and white matter and to appreciate that the architectural arrangements of the cerebral cortex differ from those of the basal ganglia, the thalami, the hippocampus, the cerebellum and the brainstem. Indeed, it is often possible to identify from which subcortical area of the brain a section has been taken by noting the size, shape and pigmentation of neurons; unfortunately, this is rarely possible in the cerebral cortex. The use of hematoxylin/van Gieson (H/VG) helps to distinguish between collagen and glial fibrils, and is particularly helpful in certain mixed tumors (gliosarcomas), where there is involvement of the meninges by tumor, and when assessing the structural components of the wall of an abscess. A particularly useful general stain is the combined cresyl violet and Luxol fast blue technique. Cresyl violet stains neurons and their Nissl granules, whereas the Luxol fast blue stains myelin a rich blue color.

Specialized techniques are, however, essential for the identification of specific structural abnormalities such as those affecting axons and myelin.

Table 1.1 Histological techniques in neuropathology

Types of preparation	Stain	Color reaction and application
Smears	Polychrome methylene blue; toluidine blue	Blue: rapid diagnosis
	Hematoxylin and eosin	Pink and blue
Paraffin	Hematoxylin and eosin	Pink and blue: general purpose
	Van Gieson	Red: collagen Yellow: other tissues
	Reticulin stain	Black: reticulin
	Cresyl violet (may be used with Luxol fast blue or Palmgren)	Violet: Nissl substance of neurons
	Palmgren	Black: axons and neurons
	Bodian	
	Glees and Marsland	
	Modified Bielschowsky's method	Black: axons
	Loyez	Black: myelin
	Luxol fast blue	Deep blue: myelin
	Holzer	Blue purple: glial fibres and astrocytes
	Perls' stain	Blue: ferric iron
	Masson Fontana	Black: melanin
	Periodic acid–Schiff	Magenta: glycogen and mucopolysaccharide
Frozen	von Braunmuhl King's amyloid	Black or brown–black: neurons and axons, senile plaques and neurofibrillary tangles
	Cajal	Black: astrocytes
	Marchi	Black: degenerating myelin
	Oil red O	Red: degenerating myelin
	Acidified cresyl violet	Purple–brown: metachromatic leukodystrophy
Cerebrospinal fluid	Leishman	Blue/pink cytology
	Hematoxylin and eosin	
	May–Grünwald–Giemsa	
	Southgate's mucicarmine	Pink: mucin

Commonly used techniques for axons are the silver impregnation methods of Palmgren, Bodian, and Glees and Marsland. The basic principles of how to identify abnormalities in myelin are somewhat confusing, but in essence there are two principal types of staining reaction. First, loss of myelin can be identified by negative staining; demyelinated areas are pale when stained with Luxol fast blue, hematoxylin lakes or H&E, or H/VG; secondly, the breakdown products of myelin can be stained positively by either the Sudan stains (oil red O) or by the Marchi technique (osmium). Both of these are applicable to frozen sections, and material that has been impregnated by the Marchi method can be embedded in paraffin wax.

There are many occasions when pigment needs to be identified. In most instances this can be resolved by the use of Perls' stain which demonstrates hemosiderin, and the Masson Fontana technique which identifies melanin.

In patients with diffuse brain damage, for example cardiac arrest, hypoglycemia or some other generalized disease process, it is desirable to examine large sections of brain so that the precise anatomical distribution of the damage can be defined. Most laboratories prefer large paraffin sections to celloidin-embedded sections on the grounds of cost, health and safety, considerations about handling and processing and the ability to investigate using immunohistochemical techniques.

The cytology of CSF has become of increasing value in recent years because of the development of improved techniques, e.g. cytospin, liquid-based cytology and embedding in agar. The most important prerequisites for good cytology are fresh specimens correctly handled and prepared. Considerable experience, however, is required to differentiate reactive from tumor cells, but in any patient where the CSF cell count is raised cytological examination should be undertaken, with the aim of identifying precisely the nature of the nucleated cells. Cytospin specimens are usually stained routinely by the Leishman or May–Grünwald–Giemsa methods, but various other techniques can be used, such as H&E and Southgate's mucicarmine for the identification of mucin-secreting metastatic carcinoma and by the periodic acid–Schiff technique. Various antibodies are now being used to help in the identification of nucleated cells, particularly when tumor cells are present in the CSF (Table 1.2).

Fresh samples of CSF should always be handled in exhaust-ventilated cabinets for health and safety reasons with the premise that all specimens are potentially infectious and constitute a hazard to laboratory staff. Standard operating procedures are required for the handling of biohazardous samples such as tuberculous meningitis, the cytospin preparations being fixed in 10% formol saline for between 10 and 15 min prior to staining. Immunohistochemical techniques are widely used to characterize the proteins of various cells within the developing and normal CNS. It is within the area of neuro-oncology that an almost exponential use of immunohistochemistry to classify brain tumors has developed, although one should always remember that the antibody staining is not marking particular tumors but rather acting as sign posts which, when taken into consideration with other information, including examination of sections stained with H&E, might provide a confident diagnosis of a particular tumor type.

Immunohistochemical methods are now used routinely to overcome some of the difficulties associated with the classical staining methods. As a consequence the silver techniques used for the selective impregnation of astrocytes, oligodendrocytes and microglia have largely been superseded (Table 1.3).

S-100 protein is found in substantial amounts in glial cells and cells derived from the neural crest. However, S-100 protein is not brain specific but is a useful general marker indicating an origin from the embryonic neural crest.

Neurons and their axons may be identified by antibodies raised to *neurofilaments* and antibodies raised to *synaptophysin* have been used as a marker of synaptic vesicles in neurons. In appropriately or lightly fixed material synaptic vesicles containing various neurotransmitter substances and all their associated enzymes maybe identified as may certain neuropeptides such as *substance P, somastostatin* and *vasoactive intestinal peptide.*

Glial fibrillary acidic protein (GFAP) is a major component of astrocytic fibres and is the subunit of the 8–9 nm intermediate filament of astrocytes, and with antisera to the protein there is intense immunohistochemical staining of the cell bodies and their processes. To all intents and purposes, GFAP is confined to astrocytes in normal mature brain and is a very useful marker for identifying normal, reactive and tumor astrocytes. Although, GFAP is now most widely used to identify astrocytes, glutamine synthetase, which is confined to astrocytes in the CNS, is an alternative antibody. Since both oligodendrocytes and myelin are usually rich in the glycolipid galactocerebroside, antisera raised against this component have been applied extensively to the investigation of white matter. Because of the particular importance of oligodendrocytes in demyelinating diseases, antibodies to *myelin basic protein* and *myelin-associated glycoprotein* have been used extensively in the study of myelinogenesis and demyelination. Myelin basic protein is the most extensively studied brain-specific membrane protein, and has been localized in myelin with fluorescent-labeled antibodies and, more specifically, to the major dense line by electron microscopy. In contrast, myelin-associated glycoprotein appears to be localized to the cell bodies of oligodendrocytes. Increasing use is being made of antibodies raised against several enzymes which

Table 1.2 Immunohistochemistry in neuropathology: cerebrospinal fluid in health and in certain diseases

	Normal	Acute pyogenic meningitis	Tuberculous meningitis	*Acute virus infection with meningo-encephalitis	General paralysis of the insane	Tabes dorsalis	Multiple sclerosis	Subarachnoid hemorrhage	Complete spinal block (Froin's syndrome)
Pressure (horizontal posture)	60–150 mm H_2O	Probably to 200 mm or more	Increased to as much as 300 mm or more	Increased sometimes to 250 mm	Normal	Normal	Normal	Raised often to 300 mm or more	Low: CSF may have to be actively withdrawn
Appearance	Clear and colorless	Turbid or frankly purulent	Clear or slightly opalescent. A fine fibrin coagulum may form on standing	Clear or slightly opalescent	Normal	Normal	Normal	Frankly bloodstained: on centrifugation, supernatant is yellow	Yellow, opalescent and tends to clot
Cell content per μL	0.4 leukocytes (all lymphocytes)	Markedly raised 500–5000 polymorphs at first, mononuclears* later	Increased up to 500 mononuclears; some polymorphs at first	Increased 50–500 mononuclears; some polymorphs at first	Up to 100 mononuclears	Up to 50–100 mononuclears	Slight increase to 20–100 mononuclears	Many red cells and some leukocytes	Slight increase of mononuclears
Protein (g/L)	0.15–0.45	0.5–2.0 average; up to 10 g	0.5–0.3 usually; if spinal block present, may rise to over 10 g	0.5–2.0; 0.5–1.0 in paralytic polio	0.5–1.0 Oligoclonal IgG	0.3–0.6 Oligoclonal IgG	0.3–0.6 Oligoclonal IgG	Normal in the early stages. Slight rise later	More than 30 g
Glucose (mg/100 mL; mmol/L)	50–80 (2.8–4.4)	Absent or greatly reduced	Decreased to 20–30 (1–1.5)	Normal	Normal	Normal	Normal	Normal	Normal
Bacteriology	Sterile	Causative organisms present; type confirmed by culture	Tubercle bacilli in fibrin coagulum or in deposit. Positive cultures usually obtained	Sterile	Sterile	Sterile	Sterile	Sterile	Sterile
Wassermann	Negative	Negative	Negative	Negative	Positive	Positive in 80% of cases	Negative	Negative	Negative

* Mononuclears is used here to indicate lymphocytes and monocytes.

Table 1.3 Immunohistochemistry in neuropathology

Antigen	Types of cell identified
S-100 protein	Glia and cells derived from neural crest
Glial fibrillary acidic protein (GFAP) Glutamine synthetase	Astrocytes
Galactocerebroside Myelin basic-protein Myelin-associated glycoprotein	Oligodendroglia and myelin
Fibronectin	Fibroblasts
Factor VIII-related antigen CD34	Endothelial cells
Anti-human HLA-DP DQ DR antigen CD68	Macrophages and microglia
Prolactin Growth hormone ACTH Follicle-stimulating hormone Luteinizing hormone Thyroid-stimulating hormone	In anterior pituitary
Neurofilaments Synaptophysin	Neurons, axons and synapses
Cytokeratin Epithelial membrane antigen	Cells of epithelial tissues
Vimentin	Cells of mesenchymal and glial origin
Desmin Myosin	Cells of myogenic origin
Chorionic gonadotrophin α_1-Fetoprotein	Cells of trophoblastic origin
Carbonic anhydrase C Leukocyte common antigen T and B cells	Choroid plexus Lymphocytes
Anti-human melan-A Anti-human melanosome	Melanoblasts

are either specific for the myelin membrane, e.g. carbonic anhydrase and the soma of the oligodendrocyte (glycerol phosphate dehydrogenase).

The immune system in the CNS has been studied traditionally by its metallophil-staining reactions, a feature that suggests a relationship between microglia and macrophages. These staining reactions, however, are variable and so the increasing availability of antibodies for identifying microglia and phagocytic cells provide useful information about the cell types in normal, reactive and neoplastic conditions. Reactive microglia are well seen in CR3/43 and macrophages are readily identified by CD68. Antibodies against fibronectin for fibroblasts and factor VIII-related antigen and CD34 for endothelial cells are also available. In the study of tumors the ability to identify *vimentin filaments, desmin* and *myosin* in cells of mesenchymal origin may be helpful.

The application of various conventional stains to the cells of the anterior lobe of the pituitary gland is not a satisfactory means of correlating morphological features with secretory activity. The introduction of immunohistochemistry has allowed the specific localization of pituitary hormones, e.g. *prolactin, growth hormone* and *adrenocorticotrophic hormone* (ACTH) in tissue that has been fixed in formalin and embedded in paraffin wax. Surgical biopsies are often small, and it is sometimes difficult to distinguish between metastatic carcinoma and some types of malignant neuroepithelial tumor. Antibodies for identifying metastatic carcinoma, such as the cytokeratins and epithelial membrane antigen, may aid in establishing the diagnosis. It is now possible to guide the clinicians as to the likely origin of certain metastatic carcinomas, e.g. *anti-thyroid transcription factor* (anti-TTF1) for an origin in bronchus, *thyroglobulin* for an origin in thyroid, and *melanan* A or *HMB-45* for melanoma. Likewise, the presence of *chorionic gonadotrophin* and α_1-fetoprotein are important in the identification of cells of trophoblastic origin in germ-cell tumors arising in the region of either the hypothalamus or the pineal gland.

It is probably true to say that at present there are no specific immunocytochemical probes for ependyma, although antibodies to *carbonic anhydrase C* may be used to identify the choroid plexus.

A small number of lymphocytes are commonly present in the CSF of normal subjects, and in many disease processes the numbers of lymphocytes and monocytes increase and in certain circumstances there is infiltration by plasma cells. All leukocytes react with antibodies to *leukocyte common antigen*, and further classification can be obtained by using antibodies specific for *T and B lymphocytes.* If lymphoid tumors are suspected, myelomas and B-cell lymphomas can be further classified using antibodies to κ and λ light chains and immunoglobulin heavy chains. Refinement and diagnosis is now greatly enhanced by the use of *in situ* hybridrization, various molecular techniques and flow cytometry.

CHAPTER 2

STRUCTURAL AND FUNCTIONAL NEUROANATOMY

Ian Bone and Donald M Hadley

INTRODUCTION

The purpose of this chapter is to introduce the pathologist to the essentials of structural and functional neuroanatomy, so that relationships between nervous system structure and symptoms and signs of disease can be more fully understood. Knowledge of functional anatomy ensures that the pathologist, when carrying out an examination, concentrates attention on clinically relevant regions of the central and/or peripheral nervous systems. Precise anatomical localization of symptoms and signs had previously been dependent upon clinicopathological correlations carried out by earlier generations of clinicians and pathologists usually after surgery or death.

In the 1970s Godfrey Hounsfield and his team revolutionized radiology and pathological localization when they developed computed tomography (CT) and for the first time intracranial lesions could be imaged directly and non-invasively. Magnetic resonance imaging (MRI), magnetic resonance spectroscopy (MRS) and developments in functional imaging: functional MRI (fMRI), positron emission tomography (PET) and single photon emission computed tomography (SPECT), have over the last two decades, corrected many of the earlier dogmas of neurological localization.

Since the development of CT and MRI, plain skull radiographs are now only occasionally used to (1) assess conditions that affect the density of the skull, (2) assess causes of bony remodeling, (3) show gross facial or skull fractures and (4) identify or exclude radio-opaque foreign bodies such as before MRI or following a penetrating injury.

CT uses X-rays to construct sections of the brain or spine based on their attenuation by the tissues they traverse. This attenuation is proportional to the electron density of the tissue. Since most lesions either increase the intra- or extracellular water or change the cellular density of tissues they can be visualized by changes in electron density. This is depicted in a gray scale of Hounsfield units (H) which range from the highest attenuation (brightest) of $+1000$ H for calcium or cortical bone to the darkest of -1000 H for air. Normal gray matter is ≈ 45 H, white matter is ≈ 30 H, cerebrospinal fluid ≈ 8 H and fat ≈ -70 H (Fig. 2.1).

MRI depends on the way protons (or other nuclei which have an odd number of protons or neutrons and therefore possess the quantum quality of 'spin') absorb and then retransmit pulses of electromagnetic radiation in the radio-frequency range when prepared in a very homogenous strong magnetic field routinely now between 1.0 and 3.0 T. The returned signal encodes positional information and reflects multiple tissue parameters related to the

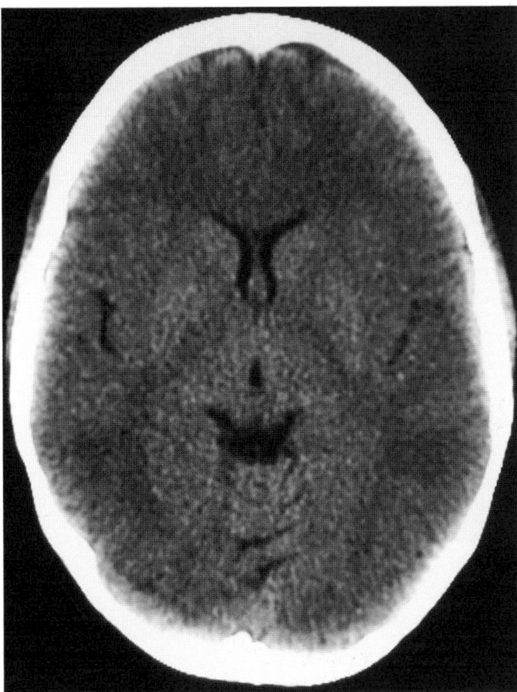

Figure 2.1 Normal computed tomography (CT) section through the basal ganglia and occipital lobes showing the low attenuation cerebrospinal fluid (CSF) in the cisterns and ventricles with reasonable gray matter and white matter differentiation and high attenuation in the skull vault.

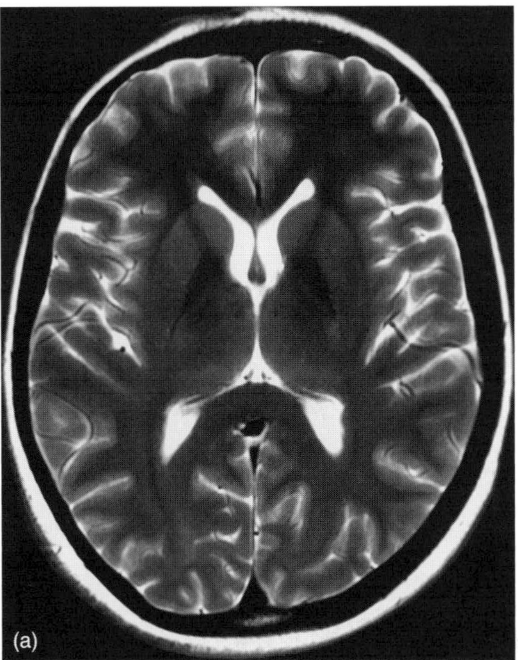

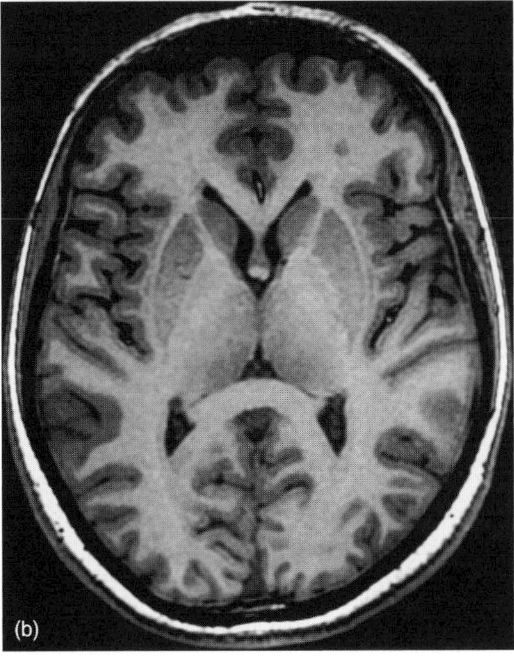

Figure 2.2 Normal magnetic resonance image (MRI). (a) T2-weighted axial section and (b) T1-weighted sagittal sections show the excellent tissue differentiation and flexibility of scan plane.

number of free water protons and their molecular environment. The most important of these are the proton density, T2 relaxation time, T1 relaxation time and diffusion. By manipulating the radiofrequency pulses these individual characteristics in different tissues can be highlighted to provide contrast between lesions and the normal background. As the CNS is between 80 and 85% water and the hydrogen nucleus is a proton MRI has been developed into a sensitive technique for imaging the brain and spine (Fig. 2.2). In MRS, instead of using the magnetic resonance signal to construct a cross-sectional image from the protons associated with water these can be suppressed and the tiny signal from protons in other molecules can be collected from one or more tissue volumes and can be displayed graphically (Fig. 2.3).

fMRI evolved from the observation that the magnetic resonance signal from blood oxyhemoglobin

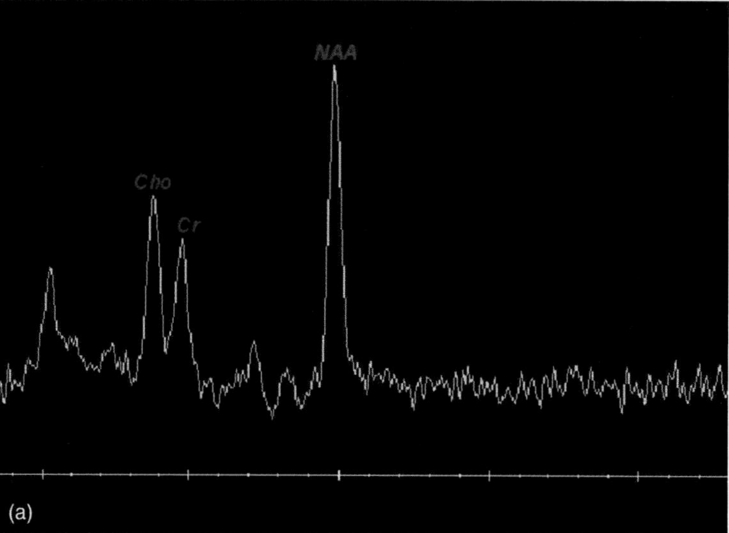

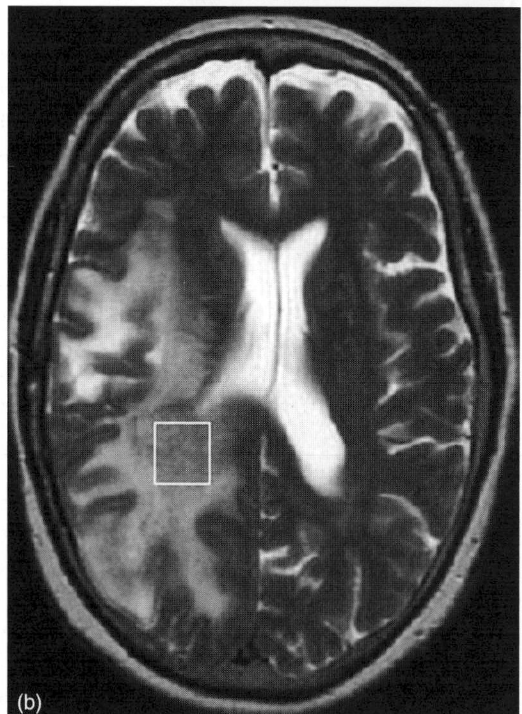

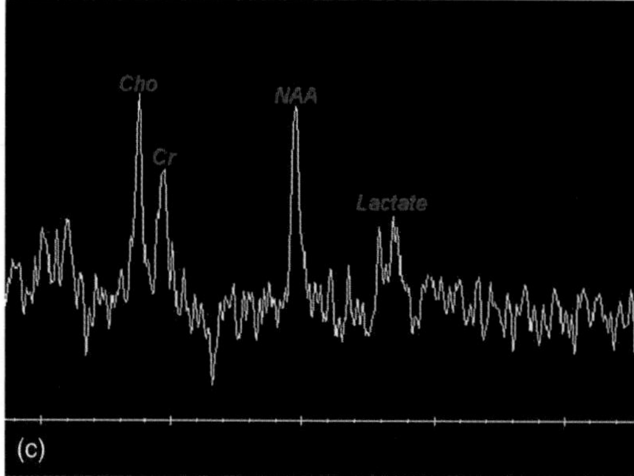

Figure 2.3 Magnetic resonance spectroscopy (MRS). (a) Normal proton spectrum of brain showing the key metabolites of *N*-acetyl-aspartate containing compounds (NAA), creatine (Cr) and choline (Cho). (b) A mass lesion surrounded by vasogenic edema on a T2-weighted section showing the volume element sampled by MRS. (c) A typical spectrum from a glioblastoma with reduced NAA confirming a reduction in normally functioning neurons, a raised choline indicating an increased membrane turnover and little change in creatine. The lactate peak indicates anaerobic respiration.

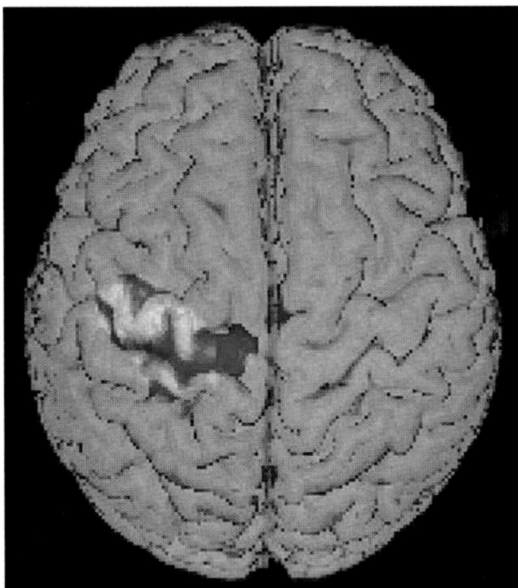

Figure 2.4 fMRI showing the difference in oxygenation of blood draining the area activated by a right hand opening and closing paradigm superimposed on the structural three-dimensional image highlighting the left precentral gyrus and a small part of the post-central gyrus.

was subtley different from that of deoxyhemoglobin. In activated areas of the brain, so long as the coupling between perfusion and metabolism is retained, there is normally an increase in perfusion additional to the tissue requirements. This net additional oxyhemoglobin in the veiniolar bed compared to 'resting' brain can be measured by subtraction and after several filtering and correction techniques can be displayed on a structural image (Fig. 2.4). As the signal change is very small the activation paradigms usually have to be repeated many times to improve the signal-to-noise ratio. This results in relatively long imaging times and requires considerable patient co-operation.

Intravenous contrast agents are used in both CT and MR examinations to assess the vascularity of lesions and the state of the blood–brain/blood–spine barrier. With CT, iodinated contrast agents show increased attenuation in blood vessels immediately after administration and patterns of increased attenuation in areas of blood–brain barrier/blood–spine barrier breakdown a short time after the injection (Fig. 2.5). Gadolinium-based compounds are used in MR in a similar way and result in an increased signal particularly on T1-weighted images by shortening the T1 relaxation time of adjacent water protons when the proton becomes closely associated with the gadolinium on a molecular scale (Fig. 2.6).

Nuclear medicine studies include SPECT and PET, both making use of the radiation emitted from an administered radioligand which is designed to act as a tracer for a particular function or receptor to form a cross-sectional image of its distribution or binding. Both produce mainly functional data. With SPECT (Fig. 2.7, page 22) the emitted gamma radiation is measured directly while with PET the radioligands utilized emit positrons which travel a few millimeters before colliding with an electron resulting in the emission of two high-energy photons travelling at approximately 180° to each other and are detected by radiation detectors linked in coincidence circuits. This is then reconstructed into an image. In general the resolution of PET is superior to SPECT. Radioligands specific for each have been developed and the choice depends on the function to be measured or imaged but cost and availability limit the use of PET.

By using these multiple imaging modalities structural and functional information and often a combination of both can now be obtained to assist in the patient's assessment. In no other area of the body are so many imaging modalities available. This has advanced our understanding of the normal and abnormal central nervous system, but this increase in sensitivity has unfortunately not been matched by an increase in specificity and basic radiological interpretation and pattern recognition is still the key to a differential diagnosis. Nowhere is this more evident than in the study of higher cortical function. Whereas previously specific areas had been associated with particular tasks, it is now realized that there is a complex integration of function rendering pinpoint clinical localization an outmoded goal. Also, the face of clinical psychiatry has changed greatly in recent years, from the analytical to the organic or neurobehavioral and pathologists can expect in the future to be asked to explore once more the anatomical substrate of disorders such as schizophrenia.

In the peripheral nervous system the classification of nerve and muscle disease has been greatly

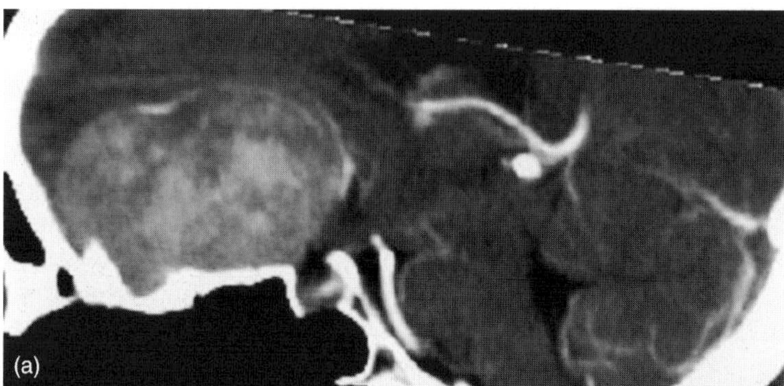

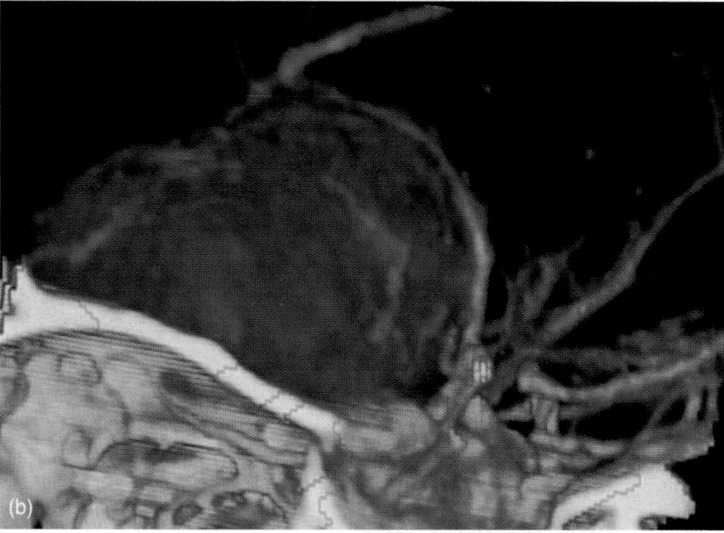

Figure 2.5 Subfrontal meningioma CT in a 62-year-old woman. (a) Sagittal reformat after intravenous contrast shows the enhancing tumor. (b) Three-dimensional volume rendered image shows the tumor and the displaced anterior cerebral arteries.

advanced by the development of improved electrophysiological techniques: evoked responses, nerve conduction and electromyography studies. These can demonstrate early or presymptomatic disease often before the development of abnormal neurological signs. Advances in neurophysiology localize with greater precision, to nerve root, plexus, peripheral nerve, neuromuscular junction or muscle as well as inform on the putative pathological process (e.g. axonal or demyelinating neuropathy). Genetics studies have also brought greater clarity to diagnostics with many central and peripheral nervous system disorders having a specific mutation or deletion.

These advances in diagnostic testing have profoundly enhanced our understanding of the importance and limitations of functional neuroanatomy. This chapter will deal more specifically with signs and symptoms of central nervous system (CNS) disease, so that the taxonomy of neurological disease (e.g. apraxia, dystonia, aphasia) will come to have meaning in terms of the possible sites of origin of such symptomatology.

THE CEREBRAL CORTEX

The cerebral cortex was, until the mid-nineteenth century, regarded as being functionally homogeneous – the seat of the soul and mind. Pierre Paul Broca (1861) first demonstrated localized dysfunction when describing impaired language (dysphasia) in two patients with a lesion in the posterior third of the left third frontal convolution. These early observations in patients with neurosyphillis were supported and added to by subsequent

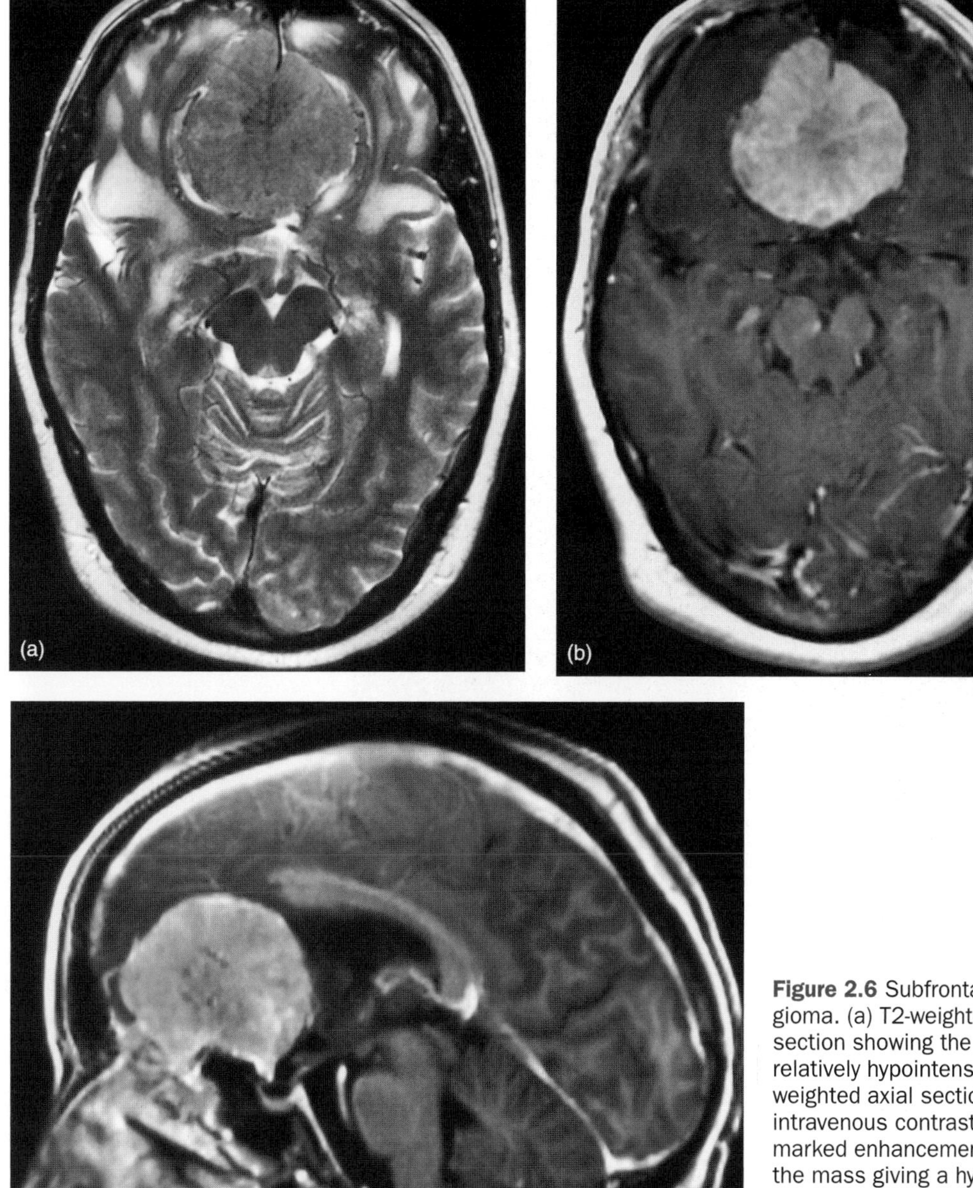

Figure 2.6 Subfrontal meningioma. (a) T2-weighted axial section showing the mass as relatively hypointense. (b) T1-weighted axial section after intravenous contrast shows marked enhancement with the mass giving a hyperintense signal. (c) T1-weighted post-contrast sagittal section.

observations in patients with cerebrovascular disease, brain tumors or focal epilepsy. John Hughlings Jackson, a nineteenth century British neurologist confirmed laterality of function in aphasia and introduced the 'hierarchical' theory – that functions such as thought and memory were less affected by focal disease requiring a more diffuse process. By the end of the nineteenth century the concept of brain localization was sufficiently well established to allow Victor Horsley and others to operate on

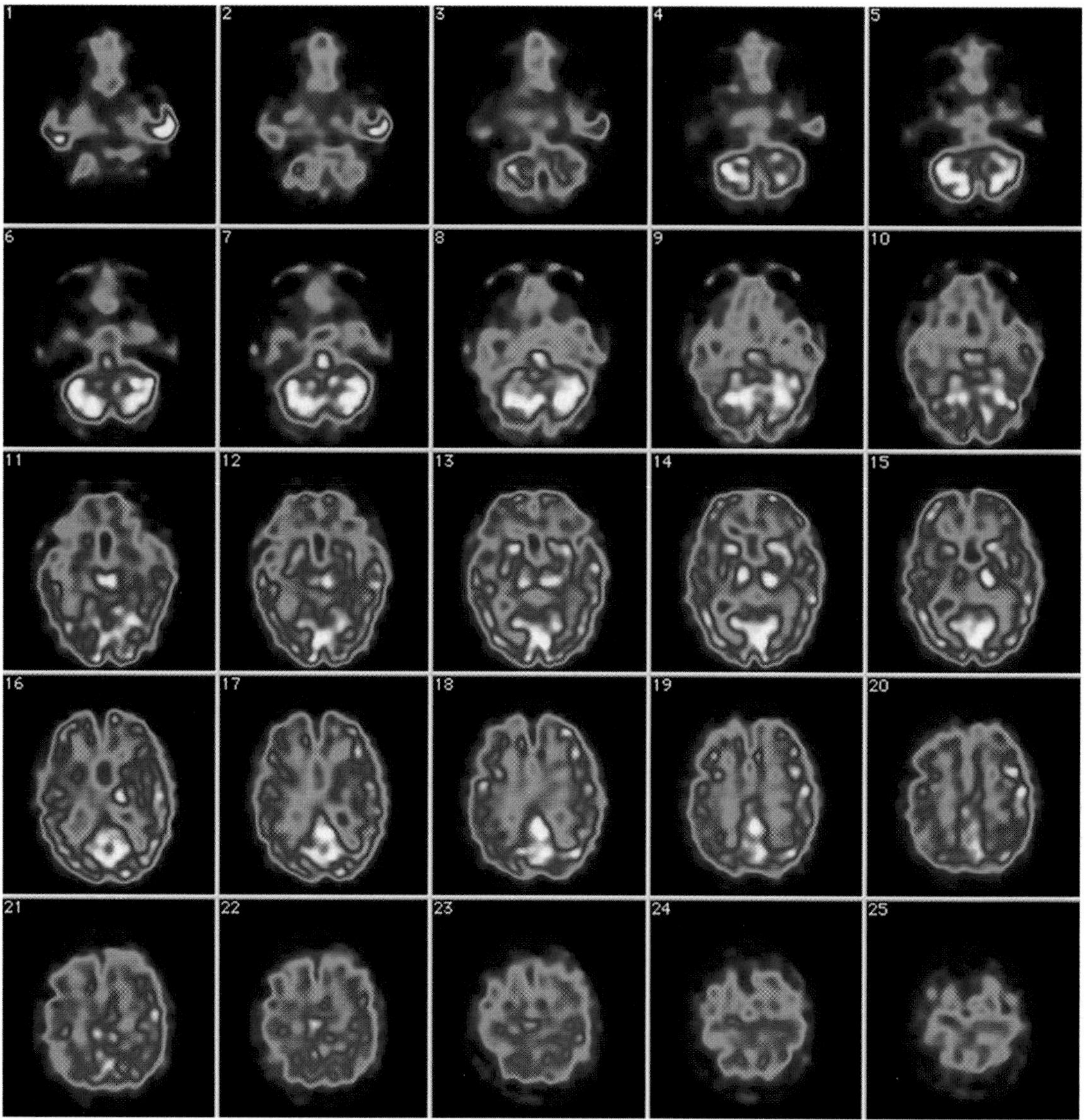

Figure 2.7 ^{99m}Tc-HMPAO perfusion SPECT showing markedly reduced perfusion in the frontal and temporal lobes in addition to atrophy typical of frontal–temporal dementia.

the brain solely on the basis of clinical localization. In time it was recognized by Geschwind (1965) and others that subcortical disease could 'disconnect' one area of cortical function from the next. The appreciation of these *disconnection syndromes* led to the acceptance that, whereas certain skills were localized to specific sites within the cerebral cortex, connection between these sites is essential for normal integrated cortical function. The advent of PET and subsequently fMRI continue to explore the complex field of higher cortical function.

The cerebral hemisphere may be divided into frontal, parietal, temporal and occipital lobes (Fig. 2.8). The *frontal lobe* extends from the frontal pole backwards to the central sulcus (fissure of Rolando), and downwards on the lateral surface of the hemisphere to the lateral fissure. The *parietal lobe* extends from the central sulcus to the parieto-occipital

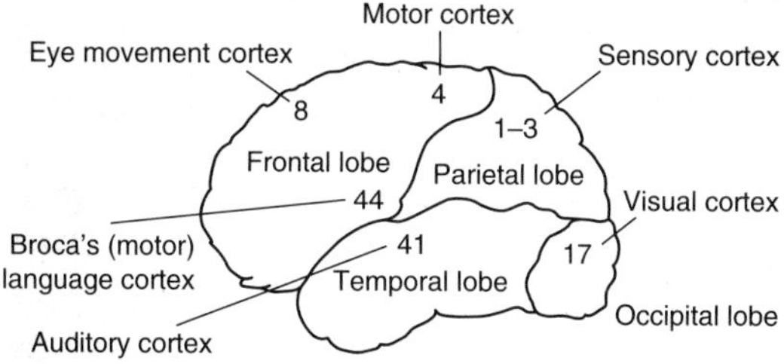

Figure 2.8 The lateral aspect of the cerebral hemispheres.

fissure, and again laterally to the lateral cerebral fissure. The *temporal lobe* lies inferior to the lateral cerebral (Sylvian) fissure and extends back to the parieto-occipital fissure. The *occipital lobe* has a pyramid-like configuration and lies behind the parieto-occipital fissure. Each of these lobes can be divided into specific subdivisions. Within the lateral fissure lies an important buried island or *insula* of cerebral cortex. A further deeply situated constituent of the cerebral hemispheres is the *rhinencephalon*, the phylogenetically old portion of the cerebral hemispheres comprising the olfactory bulb and tract, the anterior perforated substance and the piriform area, these structures being associated with the perception of smell – olfactory sensation. Further deeper structures such as the *fornix* and *hippocampal formation* play an important role in modifying behavior responses and memory processing.

Histologically, the cerebral cortex appears to be made up of six definable layers (Fig. 2.9). These layers are not of homogeneous thickness throughout the cerebral cortex, but show considerable regional variation; for example, in that part of the neocortex that receives major sensory projections, the granular layer is more prominent than the pyramidal layer (*granular cortex*), the opposite being the case in areas from which major motor projections emanate (the *agranular* or *pyramidal cortex*). Based on these subtle differences in cytoarchitecture, Brodmann (1909) and Von Economo (1927) divided the cerebral cortex into specific regions, implying that each discrete area had a specific and unique function. Brodmann's classification is commonly used today and the areas defined by him have been used as a reference base for the localization of physiological and pathological processes. Ablation or stimulation of these regions, electrically or with

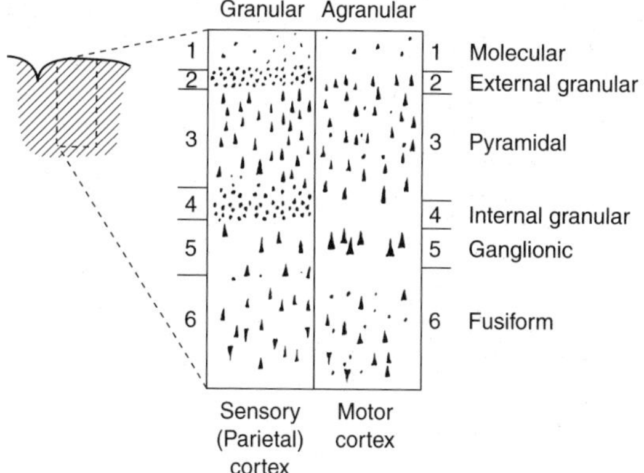

Figure 2.9 The structure of the cerebral neocortex with diagramatic representation of its layers.

(a)

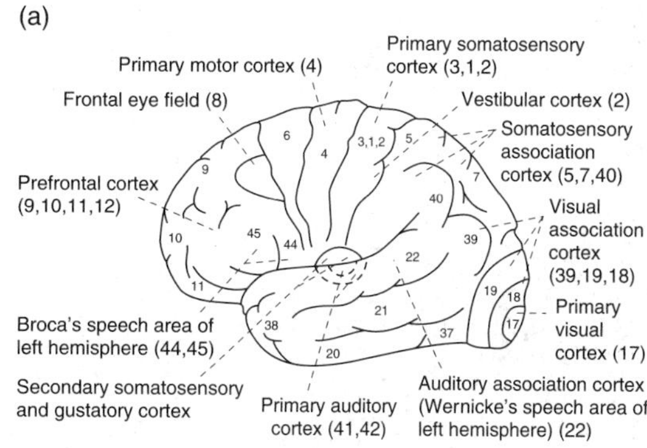

(b)

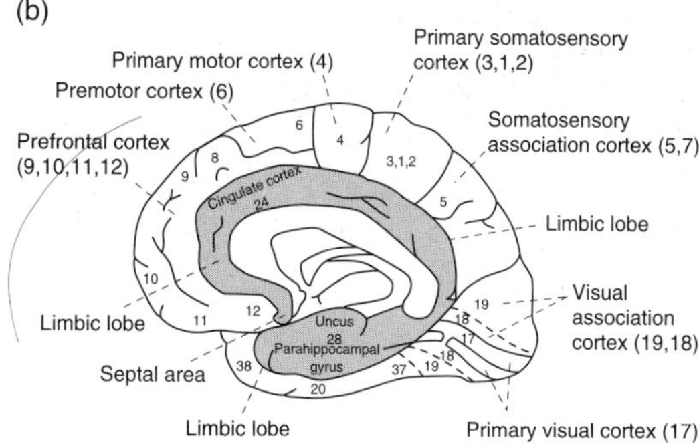

Figure 2.10 The cerebral hemispheres (Brodman areas).

chemicals in experimental animals, has confirmed their functional importance, as have recent fMRI studies. Important Brodmann areas are illustrated (Fig. 2.10). For example, area 4 is a primary motor cortex, whereas area 8 is concerned with the control of eye movements and pupillary responses, and area 17 is the striate or primary visual cortex surrounded by areas 18 and 19, the visual association cortex.

Studies in patients with lateralized hemisphere disease confirmed Hughlings Jackson's belief that there is a *major* or *dominant* cerebral hemisphere which is functionally distinct from the opposite or *minor* hemisphere. In all right-handed and approximately 95% of left-handed persons, the left hemisphere appears dominant in that in it reside the verbal, linguistic, calculating and analytical functions, whereas the non-dominant or minor hemisphere is concerned with visual, spatial and perceptual skills. Hemisphere dominance appears to be established within the first 3–5 years of life, although in trauma and disease dominance can switch in later childhood. Such *plasticity* diminishes with age through adolescence and adult life. In early childhood hemispherectomy for intractable seizures or extensive traumatic brain injury does not have the catastrophic outcome that would normally be anticipated. Anatomical differences are evident in the structure and symmetry of the dominant and minor hemispheres. This is most evident in the upper surface of the temporal lobe, where Heschl's gyrus (the primary auditory cortex, Brodmann area 41) is found, in the majority of brains, to be larger in the left (dominant) cerebral hemisphere.

The degree of disability and symptomatology that a patient may manifest in cortical disease is variable, being influenced by the tempo of the illness as well as the nature of the disease process and the capacity of the cerebral hemispheres to show plasticity. This means that functional recovery following a lesion may occur as a consequence of cortical neuronal reorganization, possibly through secondary or supplementary areas within the cerebral cortex that can 'take over' function in the face of focal disease. It therefore follows that the size and site of lesion do not always predict deficit. In cerebrovascular disease, infarct volume in the dominant hemisphere does predict disability and handicap but not so in the non-dominant hemisphere (Fig. 2.11).

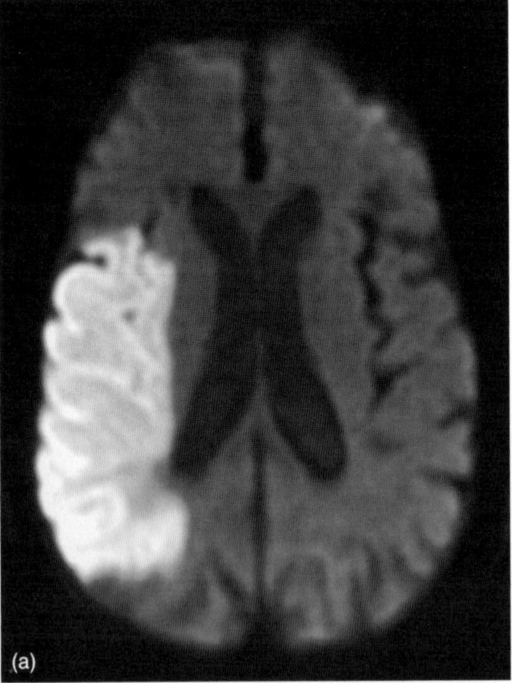

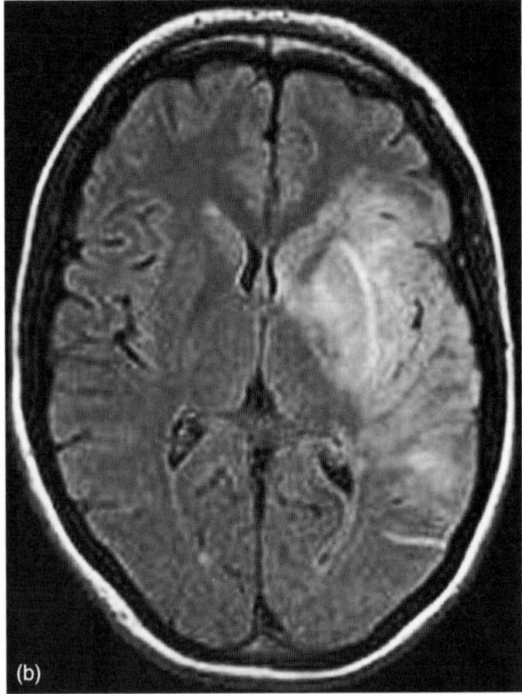

Figure 2.11 Middle cerebral artery infarcts. (a) Dominant hemisphere: acute >3 h showing restricted diffusion on this b1000 diffusion-weighted MRI. (b) Non-dominant hemisphere fluid attenuated inversion recovery (FLAIR) MR section showing a hyperintense infarct.

Symptoms of frontal lobe disease

In normal health the frontal lobes are responsible for contralateral movement in the face, arms, legs and trunk. The dominant hemisphere contains the center for the expression of language (Broca's area). The frontal lobes also control contralateral head and eye turning, inhibition of bladder and bowel voiding (Fig. 2.12) and play an important part in the maintenance of personality and initiative.

(a)

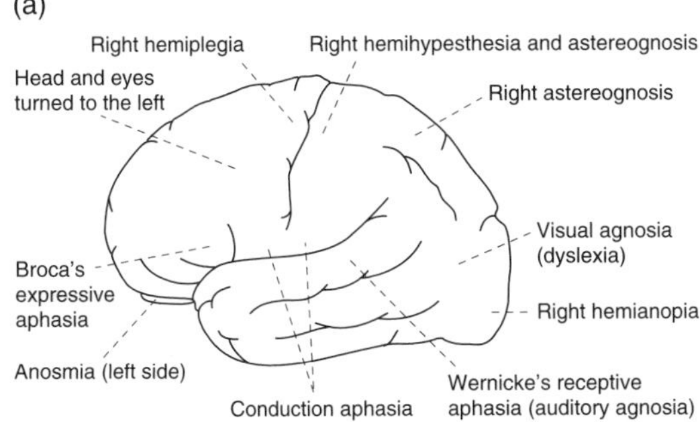

(b)

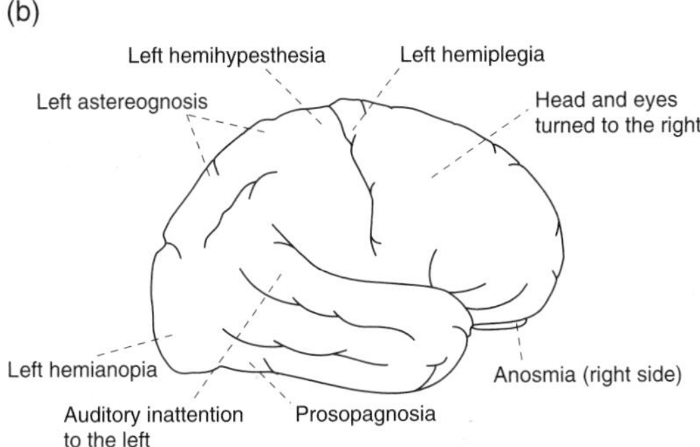

(c)

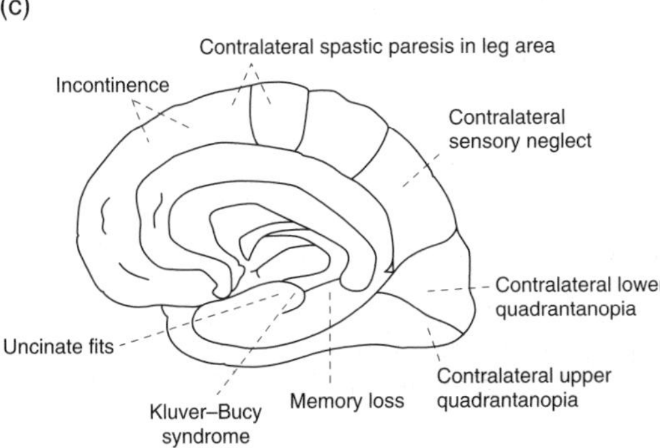

Figure 2.12 Cerebral hemispheres. Left and right lateral and medial surfaces.

The *motor cortex* (Figs 2.4 and 2.12) lies anterior to the central sulcus, with the areas responsible for movement in the face, arms and trunk on the lateral surface and those serving movement in the legs on the medial surface. It can be seen (Fig. 2.13) that certain functions, such as hand or lip movements, have a greater area of cortical representation (the homunculus). This representation ensures that refined and sophisticated movements are better served whilst cruder movements such as at a large joint require only a small area of cortex to execute (Hughlings Jackson's 'hierarchical' theory once more).

Damage to the motor cortex results in contralateral *hemiplegia*. If the medial cortex is affected primarily, as in occlusion of the anterior cerebral artery or by compression from a parasagittal tumor, paralysis is evident in the leg, with sparing of the trunk, upper limb and face. If the lateral surface only is affected, as in occlusion of the middle cerebral artery, then paralysis is present in the face, arm and trunk, with relative sparing of the leg (brachio-facial paralysis). In recovering destructive disease there is also a tendency for more complex functions with greatest cortical representation to improve more slowly. For instance, a patient recovering from occlusion of a middle cerebral artery may regain movement at the shoulder, elbow and wrist but no useful fine hand movement.

When *Broca's area* (Brodmann area 44) (Fig. 2.14) is diseased in the dominant hemisphere, there is a loss of expressive language, the patient being able to comprehend and carry out commands, but not to produce meaningful language. This form of disturbance is referred to as *expressive dysphasia* or alternatively, because of its hesitant almost telegraphic nature, *non-fluent dysphasia*. Damage to the *paracentral lobule* on the medial surface of the frontal lobe results in '*frontal incontinence*'. Here, the normal cortical inhibition of a full bladder and bowel is lost, resulting in loss of sphincter control.

Disease of the *prefrontal areas* (the substantial part of the frontal lobes anterior to the motor cortex, as well as the undersurface/orbital surface of the frontal lobes) produces predominant disturbances in behavior. When the *orbitofrontal cortex* is affected, disinhibition, inappropriate jocularity, emotional lability and distractibility occur. When

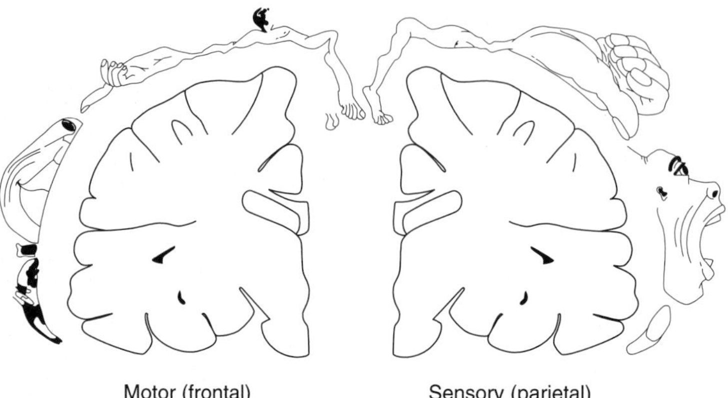

Figure 2.13 The motor and sensory homunculus.

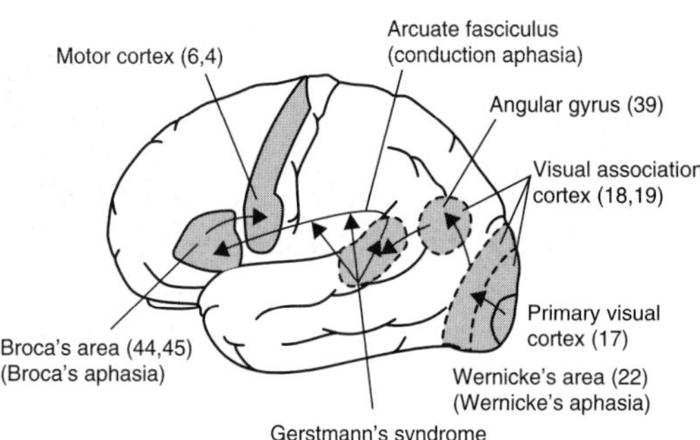

Figure 2.14 The cerebral hemispheres: language, vision and Gerstmann syndrome.

the *lateral surfaces of both frontal lobes* are affected, apathy, indifference and perseveration (the repetition of motor or language tasks) are evident. When the *medial surface* of the prefrontal cortex is affected the patient become akinetic, lacking spontaneous movements and gestures and with sparse verbal output; this state is often referred to as *akinetic mutism*, and is associated with frontal incontinence of bladder and bowel.

Frontal lobe dysfunction may be associated with the presence of *primitive reflexes*. These reflexes are normally apparent in very early infancy and then diminish. In disease they are 'released' from cortical inhibition and derive at the brainstem level. These reflexes may take the form of a *grasp reflex*, in which the patient may clutch the examiner's hand and tighten upon it, or a *snout reflex* when, if the mouth is tapped with a tendon hammer, pouting movements of the lips are made. The *palmomental reflex* is elicited by stroking the palm of the hand and observing contraction of the ipsilateral mentalis muscle. Finally, frontal lobe disease affecting the *corpus callosum* can result in a 'disconnection' between the desire to walk and the execution of the task. This results in an *apraxia* of gait, the patient appearing to have normal power in the limbs but being unable to initiate movement of them when attempting to walk.

Unilateral disease of the frontal lobe may be caused by cerebrovascular disease (anterior cerebral artery embolism), infection (e.g. pyogenic brain abscess) and tumor. Bilateral frontal lobe disease may be caused by large subfrontal tumors (Fig. 2.15), tumors of the corpus callosum, hydrocephalus, degenerative disorders such as Pick's or frontotemporal dementia, and hematomas or vasospasm from anterior communicating artery aneurysm rupture.

Symptoms of parietal lobe disease

The *main sensory cortex* lies behind the central sulcus (Fig. 2.8, page 23) and manifests a similar representation of body areas as the motor cortex – *the sensory homunculus* (Fig. 2.13). The dominant hemisphere contains part of the receptive language area (*Wernicke's area*) as well as being implicated in other language-related skills. The fibers of the *optic radiation* responsible for perception of vision in the lower homonymous visual fields pass deep through the parietal lobe. In disease affecting the sensory cortex there is *contralateral loss of discriminatory sensation*, with impaired awareness of touch, shape

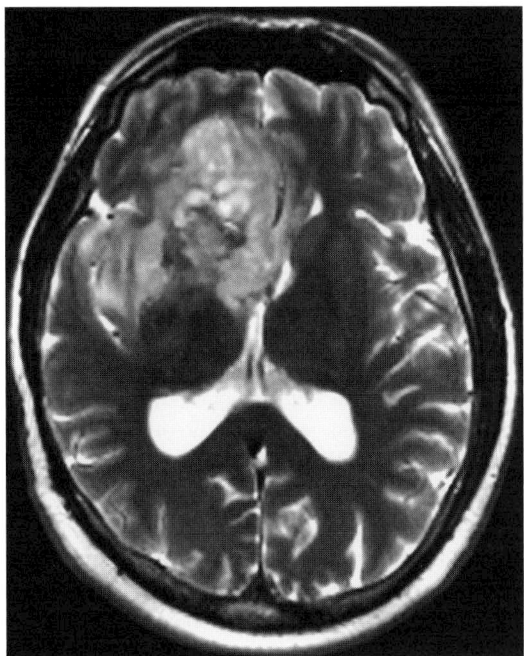

Figure 2.15 T2-weighted MRI section showing a large right sided frontal intrinsic neoplasm extending through the genu of the corpus callosum into the paramedial aspect of the right frontal lobe in a 43-year-old man. This was found to be a glioblastoma (WHO IV).

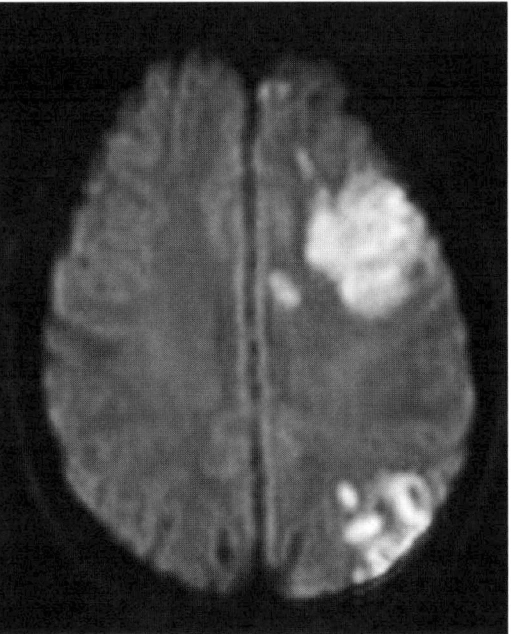

Figure 2.16 FLAIR MRI section showing boundary zone infarctions involving the left parieto-occipital cortex and underlying white matter in addition to the left frontal lobe.

and form. Disease of the dominant hemisphere results in an inability to appreciate or understand spoken language. This is referred to as a *receptive dysphasia*, or sometimes, because spoken language is rapid and nonsensical, *fluent dysphasia*. There is also impaired calculation (*acalculia*), impaired handwriting (*dysgraphia*) and disturbed reading ability (*dyslexia*). These features in conjunction with right/left disorientation and an inability to identify fingers on the patient or examiner's hand (*finger agnosia*) constitute Gerstmannsyndrome and is most commonly seen in middle cerebral artery territory infarction (Fig. 2.14).

In non-dominant hemisphere disease loss of spatial orientation and body image occur. This will result in neglect of the immediate environment (extrapersonal) which can be tested for by asking the individual to carry out simple constructional tasks such as bisecting a drawn line or copying a simple cartoon (*constructional apraxia*). Also there may be neglect to simultaneous bilaterally presented visual stimuli (*visual inattention*). Intrapersonal neglect can take the form of difficulty with dressing (*dressing apraxia*) or denial of unilateral defects such as hemiparesis (*anosognosia*) or a lack of concern for them (*anosodiaphoria*). Visual field loss, in the form of a lower quadrantanopia, will occur if the *optic radiation* is damaged.

Bilateral parietal lobe disease is rare, though it can occur as the result of a hypotensive episode with bilateral arterial boundary zones ischemia. Unilateral disease is most frequently due to middle cerebral artery territory ischemic cerebrovascular disease (Fig. 2.16), usually large-vessel thromboembolic occlusive disease from the heart, aortic arch or carotid system. Lobar hematomas may present in the parietal region (amyloid angiopathy) as may pyogenic or fungal infection, primary and metastatic tumors.

Symptoms of temporal lobe disease

The temporal lobe comprises a lateral and 'buried' insular cortex as well as the deep limbic lobe, including part of the rhinencephalon, hippocampus and associated structures (Fig. 2.8, page 23). The *lateral cortex* serves some memory function and posteriorly is implicated in the reception of language. The *auditory cortex* lies buried in the insula. *Limbic structures* are important in the perception of smell and taste, emotion, affect and memory processing. The *optic radiation* from the upper contralateral homonymous fields again passes deep through the temporal lobes. Disease of the dominant temporal lobe will result again in a *receptive* or *fluent dysphasia*, with impaired verbal memory. Disease of the minor temporal lobe will result in impaired visual memory. Unilateral damage to the auditory cortex will not result in hearing loss, as hearing has bilateral cortical representation. Bilateral lesions are rare but may result in *cortical deafness*. Disease of the limbic system may result in aggressive or antisocial behavior, and may be associated with the inability to establish new memories. Damage to the optic radiation will result in an upper homonymous quadrantanopia.

Unilateral temporal lobe disease may occur as a consequence of vascular or neoplastic processes. Pyogenic abscess may result from extension of localized infection in the middle ear or mastoid. Unilateral and bilateral temporal lobe disease may occur in herpes-simplex virus encephalitis (Fig. 2.17), limbic encephalitis (paraneoplastic), vascular disease or Wernicke–Korsakoff syndrome, where limbic structures are affected. The most common condition affecting temporal lobe function is *epilepsy*. This usually gives rise to positive phenomena, such as memory disturbance, déja vu or jamais vu, transient hallucinations of smell and taste and formed visual hallucinations. Where awareness is retained attacks are termed *simple partial seizures*, where lost, *complex partial seizures*. The term *psychomotor seizure* is reserved for temporal lobe attacks associated with primitive limb or truncal movements. In persons with temporal lobe epilepsy, between seizures (*interictal*), certain features have been described that are purported to have origins within the temporal lobe; hypergraphia

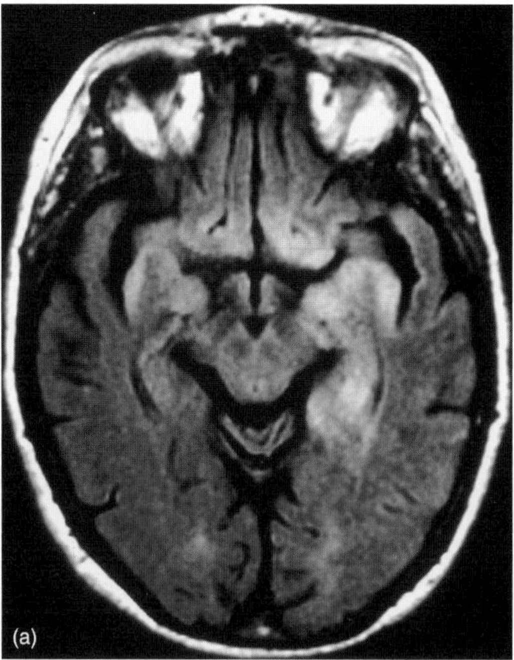

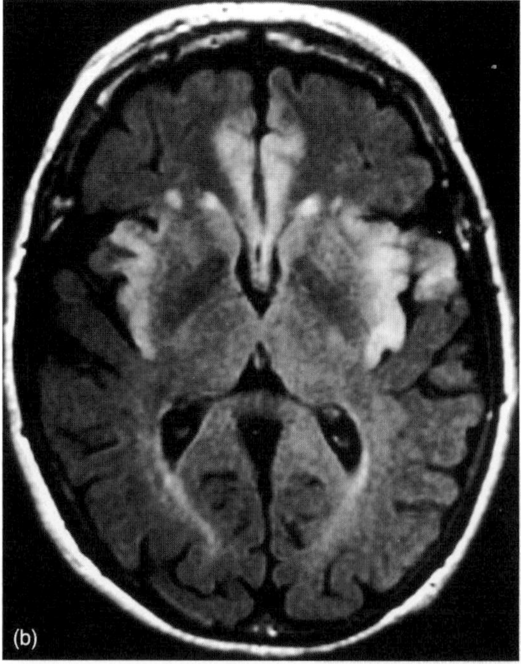

Figure 2.17 Herpes simplex encephalitis at two levels of MRI FLAIR sequence: (a) and (b) show the hyperintensity in the medial aspects of the temporal lobes, the insular cortex and the frontal cingulate regions bilaterally, worse on the left.

(rapidity of handwriting), paranoid ideation, hyposexuality and excessive religiosity. Whether these are true associations or represent reporting bias is uncertain. However, the concept of an epileptic personality is unfounded and unnecessarily stigmatizes sufferers.

Diseases of the occipital lobe

The occipital lobe (Fig. 2.8, page 23) is concerned with the perception of vision (the *visual cortex*) and its interpretation (the *parastriate* or association visual cortex). A unilateral cortical lesion will produce loss of vision in the homonymous fields. The macula or central vision is represented at the occipital pole. Diseases that extend to this will result in a loss of macular or central vision. *Cortical blindness* occurs with an extensive bilateral cortical lesion affecting the striate cortex (Fig. 2.18). Here the pupillary light reflex is retained despite the absence of any conscious perception of light. This may occur in a patient who has already sustained an occipital infarct from posterior cerebral artery occlusion who then suffers a similar event on the opposite side. Simultaneous occipital infarction may be the consequence of distal basilar artery occlusion, transtentorial herniation with compression of the posterior cerebral arteries, or may occur as a result of a hypoxic ischemic event, such as status asthmaticus. *Anton*syndrome results from disease extension into the association visual cortex; here there is denial of blindness despite obvious loss.

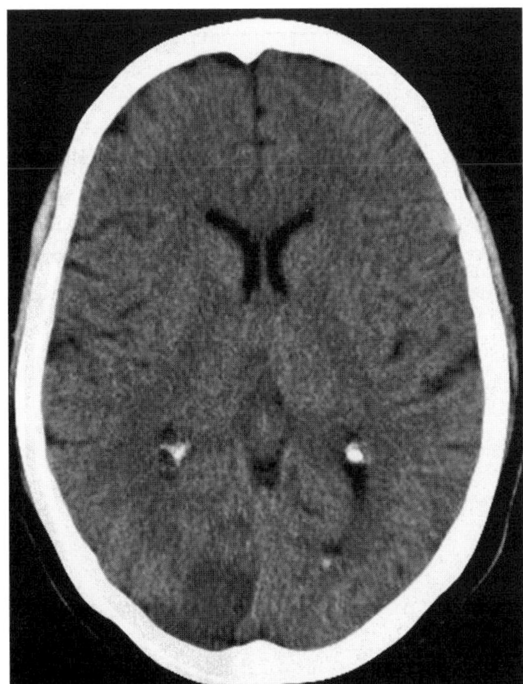

Figure 2.18 CT following traumatic vertebral dissection low attenuation segment in the right striate cortex represents an infarction.

Visual hallucinations of an unformed nature (shapes and colors) are common in migraine and here may have a retinal or an occipital cortical origin. Unformed hallucinations also occur with occipital simple or complex partial seizures. Subtle degrees of occipital dysfunction seen in degenerative or vascular disease result in patients having difficulty in naming an object – *visual agnosia* – or putting a name to a familiar face – *prosopagnosia.*

Other unusual perceptual disorders of the non-dominant hemisphere are not easily localizable to either parietal or occipital lobes. *Capgra syndrome* is an identity disorder; patients mistakenly believing that family members, for example, have been replaced by doubles impersonating them. *Reduplicative paramnesia* is a term applied when patients believe that they are simultaneously at two different locations (for example, in the ward and at home).

The disconnection syndromes

When the subcortical fiber connections between one area of the cortex and the next are damaged, a disconnection of one area from the other results. There are several forms of such disconnection syndromes. The isolation of the hearing from the language cortex results in *pure-word deafness.* Here patients can hear sounds but are unable to interpret the meaning of the spoken word. Another disconnection syndrome has already been described earlier with disease of the corpus callosum isolating a part of one hemisphere from the other. Infarction, demyelination, tumor or agenesis results in apraxia of movement, the patient having normal power in the limbs but being unable to initiate midline movement and thus unable to walk (*gait apraxia*). Another form of disconnection occurs when the sensory language cortex, Wernicke's area, is disconnected from the motor language cortex,

Broca's area. This results in a form of language disturbance termed *conduction aphasia*, a characteristic of which is impaired repetition. The arcuate fasciculus that links the two language areas is particularly susceptible to ischemia (the internal watershed between the pial and middle cerebral artery circulation).

THE THALAMUS

The thalamus is part of the basal ganglia structures that, with complex interconnections, cluster deep within the hemispheres. These paired masses of gray matter are egg-shaped and lie in relation to the lateral wall of the third ventricle. Anatomically and functionally four regions can be identified: anterior, posterior, medial and lateral. Efferent connections from the thalamus project to the frontal lobes, the hypothalamus, the cingulate gyrus, the mesial parietal cortex and the orbitofrontal cortex. Afferent connections are received from the mamillary bodies, the hippocampus, the frontal lobes, the amygdala, the hypothalamus, other basal ganglia structures and the sensory afferent pathways. These multiple connections emphasize the important role of the thalamus in attention, alertness and relaying sensory information (Table 2.1). The complex thalamic connections result in a plethora of symptoms and signs in disease. Four syndromes can be recognized, depending on the site of the lesion. Disease of the *anterior thalamic region* in the dominant hemisphere may cause dysphasia, inattention and memory impairment. Extension of disease into the *subthalamic region* may cause a movement disorder that takes the form of wild involuntary movements of the contralateral limbs (*hemiballismus*). Disease of the *medial thalamic region* results in impairment of recent memory, apathy, agitation, impaired attention and, occasionally, coma. Extension of the lesion into the midbrain region may result in impairment of ocular movements. *Ventrolateral thalamic* lesions result in sensory loss on the contralateral side of the body, often associated with paroxysmal sensory discomfort or pain. Finally, involvement of a *posterior thalamic* region results in hemianesthesia or sensory loss on the contralateral side of the body, often with visual field impairment and, again with pain.

Thalamic pain is a very specific symptom. It is unpleasant, often excruciating in quality and generally appears when the sensory loss following a thalamic lesion is recovering. The pain feels superficial and is exacerbated by touching the skin. When impairment of sensation is associated with this pain, the term *anesthesia dolorosa* is used. Thalamic pain and thalamic syndromes are rare, and although they occur with tumors they are usually more indicative of cerebrovascular disease, in particular disease affecting the small perforating blood vessels.

Whilst vascular disease is the commonest thalamic pathology, involvement is seen in many conditions such as cerebral palsy, head injury, infections, variant CJD (selectively affecting the pulvinar and dorsomedial nucleus) and frontotemporal dementia.

Table 2.1 Thalamus, geniculate bodies and their connections

Thalamic region	Afferent input	Efferent output
Anterior	Mamillary bodies	Cingulate gyrus
Dorsal medial	Amygdala, caudate, temporal cortex, olfactory, limbic regions	Dorsal lateral nucleus
Ventral anterior	Basal ganglia	Premotor and motor area
Ventral anterior	Cerebellum, basal ganglia, substantia nigra	Motor area
Lateral posterior		
Ventral lateral posterior	Touch, pressure, pain, termperature	Area 1, 2, 3, postcentral gyrus
Pulvinar	Posterior cortex, superior colliculus	Posterior cortex, areas 17–18
Lateral geniculate body	Visual projection	Area 17, occipital cortex
Medial geniculate body	Auditory projections	Area 41, temporal lobes

THE HYPOTHALAMUS AND PITUITARY GLAND

The hypothalamus is involved in the regulation of the 'internal milieu' of the body – its *homeostatic control.* It achieves this by means of a neuroendocrine role, in collaboration with the pituitary gland, as well as by its influence upon the autonomic nervous system. Through these pathways body temperature is regulated, the cardiovascular system controlled, and food and water intake balanced.

The hypothalamus also lies in the lateral wall of the third ventricle, being separated from the thalamus by a short sulcus. The hypothalamus can be divided into four regions: anterior, posterior, medial and lateral, with specific nuclei lying in each (Fig. 2.19). There are projections to the midbrain and to the reticular formation, these being responsible for alertness and arousal. There are also connections to the limbic system, important in behavior and memory; and, finally, links to the sympathetic and parasympathetic nuclei of the brainstem and spinal cord, controlling autonomic function. The precise relationship of a particular function to a specific area of the hypothalamus remains uncertain, and is compounded by the identification of multiple neuropeptides found within these regions and active in the control of body temperature, cardiac and respiratory function, fluid balance, behavior, reproductive function and circadian rhythm. The hypothalamic control of vegetative function is to a greater extent mediated through the pituitary gland, the control of hormonal secretions from the anterior pituitary being regulated by hypothalamic releasing factors (Table 2.2). Bilateral hypothalamic disease is usually a prerequisite for the development of symptoms. Involvement of the *anterior hypothalamus* will result in cachexia, diabetes insipidus and hypothermia. *Posterior hypothalamic* involvement will produce hypothermia, coma and apathy. Involvement of the *medial hypothalamic* structures results in excessive water intake, inappropriate secretion of antidiuretic hormone (ADH), obesity, memory impairment and aggression. Involvement of the *lateral hypothalamus* results in reduced water intake, dehydration, emaciation and apathy. The identification of specific neuropeptides that control body temperature, food intake and emotion has greatly enhanced understanding of these disorders. Hypothalamic peptides also play an important role in controlling the release of anterior pituitary hormones. The hypothalamus may be damaged by trauma, metabolic and vascular disease or, rarely, by neoplasm.

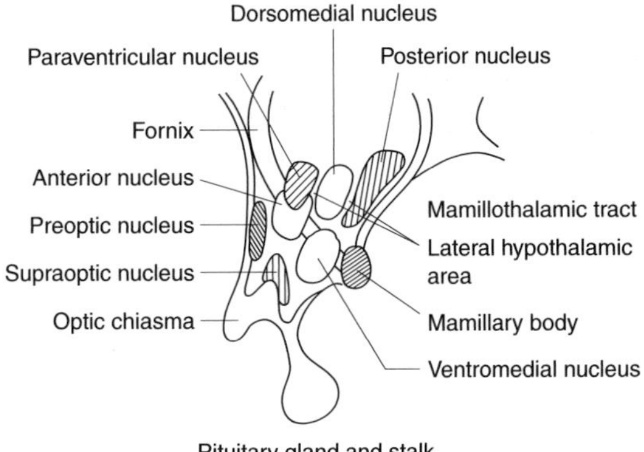

Figure 2.19 The hypothalamic nuclei and their relationship to surrounding structures.

Lesions that affect the pituitary gland may present hormonally with either decreased or increased pituitary hormone production (Table 2.2). Increased production is associated with *pituitary adenomas.* Excess *growth hormone* causes gigantism in children and acromegaly in adults. Increased *prolactin* causes delayed puberty in children and, in adult females, amenorrhea, galactorrhea and infertility. In males it may be associated with impotence, infertility and, rarely, galactorrhea. Increased *thyrotropin* results in hyperthyroidism, and increased *luteinizing hormone* and *follicle-stimulating hormone* will produce precocious puberty in children and, in adults, infertility, hypogonadism and the polycystic ovary syndrome. Adenomas that do not result in excessive hormone secretion are termed 'silent' or 'non-functioning' and present with generalized pituitary failure – *pan-hypopituitarism.*

An expanding lesion in the pituitary gland will often give rise to headache due to stretching of the diaphragma sella (Fig. 2.20). Because of the proximity to the optic chiasm, visual field defects are commonly associated with large pituitary tumors, the usual presentation being that of a *bitemporal hemianopia.* Visual field defects are not always

Table 2.2 The pituitary hormones

Part of the pituitary	Hormone	Major target organ	Physiologic effects
Anterior	Growth hormone		
	*Growth hormone releasing hormone	Liver, adipose tissue	Promotes growth, control of protein, lipid and carbohydrate metabolism
	Thyroid stimulating hormone	Thyroid	Stimulates secretion of thyroid hormones
	*Thyropropin releasing hormone		
	Adrenocortiotropic hormone	Adrenal gland	Stimulates secretion of
	*Corticotropin-releasing factor	(cortex)	glucocorticoids
Posterior	Prolactin	Mammary gland	Stimulates lactation
	*Prolactin inhibiting factor		
	Luteinizing hormone	Ovary and testis	Control of reproductive function
	*Gonadotropin releasing factor		
	Follicle-stimulating hormone	Ovary and testis	Control of reproductive function
	Antidiuretic hormone	Kidney	Conservation of body water
	Oxytocin	Ovary and testis	Stimulates milk ejection and uterine contractions

The anterior pituitary synthesizes and secretes six major hormones. That individual cell groups secreted a single hormone supported the one-cell – one-hormone theory. Now considered that the presence of more than one hormone in the same cell favors plurihormonality. Secretion is influenced by hypothalamic releasing hormones, which are indicated by asterisks.

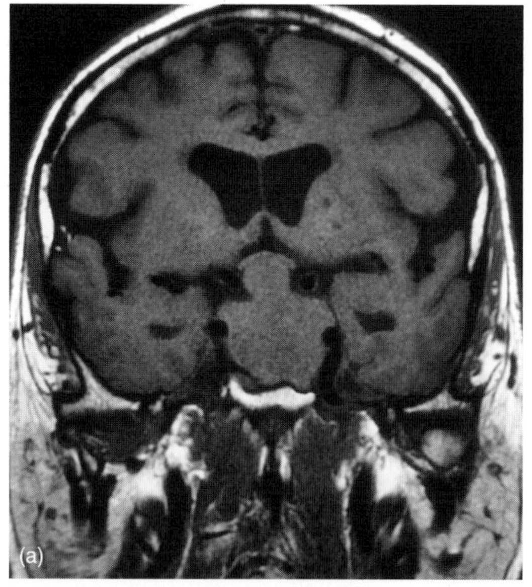

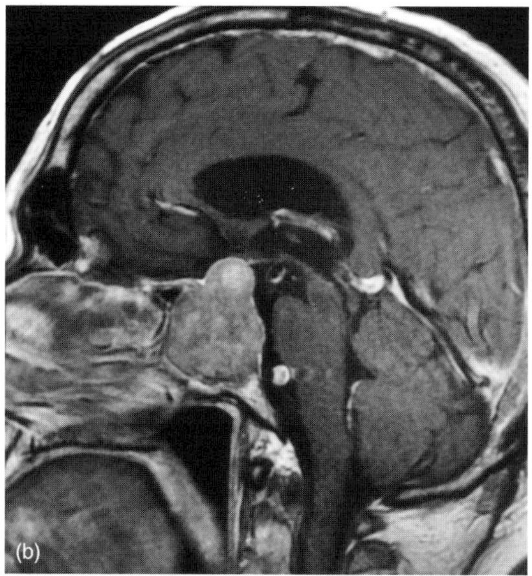

Figure 2.20 Pituitary macroadenoma on (a) T1-weighted coronal section and (b) T1-weighted sagittal section after intravenous contrast showing marked enhancement of the adenoma which has expanded out of the enlarged and eroded sella to fill the sphenoid sinus and suprasellar cistern to compress the optic chiasm.

associated with compression but can result from intermittent displacement or vascular shunting.

Whilst tumors account for most pituitary lesions, inflammatory conditions (lymphocytic hypophysitis) and developmental disorders (Rathke's cleft cyst) also occur.

THE BASAL GANGLIA

The deep subcortical paired masses of gray matter are referred to collectively as the basal ganglia (Fig. 2.21) and include the *corpus striatum*, consisting of the putamen and caudate nucleus, the *substantia nigra*, the *globus pallidus* and the *subthalamic nuclei*. The basal ganglia are responsible for the control and modulation of movements as well as the maintenance of posture. The anatomical connections are complex and circuitous, there being multiple interconnections as well as afferent and efferent projections from all parts of the cerebral cortex. The majority of striatal efferents project to the globus pallidus, the rest to the substantia nigra. The globus pallidus projects to the hypothalamus and to the subthalamic nuclei (Fig. 2.22).

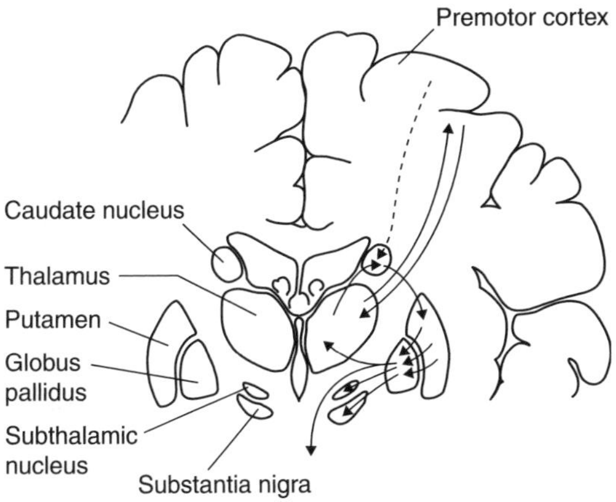

Figure 2.21 The basal ganglia and their principal connections.

The observation that certain drugs can produce symptoms identical to those found in disease of the basal ganglia has served to clarify the neurochemical basis of many movement disorders, and delineate the central role of certain specific neurotransmitters. The major two neurotransmitters within the basal ganglia are *acetylcholine*, synthesized in striatal cells, and *dopamine*, synthesized by cells of the substantia nigra. In disease of the basal ganglia two types of symptom are noted: *negative symptoms*, in which there may be a loss or slowness of movement or impairment of posture, and *positive symptoms*, which take the form of involuntary movements. Advances in functional imaging have further enhanced understanding of pre- and post-synaptic neurotransmission. SPECT by deploying specific ligands is a sensitive and specific diagnostic tool in tremor evaluation (Fig. 2.23).

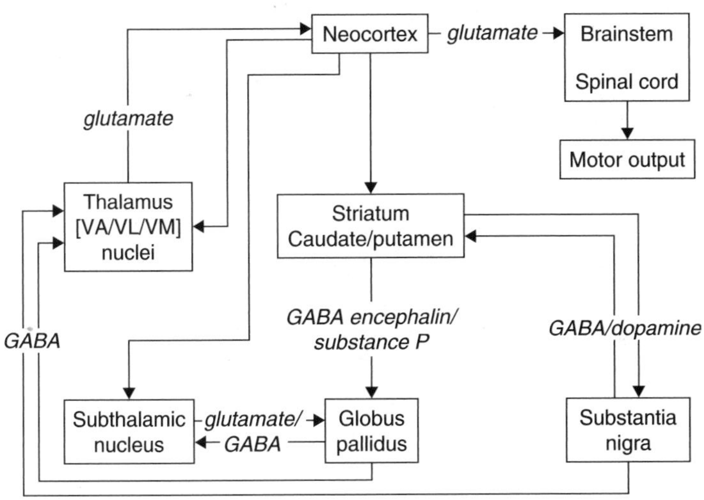

Figure 2.22 Connections of the basal ganglia and their neurotransmitters. VA = ventral anterior nucleus, VL = ventral lateral nucleus, VM = ventral medial nucleus.

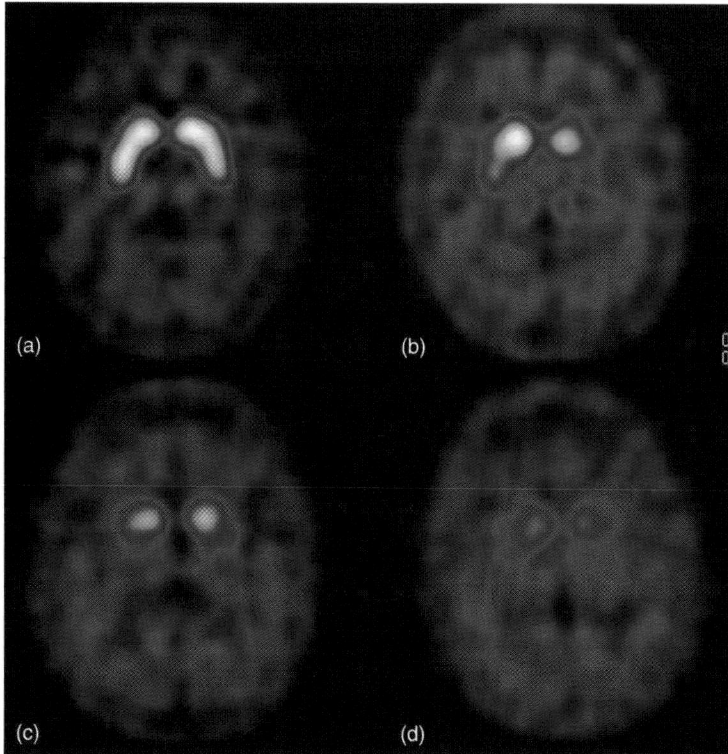

Figure 2.23 SPECT scan with ^{123}I-FP-CIT visualizing the D2 transporters in the striatum. (a) Patient with essential tremor: normal uptake. (b) Early Parkinson's disease: stage 1. (c) Worse disease: stage 2. (d) Severe disease: stage 3.

Particular types of such movement disorder are associated with a distinct anatomical region.

Chorea

Choreiform movements are brief, sudden involuntary movements of an irregular nature, appearing like jerks or fidgeting. These movements are classically encountered in Huntington's and Sydenham's choreas, although they may occur in a host of metabolic, degenerative and drug-induced disorders. Pathological studies suggest that choreiform movements are associated with disease affecting the caudate nucleus and putamen.

Athetosis

Movements that are uncontrolled, slow, and writhing characterize athetosis. These often seem to blend into single sinuous movements. The distal musculature of extremities (hands and feet) is involved but also face, neck and tongue muscles are affected. Athetoid movements are a frequent feature of cerebral palsy and co-exist with chorietic movements. These movements are encountered in Wilson's disease, and other neonatal disorders: kernicterus and perinatal hypoxia. Damage to the cerebral cortex is essential in combination with involvement of the globus pallidus and substantia nigra.

Dystonia

These can be defined as sustained muscle contractions, often with a twisting and repetitive quality. Dystonia is classified as *primary* where there is no clear cause and secondary when it arises after birth injury, trauma, toxins, drugs or stroke. The movements may be *segmental* confined to a single or group of muscles (blepharospasm, cervical or oromandibular dystonia and writer's cramp) or *generalized.* The latter where primary is often inherited (early-onset generalized, Dopa-responsive and paroxysmal dystonias). Genetic advances have identified dystonia genes – *DYT 1*, for example. When structural lesions are found these usually reside in the contralateral striatum, especially the putamen.

Hemiballismus

These wide-amplitude violent flinging or flailing movements appear to affect proximal limb muscles. They are rarely bilateral and can result in self-injury. Such movements are associated with lesions in the contralateral subthalamic nucleus and may be encountered in tumors, demyelination or acutely in cerebrovascular disease.

Tremor

Tremor is not necessarily a symptom of basal ganglia disease. It can occur physiologically as well as in certain metabolic and cerebellar disorders. It may also occur in peripheral neuropathies, especially demyelinating ones. Tremor, however, is a consistent finding in parkinsonism, whether idiopathic or drug-induced. *Parkinson's disease* is a consequence of striatal dopamine deficiency and results in degeneration of the pigmented neurons in the pars compacta of the substantia nigra. The tremor characteristically occurs at rest, is coarse in quality and is associated with rigidity and paucity of movement (bradykinesia). The distinction between late onset benign *essential tremor* and Parkinson's disease can be clinically difficult and SPECT imaging has proved helpful (Fig. 2.23). Tremor can also be a feature of other neurodegenerative disorders often mistaken for Parkinson's disease, *progressive supranuclear palsy, multi-system atrophy* and *diffuse Lewy body disease*. These conditions are associated with rigidity, bradykinesia, eye movement disorders and autonomic failure. The myriad diagnostic difficulties are exemplified by the final diagnostic outcomes of the United Kingdom Parkinson's Disease Society Tissue Bank.

THE BRAINSTEM

The relationship of the brainstem to the cerebral hemispheres and cerebellum is shown in Fig. 2.24. The brainstem is classically divided into midbrain, pons and medulla. Each of these regions contains cranial nerve nuclei as well as ascending and descending pathways. Knowledge of the anatomy of the brainstem is essential in clinical neurology, not only in order to localize disease to a specific level, but also to help distinguish intrinsic brainstem disease from an extrinsic compressive process.

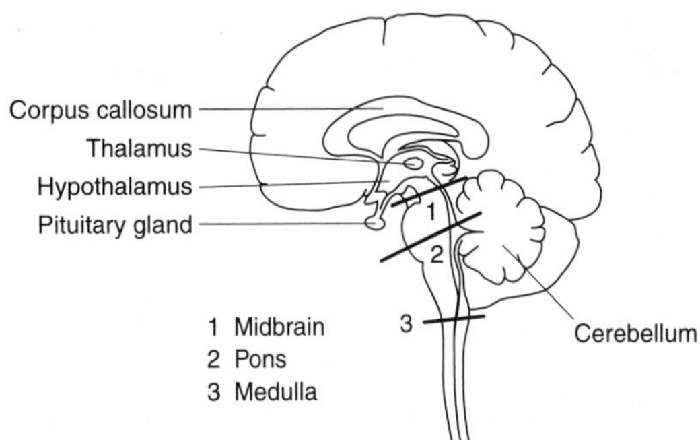

Figure 2.24 Midsagittal section of the brain showing relationship between brainstem and cerebellum.

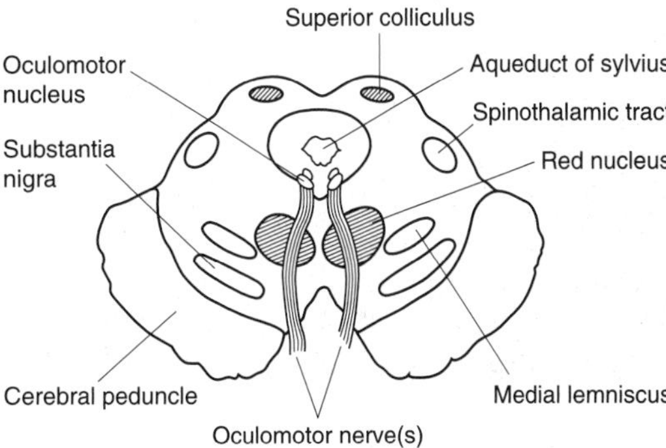

Figure 2.25 Section through the midbrain.

The midbrain

The midbrain lies between the pons and the cerebral hemispheres, the dorsal aspect being made up of the paired *superior* and *inferior colliculi* (Fig. 2.25). The *cerebral peduncles* converge upon one another, entering the pons at its upper surface. The *IIIrd* and *IVth cranial nerve nuclei* and their emergent nerves, as well as part of the interconnecting *medial longitudinal fasciculus* that coordinates ocular movements, lie within the midbrain associated with the ascending sensory and descending motor pathways. Symptoms of midbrain disease take the form of contralateral spastic hemiplegia if a cerebral peduncle is diseased, *diplopia* if destruction of the IIIrd and/or IVth cranial nerve nuclei occurs, and impairment of vertical eye movements and convergence if the superior colliculus is damaged. There are three specific midbrain syndromes usually encountered in cerebrovascular disease: *Weber syndrome* takes the form of an ipsilateral complete IIIrd nerve palsy associated with contralateral hemiplegia; *Benedikt syndrome* results from damage to the red nucleus and the IIIrd nerve fasciculus, giving tremor and cerebellar signs contralateral with an ipsilateral IIIrd nerve palsy; *Parinaud syndrome* results from damage to the superior colliculus, with impaired upward gaze and convergence. This syndrome may be seen with posterior third ventricular tumors, pineal region tumors and hydrocephalus.

The pons

As well as containing descending motor and ascending sensory pathways, the pons (Fig. 2.26) is linked to the cerebellum by the *anterior* and *middle cerebellar peduncles*. It contains the *Vth to the VIIIth cranial nerve nuclei* and their emergent nerves, as well as the continuation of the pathway linking the nuclei involved in coordinated ocular movements in the *medial longitudinal fasciculus*. The vestibular and cochlear nuclei of the VIIIth nerve lie at about the pontomedullary junction. Three pontine syndromes are recognized, usually associated with vascular disease. In *dorsolateral infarction* an ipsilateral Horner syndrome is associated with contralateral loss of pain and temperature from limbs and body, usually with sparing of the face. Ipsilateral cerebellar ataxia is also present, and impaired lateral ocular gaze to the side of the lesion is common. Other associated features, such as deafness and nystagmus, may occur if these specific cranial nerve nuclei are affected. The corticobulbar and corticospinal tracts are spared. *Paramedian infarction* may affect the VIth nerve and the associated VIIth nerve fibers as they sweep around the VIth nerve nucleus. The medial lemniscus may also be affected, with loss of touch and proprioception on the opposite side of the body. Finally, *basilar infarction*, if unilateral, will result in a contralateral hemiplegia associated with VIth and VIIth nerve palses (Millard–Gubler syndrome). Bilateral basilar infarction will result in quadriplegia.

Medulla oblongata

The medulla oblongata is a pyramid-shaped section of the brainstem connecting the pons with the spinal cord (Fig. 2.27). The lower part contains the floor and body of the *fourth ventricle*. As well as ascending sensory and descending motor pathways, the medulla oblongata contains the *IXth to the XIIth cranial nerve nuclei* and their emerging nerves. It also contains specific centers for vital function involved in respiration and cardiac control. Two vascular syndromes are recognized: *dorsolateral infarction* (Wallenberg syndrome or lateral medullary syndrome) is usually the consequence of occlusion of the posterior inferior cerebellar artery. It results in an ipsilateral Horner syndrome with contralateral loss of pain and temperature perception. Ipsilateral facial sensation is usually affected. Vertigo and vomiting are common, ipsilateral ataxia is usually present, and the IXth and Xth cranial nerves are occasionally affected.

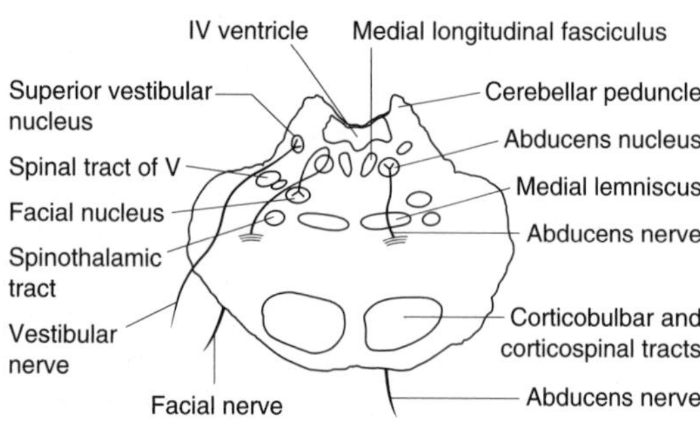

Figure 2.26 Section through pons.

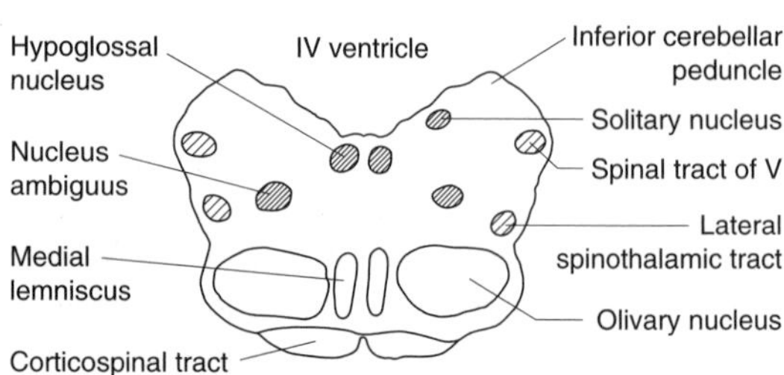

Figure 2.27 Section through the medulla oblongata.

Paramedian or *basilar infarction* usually occurs as a consequence of basilar artery occlusion. Here, bilateral damage to the medulla results in the patient being mute and quadriplegic, often with impaired sensation in the medial lemnisci and relatively spared lateral spinothalamic pathways. This results in the so-called '*locked-in syndrome*', in which the patient is quadriplegic and unable to communicate, although fully conscious.

Throughout the brainstem runs the *reticular formation*, consisting of scattered groups of neurons responsible for activation of the thalamus and cortex. The reticular formation plays a major role in the maintenance of consciousness and its integrity is essential for arousal from sleep, wakefulness and attention. Impaired function results in comatose states. The reticular formation may be damaged by vascular disease, but is also influenced by drugs and anaesthetic agents.

The brainstem is susceptible to compression at any point in its course. This may occur as a consequence of a fusiform aneurysm in the posterior fossa or the cerebellopontine angle, an ectatic basilar artery and tumors lying in the posterior cranial fossa. The latter usually present initially with cranial nerve dysfunction, such as loss of sensation in the face in the case of a trigeminal schwannoma, or impaired hearing in the case of an acoustic schwannoma (neuroma), long before secondary brainstem compression occurs with resultant central brainstem symptomatology. Advances in imaging have made such separation on clinical grounds alone unnecessary. The clinician should, however, always be aware that the development of subtle unilateral hearing loss or disturbed facial sensation might be the initial presentation of an extrinsic tumor that eventually causes complex brainstem symptomatology. Extra-axial lesions (outside the brainstem) may cause multiple contiguous cranial nerve palsies, often too far apart (in the brainstem) to be caused by an intra-axial lesion. Intra-axial lesions (within the brainstem) tend to cause long tract signs (motor and sensory changes) in addition to cranial nerve palsies. Typically, these are 'crossed'. For example, right-sided facial weakness with weakness of the left arm and leg.

Specific constellations of cranial nerve involvement inform on localization at discrete sites other than the brainstem alone. Clusters of contiguous cranial nerve disturbance generally indicate extra-axial disease. These diagnostic syndromes together are listed (Table 2.3).

Table 2.3 Combination of cranial nerve palsies and their localization

Anatomical site	Cranial nerves affected
Superior orbital fissure (anterior cavernous sinus)	3, 4, 6 and 5 (1st division)
Posterior cavernous sinus	3, 4, 6, and 5 (1st and 2nd division)
Apex of petrous temporal bone	5 and 6
Internal auditory meatus/cerebellar pontine angle	7 and 8
Jugular foramen	9, 10 and 11
Below skull base (retropharangeal space)	9, 10, 11, 12 and sympathetic

THE CEREBELLUM

The cerebellum is located in the posterior cranial fossa behind the pons and medulla and is connected to these structures by *three paired peduncles*. The cerebellum is composed of a small unpaired median portion referred to as the *vermis* and the two large paired *cerebellar hemispheres*. Deep within the cerebellum are located groups of nuclei: the *dentate*, *emboliform*, *globus* and *fastigial* nuclei. The cerbellar efferent and afferent connections are complex. The function of the cerebellum is to modulate motor activity, controlling and smoothing out movements and maintaining stance, posture and gait. The major symptom of cerebellar disease is *ataxia*. This implies a disturbance in the smooth performance of voluntary motor acts. This results in movement that is no longer continuous and coordinate but rather broken up into small jerky components, with abnormal excessive excursions. Patients experience problems in performing rapid alternating tasks with their limbs, unsteadiness of the feet while walking, and the necessity to walk

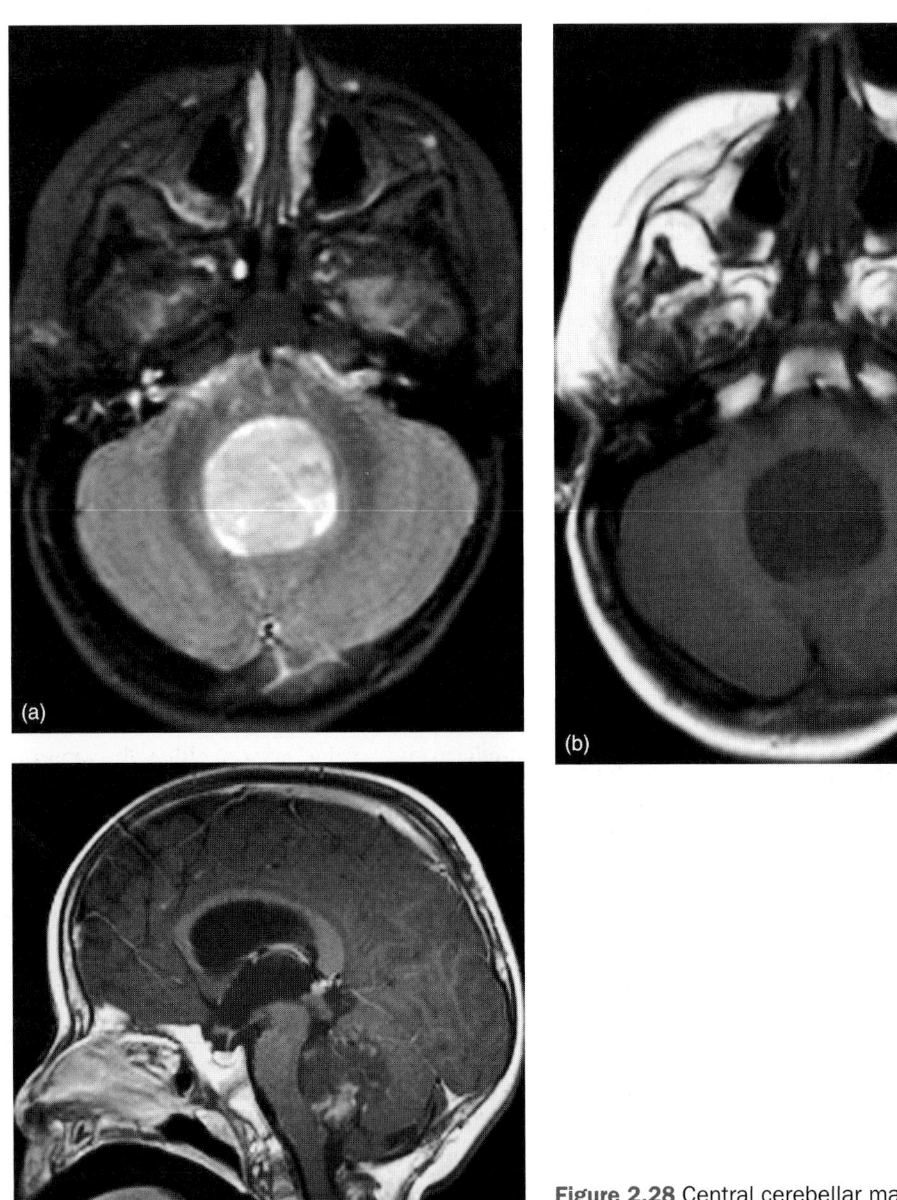

Figure 2.28 Central cerebellar mass involving and effacing the IV ventricle in a 6-year-old. (a) T2-weighted and (b) T1-weighted axial sections with (c) T1-weighted post-contrast sagittal section. Appearances are typical of a medulloblastoma.

and turn with the feet placed widely apart. Slurring of speech occurs as a consequence of poor motor control of articulatory movement (*dysarthria*). Tremor is present, as is disturbance of smooth eye movement, and nystagmus (jerks of eye movement) is commonly encountered. Certain specific cerebellar syndromes are recognized: *anterior cerebellar lobe* involvement results in the patient walking with a broadened gait but with no evidence of limb incoordination, disturbance of speech or ocular movements. Such cerebellar dysfunction is often found as a consequence of nutritional or alcohol indiscretion. It may also result from long-term drug treatments.

Posterior cerebellar vermis syndrome takes the form of a more profoundly disturbed gait, with an inability to stand without swaying. Again there is no evidence of limb ataxia and no disturbance of ocular movement. This syndrome may also be associated with alcohol and drug abuse, but is also encountered in cerebrovascular disease.

Finally, a *cerebellar hemisphere syndrome* occurs with unilateral cerebellar disease. This results in marked incoordination of the ipsilateral limbs, unsteadiness of gait with a tendency to lurch to the diseased side, slurring or dysarthria of speech, and nystagmus with fast beats to the affected side. This hemisphere syndrome may be encountered with cerebellar tumors, infarction or hematoma (Fig. 2.28).

A further syndrome is recognized in which all features of cerebellar function are involved. In this so-called *pan-cerebellar syndrome* there is marked disturbance of gait and balance, ataxia in all four limbs, disturbed ocular movements and dysarthria. A pan-cerebellar syndrome is encountered in certain degenerative disorders and may also occur as a non-metastatic manifestation of malignancy (paraneoplastic syndrome). Cerebellar disease may be the consequence of developmental disorders such as cerebellar hypoplasia, vascular disease (either ischemic or hemorrhagic) and tumors arising from midline structures such as medulloblastoma, or from the hemispheres – glioma, hemangioblastoma or metastases. There is also a large group of degenerative, hereditary and metabolic disorders such as sporadic acquired cerebellar degeneration, the familial spinocerebellar degeneration (associated with specific ataxia genes – SCA mutations) and certain inborn areas of metabolism. Infective disorders, in particular viral infection in childhood with varicella zoster, may give rise to a self-limiting 'cerebellitis'.

Finally, cerebellar symptoms and signs, in conjunction with brainstem dysfunction, are commonly encountered in demyelinating disease, either in the form of acute disseminated encephalomyelitis or, more commonly, in multiple sclerosis.

RAISED INTRACRANIAL PRESSURE

The skull is a rigid structure and its contents – blood, brain and cerebrospinal fluid – are incompressible. An increase in one constituent or an expanding mass within the skull will result in *increased intracranial pressure*. The primary causes of raised intracranial pressure are many, and are compounded by the development of brain edema, which may arise around an intrinsic lesion within brain tissue or in relation to traumatic, ischemic or toxic brain damage. The clinical effects of raised intracranial pressure are the development of headache, vomiting and papilloedema as well as the shift of structures within intracranial compartments. The pathologist should be aware of the clinical features of *brain shift syndromes* (Fig. 2.29). Four specific types of herniation syndrome are recognized. *Subfalcine* midline shift occurs with unilateral space-occupying lesions and seldom produces any clinical effects, although compression of the ipsilateral anterior cerebral artery with infarction of the medial aspect of the frontal lobe has been documented. *Transtentorial herniation* (lateral) with a unilateral expanding lesion causes

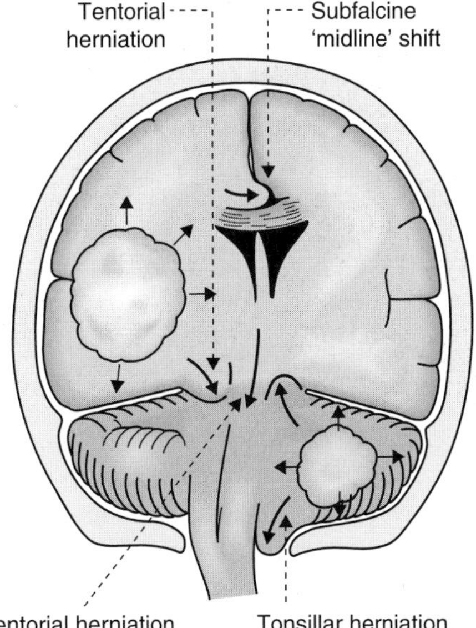

Figure 2.29 Brainstem herniations.

tentorial or uncal herniation, with the medial part of the temporal lobe passing through the tentorial hiatus. This results in compression of the IIIrd cranial nerve in its intracranial course, and manifests clinically as an ipsilateral dilated pupil unreactive to light, associated with ptosis and downward and outward deviation of the eye. Lateral shift at the tentorial hiatus may result in compression of the ipsilateral cerebral peduncle (*Kernohan's notch*). Clinically, this will result in hemiparesis *ipsilateral* to the mass lesion causing herniation, and is consequently regarded as 'a false localizing sign'.

Tentorial herniation (central) results in buckling of the midbrain, with distortion and stretching of the perforating blood vessels. This leads to deterioration of conscious level, and initially small pupils that then become intermediate in size and unreactive to light and to accommodation. Compression on the upper midbrain may result in impairment of upward gaze, convergence and pupillary enlargement (*Parinaud syndrome*), and downward compression on the pituitary stalk and hypothalamus may result in diabetes insipidus. *Tonsillar herniation* caused by an infratentorial expanding mass will cause the cerebellar tonsils to prolapse or herniate through the foramen magnum. This will result in neck stiffness, often with a head tilt, depression of consciousness and disturbance of vital respiratory and cardiac function (Chapter 4).

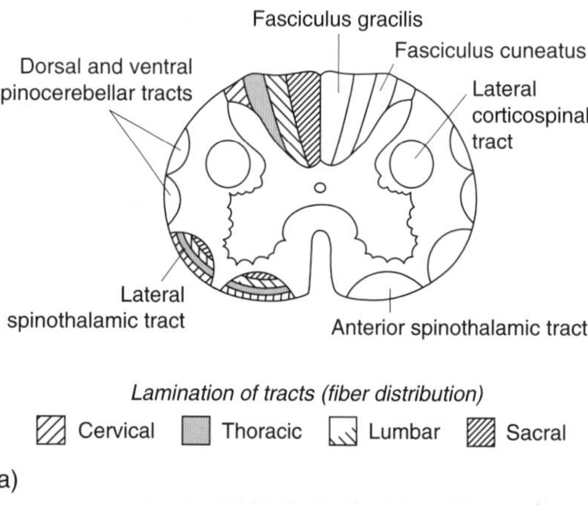

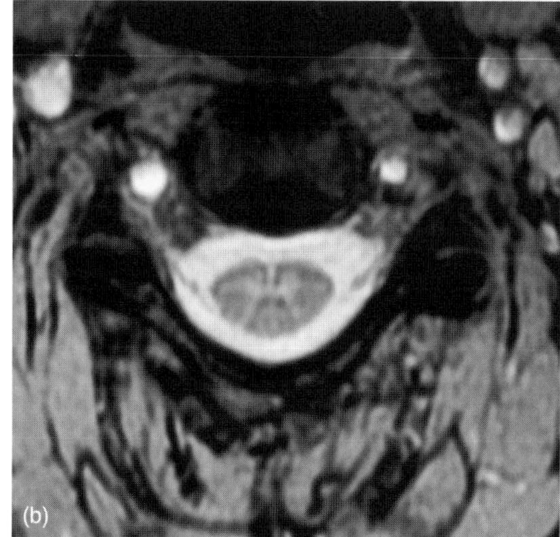

Figure 2.30 (a) Schematic representation of spinal cord pathways. (b) 3T high definition axial T2-weighted section of the cervical cord at CV4. The medullary gray matter and cervical roots are well delineated.

THE SPINAL CORD

The spinal cord extends from the level of the cranial border of the atlas, where it is continuous with the medulla, to the first lumbar vertebra. In fetal life the spinal cord extends beyond this to the end of the sacrum, but as elongation of the vertebral column occurs during life the spinal cord retreats, although still remaining connected to the sacrococcygeal region by the *filum terminale*. The cross-sectional anatomy of the spinal cord is shown in Fig. 2.30. There is variability in the size of fiber tracts at specific levels and, therefore, the cross-sectional appearance of the spinal cord is variable, depending on whether this be at cervical, thoracic or lumbar levels. Also, the *inter-mediolateral gray column* giving rise to preganglionic sympathetic autonomic fibers extends only from T1 to L2. A laminar cytoarchitecture of nine layers within the central gray matter of the spinal cord is recognized. This comprises sensory neurons dorsally and motor neurons ventrally. The *major ascending tracts* carry sensation to the thalamus and cerebral cortex, finely myelinated or unmyelinated sensory fibers passing through the dorsal root, terminating in neurons in the dorsal horns and then crossing over the next few segments to form the *lateral* and *anterior spinothalamic tracts*, conveying the sensations of pain, temperature and light touch to consciousness. The more heavily myelinated fibers in the dorsal roots pass into the dorsal horns and then ascend in the *posterior columns*, ending in the nucleus gracilis and nucleus cuneatus on the dorsal surface of the medulla, then decussating within the medulla to form the medial lemnisci and passing up to the ventral nucleus of the thalamus and on to the primary sensory cortex. These fibers carry discriminatory sensations (vibration, weight, proprioception, pressure). Other ascending pathways include the dorsal and ventral spinocerebellar tracts, which convey unconscious proprioceptive information from the trunk and lower half of the body to the cerebellum.

The descending pathways all exert their influence on α and γ motor neurons lying in the ventral layers of the central gray matter of the anterior horns of the spinal cord. The major pathway is the corticospinal tract, arising predominantly from the primary motor cortex, passing down through the internal capsule into the cerebral peduncle of the midbrain and the basis of the pons, with projections to motor cranial nerve nuclei (corticobulbar fibers) before descending to the pyramidal decussation in the lower part of the medulla, arm fibers decussating before lower limb fibers. It follows from this that any disorder of the spinal cord will result in a combination of motor, sensory and autonomic dysfunction. Also important in the understanding of diseases of the spinal cord is an awareness of its complex blood supply. Paired *posterior spinal arteries* arise from the posterior inferior cerebellar artery and pass on the dorsal aspect of the spinal cord, where they form a plexus which is joined in its course down the spinal cord by approximately 12 unpaired radicular feeding arteries. This rich circulation protects the posterior part of the spinal cord from vascular disease. The *anterior spinal artery* is a single vessel formed by two branches of the vertebral artery running together. The anterior spinal artery lies in the median fissure of the spinal cord and receives approximately seven to ten unpaired radicular branches during its course, these arising in the cervical region as well as from intercostal blood vessels. The anterior spinal artery is at its narrowest in the lower dorsal region, and its largest radicular vessel, the *artery of Adamkiewicz*, enters between T10 and T12. This blood supply can be easily compromised, most often at a mid-dorsal level, which is the watershed area and thus vulnerable to damage by prolonged hypotension.

Disorders of the spinal cord

Localization to a specific level of the spinal cord is dependent upon knowledge of the segmental innervation of limb reflexes, the level of decussation of the spinothalamic fibers and the assessment of motor and sensory levels. By careful clinical examination, it is possible to delineate certain specific spinal cord syndromes synonymous with particular disease processes. The history and clinical examination may help distinguish extrinsic or *extramedullary* lesions from intrinsic or *intramedullary* pathology. In the former, *root pain* is a common initial symptom and cord compression, when it occurs, appears selective, compromising motor before sensory pathways. Also, disturbance of bladder and bowel function is a late feature. In intramedullary spinal cord disease there is often a sparing of lower lumbar or sacral sensory modalities (*sacral sparing*), which reflects the lamination of fibers within the spinothalamic pathways, in that sacral and lumbar segments lie to the outside whereas thoracic and cervical segments lie to the inside and are thus more susceptible to intrinsic pathology. In intramedullary lesions bladder and bowel dysfunction commonly occur early, and motor and sensory upsets tend to occur in conjunction.

The spinal cord syndromes

Spinal cord syndromes are outlined in Fig. 2.31.

Complete transection

Complete transection of the spinal cord will result in loss of power below the level of transection. If this is in the cervical region, quadriplegia ensues; if in the thoracic region, paraplegia. Below the level of transection all sensory function to pain and temperature as well as discriminatory sensation is lost, and a clear level of sensory loss can be documented on the trunk. Bladder and bowel function is also lost, the bladder becoming automatic, unable to be emptied at will but emptied by means of manual compression. Disturbances of blood pressure and temperature control are common. Complete cord transection

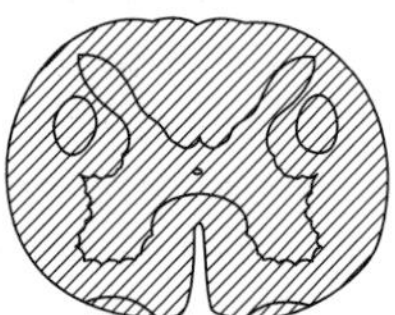

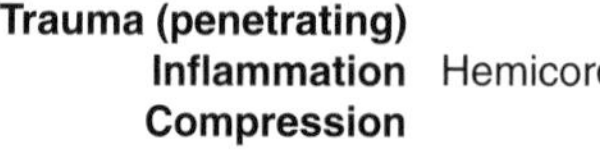

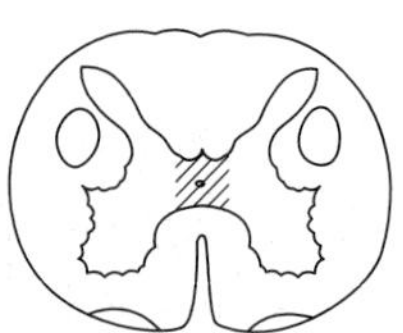

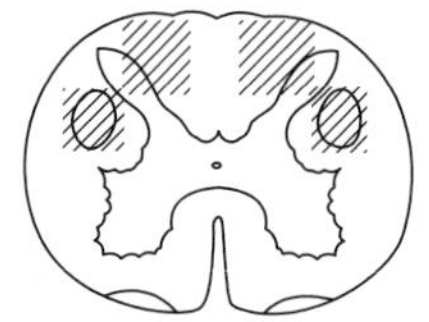

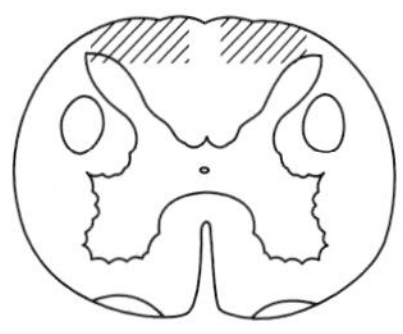

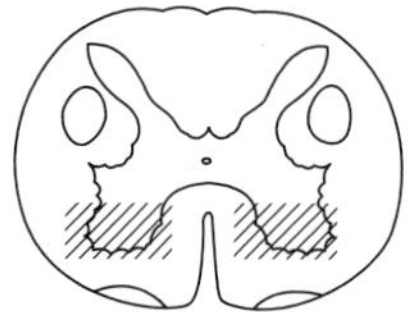

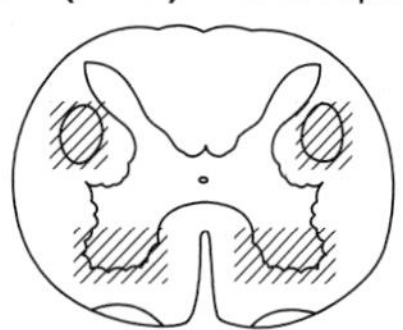

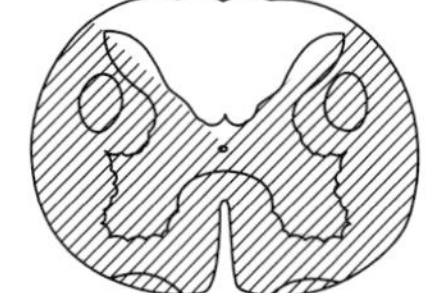

Figure 2.31 Spinal cord syndromes.

is usually the consequence of trauma, but may occur following inflammation in transverse myelitis, or is the end result of an untreated compressive lesion.

Hemicord or Brown–Séquard syndrome

Here, one side of the spinal cord is diseased but the other is spared. Reflex, motor and sensory dysfunction is evident. There is loss of discriminatory sensation on the same side of the body, and limb paresis with loss of spinothalamic function (i.e. temperature and pain perception) on the contralateral side. This syndrome is encountered with penetrating injuries to the spinal cord as well as inflammatory and compressive lesions.

Central syndrome

Lesions within the center of the spinal cord first affect the decussating fibers of the spinothalamic pathways conveying pain and temperature. This results in a loss of those modalities of sensation, with retention of discriminatory or dorsal column sensation. This is referred to as *dissociated sensory loss*, and often takes the form of a cape-like distribution affecting the arm, shoulder and trunk, with sparing of the face, abdomen and lower limbs. This means that an upper and lower segmental level can be defined. As the central cord lesion progresses, anterior horn-cell involvement ensues, with wasting and paralysis and loss of reflexes. Extension into the dorsal columns will eventually result in the loss of discriminatory sensation, and extension into the corticospinal tracts will result in spasticity and upper motor neuron paresis of limbs distal to the lesion. This syndrome is classically encountered in *syringomyelia*, but it may occur with any intramedullary tumor and has been reported following severe hyperextension neck injuries.

Selective involvement of specific ascending and descending pathways

Tabes dorsalis predominantly affects the dorsal columns and posterior root entry regions. This results in a loss of discriminatory sensation as well as pain and temperature perception in the absence of paralysis. *Posterolateral degeneration* (subacute combined degeneration of the spinal cord) is classically the result of vitamin B_{12} deficiency. Here the dorsal columns conveying discriminatory sensation are involved, but also the corticospinal pathways, resulting in spasticity. Peripheral nerve involvement is also encountered, accounting for loss of limb reflexes.

The anterior horn region of a spinal cord may be specifically involved. This classically occurs in poliomyelitis, where wasting and loss of reflexes occur in a segmental distribution with no impairment of sensory function. A similar, although more chronic, and generally symmetrical picture is encountered in the progressive muscular atrophy form of motor neuron disease, as well as in other rarer forms of motor neuron diseases (spinal muscular atrophies). *Combined anterior horn cell* and *corticospinal tract dysfunction* is seen in amyotrophic lateral sclerosis (classic motor neuron disease). Here, segmental wasting and weakness is associated with hyper-reflexia.

Finally, *vascular syndromes* of the spinal cord are commonly encountered, in particular the *syndrome of infarction in the anterior spinal artery* territory. Here, the anterior two thirds of the spinal cord are affected, with preservation of posterior function, paralysis being associated with loss of spinothalamic sensation but retention of dorsal column sensation.

The causes of spinal cord disease are multiple. Compression may be secondary to degenerative disease of the cervical or thoracic spine, or may be the consequence of lesions such as neurofibroma, meningioma and metastatic carcinoma. It may also result from direct trauma to the spinal cord, or inflammatory processes such as transverse myelitis or multiple sclerosis. The spinal cord may be affected in a variety of nutritional and metabolic disorders, as well as by infection such as tuberculous spinal compression, HIV myelopathy or spinal abscess. The spinal cord is also susceptible to radiation injury, such as after radiotherapy, and other physical insults including hypothermia and electrocution.

DISORDERS OF PERIPHERAL NERVES

The function of the peripheral nervous system is to convey information to and from the central nervous system with regard to motor, sensory and autonomic activities. The *axon* is an elongation of the neuron, either lying within the central nervous system, in the a and g neurons of the spinal anterior horn, or else in an outlying ganglion such as the dorsal root ganglion, whose peripheral and central axons are responsible for conveying sensory information to the spinal cord. Peripheral nerves can be divided into those insulated by a myelin sheath and those that are unmyelinated. Diseases of the peripheral nervous system are selective, in that they may affect motor, sensory or autonomic fibers or else they preferentially affect myelinated or unmyelinated fibers, sparing others. The clinical features of *peripheral neuropathy*, the commonest disorder of the peripheral nervous system, are those of distal motor weakness and/or distal sensory loss accompanied by a loss of deep tendon reflexes. In some of the hereditary neuropathies, peripheral nerves are palpable and skeletal abnormalities such as pes cavus occur in association. The commonest causes of peripheral nerve damage seen in clinical practice in western countries are diabetes mellitus, alcohol abuse and nutritional disturbance. Neuropathy may also occur as a non-metastatic syndrome, in association with collagen vascular disease and as the consequence of a host of drugs and toxins.

There are specific circumstances when *nerve biopsy* is essential to direct appropriate management. This is particularly the case in the chronic, inflammatory demyelinating neuropathies and in neuropathy due to vasculitic disease. A nerve biopsy is not routinely performed in the evaluation of peripheral nerve disease, but only in highly specific circumstances where a combination of clinical presentation, electrophysiological investigations and ancillary laboratory tests suggest it is appropriate.

DISEASES OF MUSCLE

Disease of skeletal muscle may present with obvious wasting and/or weakness, or give rise to more subtle symptomatology, taking the form of aches and pains in muscles induced by exercise in the context of normal muscle bulk and strength on formal examination. There is an increasing recognition of *mitochondrial disorders*, which may present without muscle symptomatology and yet muscle histology may prove to be diagnostic. The *muscular dystrophies* are genetically determined myopathies in which progressive degeneration, wasting and weakness occur; the pathogenesis is unknown. Muscular dystrophies may have sex-linked, autosomal dominant or autosomal recessive inheritance whilst earlier diagnosed clinically on the topography of weakness, age of onset and the presence or absence of associated features such as contractures, muscle hypertrophy, cardiomyopathy. Molecular testing has revolutionized the diagnostic approach. The phenotype of a specific genotype can be surprisingly variable and thus misleading.

Inflammatory myopathies often present in childhood as *dermatomyositis*, or in adult life as *polymyositis*. These conditions are usually acute or subacute in onset, predominantly affecting proximal muscle groups often associated with weakness of neck flexion and, often, difficulties in swallowing. Skin and joint features may be characteristic. Muscle enzymes (creatinine kinase) are profoundly elevated and the diagnosis can be confirmed by muscle biopsy, which is essential in view of the complexity of treatment in those patients resistant to initial conventional treatment.

Metabolic myopathies are often easily diagnosed clinically in view of the associated features, e.g. thyrotoxicosis, acromegaly, hypoparathyroidism. Other more subtle metabolic myopathies such as those of phosphorylase (McArdle's disease) and acid maltase deficiency require biopsy for confirmation. Advances in histocytochemistry has led to the recognition of many complex disorders of carbohydrate, lipid and protein metabolic pathways in muscle. Finally, the *mitochondrial disorders* may present with a variable phenotype of neurological features, including myoclonic epilepsy, stroke-like syndromes and a relatively non-progressive polymyopathy. In these conditions a muscle biopsy with deletion/mutation studies are essential for diagnosis.

CHAPTER 3

THE CENTRAL NERVOUS SYSTEM AND ITS REACTIONS TO DISEASE

David I Graham

MICROSCOPY OF THE NORMAL NERVOUS SYSTEM

The neuron

A neuron consists of a cell body (perikaryon) and its processes. Neurons vary considerably in shape and size, ranging from the small granule cells of the cerebellum that measure about 5 μm in diameter to the larger motor cell in the ventral horns of the spinal cord that measure up to 120 μm in diameter. Each possesses a single axon that also varies considerably in length, ranging from a few millimeters to up to 90 cm. The number of its dendrites varies from one to as many as 80, according to the type of neuron. Whatever their size or function, neurons share certain features: they have a high metabolic rate, they are vulnerable to lack of oxygen and/or glucose, and in postnatal life they lose the ability to multiply.

Large neurons have vesicular nuclei, prominent nucleoli and a coarsely granular cytoplasm (Fig. 3.1). These basophilic granular masses (Nissl substance) are composed of RNA-rich stacks of rough endoplasmic reticulum and intervening groups of polyribosomes (Fig. 3.2a and b). Mitochondria and Golgi apparatus are usually highly developed. Neurofibrils are present in all neurons and are of

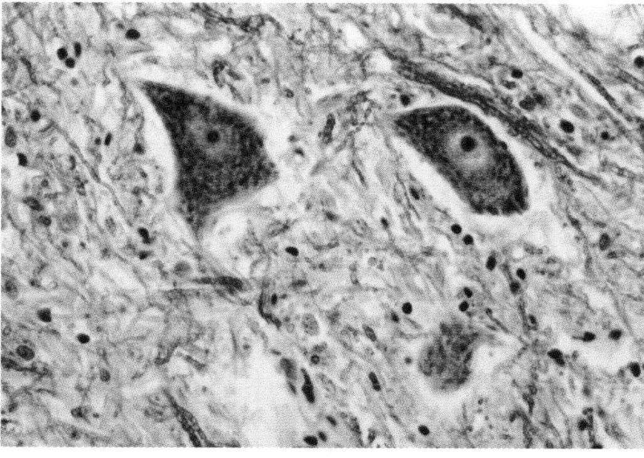

Figure 3.1 Normal neuron. Ventral horn cells from human lumbar spinal cord. The nucleus is round and centrally placed, and contains a prominent nucleolus: the cytoplasm contains large numbers of Nissl bodies that extend into dendrites. Luxol fast blue/cresyl violet.

two principal types, 20–30 nm neurotubules, and 6–10 nm neurofilaments, both of which resemble similar structures in axons and dendrites. There are organized mechanisms that transport material within axons both away from (*anterograde*), which has fast and slow components and towards (*retrograde*) the perikaryon. Fast anterograde flow (up to 1000 mm per day) transports mitochondria and neurosecretory vesicles: the slow component (up to 5 mm per day) conveys components of the cytoskeleton. Retrograde flow (about 200 mm) transports

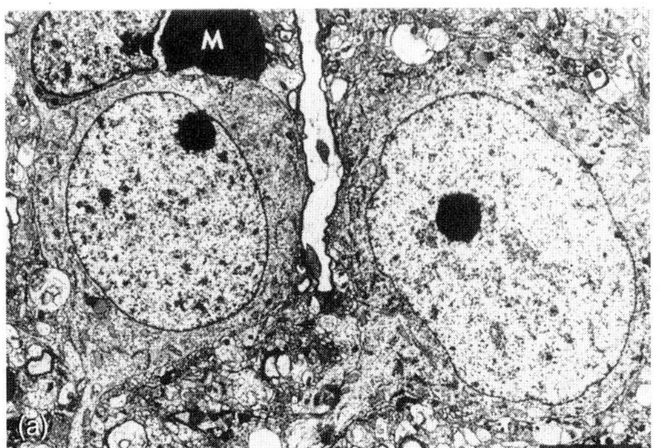

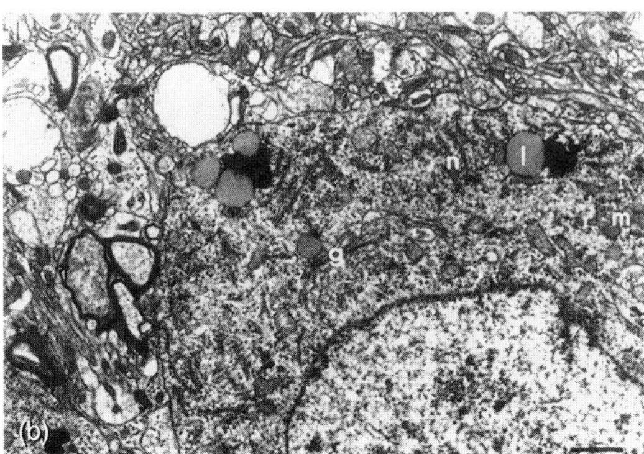

Figure 3.2 Normal neuron in human cerebral cortex. (a) The pale cytoplasm contains membranous organelles and Nissl substance. An electron-dense perineuronal microglial cell (M) lies in close relation to one neuron. (b) The pale central nucleus is surrounded by cytoplasm containing mitochondria (m), Golgi apparatus (g), Nissl substance (n) and lipofuscin granules (l). Transmission electron micrograph. Bar (a) 5 μm (b) 1 μm. (Courtesy of Dr W.L. Maxwell, Laboratory of Human Anatomy, University of Glasgow, UK.)

lysosomes and a heterogeneous collection of small vesicles that are either disposed of or are recycled in the perikaryon.

Neurotransmitters are transported to the *boutons terminaux* which form *synapses* on dendrites and perikarya of other neurons. The cytoplasm of synapses contains mitochondria and neurofibrils similar to and continuous with those in the perikaryon, but the characteristic organelle of the bouton is the *synaptic vesicle* (Fig. 3.3) in which the neurotransmitter is stored. In catecholaminergic excitatory fibers the synaptic vesicles usually have a dense osmiophilic core but in inhibitory neurons the vesicles are clear and agranular. Larger vesicles are seen in some neurons, and in the hypothalamus take the form of neurosecretory granules associated with peptide hormones and their carriers. Although, neurotransmitters exhibit great diversity in many of their properties, all are stored in vesicles in nerve terminals and are released to the extracellular space. In some terminals more than one type of transmitter substance is released.

Lipofuscin is a cytoplasmic organelle which measures about 1 μm diameter (Fig. 3.2b) and is the type of lysosome (residual body) in which nonmetabolizable substances accumulate: it stains bright red with Sudan dyes and is positive for periodic acid–Schiff reagent. It is membrane-bound and usually has an electron-dense and an electron-light component, which is presumably responsible

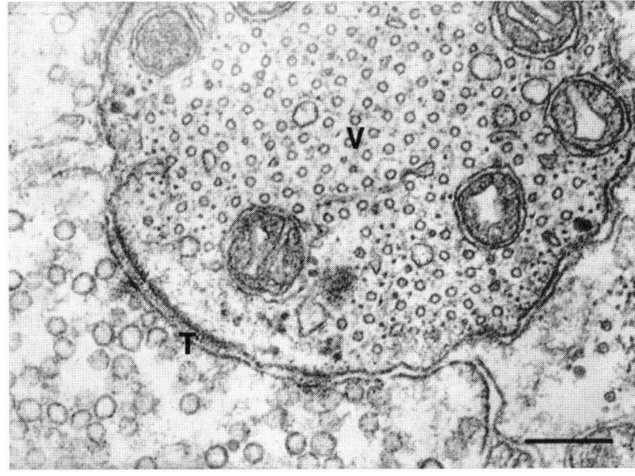

Figure 3.3 Synapse. Clear round synaptic vesicles (V) predominate in the presynaptic element and there is prominent post-membranous thickening (T) in the postsynaptic element. Bar = 0.5 μm.

for its light yellow color. The normal organelle that is particularly conspicuous in certain neurons, such as those in the olivary nuclei (Fig. 3.4) and the ventral horns of the spinal cord, increases with age, and an increased number of lipofuscin granules are seen in certain pathological conditions, such as aging and dementia. It is also found in many somatic cells, e.g. the skeletal and cardiac muscle, and liver. In certain sites, e.g. the substantia nigra and locus caeruleus, granules of *neuromelanin* are normal cytoplasmic constituents (Fig. 3.5).

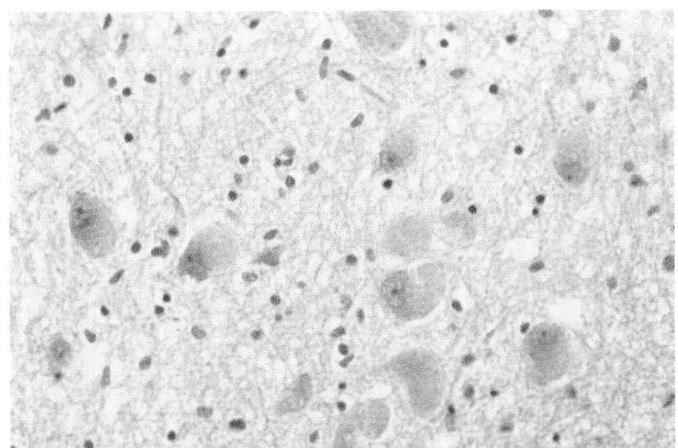

Figure 3.4 Lipofuscin. Olivary nucleus of elderly subject.

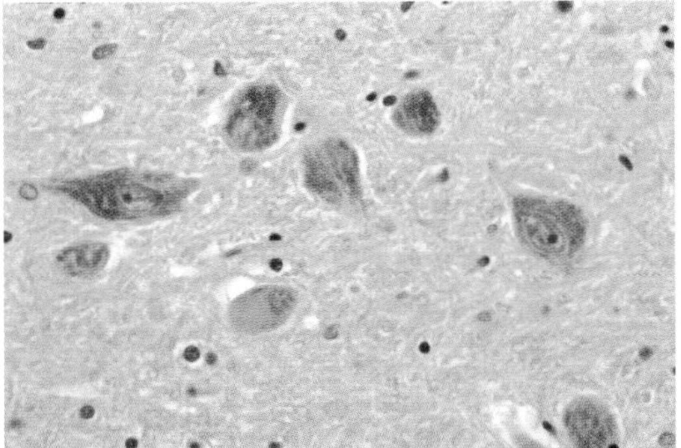

Figure 3.5 Neuromelanin. Normal neurons of substantia nigra.

The neuroglia

Astrocytes

Traditionally, two types of astrocytes are recognized, *protoplasmic* and *fibrillary* (fibrous). Only their round or ovoid 8–10 μm nuclei can be recognized in routinely stained sections, and special techniques (e.g. immunohistochemistry) are required to stain their processes which, by electron microscopy, contain glycogen and large amounts of 9 nm intermediate filaments. *Fibrillary astrocytes* are widely distributed throughout the white matter of the central nervous system (CNS), and their numbers increase with age. They occur in the white matter of the CNS as a thick layer beneath the pia (Fig. 3.6a and b). A similar layer is seen beneath the ependyma and between these two surfaces, fibrillary astrocytes are intimately associated with neurons and myelinated fibers, and there is a close association with the microvasculature, the basement membrane of all capillaries being enveloped by the foot processes of astrocytes. *Protoplasmic astrocytes* are largely confined to gray matter (cortex, basal ganglia and thalami), where they closely

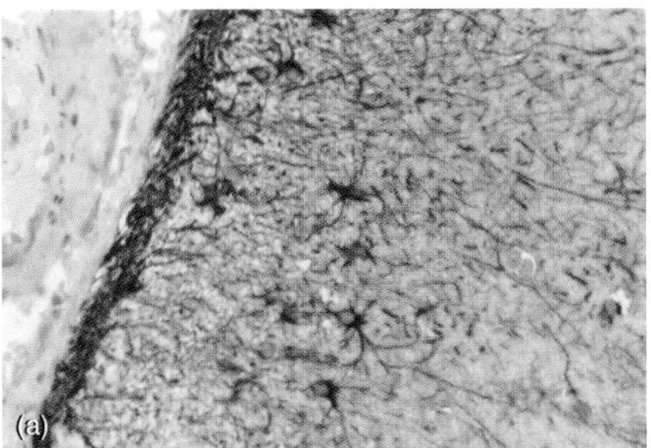

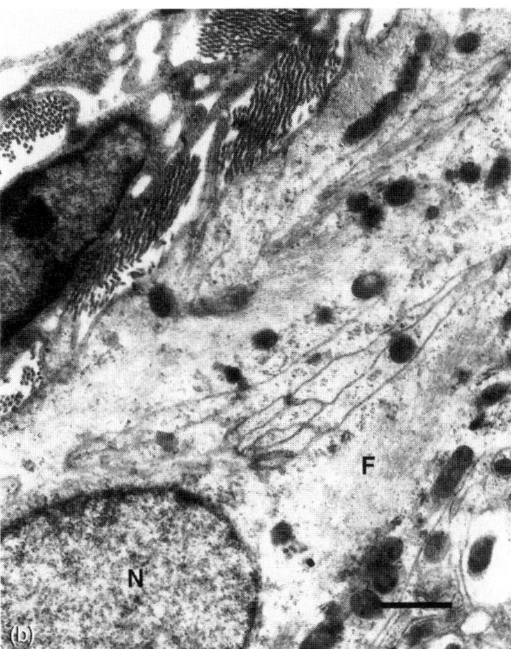

Figure 3.6 Astrocyte. (a) There is a felt work of normal astrocytes beneath the pia mater. (b) An astrocyte in the glia limitans from the human cerebral cortex. The nucleus (N) has a characteristic electron-dense rim. Bundles of intermediate filaments, (F) occur in the cytoplasm among other organelles. (Courtesy of Dr W.L. Maxwell, Laboratory of Human Anatomy, University of Glasgow, UK.) (a) Immunohistochemistry glial fibrillary acidic protein. (b) Transmission electron micrograph. Bar = 1 μm.

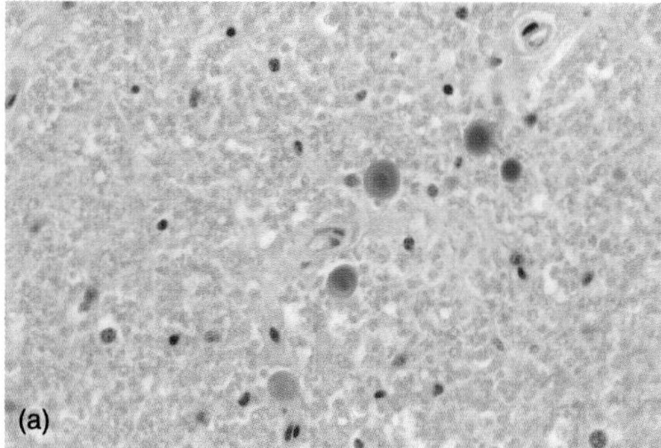

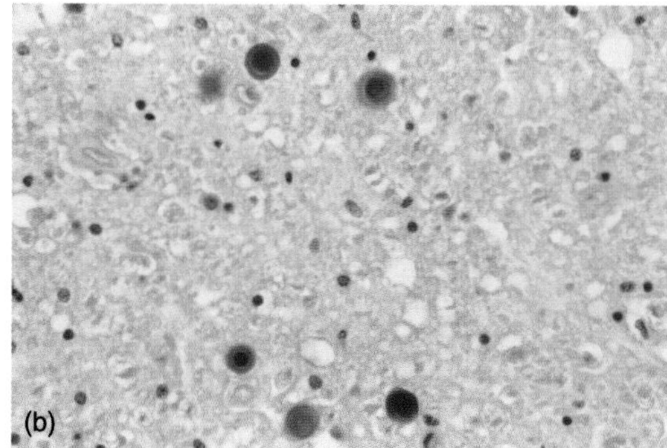

Figure 3.7 Corpora amylacea in subpial white matter. (a) H&E. (b) PAS.

invest neurons and their processes except at synapses. The processes of protoplasmic astrocytes are short and stout and they branch more often than the long, fine processes of the fibrillary astrocytes. The Bergmann cells found in the granule layer of the cerebellum near the Purkinje cells are a variant of astrocytes.

Multiple functions have been ascribed to astrocytes, in addition to that of a structurally supportive role. Thus, during fetal development the radial glia guide migrating neurons to their permanent positions in the cerebral and cerebellar cortex. There is also an increasing awareness of the metabolic functions of astrocytes because of the close functional relationships that exist between them and neurons: these include regulation of the ionic composition of the extracellular fluid and their influence on calcium and neurotransmitter metabolism. Another major role is healing and repair after damage to the CNS.

Corpora amylacea are 10–15 μm diameter rounded, laminate bodies that are often present in the periventricular and subpial white matter, and in the spinal cord, particularly of elderly subjects. They stain gray or grayish blue in H&E preparations and are PAS-positive (Fig. 3.7a and b). They are thought to represent end-stage degeneration of astrocytes.

Oligodendroglia

There are two main types of oligodendroglia. In gray matter they are closely related to neurons, when they are referred to as *perineuronal satellite cells*: in white matter they are lined up between myelinated fibers as the *interfascicular glia*. The cytoplasm of normal oligodendrocytes is more electron-dense than that of astrocytes (Fig. 3.8). They contain the usual organelles apart from cytoplasmic filaments.

Myelin in the CNS is formed and maintained by oligodendrocytes. It consists of the compaction of the oligodendrocyte cell membrane, the resulting laminated structure of many successive layers of protein and lipid wrapped around the axon, having a characteristic ultrastructural feature with appearance and periodicity in which the major dense period line is formed where the cytoplasmic components of the cell membranes fuse, and the interperiod line from the fusion of the outer surfaces of the oligodendroglial membrane. Schwann cells subserve the same function in peripheral nerves (Fig. 3.9). A unique feature of the oligodendrocyte is that it myelinates a single internode of up to 10–15 axons: this contrasts with the Schwann cell (see Chapter 18), which can only form a single internode of myelin. There is some relationship both in the CNS and PNS between the thickness of the myelin sheaths formed by oligodendrocytes and Schwann cells, respectively, and the diameter of the axon, and the length of the internode. Thus, in general, large-diameter axons have thick myelin sheaths and small-diameter axons thin myelin sheaths, whereas the internodes and large-diameter axons are longer than those on small diameter axons. The constituents of myelin include cholesterol, phospholipids and cerebroside in a ratio of 2:2:1, and there are large amounts of *Folch–Lees phospholipid* and *myelin basic protein*. Myelin

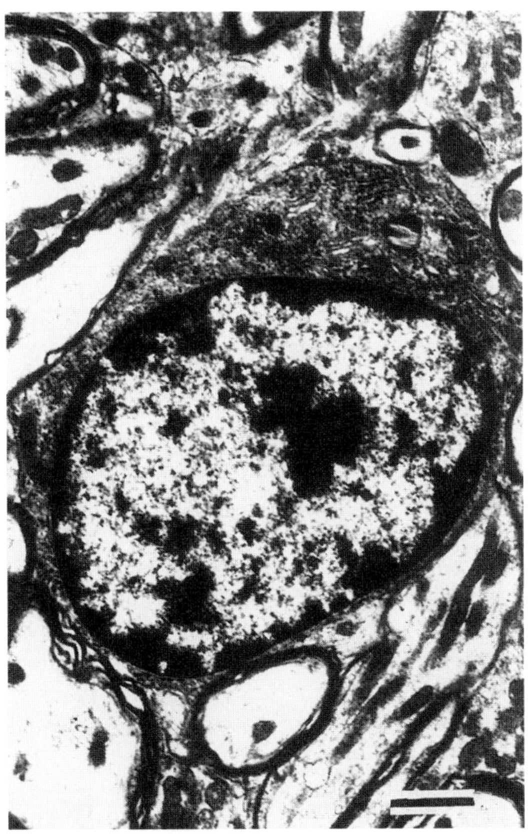

Figure 3.8 Oligodendrocyte from the white matter in man. Punctate heterochromatin occurs within the nucleus. The cell cytoplasm forms a thin, electron-dense perinuclear sheath. Transmission electron micrograph. Bar = 1 μm. (Courtesy of Dr W.L. Maxwell, Laboratory of Human Anatomy, University of Glasgow, UK.)

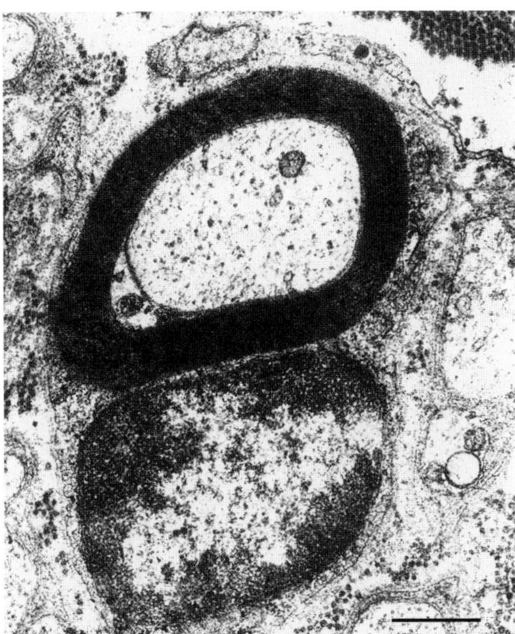

Figure 3.9 Myelinated fiber from a peripheral nerve. Note the pale axoplasm, the myelin sheath and the associated Schwann-cell nucleus. Transmission electron micrograph. Bar = 1 μm. (Courtesy of Dr W.L. Maxwell, Laboratory of Human Anatomy, University of Glasgow, UK.)

acts as an insulating material and prevents excitation of the axolemma other than at the *nodes of Ranvier*. At the nodes, the myelin sheaths at either side form end loops of cytoplasm and attachment zones between the sheath and axon. These form the glial–axonal junction (Fig. 3.10a and b). Conduction of a nerve impulse is mediated through polarization and repolarization at the nodes of Ranvier, the impulse passing in a *saltatory fashion*.

Ependyma

The ventricles and the central canal of the spinal cord are lined by ciliated cuboidal or columnar cells known as ependymal cells (Fig. 3.11a and b). At the base of the cilia of the ependymal cells are small bodies known as *blepharoplasts*. The blepharoplast stains with phosphotungstic acid hematoxylin (PTAH) and corresponds to the basal corpuscle seen with the electron microscope. The ependyma is normally a continuous layer, although both tight and gap junctions exist between the cells, but with increasing age it becomes discontinuous and there is thickening of the subependymal layer of astrocytes. It seems highly likely that a primary function of the ependymal cells is related to circulation of the CSF.

Choroid plexus

These are vascular structures (Fig. 3.12a and b) in the lateral, third and fourth ventricles. They are covered by non-ciliated cuboidal cells and are the major source of CSF, the circulation of which is dealt with in Chapter 4. A small quantity of CSF is formed by exudation through the ependyma.

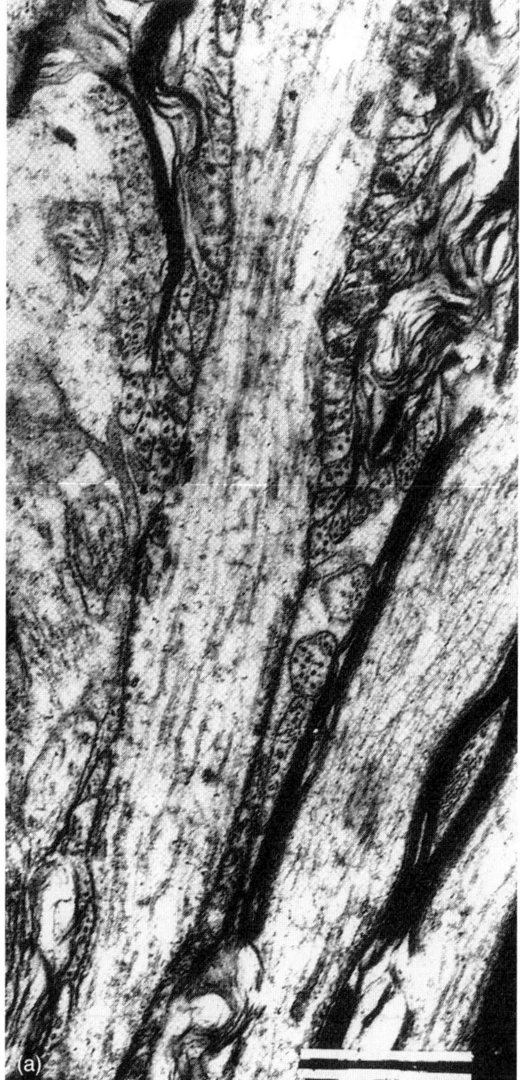

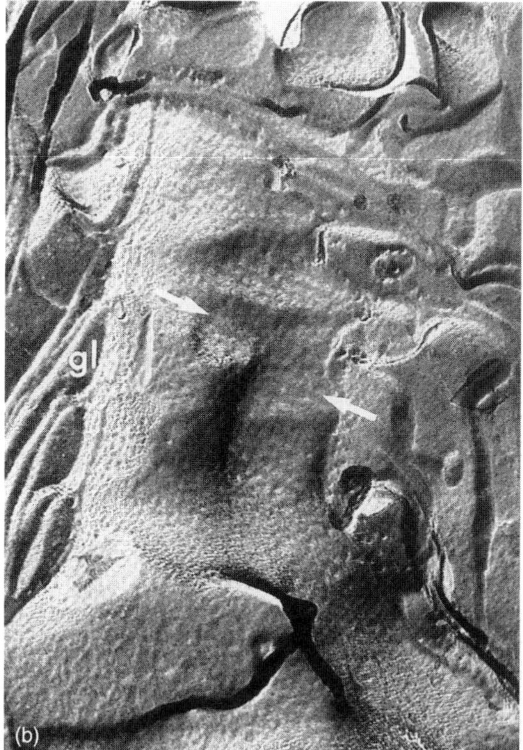

Figure 3.10 Node and paranode. (a) This is a longitudinal section of a central myelinated nerve fiber to illustrate the structural features of the nodal and paranodal regions. Transmission electron micrograph. Bar = 1 μm. (b) Central myelinated nerve fiber of a non-human primate. The glial end loops (gl) closely abut the axolemma. Helical particulate arrays (arrows) occur on the axolemma at the sites of the glial–axonal junctions. (Courtesy of Dr W.L. Maxwell, Laboratory of Human Anatomy, University of Glasgow, UK.)

The neuropil

This term is used to designate the intercellular matrix in the CNS. In H&E stained sections it appears as 'ground substance' (Fig. 3.5), whereas electron microscopy has established that it consists of a dense complex of glial and neuronal processes together with some myelin. Between the membranes of adjacent cells there is a potential extracellular space, which is estimated by electron microscopy to be 20 nm wide, and it is in this space that the movements of ions are believed to occur.

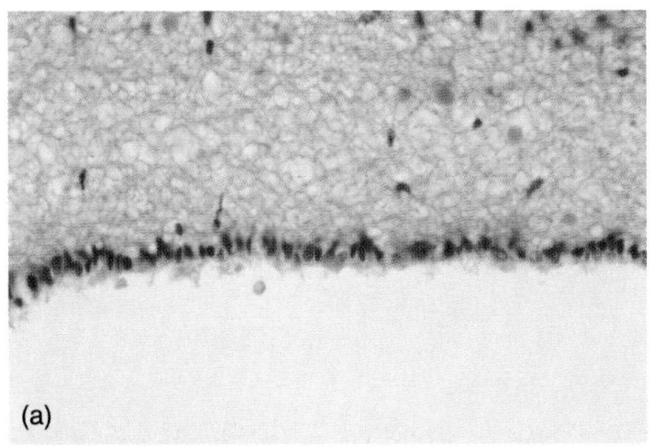

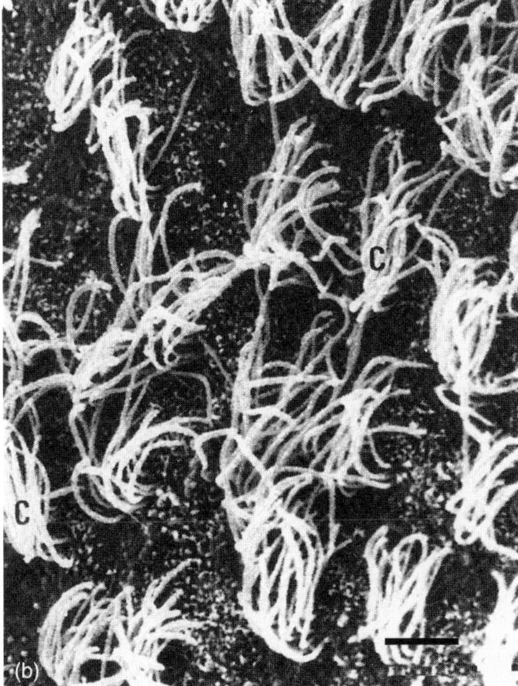

Figure 3.11 Ependyma from a human lateral ventricle. (a) Normally the ventricular system is lined by a continuous layer of cuboidal cells that separate CSF from brain tissue (H&E). (b) There are numerous cilia. Scanning electron micrograph. Bar = 10 μm. (Courtesy of Dr W.L. Maxwell, Laboratory of Human Anatomy, University of Glasgow, UK.)

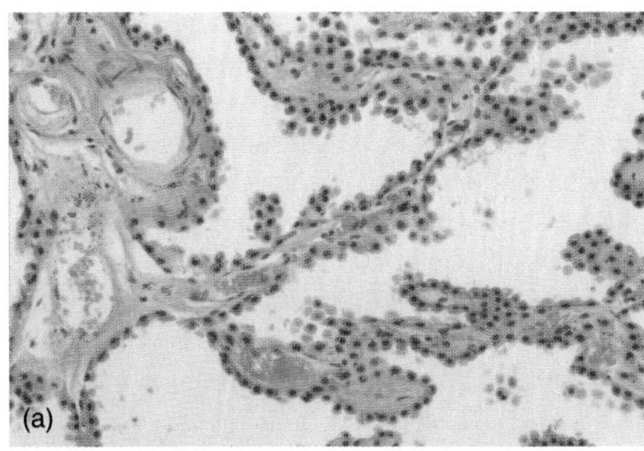

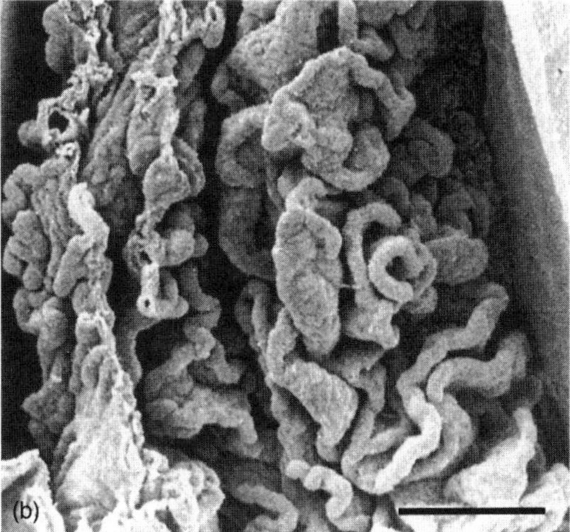

Figure 3.12 Human choroid plexus. (a) A papillary structure that is covered by non-ciliated cuboidal cells on a fibrovascular core (H&E). (b) The surface has a highly convoluted appearance. Scanning electron micrograph. Bar = 5 mm. (Courtesy of Dr W.L. Maxwell, Laboratory of Human Anatomy, University of Glasgow, UK.)

Blood vessels of the brain and the blood–brain barrier

The blood supply to the brain is derived from blood vessels lying in the subarachnoid space that ultimately perforate its surface (see Chapter 5). The traditional view is that the *Virchow–Robin space* seen around the larger blood vessels as they enter the brain represents an extension of the subarachnoid space, but it has now been demonstrated that there is a structural barrier between the subarachnoid and Virchow–Robin spaces. There is no space around capillaries, where the basement membranes of the endothelial cells, perivascular astrocytes and pericytes fuse to form the basement membrane of the capillaries (see Fig. 4.12). A potential space, however, remains at arteriolar level because, in cases of pyogenic or carcinomatous meningitis, cells may accumulate and separate the perivascular astrocytes from the endothelial cells.

In contrast with several other tissues of the body, the rate at which various substances pass from the blood stream into the CNS is usually slow, reflecting the activity of membrane pumps. This selective permeability is referred to as the *blood–brain barrier* and numerous dyes such as trypan blue, have been used to study it. Current views attribute the blood–brain barrier to the relative impermeability of the specialized endothelium of the capillaries. Capillaries in the brain, unlike those in the remainder of the body, have circumferential tight junctions (*zonula occludens*) which prevent or retard the passage of large and small molecules from the blood to the intraventricular (blood–CSF barrier) or interstitial space. Some substances do, however, pass through the endothelium in pinocytotic vesicles, the number of which increases considerably under certain conditions, and by active transport systems.

There are sites where the blood–brain barrier is deficient – the *area postrema* on the floor of the fourth ventricle, the pineal gland, the choroid plexus and the ganglia of the dorsal spinal nerve roots. It may be that toxins and some neurotropic viruses gain access to the CNS at these apparently more permeable sites.

Artefacts

Pathologists must be aware of these so that they are not interpreted as evidence of structural damage to the brain. Provided refrigeration has been adequate, *post mortem autolysis* is not usually too advanced to preclude reasonable light microscopy. An exception to this is when the patient has been maintained on a life support system. Once a patient is clinically '*brainstem dead*', the brain undergoes *in vivo* autolysis since there is no cerebral blood flow. At post mortem the brain, the so-called 'respirator brain', may be increased in weight; it becomes semifluid in consistency and hardens poorly or not at all in formalin. The tissue is usually discolored and there is loss of definition between gray and white matter and disintegration of tissue, particularly in the deep gray matter, in the corpus callosum and in the cerebellum (Fig. 3.13). Fragments of the latter may be found around the spinal cord. Histologically, the neurons have large, pale nuclei with indistinct nucleoli and their cytoplasm is frequently vacuolated, an appearance that is referred to as *hydropic cell change*. These changes are particularly severe in the granule cells of the cerebellum: in contrast, Purkinje cells are relatively well preserved.

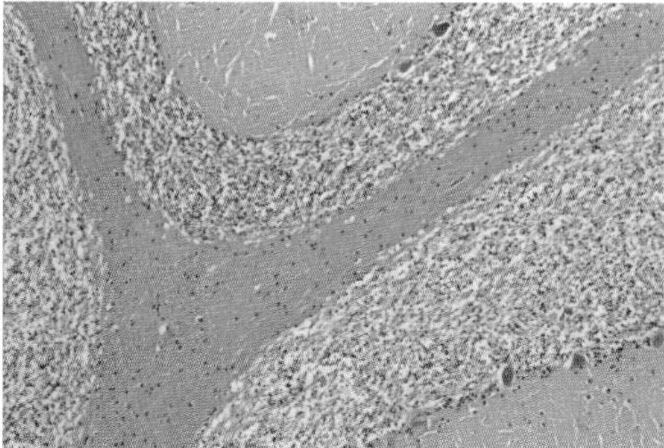

Figure 3.13 Post-mortem autolysis in cerebellum. Note so-called 'gray line' representing autolysis of the internal granule cell layer. H&E.

Another artefact is '*Swiss cheese change*' when smooth-walled cysts occur in the deep white matter of the brain (Fig. 3.14a and b). These cysts are formed by gas-producing organisms that continue to proliferate after death and before adequate refrigeration or fixation. Organisms can be identified histologically in the cysts in the absence of any inflammatory reaction.

Histological artefact is seen in most surgical specimens that are placed in 10% formalin immediately after removal. The neurons near the surface of the specimen are shrunken, their nuclei stain deeply with basic dyes and their axons and dendrites are twisted in a corkscrew fashion. This is referred to as *dark cell* change (Fig. 3.15), which can easily be confused with the *ischemic cell process* (see below), an important vital reaction. This artefact can be prevented, or at least reduced, by minimizing handling of fresh unfixed brain tissue. In experimental animals it can be obviated by perfusion fixation and leaving the brain in the skull for several hours after fixation before its removal. Other common artefacts include swollen hydropic cells and '*perineuronal*' and '*perivascular spaces*', which are probably due to shrinkage occurring during tissue processing (Fig. 3.16). They are commonly seen

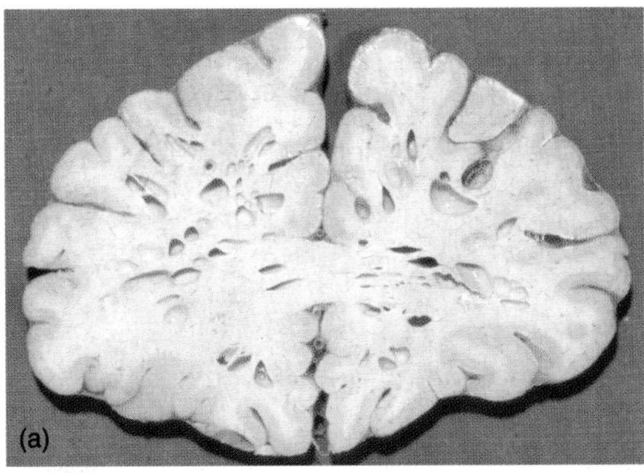

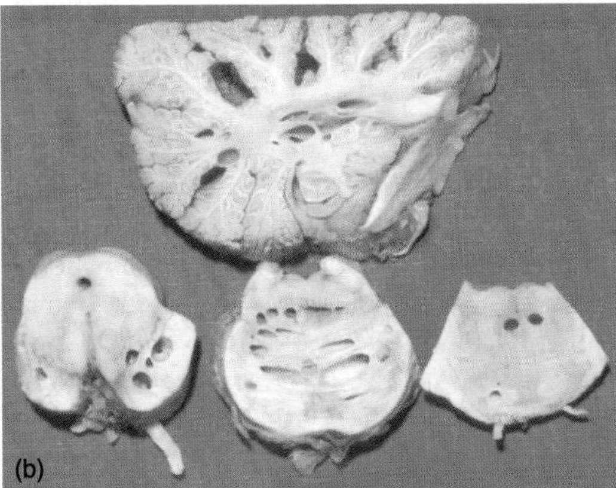

Figure 3.14 Post-mortem autolysis. 'Swiss cheese change'. There are multiple smooth-walled variably sized cysts. (a) Frontal lobes at level of genu of the corpus callosum. (b) Cerebellum and brainstem.

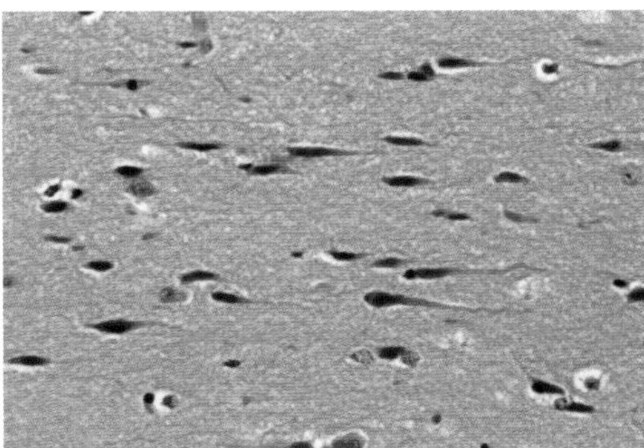

Figure 3.15 Artefact. Dark-cell change due to handling prior to fixation. H&E.

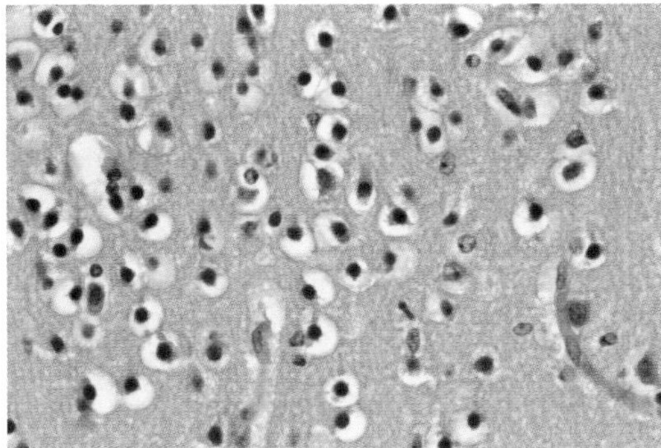

Figure 3.16 Artefact due to processing. Note the perineuronal and perivascular spaces. H&E.

in paraffin sections, particularly pediatric material, and can be reduced only by prolonging the duration of each stage of dehydration, clearing and impregnation with paraffin wax. Another artefact is the formation of *mucocytes*, which appear as metachromatic bodies in the white matter of frozen sections, although they may also be seen in paraffin embedded tissue.

REACTIONS OF THE NERVOUS SYSTEM TO DISEASE

A wide range and variety of physical, chemical and biological agents are associated with cellular injury, major examples of which include trauma, thermal injury, poisons, hypoxia–ischemia, drugs, infectious organisms and ionizing radiation. Some of these effects are reversible, others are irreversible the response of the cells depending on the duration of injury, the nature of the injurious agent, the susceptibility of the cell and the tissue in which it lies, the ability of the cell to counter the noxious agent and its ultimate ability to regenerate. Regardless of the nature of the noxious agent there are only a relatively small number of mechanisms by which cellular injury occurs: these include mechanical disruption by trauma, membrane damage by lipid peroxidation or free radical production, deficient metabolism of glucose or hormones, failure of membrane functional integrity such as occurs when there is damage to ionic pumps, and disruption of metabolic pathways such as those involved in the respiratory chain or in protein synthesis.

In addition to the specific changes that occur in neurons, astrocytes and other cell types in the CNS in response to various diseases, *necrosis* and *programmed cell death* can be identified histologically. Necrosis refers to death of cells or tissues irrespective of its cause in the living organism. Coagulative necrosis is the most common form of necrosis in which proteins coagulate and metabolic activity ceases. At first, there will be no abnormal staining but subsequently there will be progressive loss of nuclear staining until it ceases to be haematoxiphilic and this is usually accompanied by loss of cytoplasmic detail. The equivalent process in the CNS is called *colliquatitive necrosis*. Programmed cell death is the normal process by which modeling of organs occurs it being estimated that there is about 50% loss of neurons in the normal developing brain. In addition, it is a mechanism for continuing control of organ size maintaining normal size in the face of cell turnover or reduction during atrophy. Apoptosis is the term used when the nuclei of the dead cells break into small membrane-bound fragments called *apoptotic bodies* a feature that is increasingly being recognized in AIDS, various neurodegenerative disorders e.g. Alzheimer's disease and Parkinson's disease, after trauma, and in many tumors.

Neurons

Structural changes resulting from hypoxia

Neurons are more vulnerable to a lack of oxygen than the neuroglia, whereas microglia and capillaries are the least vulnerable. Neurons are particularly susceptible to hypoxia since they have an obligative aerobic glycolytic metabolism. The respiratory quotient of the brain is almost unity and glucose is the principal source of energy by oxygenation.

The identification of alterations in neurons attributable to hypoxia may be difficult in the human brain because of the frequent occurrence of histological artefacts (see above). They are due partly to post mortem handling and to the slow penetration of fixative. Although these artefacts will obscure the earliest stages of hypoxic neuronal changes, the later stages of the same process after a survival of days or weeks are easily recognisable as loss of neurons and a glial reaction. The use of perfusion-fixed material in experimental animals, and selective human material, has shown that there is an identifiable sequence of events, namely the *ischemic cell process*, which is the neuropathological common denominator in all types of hypoxia (see Chapter 5).

The earliest histological feature of hypoxic damage to neurons is *microvacuolation* when the perikaryon of an essentially otherwise normal neuron becomes vacuolated. Most of the vacuoles are swollen mitochondria, although some may be due to dilation of endoplasmic reticulum. This rather subtle change is difficult to identify in human material but has been recognized in experimental animals after only 5–15 min of hypoxia. If the neuron is irreversibly damaged, there is a gradual transition from the stage of microvacuolation to that of *ischemic cell change* in which the cell body and nucleus become shrunken and triangular in shape. The cytoplasm stains intensely with eosin and forms bright blue to dark mauve with the combined Luxol fast blue and cresyl violet technique; the nucleus stains intensely with basic aniline dyes (Fig. 3.17a left and right). The next stage of ischemic cell change is the development of small dense granules lying on or close to the surface of the neurons known as *incrustations*. These are electron-dense profiles of the neuronal cytoplasm (Fig. 3.17b) which are formed into projections from the cell surface, which is indented and distorted by clear, swollen astrocytic processes. Such appearances have been seen between 30 and 90 min after an episode of hypoxia in experimental animals, and they may persist for 48 h. Finally, the neuron undergoes *homogenizing cell change* when the cytoplasm becomes progressively paler and homogeneous and the nucleus smaller. This type of change is most commonly seen in the Purkinje cells of the cerebellum (Fig. 3.18), where it may be seen in a few hours after hypoxia and persist for 10 days or longer. The end stage of hypoxic cell damage (*ghost cell change*) is a shrunken, pyknotic and fragmented nucleus without recognizable cytoplasm.

The time course of ischemic cell change is relatively constant for neurons according to their size and site, so that the interval between an hypoxic episode and death, if between 2 and 24 h, can be

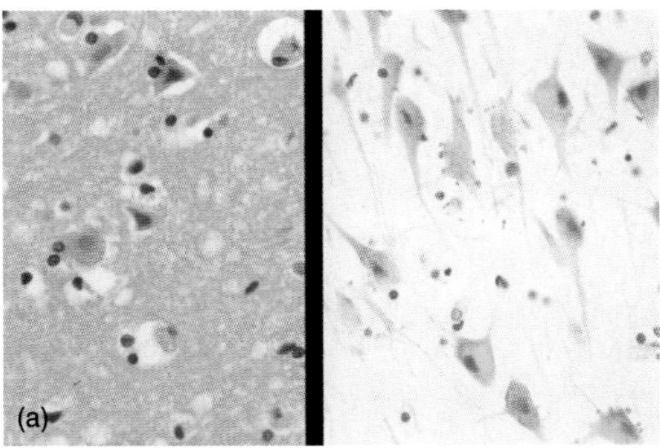

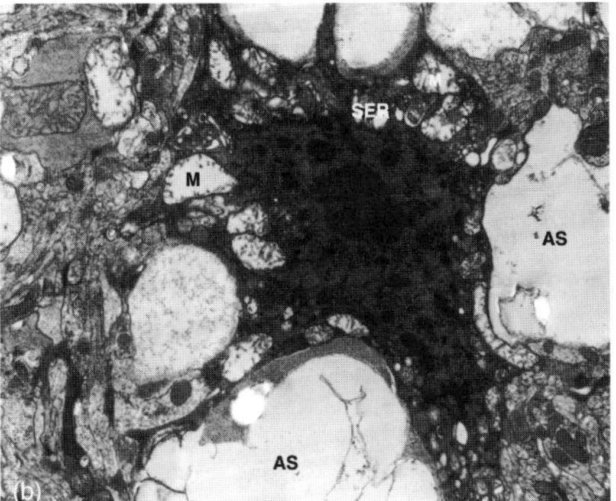

Figure 3.17 Ischemic cell process. (a) Ischemic cell change in cortical neurons. The cell bodies are shrunken and the nuclei triangular. The cytoplasm is intensely eosinophilic (left) and luxophilic (right). Incrustations project from the surface of the neurons. (b) Electron micrograph of a neuron showing ischemic cell change with early incrustation formation. The incrustations are electron-dense portions of the perikaryon and dendrites distorted by swollen astrocytic profiles (AS) and appear as mitochondria with disrupted cristae (M) and profiles of smooth endoplasmic reticulum (SER). (a) H&E – left; LFB/CV – right. (b) Transmission electron micrograph. Bar = 1 μm.

assessed with reasonable accuracy. The ischemic cell process is energy-dependent, and occurs only if the patient has been resuscitated for a sufficient length of time after the period of critical hypoxia. It therefore does not occur after the onset of brainstem death due to a raised intracranial pressure. In such circumstances any evidence of ischemic cell change must be interpreted as having preceded the onset of brainstem death.

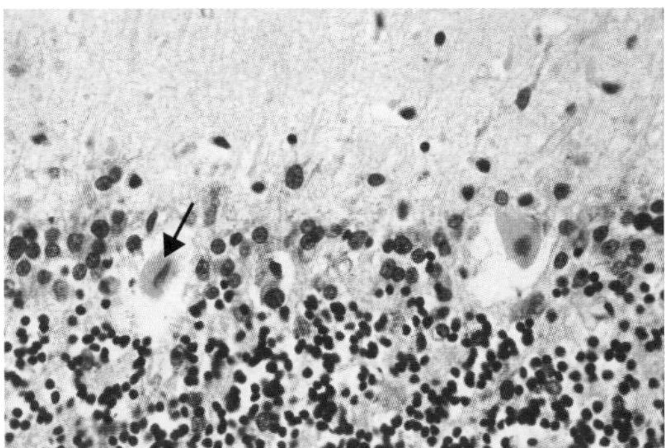

Figure 3.18 Ischemic cell process. Homogenizing cell change (arrow) in Purkinje cell in the cerebellum. LFB/CV.

So-called 'pink' neurons are a common feature in neuropathological practice being particularly obvious with autolysis. Due to a prolonged interval between death and autopsy and fixation it is also possible to misinterpret the pink staining cytoplasm of various inclusions for hypoxic damage. Under these circumstances the neuropathologist is often asked to describe the features of hypoxic brain damage. The presence of incrustations is incontrovertible evidence that the ischemic cell process has indeed been initiated: in its absence the neuropathologist should be cautious in accounting for the presence of pink neurons.

Changes in the neuroglia and blood vessels resulting from hypoxic brain damage are proportional to the severity of neuronal destruction. Thus, if selective *neuronal necrosis* is mild, so also is the reaction; if, however, it is severe, then the reaction is intense and the tissue comes ultimately to be represented by a firm, shrunken scar.

Neuronophagia

In this process macrophages engulf, and eventually digest, irreversibly damaged neurons (Fig. 3.19). The macrophages, which appear to be both microglial and monocytic in origin, are stimulated to react in this way when neurons undergo rapid death as, for example, in viral infections and in hypoxic brain damage. The clustering of the macrophages indicates the position of the dead neuron, which may still be recognisable by its outline. Neuronophagia is less evident in conditions in which necrosis is less acute.

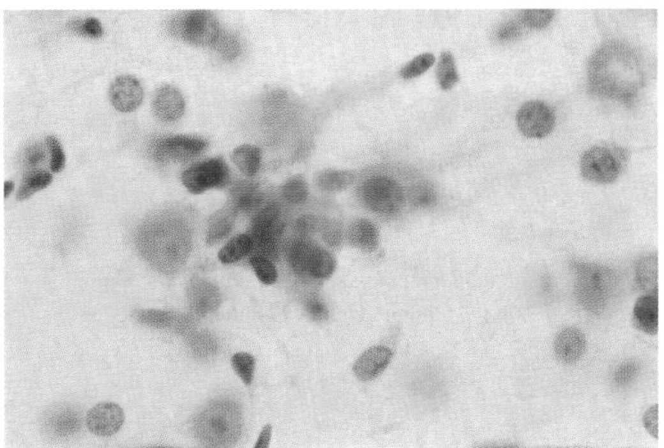

Figure 3.19 Neuronophagia. Macrophages surround necrotic neurons. Cresyl violet.

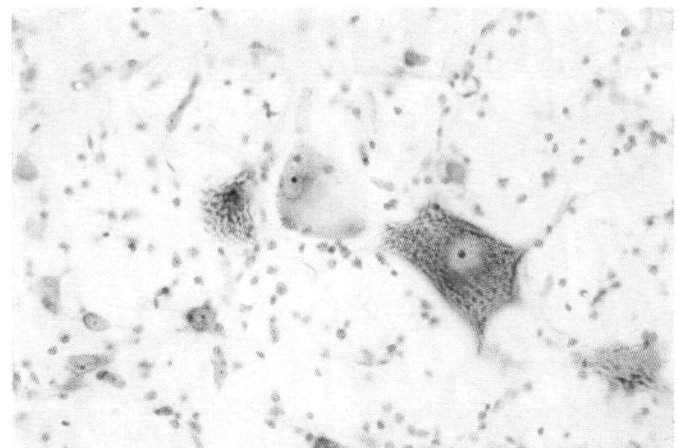

Figure 3.20 Central chromatolysis. Neurons in the tegmentum of the brainstem have become more round, the nuclei eccentric and there is loss of Nissl bodies from the central part of the perikaryon. LFB/CV.

Transneuronal degeneration

This process takes place when the neuron becomes *deafferentated*, from which can be inferred that the normal appearance of a neuron is the product of a number of factors, one of which is its synaptic input. The rate at which neurons undergo transneuronal degeneration is dependent upon age, it being lower with advancing years, and the degree of deafferentation. Affected neurons undergo one or two processes. Most commonly, they become atrophied, eventually dying and being replaced by gliosis. This type of degeneration is seen at a number of sites, *viz.* in the lateral geniculate body after the loss of an eye or lesions in the optic nerve, and in the gracile and cuneate nuclei after loss of sensory fibers in the posterior columns of the spinal cord. A second, and less common, type of transneuronal degeneration is seen in the cells of the inferior olivary nucleus, which undergo an initial phase of enlargement associated with vacuolation of the cytoplasm and a fibrillary gliosis. If many neurons are affected, the olives undergo hypertrophy, a finding that is particularly common after lesions of the central tegmental tract.

Reactions to axonal transection

These include both the central somal response of central *chromatolysis* and the peripheral axonal response of *Wallerian degeneration*. The two processes are often discussed separately, but they constitute basic reactions to the same injury.

Central chromatolysis

This term describes a process that is characterized by swelling of the cell body, displacement of the nucleus to the periphery of the cell, folding of the nuclear membrane and enlargement of the nucleolus (Fig. 3.20). At the same time there is dispersion of the Nissl substance (chromatolysis), a change that is particularly marked in the centre of the cell body. Electron microscopy has shown that the chromatolytic change is due to fragmentation and dispersion of the granular endoplasmic reticulum and the ribosomal rosettes. Other ultrastructural changes include an increase in the amount of neurofilamentous material and lysosomal bodies.

The chromatolytic reaction occurs in both central and peripheral neurons, and may be followed by recovery of the neuron with or without axonal regeneration, or may proceed to degeneration and ultimate death of the neuron. Changes tend to develop more rapidly and to a greater degree if the axonal damage is close to the cell body. Chromatolysis may be identifiable within a day or so of injury, and changes may persist for weeks or months. They are particularly obvious in the perikarya of neurons whose axons project out of the CNS into cranial or peripheral nerves, e.g. the motor neurons in the brainstem and spinal cord. Whereas such neurons may recover, neurons whose projections lie entirely within the CNS tend eventually to degenerate and die.

There is considerable biochemical evidence that chromatolysis is accompanied by a net increase in the amount of RNA and protein synthesis, features which are very strongly suggestive of a *regenerative process* rather than a degenerative one. In general, however, although the severity of chromatolysis appears to be a measure of initial cell injury, its significance in terms of cell function is not clear.

Axonal degeneration (Wallerian degeneration)

After an axon is disrupted, the severed ends of both the proximal and distal stumps swell to form *axon bulbs* (see Chapter 8). The swellings, which are due to the accumulation of neurofilaments, microtubules, mitochondria and dense bodies, are attributed to anterograde and retrograde axoplasmic flow, which continues in spite of the axonal damage. Axonal bulbs can be seen by electron microscopy in experimental preparations within hours of injury, but usually they are not identifiable by light microscopy much before 8 h: by immunohistochemistry using an antibody to β-amyloid precursor protein (β-APP) damage to axons can be identified within 2 h of injury. They are commonly seen adjacent to infarcts or in certain types of head injury, as homogeneous eosinophilic bodies: they are much more readily apparent in sections stained for axons by silver impregnation although the vagaries of these techniques usually means that not all damaged axons are highlighted, and then only after some 18–24 h after injury. The proximal bulbs may reach a size in excess of 50 μm in diameter, and it is from such swellings that regeneration of fibers occurs in the peripheral nervous system. In contrast, the distal portion of the transected axon undergoes progressive degeneration and by 3–4 days the whole length of the axon is irregularly fusiform. Later, fragmentation occurs, a feature that can be easily seen in silver impregnation preparations. Most of the axonal debris has been removed by phagocytosis within about 1 month of injury. Commensurate with axonal bulb formation are degenerative changes within the terminal innervation fields of the affected axons. Again, these may be seen in silver impregnation preparations, which show the characteristic argyrophilic terminals of degenerating *boutons termineaux*. The degenerating terminals are removed rapidly by phagocytosis, and consequent neurogenic atrophy in muscle (see Chapter 18) are important sequelae of axonal transection.

As the distal part of the axon degenerates, so also does the myelin: this is referred to as *Wallerian degeneration*, during which myelin breaks down into ovoid bodies. Within the PNS most of the breakdown products of myelin are removed by macrophages within weeks. In contrast, the process within the CNS is very much slower, demonstrable macrophages remaining within the affected tissue for many months or even years. Once myelin debris has been phagocytosed its staining properties change, largely due to the *production of cholestral esters*, which stain red with sudan dyes and black with osmium in the Marchi technique (Fig. 3.21a–c). Loss of myelin can also be demonstrated by the Heidenhain method, which stains normal myelin black: zones where myelin has been lost do not stain (see Fig. 10.8).

Regeneration and recovery of function

If the optic nerve or spinal cord in humans is severed, irreversible blindness and paraplegia ensue, respectively. Not so in the frog or fish, for within weeks the frog's vision will be restored. For many years it has been taught that, although axons in the CNS of adult mammals are capable of regeneration, growth ceases by 2 weeks, thereby apparently confirming the early work of Cajal. However, studies have demonstrated that under certain experimental circumstances, in both the adult and the fetal mammalian brain, axons can regenerate to form synapses and recover some function. The capacity for regeneration depends on age, being much less in old than in young animals, and on the nature of the system damaged, being greater in noradrenergic fibers and dopaminergic and cholinergic neurons than in serotonergic and GABAergic neurons. Apart from these special circumstances, regeneration is thought to be abortive, either because of the concomitant development of a glial or collagen scar at the site of injury which acts as an impenetrable barrier to the passage of regeneration axons, or because trophic or growth factors are absent from the adult CNS.

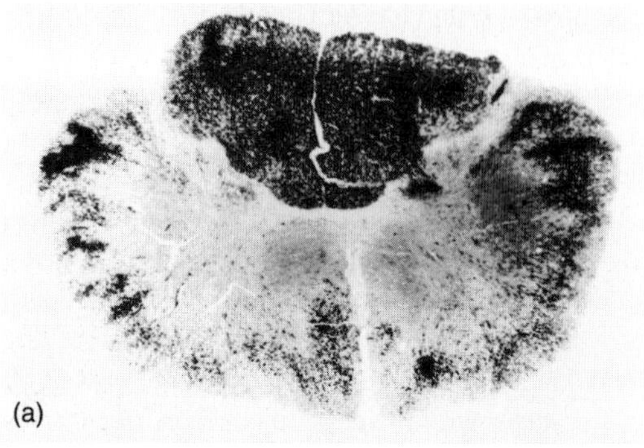

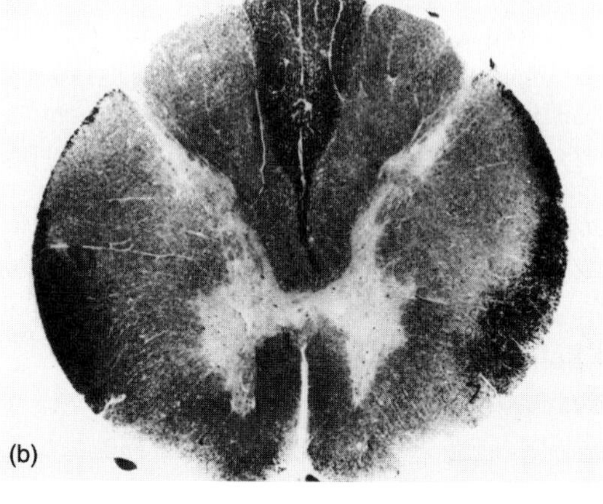

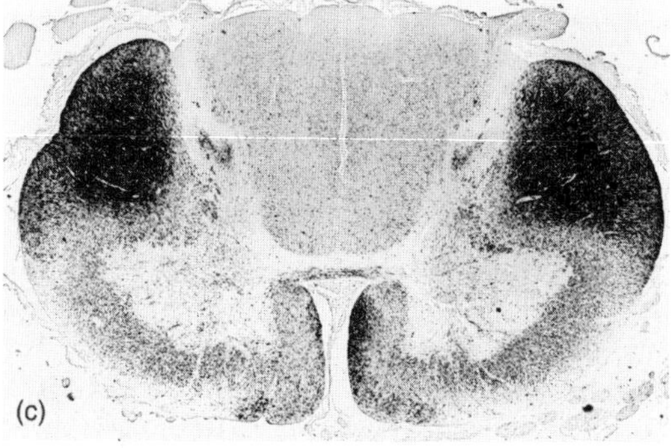

Figure 3.21 Wallerian degeneration. (a) Degeneration in both ascending and descending fiber tracts at level of spinal cord injury. (b) Ascending degeneration above lesion. Note there is degenerating myelin in the spinocerebellar and gracile tracts of the posterior columns. (c) Descending degeneration below lesion. Note there is degenerating myelin in the corticospinal tracts of the lateral (crossed) and anterior (uncrossed) columns. (a), (b) and (c) Marchi preparation.

There has been considerable interest in the last few years in the capacity of transplants to survive and form connections when grafted to adult central or peripheral nervous systems. At the present time only embryonic or early postnatal donor tissue from the CNS can survive, and there is no evidence of immunological rejection of the CNS tissue transplanted into brain. If hippocampal primordia is transplanted into the hippocampal region of adult rat hosts, the grafts differentiate and send mossy fibers to the host brain and receive mossy fibers from it. Dopamine deficiency in animal models of Parkinson's disease has been reversed by the transplantation of fetal substantia nigra or fetal adrenal medulla into the lateral ventricle adjacent to the dopamine-deprived caudate nucleus. These encouraging experiments give some credence to the belief and hope that transplantation in the future may be a form of therapy for paraplegia and degenerative disorders such as Parkinson's disease.

More recently, the phenomenon of neurogenesis has been investigated as a natural means by which repair and regeneration might be achieved by the migration of *neural stem cells* from the subventricular zone of the hippocampus and body of the striatum, to sites of damage. It has been suggested that this might occur throughout natural life and while one paradigm might be to provide such donor cells, an alternative strategy might be to induce and accelerate the potential for neural stem cells to proliferate within the patient.

It is well recognized that some recovery of function may continue to appear in neurologically damaged patients after initial injury. Because actual regeneration of the originally damaged axons is unlikely to have occurred, the functional improvement has been attributed to *plasticity*. This is attributed to an adaptation whereby a deafferented neuron becomes reinnervated.

Pigment in the nervous system

Variable amounts of *melanin* are found in the meninges. Although, some of the melanin-containing cells are probably melanophores, others appear to be melanoblasts and are thought to be the origin of the rare examples of primary melanoma of the meninges.

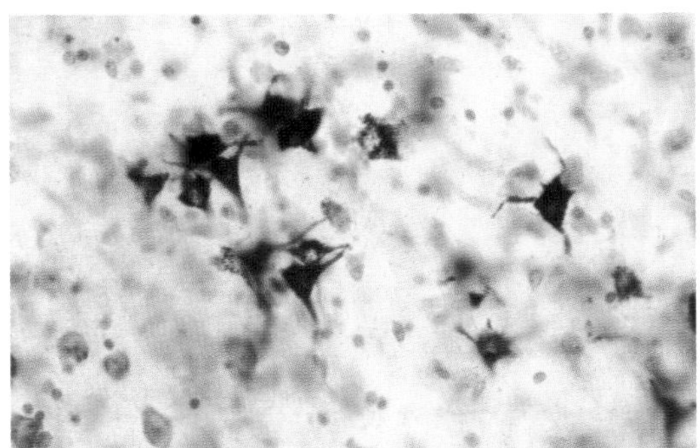

Figure 3.22 Ferruginated neurons. Cresyl violet.

Increased amounts of lipofuscin (the so-called aging pigment) are seen in many nuclei and neuromelanin is found in some nuclei of the brainstem, e.g. the locus caeruleus, the substantia nigra and the dorsal motor nucleus of the vagus. Whereas the melanin in the locus caeruleus appears at an early stage in fetal development, pigmentation of the substantia nigra is delayed until about the age of 2 years.

Neurons in the vicinity of old infarcts often become encrusted with iron and calcium (ferrugination) (Fig. 3.22).

Other alterations in neurons

A variety of structural abnormalities occur within neurons, and some are characteristic of specific diseases. Although many of these will be described in greater detail in ensuing chapters, brief descriptions of the more common types will be given here.

Neurofibrillary tangles and amyloid deposits

This type of degeneration is easily identifiable by light microscopy in frozen or paraffin sections stained by silver impregnation techniques or by immunohistochemistry. It is much less easy to see them in H&E stained preparations (Fig. 3.23). They appear as a skein (tangle) of thick neurofibrils in the perikaryon of affected neurons (Fig. 3.24a). Ultrastructurally, the tangles consist of paired helical filaments with a characteristic periodicity. Occasional tangles may be seen in the cerebral cortex in normal old age, but they are abundant and widely distributed in Alzheimer's disease (see Chapter 17) and in cases of Down syndrome surviving into adulthood: they also occur in the brainstem in postencephalitic parkinsonism and in the parkinsonism–dementia complex of Guam.

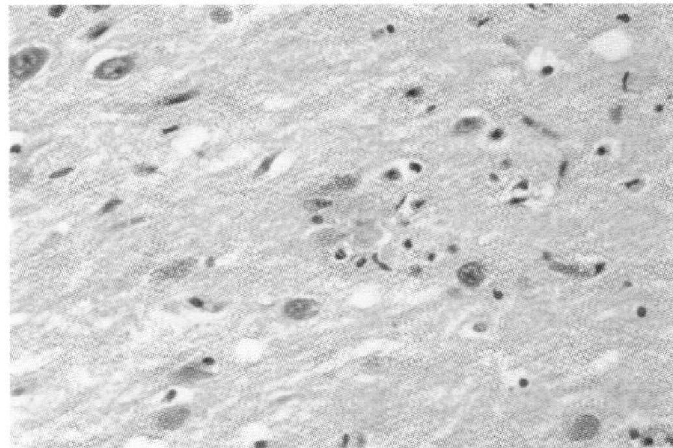

Figure 3.23 Amyloid plaque in non-demented elderly subject. In addition to the amyloid it is possible to identify both neurofibrillary tangles and vacuolar degeneration in some of the adjacent neurons.

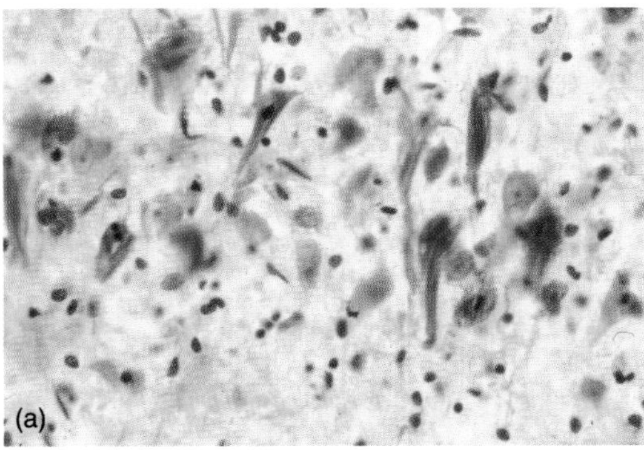

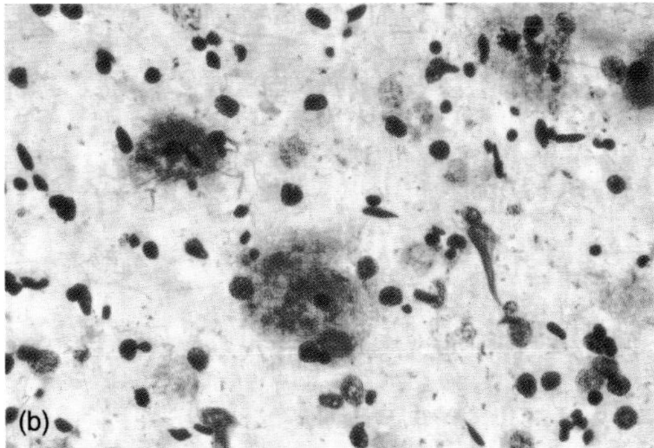

Figure 3.24 Neurofibrillary tangles and amyloid plaques. (a) Neurofibrillary tangles in hippocampus of elderly non-demented subject. (b) Amyloid plaque adjacent to (a). (a) and (b) silver impregnation.

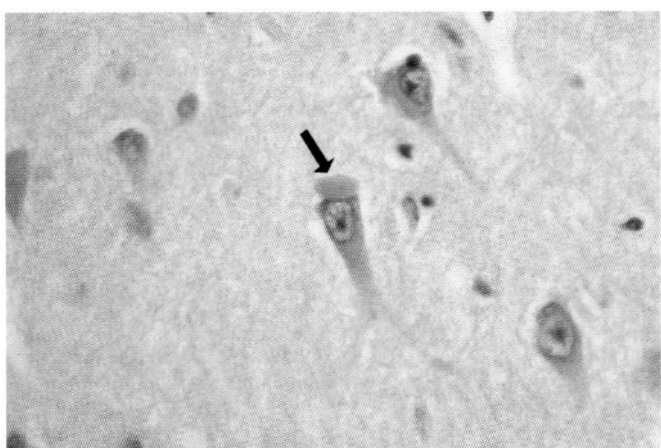

Figure 3.25 Hirano body. There is an elongated eosinophilic body beside a neuron in the hippocampus (arrow). H&E.

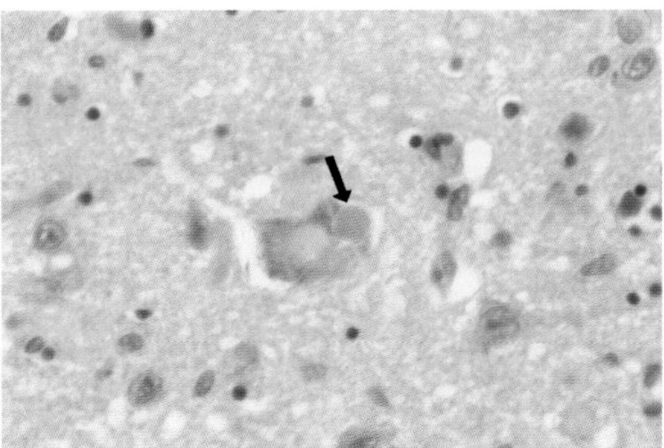

Figure 3.26 Lewy body in Parkinson's disease. There is a rounded concentric hyaline inclusion (arrow) in the perikaryon of a pigmented neuron of the substantia nigra. H&E.

The amyloid which may be seen in H&E stained preparations is easily demonstrated by silver impregnation (Fig. 3.24b) or immunohistochemically.

Granulovacuolar degeneration

This refers to one or more 3–4 μm diameter vacuoles in the cytoplasm of neurons, particularly in the pyramidal cells of the hippocampus. Within each vacuole there is a centrally placed 0.5–1.5 μm diameter hematoxyphilic and argyrophilic inclusion. This degenerative change is rare before the age of 65 years, but thereafter it increases in frequency even in non-demented elderly subjects. It is particularly apparent in Alzheimer's disease (see Chapter 17), and its occurrence has also been described in certain nuclei of the brainstem in progressive supranuclear palsy.

Hirano bodies

In sections stained with H&E, these bodies are elongated eosinophilic structures that measure from 10–30 μm in length and between 8 and 15 μm in diameter (Fig. 3.25). Ultrastructurally, they consist of filamentous aggregates and can be found at all ages and in various conditions. They are seen frequently, however, in Alzheimer's disease.

Cytoplasmic inclusions in Pick's disease

The Pick body, which is said to be characteristic of Pick's disease, consists of a hyaline eosinophilic mass of material that distends the cytoplasm of affected neurons and displaces the nucleus to the periphery. It is argyrophilic and on electron microscopy is a mass of neurofilaments and microtubules.

Lewy bodies

These are hyaline, eosinophilic concentrically laminated inclusions, often with a central core, with surrounding pale peripheral rims (Fig. 3.26). They may be single or multiple, and occur characteristically in the substantia nigra and locus caeruleus in patients with idiopathic parkinsonism.

Lysosomal enzyme disorders

In several metabolic disorders that affect the nervous system there is an increased number of normal cytoplasmic organelles within neurons, or abnormal cytoplasmic bodies (cytosomes) within which non-metabolizable substrates accumulate, thus leading to greatly swollen neurons often referred to as 'ballooned' neurons (see Fig. 3.27); the cytoplasmic bodies may be the primary site of the cellular defect or they may represent secondary adaptive changes. The metabolic defect in many of these cellular disorders has not been clearly defined, although they are thought to be lysosomal in origin. The better-recognized inclusion bodies of this type are the *membranous cytoplasmic body* of Tay–Sachs disease and the *zebra body* of gargoylism (see Chapter 12). In many of these conditions the affected neurons also contain large amounts of lipofuscin.

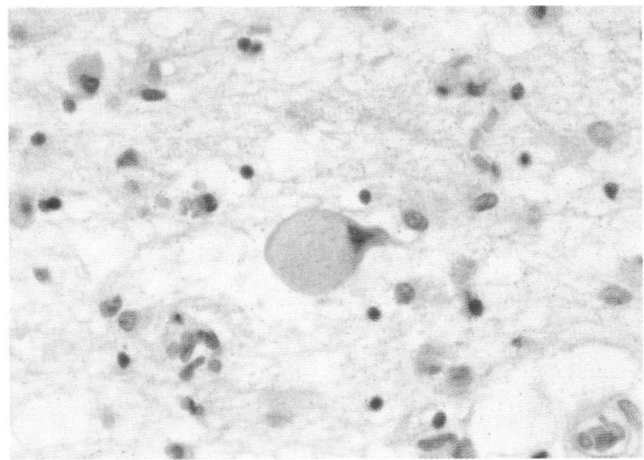

Figure 3.27 Lysosomal storage disorder. Swollen neuron in juvenile patient.

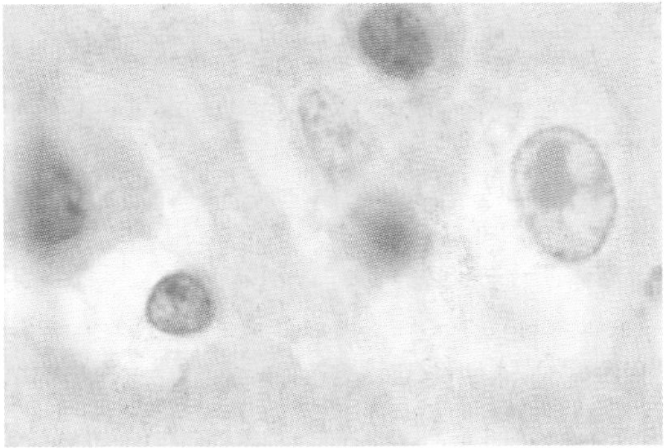

Figure 3.28 Herpes simplex encephalitis. Intranuclear bodies are present in this surgical biopsy. H&E.

Viral inclusions

These are, in general, visible by light microscopy as homogeneous pink, round or oval, intranuclear or intracytoplasmic bodies that displace the normal components of the cell and are unusually surrounded by a thin clear rim. They may be sparse or numerous, and are most often seen in herpes simplex encephalitis (see Fig. 3.28) and in subacute sclerosing panencephalitis.

The neuroglia

Astrocytes

Damage to the CNS, whatever its cause, is invariably accompanied by hypertrophy and hyperplasia of astrocytes (Fig. 3.29a–d), processes that are referred to as *astrocytosis*. The stimulus to this process is probably soluble factors derived from neurons, axons and myelin. Within 48 h of tissue damage, both fibrillary and protoplasmic astrocytes begin to divide, this resonse being associated with the production of large amounts of glial fibrillary acidic protein (GFAP) (Fig. 3.30). As the proliferation continues, astrocytic nuclei become clustered in pairs or groups of four or more. Neuronal loss is invariably accompanied by astrocytosis and hyperplasia of microglia (*gliosis*). The term gliosis is, however, used loosely to mean astrocytosis.

Characteristically, gliotic tissue is firmer than normal and tends to appear gray and translucent, as in plaques of multiple sclerosis, in relation to cystic infarcts and in the walls of syringomyelic cavities. Usually, the glial fibers are laid down in an irregular manner, but occasionally they assume a regular and parallel arrangement (*isomorphic gliosis*), as is seen most commonly, in the molecular layer of the cerebellum when there has been loss of Purkinje cells (Fig. 3.30). In areas of longstanding gliosis, in some gliomas and in certain types of leukodystrophy, *Rosenthal fibers and granular bodies* may be seen (Fig. 15.21). These are eosinophilic structures which may be round, oval or elongated, ranging in size from 10 to 40 μm in length. The nature of the center of these structures is uncertain even with electron microscopy, but their periphery consists of glial fibers which are GFAP-positive by light microscopy.

Another type of astrocytic response is seen in swollen white matter, when the cell body enlarges, becomes rounded and acquires an eosinophilic homogeneous cytoplasm, and the nucleus becomes eccentric. These cells are known as *gemistocytic astrocytes* (Fig. 3.29b) and have been found in the white matter within as little as 6 h after the onset of acute swelling due to vasogenic edema. They are seen also in relation to tumors and infarcts. If the lesion resolves, they become fibrillary astrocytes and lay down glial fibers. Giant astrocytes containing many small nuclei are occasionally encountered, particularly in relation to necrotic tumors and abscesses. Gliosis is the principal response of the CNS to injury but in certain circumstances, when there has been tissue necrosis, there is often a mixed glial and fibroblastic response referred to as a *glio-mesodermal reaction*. This is most frequently

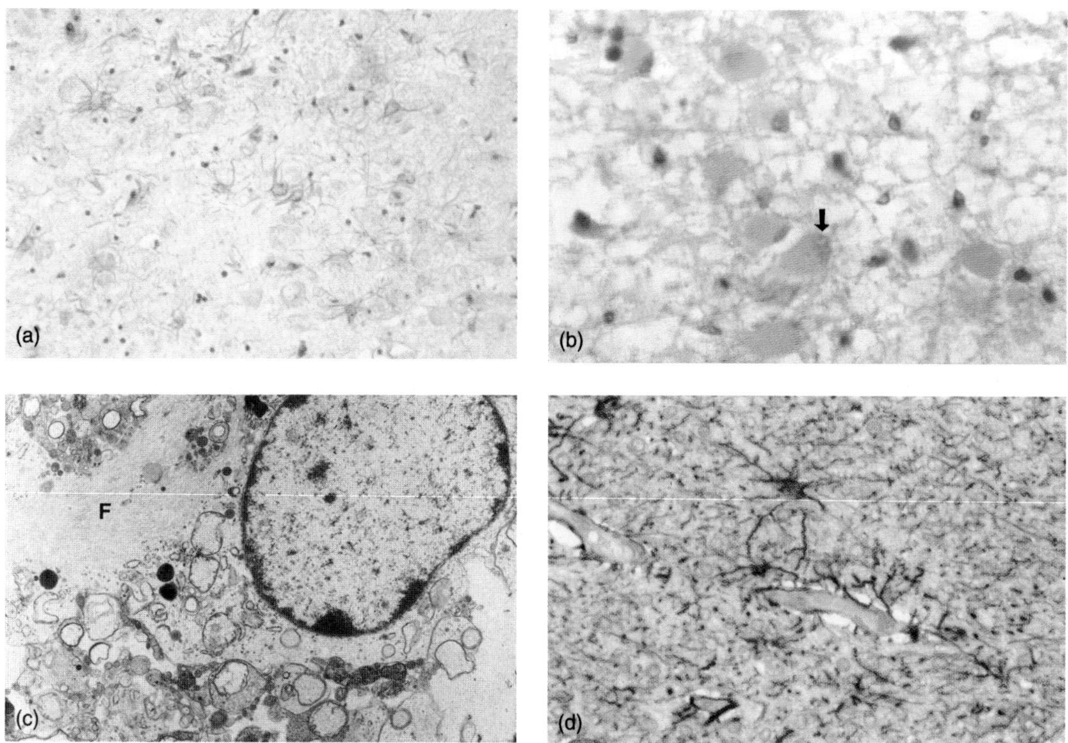

Figure 3.29 Reactive astrocytes. (a) Hypertrophy and hyperplasia of fiber-forming astrocytes. (b) Gemistocytic astrocytes in edematous white matter (arrow). (c) Fiber-forming astrocyte. The nucleus contains evenly dispersed chromatin and there are large numbers of glial filaments (F) in the perikaryon. (d) Reactive astrocyte. (a) and (b) H&E. (c) Electron microscopy ×5000. (d) Immunohistochemistry for GFAP.

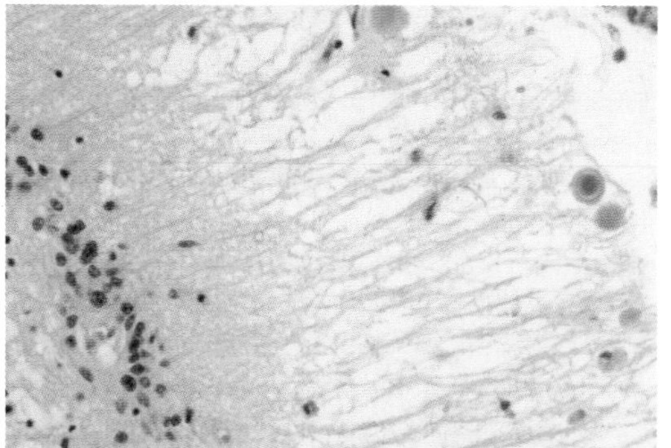

Figure 3.30 Isomorphic gliosis. Note parallel arrangement of astrocytic fibers in the molecular layer of the cerebellum. H&E.

seen as a capsule around subacute and chronic abscesses.

Neurons are more vulnerable to hypoxia than astrocytes. In a cerebral infarct, however, astrocytes undergo a sequence of changes that culminates in death, i.e. *cloudy swelling,* in which the cell and its processes swell, followed by pyknosis and disappearance of the nucleus and fragmentation of cell processes.

Alzheimer type 2 astrocytes occur principally in hepatocerebral degeneration (Wilson's disease), and in hepatic encephalopathy, particularly when associated with portocaval shunts (see Chapter 10). They have swollen vesicular nuclei, a distinct nuclear membrane and one or more prominent nucleoli (see Chapter 10). They seem to be peculiar to humans and may indeed be artefactual, since they have not been seen in similar experimental situations.

Oligodendrocytes

An increased number of oligodendrocytes around a neuron is called *satellitosis*: this is a non-specific response seen in a variety of degenerative conditions

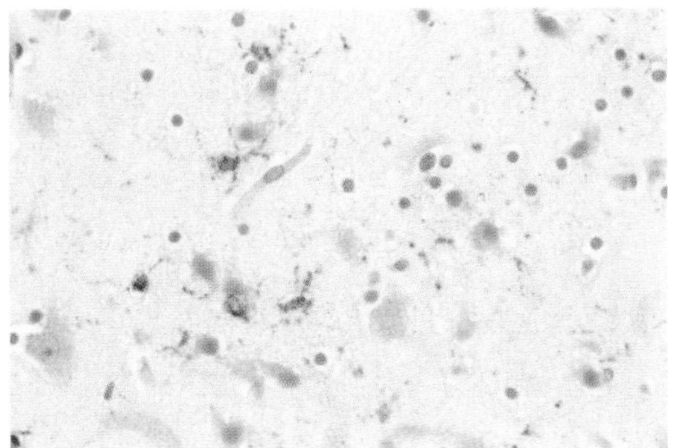

Figure 3.31 Microglia. Usual morphology and number in normal brain. H&E.

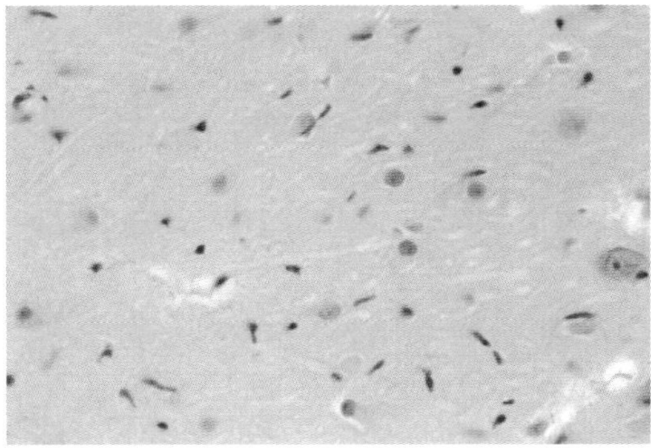

Figure 3.32 Microglia. Activated microglia in CAI sector of hippocampus in a patient who survived 4 days after cardiac arrest. H&E.

and as a normal occurrence with aging. There are, however, many conditions in which oligodendrocytes undergo *acute swelling*, but this too may be a non-specific phenomenon related to delayed fixation.

Damage to oligodendrocytes may be due to infecting lytic viruses, immunological mechanisms, specific antimetabolites, and as a bystander effect in inflammatory reactions. The resulting demyelination follows a stereotyped pattern, with only minor differences in morphology which can be related either to the mode of action of the damaging agent and/or the speed and scale of the subsequent demyelination (see Chapter 9). It is generally accepted that oligodendrocytes are not phagocytic and therefore do not play any part in the removal of effete myelin. The process of *Wallerian degeneration* has already been described (see p. 57).

Microglia

Microglia are the resident macrophages of the nervous system comprising up to 20% of the total glial cell population (Fig. 3.31). They form a relatively stable cell population, turnover being largely achieved by cells derived from the bone marrow. Normally, in a functionally quiescent stage they nevertheless can respond to injury quite rapidly phenotypically changing from ameboid to ramified resting microglia in the mature CNS, to activated but non-phagocytic microglia, to phagocytic microglia found in brain tissue damaged by trauma, inflammation or necrosis. However, resident microglia may proliferate and become activated in the absence of considerable turnover of hematogenous macrophages.

A particular feature of microglia is their ability to act as cytotoxic cells either by virtue of being phagoctytic or by the release of cytotoxic substances such as various cytokines, free oxygen intermediates, nitric oxide and excitatory amino acids. Although not fully understood, microglia, therefore, have the dual role of acting as scavengers by removing tissue debris and of having an immune regulatory/surveillance function that is protective, and they also facilitate repair/regeneration.

There are very few disorders/diseases of the CNS without involvement of microglia. They can be identified by RCA-1 lectin histochemistry or immunohistochemically by antibodies such as CD68, CR3/43 or antiferritin. *Neuronophagia* has already been described (see p. 55). In the presence of any noxious process, e.g. encephalitis or selective neuronal necrosis, microglia become elongated and their processes more apparent but confined mainly to the extremity of the cells: these cells are referred to as *rod cells* (Fig. 3.32). When brain tissue is destroyed, the microglia act as phagocytes: the cell becomes enlarged and rounded, the nucleus eccentric, and the cytoplasm filled with ingested material, which is usually the breakdown products of myelin: these cells – *lipid phagocytes* – are sudanophilic and react strongly for acid phosphatase (Fig. 3.33a, b and c). They are most commonly seen in cerebral infarcts and in recent

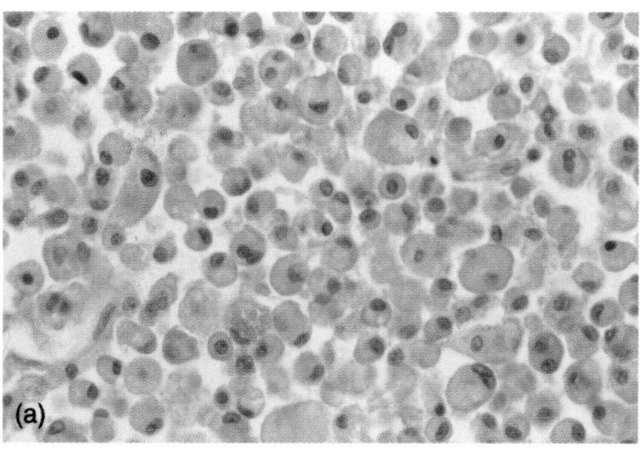

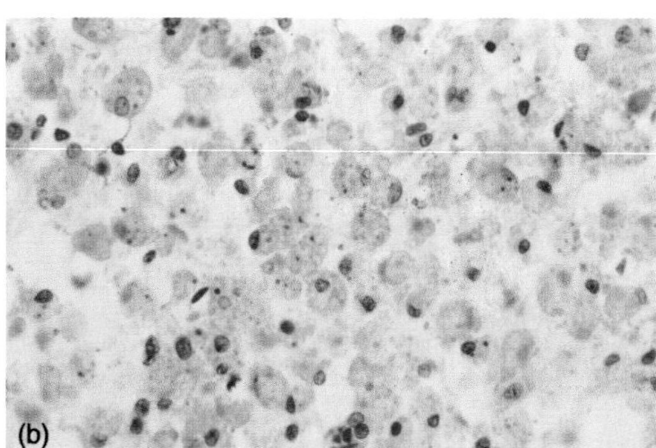

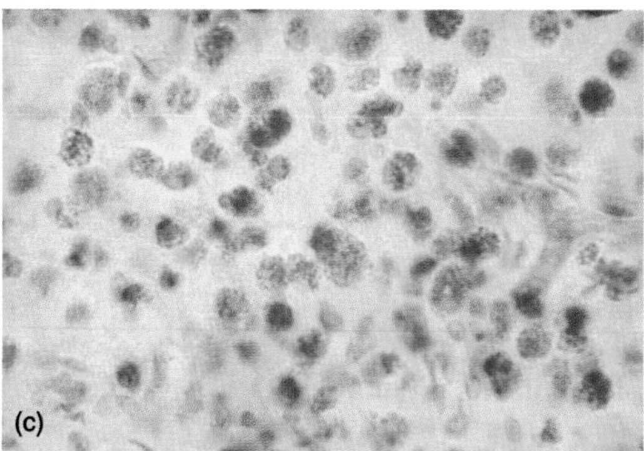

Figure 3.33 Macrophages (lipid or foamy macrophages) in center of a 7-day-old cerebral infarct. (a) H&E. (b) LFB/CV. (c) Sudan.

plaques of demyelination. Microglia also ingest the breakdown products of hemoglobin, when they are referred to as *siderophages* and stain positively with Perls' Prussian blue reaction. The ultimate fate of these macrophages remains unclear, but many appear to migrate into the perivascular spaces and then either into blood vessels or into the subarachnoid space to be absorbed through the arachnoidal villi.

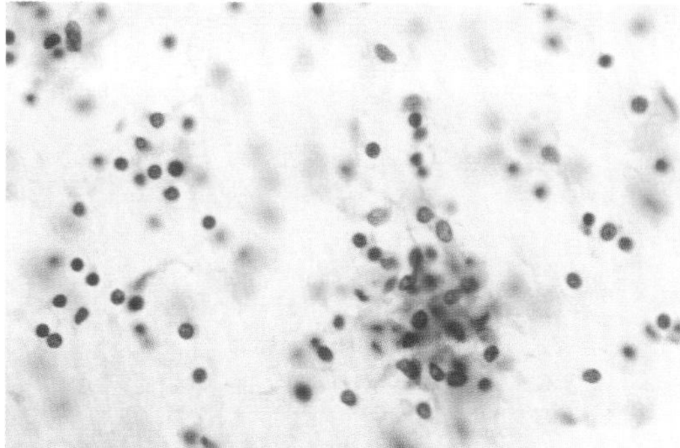

Figure 3.34 Cluster (nodule) of proliferating microglia. Cresyl violet.

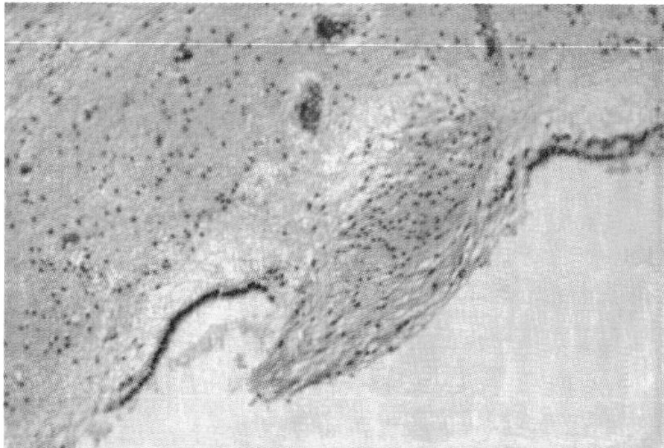

Figure 3.35 Granular ependymitis. The ependymal layer is deficient and there is proliferation of subependymal astrocytes. H&E.

Small clusters of reactive microglia are frequently seen throughout the CNS in patients with a bacteraemia, and in the white matter in patients who have sustained axonal injury as a result of trauma (see Chapter 8) (Fig. 3.34).

Ependymal cells

Ependymal cells have relatively little capacity to react to pathological conditions or to regenerate. Beneath the ependyma there is a layer of glial cells most of which are astrocytes which when activated become *subventricular glial nodules* that result in an irregular ventricular surface known as *granular ependymitis* (Fig. 3.35). Such appearances are not specific and may develop after any noxious process.

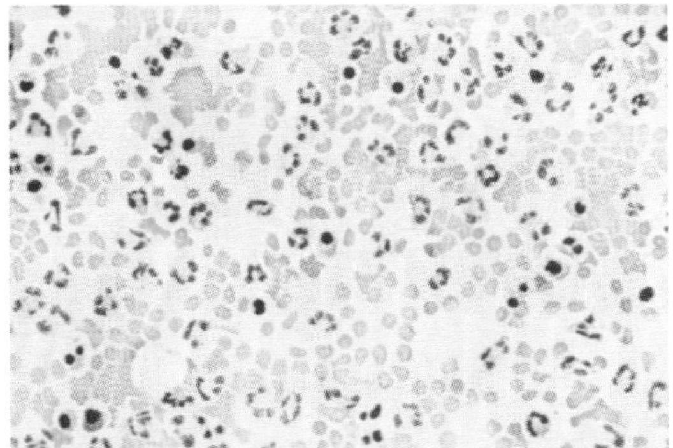

Figure 3.36 Acute bacterial meningitis. There are many polymorphonuclear leukocytes among red blood cells.

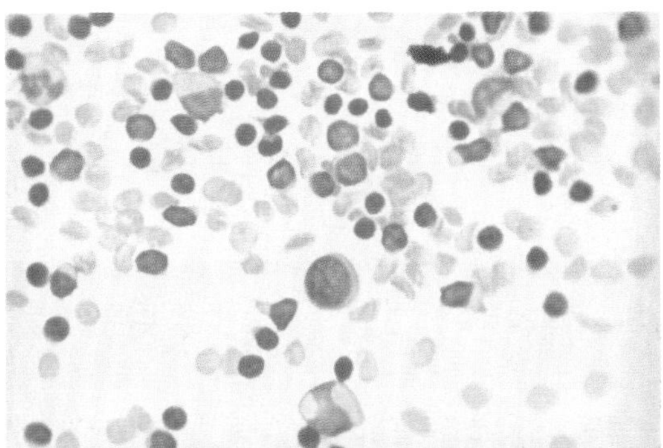

Figure 3.37 Virus meningitis. A mixed cell population with lymphocytes, 'blast-like' cells and monocytes.

The overlying ependyma may or may not be present. The subventricular zone is the source of neural stem cells.

Cerebrospinal fluid cytology

The microscopic examination of ventricular or lumbar CSF can provide valuable diagnostic information (see Table 1.2, page 13). Abnormalities of cell number and type are a particular feature of infectious and neoplastic processes. For example, in cases of acute bacterial meningitis there will be large numbers of polymorphism (Fig. 3.36), whereas in inflammation due to viral disease or tuberculosis often a mixed mononuclear response is seen (Fig. 3.37).

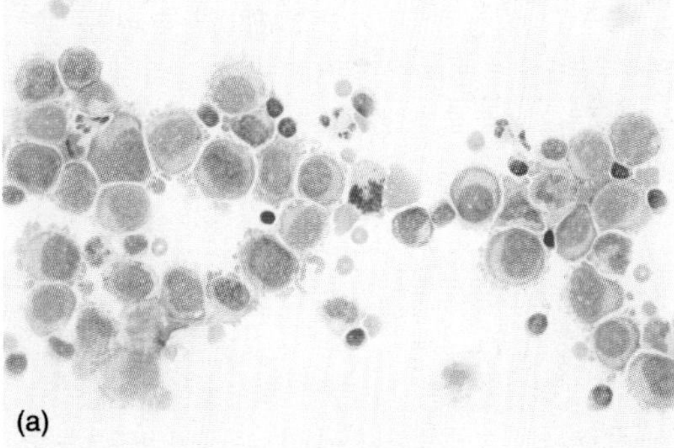

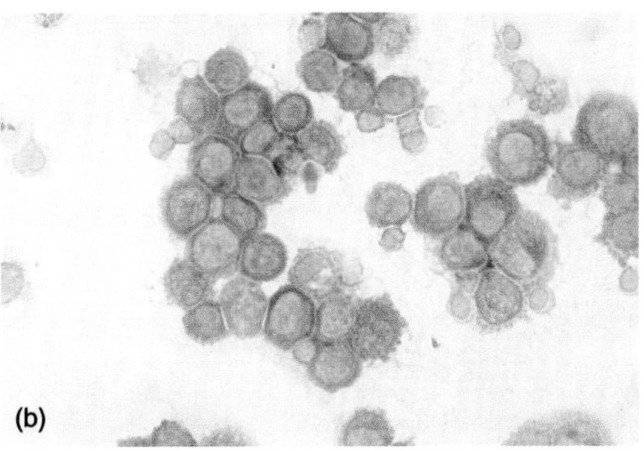

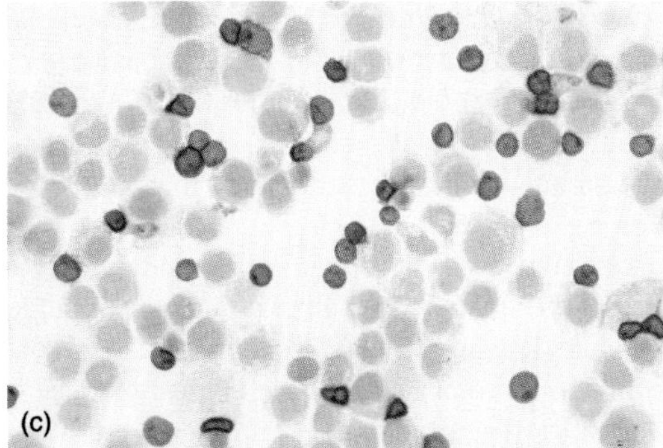

Figure 3.38 Malignant meningitis. (a) Note clumps of tumor cells and compare size with lymphocytes in preparation. (b) Same case showing immunoreactivity for carcinoma. (c) Same case showing immunoreactivity for lymphocytes. (a) Leishman, immunohistochemistry. (b) CAM 5.2. (c) Leukocyte common antigen.

Malignant meningitis due to metastatic carcinoma (Fig. 3.38a, b and c), lymphoma and meningeal spread of intrinsic tumors can also be diagnosed by careful examination of cytological preparations.

CHAPTER 4

INTRACRANIAL EXPANDING LESIONS, CEREBRAL EDEMA AND HYDROCEPHALUS

David I Graham

INTRODUCTION

After the fontanelles have closed the intracranial contents – consisting of the brain (about 70% of the intracranial volume), cerebrospinal fluid (CSF, about 15%) and blood (about 15%) – are enclosed in a rigid bony container so that any increase in the volume of one or more of these compartments will, unless compensated for by a corresponding reduction in the volume of the other components, lead to an increase in intracranial pressure (ICP). The most common cause of raised ICP in clinical practice is an intracranial expanding lesion and, as a result of distortion and herniation of the brain, this leads frequently to impaction of brain tissue in the tentorial incisura or in the foramen magnum (Fig. 4.1): this results in a *pressure gradient* between the supratentorial and infratentorial compartments of the skull, or between the intracranial and the spinal subarachnoid spaces. Such a gradient leads to rapid deterioration of the patients' clinical state (the patient is often said to have 'coned'), and may inadvertently be produced by lumbar puncture in a patient with an intracranial expanding lesion. Removal of CSF from the lumbar subarachnoid space 'opens' a 'closed' space, thus allowing downward

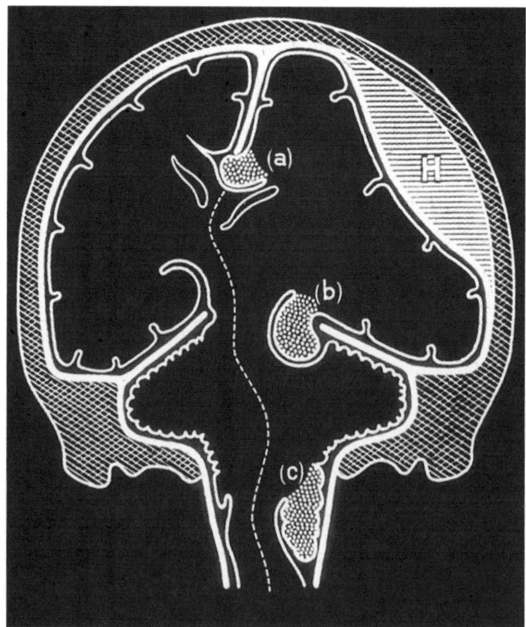

Figure 4.1 Raised intracranial pressure, showing the intracranial compartments and the result of an extradural hematoma (H) on the right hand side. In addition to a shift of the midline structures and distortion of the ventricular system, there is (a) a supracallosal hernia, (b) a tentorial hernia and (c) a tonsillar hernia.

movement of the cerebral hemispheres and of the cerebellum. If the subarachnoid space is already obliterated at the tentorial incisura or at the foramen magnum, the high ICP is not transmitted to the spinal subarachnoid space, and CSF pressure at lumbar puncture may be normal. In contrast, when there is free communication between the supratentorial, infratentorial and spinal subarachnoid spaces, as in benign intracranial hypertension, a remarkably high ICP may be well tolerated by the patient.

Introduction of continuous monitoring of ICP during life has shed considerable light on various pathophysiological concepts in patients with intracranial expanding lesions summarized in the 'four-lump' concept comprising the mass, the accumulation of CSF, vascular engorgement and cerebral edema. Such monitoring of ICP has identified that various types of *pressure waves* are common in patients in whom the ICP is rising and that critical to these events are pressure gradients between intracranial compartments and the spinal subarachnoid space. The skull is divided into three compartments – two supratentorial and one infratentorial – by the dura mater (Fig. 4.1). The falx cerebri projects downwards between the cerebral hemispheres; there is a space between its lower border and the anterior portion of the corpus callosum, but posteriorly, where the falx fuses with the tentorium, it is closely related to the splenium of the corpus callosum. The tentorium cerebelli separates the cerebral hemispheres from the cerebellum and in the midline surrounds the midbrain – the tentorial incisura. In normal circumstances, the supratentorial, the infratentorial and the spinal subarachnoid spaces are in continuity through the tentorial incisura and foramen magnum, respectively. The normal upper limit of the ICP is about 0.13 kPa (0–10 mm Hg), a moderately elevated ICP is between 0.13 kPa and 5.4 kPa (10–40 mm Hg), and a level above 5.4 kPa (40 mm Hg) is high.

The Monro–Kellie doctrine states that the brain (normal or diseased), CSF and blood are not compressible within the confines of the skull after the fontanelle and the cranial sutures have closed, and therefore any increase in the volume of one or more of these components will unless compensated for by a corresponding reduction in the volume of the other components, lead to an increase in ICP. An elevation in ICP is characterized by certain clinical signs and symptoms (Table 4.1).

Table 4.1 Neurological features associated with progressive elevation of intracranial pressure

- Reduction in level of consciousness
- Dilation of pupil ipsilateral to mass lesion
- Bradycardia, increase in pulse pressure and increased mean arterial pressure
- Cheyne–Stokes respiration

INTRACRANIAL EXPANDING LESIONS

A wide variety of pathological processes may present as intracranial expanding (space occupying) lesions. The lesion may be a malignant tumor, a hematoma, an abscess or a swollen infarct. The immediate consequences of a rise in ICP are determined by the speed at which the increase occurs and the ability of the intracranial components to compensate rather than the nature of the space occupation although the long term prognosis will be determined by the primary disease process rather than the nature of the expanding lesion itself.

Spatial compensation

Distortion and displacement of the brain usually precede any clinically significant increase in ICP because of the intrinsic compensatory mechanisms by which the total volume of intracranial contents does not necessarily increase as soon as an expanding lesion develops. This is achieved in part by a reduction in CSF volume of the ventricles becoming smaller and the subarachnoid space partially or totally obliterated. Further, the volume of blood within the cranial cavity can be reduced by compression of the major venous sinuses and in certain instances there may be a local loss of brain tissue which also contributes to spatial compensation.

The concept of spatial compensation is best understood by reference to the *pressure volume curve* (Fig. 4.2) which expresses the relationship between ICP and the volume of the intracranial contents.

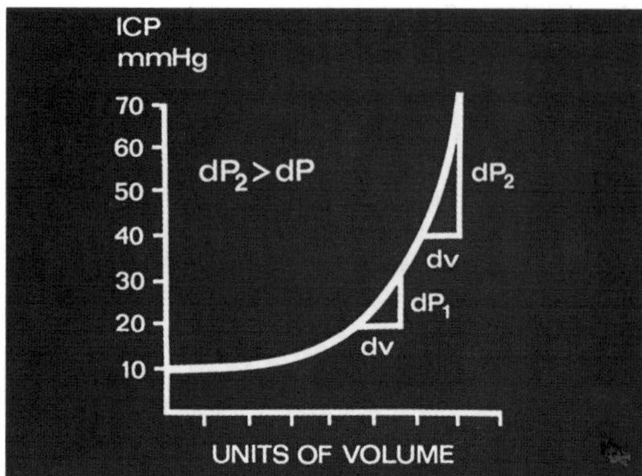

Figure 4.2 The pressure–volume curve. As the volume of a space occupying mass increases and intracranital pressure (ICP) rises, uniform increments of volume (dv) produce progressively larger increase in ICP ($-dP_1$) and ($-dP_2$). Increases or decreases in volume cause correspondingly greater changes in ICP on the steep part of the curve.

Table 4.2 Four stages associated with an increase in intracranial pressure (ICP)

1. Period of spatial compensation, any increase in one of the components is accommodated by a compensatory decrease in the other components
2. Once compensation has become exhausted, ICP rises slowly; systemic arterial pressure (SAP) may increase as ICP increases (the Cushing response), to maintain cerebral perfusion pressure
3. ICP rises rapidly and cerebral perfusion pressure may fall to a critical level
4. Cerebral vasomotor paralysis develops when ICP equals SAP, cerebral circulation ceases and brainstem death occurs

During stage 1 the addition of a small volume of the intracranial contents produces little change in ICP because of a corresponding reduction in the volume of CSF, but once the ICP begins to rise smaller increments of volume produce larger increases in ICP because the compensatory mechanisms are becoming exhausted (stage 2). A critical point occurs at the steepest part of the curve (stage 3) when a very small increase in the volume of the intracranial contents produces an abrupt and considerable rise in ICP (Table 4.2). A not uncommon reason why the clinical state of a patient with an intracranial expanding lesion may suddenly deteriorate is because the volume of circulating blood has altered particularly in response to hypercapnia as a result of respiratory problems. Conversely, rapid correction of the blood gases can have an equally dramatic beneficial effect and volatile anesthetic agents may produce cerebral vasodilation, and general anesthesia for any cause in a patient with an intracranial expanding lesion may increase the ICP.

Other factors affect the rate of increase of ICP, principal amongst which is the rate of expansion of the lesion. Thus, a rapidly expanding mass is more likely to exhaust compensatory mechanisms compared with a slowly expanding lesion. Furthermore, in older age groups when there is some pre-existing atrophy of the brain and therefore an increased volume of CSF in the ventricles and subarachnoid space the potential for spatial compensation is greater than in a younger patient.

CHANGES PRODUCED IN THE BRAIN

Focal neurological signs may occur as a result of local distortion or destruction of the brain produced by the expanding lesion. This, in turn, may result in epilepsy or a focal neurological deficit. As the mass effect becomes greater this may result in brain shift and herniation both of these consequences being more severe when the lesion expands slowly since with a rapidly fatal expanding lesion there is less time for such structural changes to occur.

Supratentorial expanding lesions

A common type of expanding lesion is one within a cerebral hemisphere but similar changes may occur as a result of an expanding lesion either in the extra or subdural space (Fig. 4.1).

As an intracerebral lesion expands so also does the hemisphere: the surface of the brain is pressed against the unyielding dura, gyri are flattened, sulci are narrowed and, as CSF is displaced from the subarachnoid space, the surface of the brain becomes dry (Table 4.3). The ventricle on the side of the lesion

Table 4.3 Neuropathological features of raised intracranial pressure due to unilateral mass lesion

- Tight dura at autopsy
- Narrowing of sulci and flattening of gyri
- Reduction in size of ipsilateral ventricle
- Midline shift
- Supracallosal hernia
- Tentorial hernia
- Compression of ipsilateral oculomotor nerve
- Tonsillar hernia
- Brainstem hemorrhage/infarction, including Kernohan notch
- Calcarine (medial occipital lobe) infarction

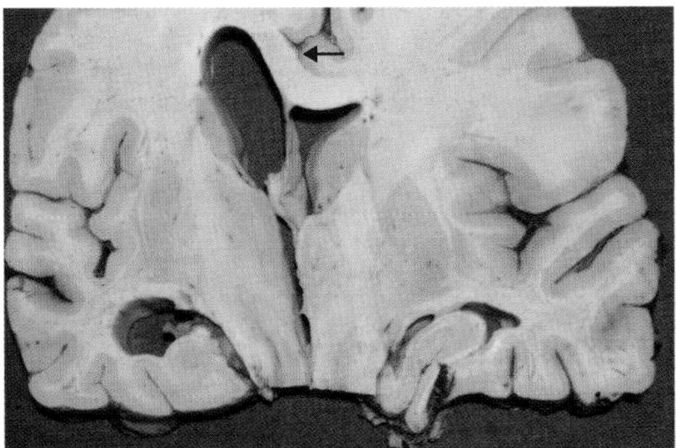

Figure 4.3 Raised intracranial pressure. Expanding lesion in right cerebral hemisphere. There is a conspicuous supracallosal hernia (arrow), a shift of the midline structures to the left and a wedge of hemorrhagic necrosis along the line of a right sided tentorial hernia (arrow head). Obstruction of the contralateral foramen of Monro has resulted in unilateral hydrocephalus.

becomes reduced in size and there is a lateral shift of the midline structures away from the lesion and there is frequently enlargement of the contralateral ventricle because of obliteration of the interventricular foramen of Monro (Fig. 4.3). If an expanding lesion has been present for some time there may be deformities on the surface of the brain where it has come into contact with bony protuberances on the base of the skull, or the cerebral cortex may actually have pushed through the dura to form small nodules on its outer surface. Continued expansion of the mass lesion results in displacement of brain tissue from one intracranial compartment to another, i.e. internal herniation develops.

A *supracallosal hernia* (subfalcine or cingulate hernia) occurs when the ipsilateral cingulate gyrus herniates under the free edge of the falx and the pericallosal arteries may be selectively displaced from the midline. As the hernia enlarges the roof of the lateral ventricle is displaced downwards and posteriorly a supracallosal hernia cannot occur until the roof of the lateral ventricle is also displaced. A small wedge of pressure necrosis may occur in the cortex of the cingulate gyrus where it is in contact with the falx and, occasionally, when the circulation within the pericallosal arteries is severely impaired because of their displacement widespread infarction may occur in the territories they supply (Figs 4.1 and 4.3).

A *tentorial hernia* (uncal or lateral transtentorial hernia), i.e. herniation of the uncus and the medial part of the ipsilateral parahippocampal gyrus through the tentorial incisura (Figs 4.1 and 4.4) is of great clinical significance because of its consequential effects on other structures. As the medial part of the temporal lobe pushes towards the midline and over the free edge of the tentorium, the midbrain is narrowed in its transverse axis, the aqueduct is compressed, and the contralateral cerebral peduncle is pushed against the opposite free edge of the tentorium. This may be sufficiently severe to cause infarction (the Kernohan lesion, Fig. 4.4) in the cerebral peduncle, leading to the potentially misleading clinical sign of a hemiparesis ipsilateral to the expanding lesion. The ipsilateral oculomotor nerve becomes compressed between the free edge of the tentorium and the posterior cerebral artery: the nerve may then become angled over the artery and, if herniation is severe, there may be hemorrhage into it (Fig. 4.4). Dilation of the ipsilateral pupil is the earliest consistent sign of a tentorial hernia and may occur before there is any impairment of consciousness. As the hernia enlarges it produces a groove on the upper surface of the adjacent cerebellar hemisphere. As with a supracallosal hernia, a wedge of pressure necrosis, often accompanied by hemorrhage, may occur along the line of a groove in the parahippocampal gyrus (Fig. 4.4). If there is no hemorrhage, the wedge of pressure necrosis may only be identifiable microscopically.

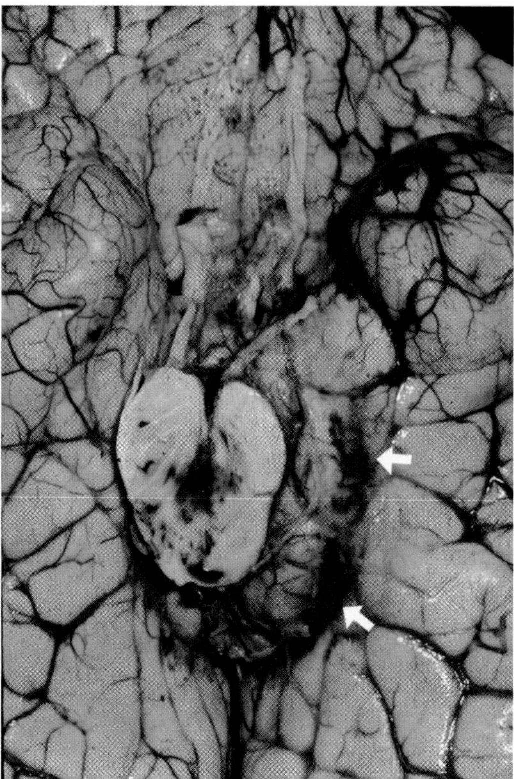

Figure 4.4 Raised intracranial pressure. Expanding lesion in left cerebral hemisphere. There is a conspicuous tentorial hernia (arrow heads). There is also compression of the ipsilateral oculomotor nerve and a contralateral peduncular lesion.

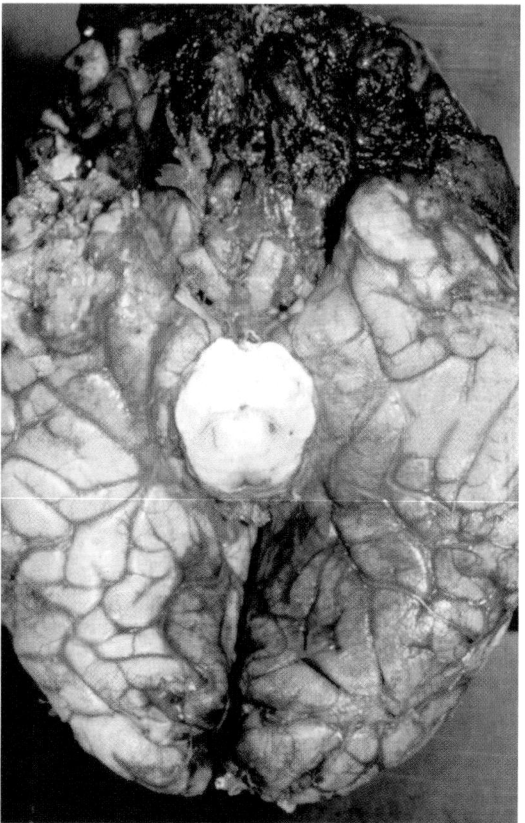

Figure 4.5 Raised intracranial pressure. Vascular complications of a tentorial hernia include hemorrhagic infarction within the distribution of both posterior cerebral arteries. This patient survived 24 h after head injury: note contusions at tips of the temporal poles and under aspects of the frontal lobes.

Clinico-pathological studies of patients in whom the ICP has been continuously monitored during life have established that where the increase in ICP has been produced by a supratentorial expanding lesion, there is always pressure necrosis in the parahippocampal gyrus if the ICP exceeds 5.4 kPa (40 mmHg). Thus, the pathologist can conclude that the ICP had been high even when it has not been monitored during life.

A tentorial hernia also produces selective compression of the posterior cerebral artery, and a common secondary effect is infarction of the cortex of the medial and inferior surfaces of the ipsilateral occipital lobe (Figs 4.5 and 4.6). In some cases infarction is more extensive and extends anteriorly along the inframedial angle of the temporal lobe involving the cortex, the subjacent white matter and the hippocampus. The infarction which may be focally hemorrhagic or anemic maybe bilateral and occasionally it may be contralateral to the expanding lesion. Other arteries may also be so compressed that infarction again usually hemorrhagic occurs in the territories they supply, e.g. compression of the anterior choroidal arteries may cause infarction of structures adjacent to the globus pallidus (Fig. 4.7); compression of the perforating arteries arising from the posterior choroidal artery may result in unilateral or bilateral infarction of the thalamus and in the splenium of the corpus callosum, whereas compression of the superior cerebellar arteries may cause infarction of the upper surface of the cerebellar hemispheres.

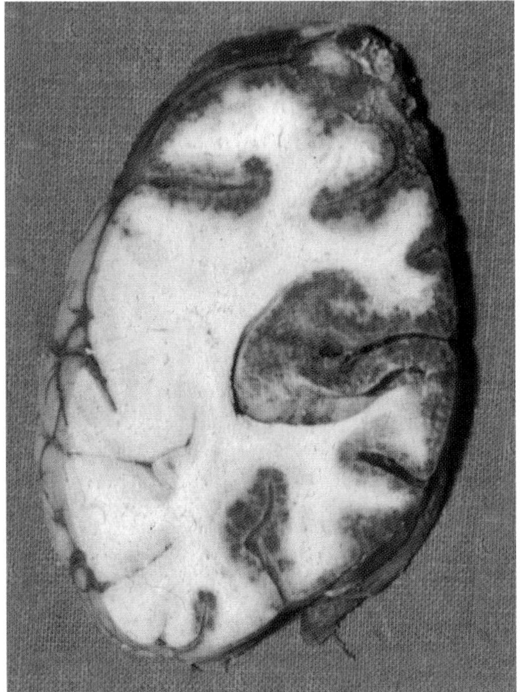

Figure 4.6 Raised intracranial pressure. Compression of posterior cerebral artery. There is hemorrhagic infarction in the cortex of the medial (calcarine) and inferior surfaces of the occipital lobe.

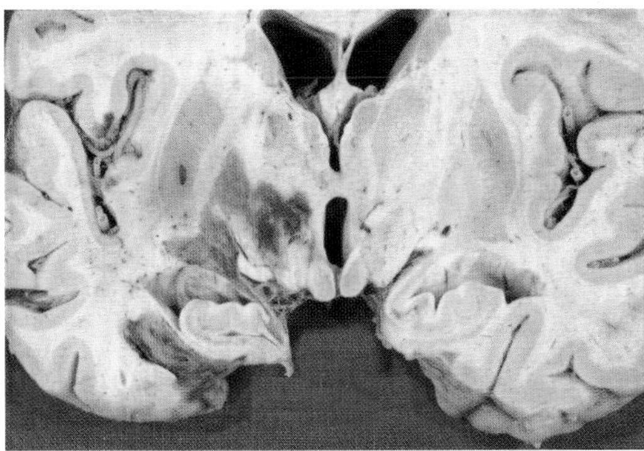

Figure 4.7 Raised intracranial pressure. There is hemorrhagic infarction in the territory supplied by the left anterior choroidal artery.

In addition to the lateral shift there may be downward movement of the brain leading to displacement of the mamillary bodies and stretching and compression of the pituitary stalk. Due to impairment of blood flow through the hypothalamo-hypophyseal portal blood vessels infarction in the anterior lobe of the pituitary gland may occur. More importantly, as a result of lateral and downward displacement of the brainstem hemorrhagic infarction may occur in the midbrain and pons (Fig. 4.4). Both types of lesion occur mainly adjacent to the midline in the tegmentum of the midbrain and in the tegmentum and in basis of the rostral pons. Whether they are due to venous obstruction, hypertension associated with the Cushing response or to mechanical shear of perforating arteries is not clear.

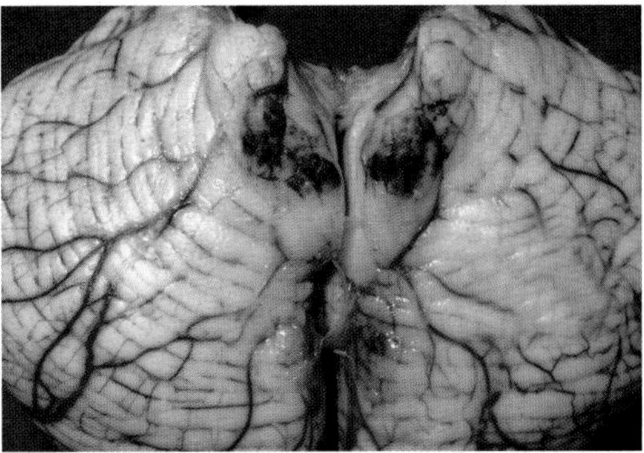

Figure 4.8 Raised intracranial pressure. The tonsils are displaced downwards and there is focal hemorrhagic necrosis affecting their tips – a tonsillar hernia.

A *tonsillar hernia* (cerebellar cone), i.e. downward displacement of the cerebellar tonsils through the foramen magnum, can occur in association with a supratentorial expanding lesion because of transmission of a high ICP from the supratentorial to the infratentorial compartment. The tentorium cerebelli is displaced downwards, the upper surface of each cerebellar hemisphere becomes concave, the volume of the infratentorial compartment is reduced and a tonsillar hernia develops, which compresses the medulla. Variation in the size and shape of the tonsils is normal so that herniation can only be said to be present if there is impaction of the tonsils at the foramen magnum, producing a depression on the ventral surface of the medulla where it has been compressed against the foramen magnum or if there is necrosis of the tips of the tonsils (Fig. 4.8).

The neuropathological features of a supratentorial extracerebral expanding lesion such as an extradural or a subdural hematoma are similar to that described for intracerebral lesions (see above). However, one difference observed is that convolutional flattening associated with a subdural hematoma is limited to the contralateral hemisphere, the blood in the ipsilateral subdural space preventing flattening of the convolutions.

When brain swelling is diffuse and bilateral the ventricles become small and symmetrical and there is not a lateral shift of the midline structures. Tentorial herniae may occur but they are relatively small and often bilateral, their size depending on the rate of brain swelling and the size of the tentorial incisura. Downward displacement of the diencephalon and the brainstem will be more severe than with a unilateral expanding lesion.

Although some 75% of patients who die in a neurosurgical intensive care unit do so from the effects of a raised ICP, evidence of there having previously been a raised ICP may be seen in patients who survive. Evidence of a previously high ICP may be seen in the form of wedge-shaped scars in the cingulate and parahippocampal gyri (Fig. 4.9) and there may also be evidence of previous infarction in the calcarine (medial occipital) cortex (Fig. 4.10) and in the territory supplied by the posterior inferior cerebellar artery (Fig. 4.11), and in the brainstem.

Infratentorial expanding lesions

A mass lesion in the infratentorial compartment (posterior fossa) distorts the aqueduct and the fourth ventricle causing obstructive hydrocephalus with increase in the size of the third and lateral ventricles. Tonsillar herniation is more severe than with supratentorial expanding lesions and may be associated with compression of the posterior inferior

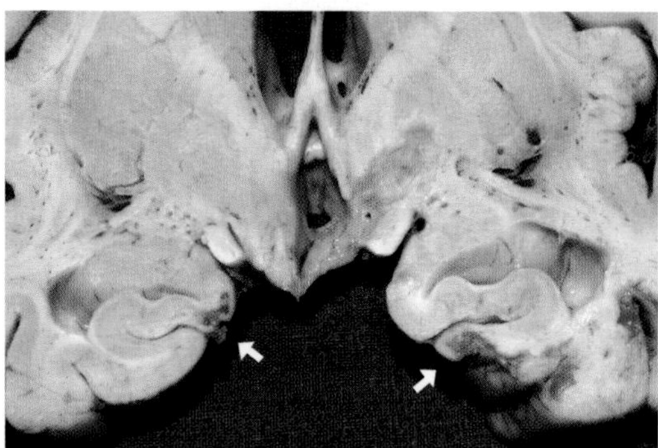

Figure 4.9 Previous episode of raised intracranial pressure. There are old scars (arrows) in each parahippocampal gyrus (cf. Fig. 4.3), and subtotal infarction within the distribution of the anterior choroidal artery.

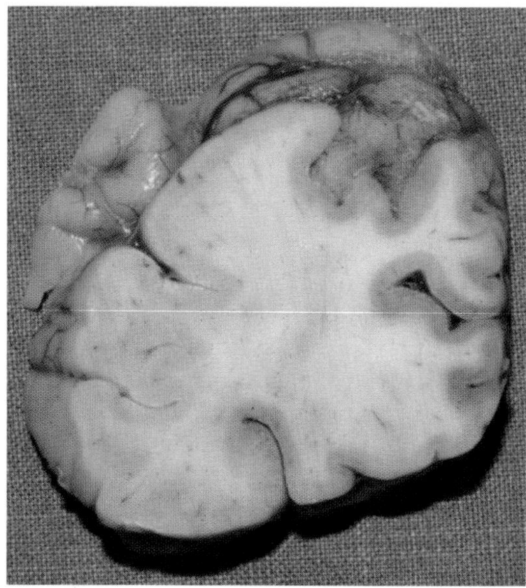

Figure 4.10 Previous episode of raised intracranial pressure. The cortex on the medial and inferior surfaces of the occipital lobe is narrowed and granular (cf. Fig. 4.6) due to compression of the posterior cerebral artery.

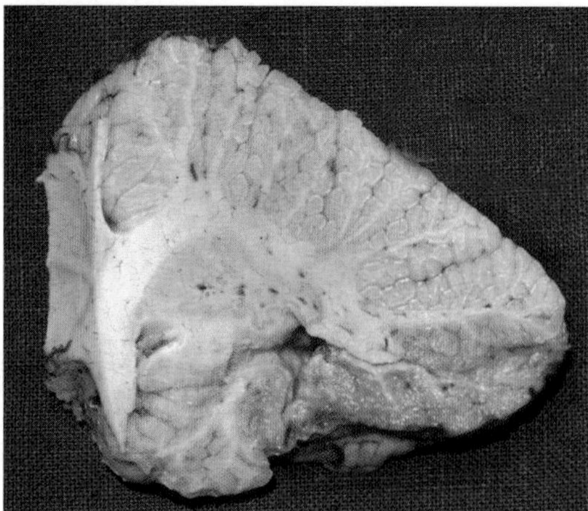

Figure 4.11 Previous episode of raised intracranial pressure. There is long standing infarction in the distribution of the posterior inferior cerebellar artery.

cerebellar arteries as a result of which infarction may occur in the inferior part of one or both cerebellar hemispheres.

Herniation of the cerebellum may also occur in an upward direction through the tentorial incisura – the so-called *reversed tentorial hernia*, and if the lesion is expanding very slowly, upward herniation of the superior vermis can produce considerable distortion of the parahippocampal gyri.

Other effects of expanding lesions

Long sustained elevations in ICP may be associated with erosion of bone, a feature that is well seen in the pituitary fossa of adults where at first there is a loss of detail of the cortex anteriorly at the lower part of the fossa. In infants and children less than 10 years of age the first sign of raised ICP is often separation of the sutures of the vault. Enlargement of the skull, thinning of the bones of the vault and prominence of the convolutional impressions also occur in children. With a result of downward pressure on the diaphragma sellae the floor of the pituitary fossa may be thinned and occasionally there may be erosion of the lesser wing of the sphenoid bone and of the roof of the orbit.

Systemic changes may occur in association with a high ICP and include subendocardial hemorrhages in the outflow tract of the left ventricle, foci of necrosis in the myocardium and hemorrhagic congestion and ulceration of the stomach, duodenum and urinary bladder.

EDEMA AND SWELLING OF THE BRAIN

The blood–brain barrier (BBB) is crucial in the regulation of fluid and various molecules from blood to brain and vice versa. The BBB consists of both anatomical (endothelial cells, pericytes and the feet processes of astrocytes) and functional (metabolic) components. By these means neurons and glial cells of the brain are isolated from the blood stream and their immediate environment is tightly controlled. The endothelial cells have tight junctions without fenestrations, a paucity of pinocytotic activity and large numbers of mitochondria. Further, the endothelial cells contain many enzymes which help to maintain the function of the BBB together with the basement membrane, pericytes and astrocytes (Fig. 4.12).

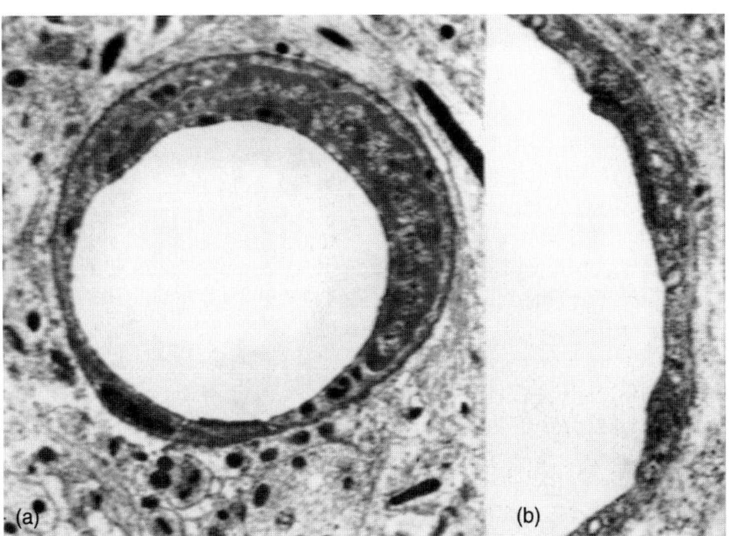

Figure 4.12 Blood–brain barrier. (a) Transverse section of small blood vessel. The luminal layer of continuous endothelium is separated from neuropil by a basement membrane. (b) Higher magnification to show tight junctions between adjacent endothelial cells. Electron micrographs (a) ×2000 (b) ×5000.

The normal BBB controls the passage of substances by a number of mechanisms that include diffusion, specific carrier systems, vesicular transport and cytoplasmic channels. In general the main ways in which the BBB may become dysfunctional ('leaky') are separation of the inter-endothelial junctions, enhancing vesicular transport and altered biochemical and structural changes of the endothelial membrane.

The term *cerebral edema* means that there is an increase in the water content of the brain tissue leading to an increase in the volume of all or part of the brain. The normal water content of gray matter is 80% of the wet weight and of white matter 68% of wet weight: the content in cerebral edema is some 81–82% and 76–79%, respectively. Enlargement of the brain may also be brought about by *congestive brain swelling* as a result of an increase in the cerebral blood volume. In either case there is ultimately an increase in the volume of one of the intracranial constituents leading to the sequence of events described in the previous section.

The effective size of many lesions may be considerably increased by associated vasodilation or edema. The various modalities of magnetic resonance imaging has allowed the identification of the various forms of congestion and edema thereby allowing treatment aimed at either removing or at least reducing the volume of expanding lesions.

Congestive brain swelling, which may affect one cerebral hemisphere, can occur remarkably rapidly, particularly in children who have sustained a head injury and in patients in whom an acute subdural hematoma has been evacuated (Fig. 4.13) or both cerebral hemispheres (Fig. 4.14). The likely mechanism is that the small blood vessels dilate and the capillary bed is flooded with stagnant blood. Particularly when arterial blood pressure is high this in turn will induce dysfunction of the BBB with the result that ICP may increase rapidly.

There are several types of cerebral edema (Table 4.4). In *vasogenic edema* the BBB is defective and water, sodium and protein molecules are extravasated into the extracellular space. It is usually unilateral and is a frequent feature of malignant (Fig. 4.15a and b) or benign brain tumors (Fig. 4.16a and b) contusions (Fig. 4.17a, b and c) and intracranial hematomas, and in relation to abscess

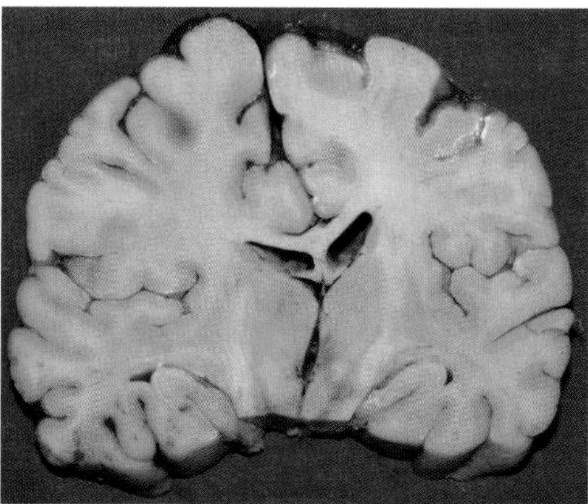

Figure 4.13 Cerebral swelling. The left cerebral hemisphere is markedly expanded, and there is a shift of the midline to the right and a supracallosal hernia. The patient died after evacuation of an acute subdural hematoma.

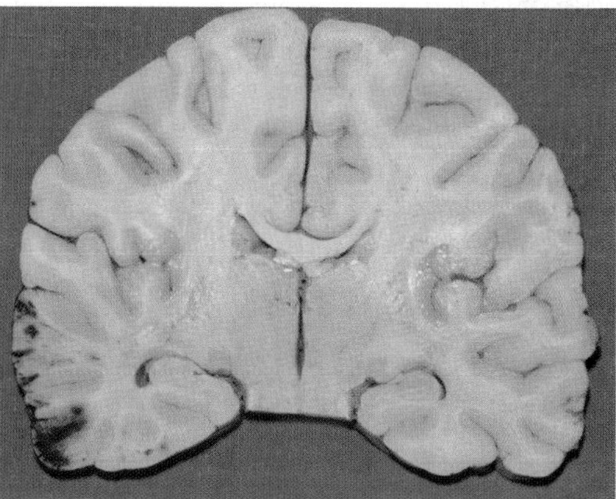

Figure 4.14 Swelling of both cerebral hemispheres. Patient died 48 h after acute head injury. Note minor surface contusions on lateral aspect of left temporal lobe. The ventricular system is symmetrically small. There is not a shift of midline structures.

Table 4.4 Types of cerebral edema

- Vasogenic
- Cytotoxic
- Hydrostatic
- Interstitial
- Hypo-osmotic

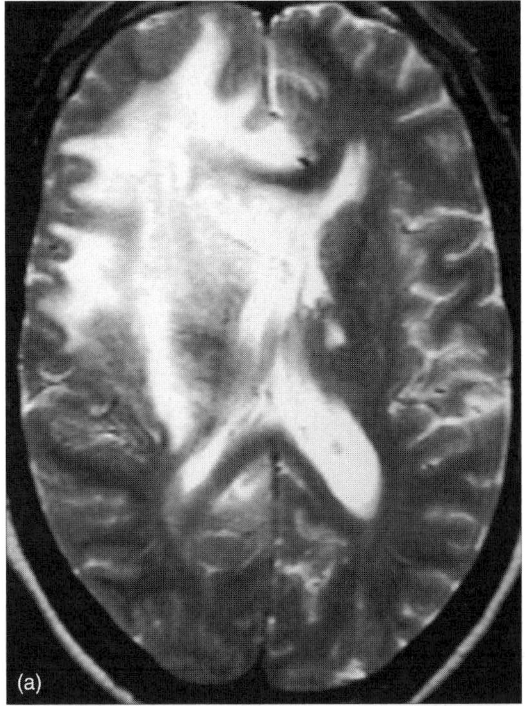

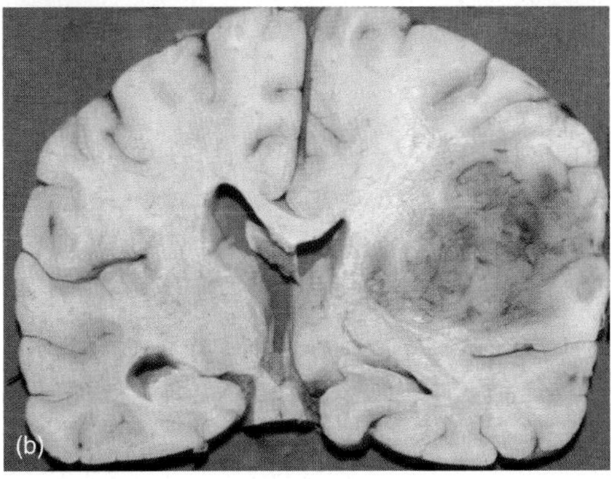

Figure 4.15 Vasogenic edema. (a) MRI T2-weighted axial image of right frontal glioblastoma. Note shift of midline structures and ventricular compression. (b) Glioblastoma in right cerebral hemisphere. There is swelling, ventricular compression and internal herniation.

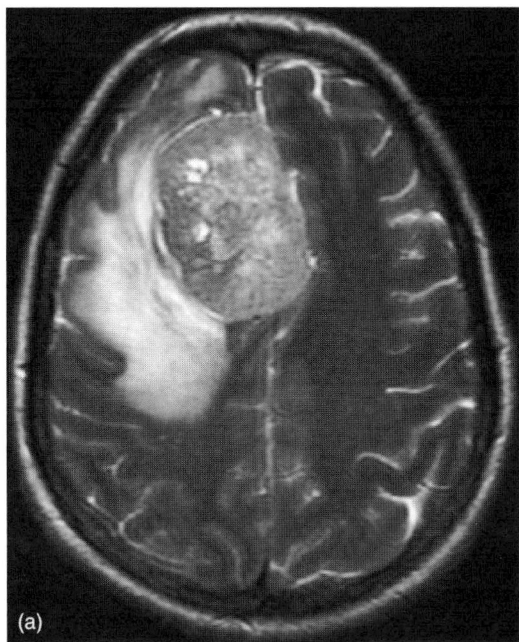

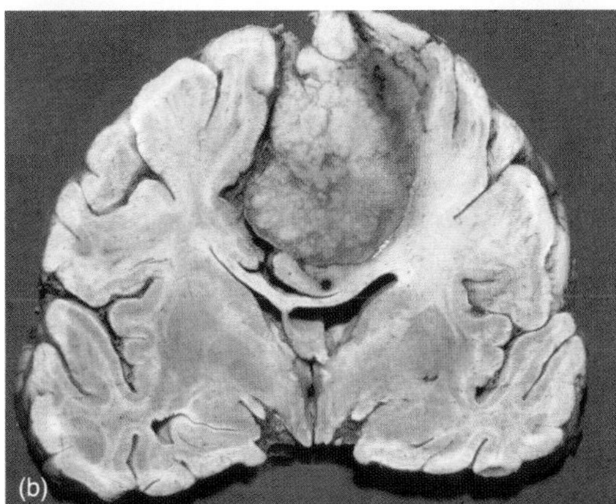

Figure 4.16 Vasogenic edema. (a) MRI T2-weighted axial image of right frontal parasagittal meningioma. (b) Meningioma in parasagittal region of right cerebral hemisphere. Note shift of midline structures and swelling of associated white matter.

formation. The edema occurs particularly in white matter and when it is extensive at the time of brain cutting may have a pale green color. Histological examination shows pallor of staining and the myelin sheaths appear rather vacuolated and pale. If the edema persists there is some destruction of myelin as shown by microcyst formation (Fig. 4.18a), the appearance of a reactive astrocytosis (Fig. 4.18b) and (Fig. 4.18c) macrophage formation. The causes of the breakdown of the BBB in this type of edema include physical disruption due to trauma, necrosis of blood vessels and in instances

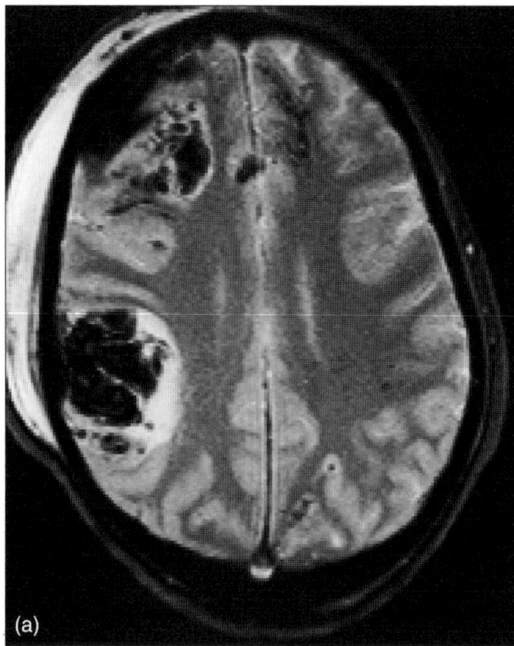

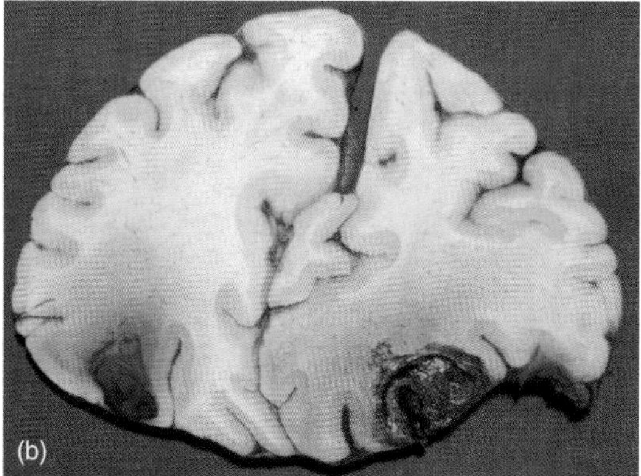

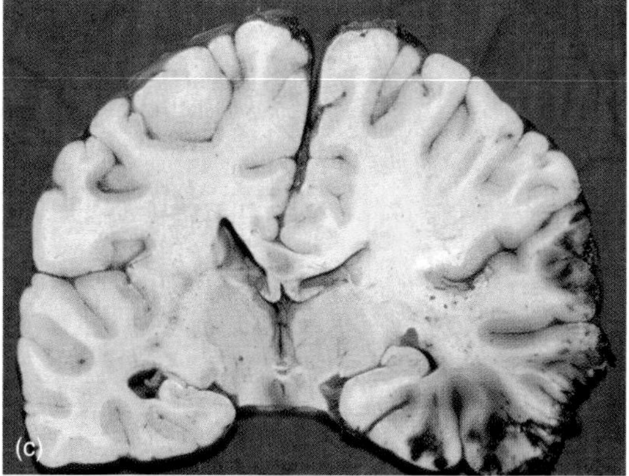

Figure 4.17 Vasogenic edema. (a) MRI gradient echo T2-weighted image of acute head injury. There are contusions in the right frontal lobes and temporal lobe. Note the edema associated with the contusions, part of which is probably vasogenic and part cytotoxic. (b) Contusions of frontal lobes. Note swelling associated with those on the right. (c) Contusions of temporal lobe. There is swelling of the right cerebral hemisphere.

where the anatomical barrier appears to be intact it is presumed that dysfunction is due to an increase in pinocytotic activity.

In *cytotoxic edema* the commonest cause of which is ischemic damage to the brain, the changes are essentially intracellular. It occurs as a result of energy failure within neurons and is therefore more prominent in gray than in white matter (Fig. 4.19).

In *hydrostatic edema* there is a sudden increase in intravascular pressure leading to flooding of the capillary bed within the brain followed rapidly by extravasation of proteinaceous fluid into the extracellular space. This type of edema is seen in hypertensive encephalopathy.

Interstitial edema occurs when fluid under high pressure is forced through damaged ependyma into the periventricular tissue as in acute obstructive hydrocephalus. *Hypo-osmotic edema* may develop when the serum osmolality is severely reduced and may explain the cerebral edema that sometimes occurs in the treatment of diabetic coma when there may be a relative reduction of serum osmolality compared with the brain tissue where the glucose level is still high.

There is no evidence to suggest that any increase in brain water content directly interferes with a patient's neurological state. Rather, it exerts its effects only when it is sufficiently severe to produce an increase in ICP. This is clearly demonstrable when steroids or mannitol are administered to a patient who is becoming decompensated from vasogenic edema around a brain tumor.

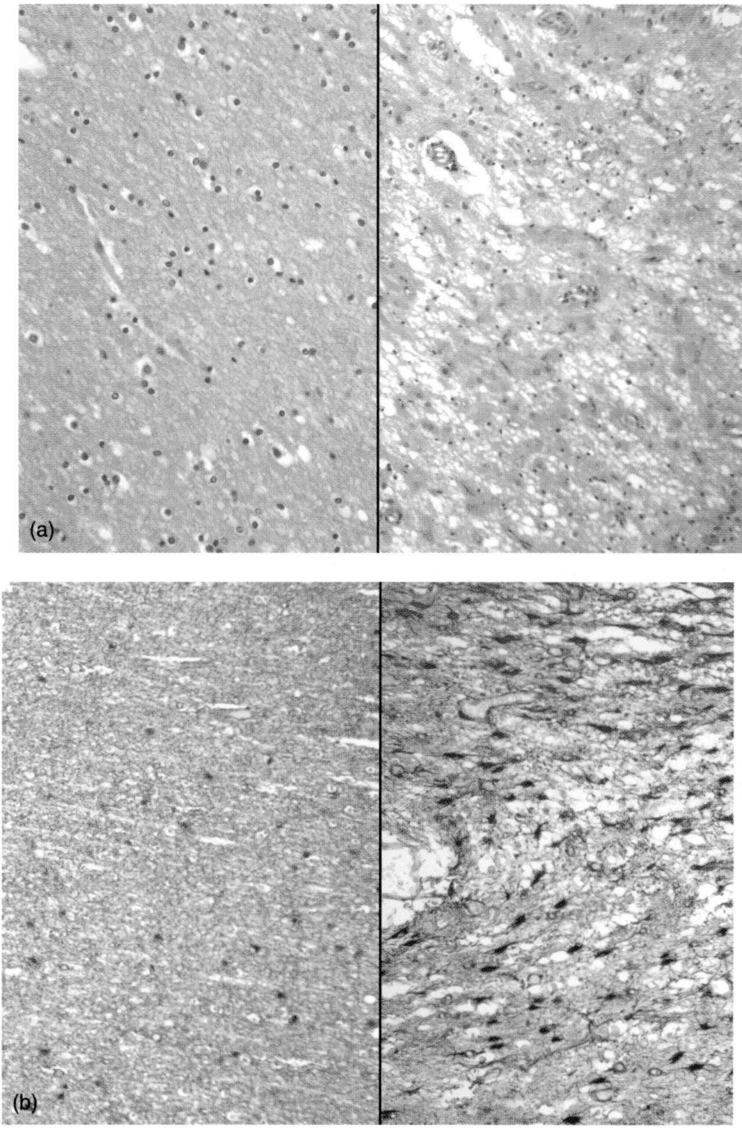

Figure 4.18 Vasogenic edema. (a) Left panel. Normal compact white matter. Right panel. There is a pallor of staining, vacuolation of myelinated fibres and reactive astrocytosis. H&E. (b) Left panel. Normal compact white matter with scattered resting astrocytes. Right panel. There is a reactive astrocytosis in the vacuolated white matter (cf. (a)). Immunohistochemistry (GFAP).

HYDROCEPHALUS

Formation and circulation of CSF

This is depicted in (Fig. 4.20a and b). The volume of CSF is between 120 and 150 mL and under normal circumstances its production and resorption are in equilibrium with a turnover of some two to five times per day. The term *hydrocephalus* means an increased volume of CSF within the cranial cavity.

CSF is produced by the choroid plexus of the lateral, third and fourth ventricles. It leaves the lateral ventricle via the interventricular foramen of

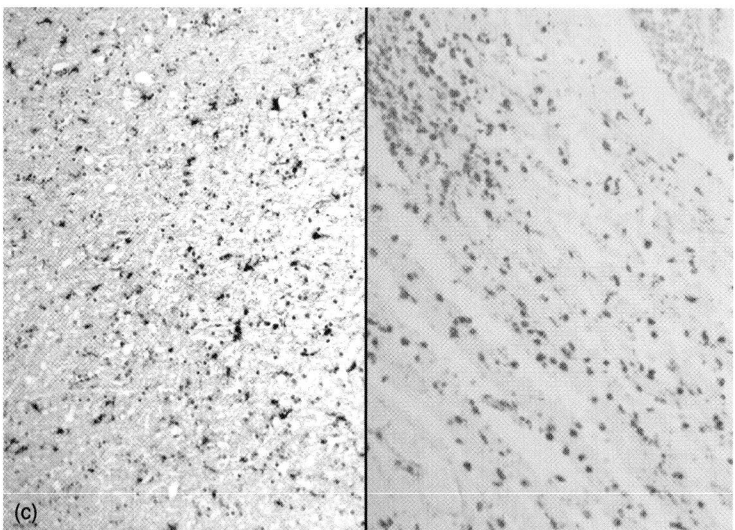

Figure 4.18 Vasogenic edema. (c) Left panel. Normal compact white matter. Right panel. There is hypertrophy of microglia and an infiltrate of macrophages. Immunohistochemistry (CD68).

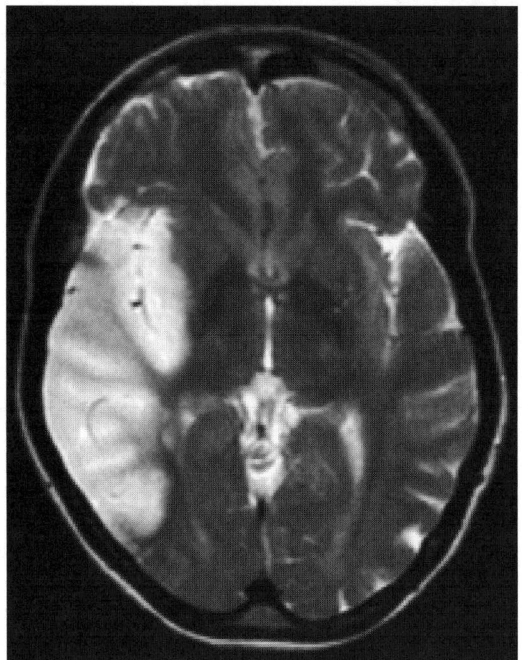

Figure 4.19 Cytotoxic edema. MRI T2-weighted image of acute infarction in distribution of right middle cerebral artery.

Monro and passes through the aqueduct of Sylvius to enter the fourth ventricle from which it exits via the foramina of Luschka (lateral) and Magendie (midline) to enter the subarachnoid space of the posterior fossa. Most CSF circulates through the posterior fossa from which it reaches the supratentorial space through the tentorial incisura to flow over the cerebral hemispheres to be absorbed via the arachnoid granulations in the superior sagittal sinus: some of the CSF passes through the foramen magnum into the spinal subarachnoid space where it is absorbed in the prolongation of the subarachnoid space along the spinal nerve roots.

Samples of CSF are usually obtained by lumbar puncture and occasionally from the cisterna magna and in neurosurgical units samples may be obtained by catheters placed in the lateral ventricles.

Types of hydrocephalus

In *internal hydrocephalus* the increased volume of CSF is within the ventricular system and, in general, the term hydrocephalus is used to denote this type of hydrocephalus. In *external hydrocephalus* the excess CSF is in the subarachnoid space. The hydrocephalus is said to be *communicating* if CSF can flow freely from the ventricular system to the subarachnoid space; if it cannot, it is *non-communicating*. In active hydrocephalus there is progressive enlargement of the ventricular system and an increase in the ventricular pressure.

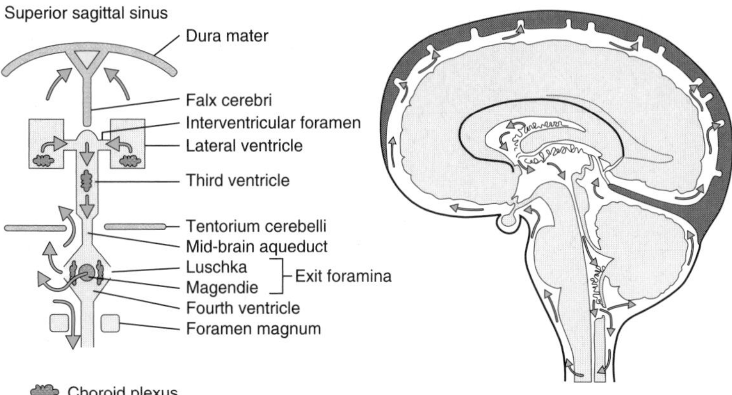

Figure 4.20 (Left and right) The formation and circulation of cerebrospinal fluid (CSF). The bulk of the CSF is produced in the choroid plexus of the lateral, third and fourth ventricles. The direction of the intraventricular flow is shown by the arrows. CSF leaves the lateral ventricles via interventricular foramina, and the fourth ventricle via the exit foramina in the fourth ventricle (Lushka and Magendie) to enter the subarachnoid space. Some descends through the foramen magnum into the spinal subarachnoid space where it is absorbed in the prolongations of the subarachnoid space along spinal nerve roots. Most circulates through the posterior fossa and then reaches the supratentorial space through the tentorial incisura. It then flows over the cerebral hemispheres to be absorbed in the superior sagittal sinus.

Hydrocephalus is said to be *arrested* when ventricular enlargement ceases and intraventricular pressure is normal. *Compensatory hydrocephalus* (sometimes referred to as *ex vacuo*) occurs when the increased volume of CSF is compensatory to loss of brain tissue.

Causes of hydrocephalus

The most common cause of ventricular enlargement is secondary to cerebral atrophy principally due to aging, neurodegenerative disease or as a consequence of structural damage due to infarction or trauma, etc. in these circumstances ICP is usually normal (Fig. 4.21a, b and c).

If there is an obstruction to the free flow of CSF hydrocephalus will develop depending upon the rapidity with which CSF accumulates. Usually, after some weeks the hydrocephalus becomes arrested because the amount of CSF absorbed is in equilibrium with the volume of CSF produced. The ependymal lining of the ventricular system becomes disrupted and interstitial edema forms in the periventricular white matter (Fig. 4.22a and b) which can be recognized on scans by reduced density. However, in any circumstance in which there is an arrest of CSF circulation, ICP can rise very rapidly and death may result from acute hydrocephalus (e.g. colloid cyst). Relief is either obtained by treating the primary pathology or by establishing ventricular drainage to remove CSF thereby allowing the ventricles to reduce in size.

In obstructive hydrocephalus it is the site of the lesion rather than its nature which is important (Table 4.5). Thus, a small lesion in a critical site adjacent to an interventricular foramen or the aqueduct in the midbrain is of much greater importance than a large expanding lesion in a frontal or occipital lobe. But the abnormality, however, need not be adjacent to the ventricular system since any process such as previous meningitis or subarachnoid hemorrhage which results in obliteration of the subarachnoid space – particularly at the level of the tentorial incisura – will restrict the free flow of CSF. Mass lesions in the infratentorial compartment of the skull are particularly important (e.g. hematomas, infarcts and tumors). However, a similar sequence of events may occur as a result of congenital abnormalities such as the Dandy–Walker syndrome, Chiari malformations and gliosis of the aqueduct. In addition, obstruction may result from abnormalities in the base of the skull, e.g. Paget's disease, achondroplasia. The consequences of an obstruction are straightforward insofar as the proximal ventricular

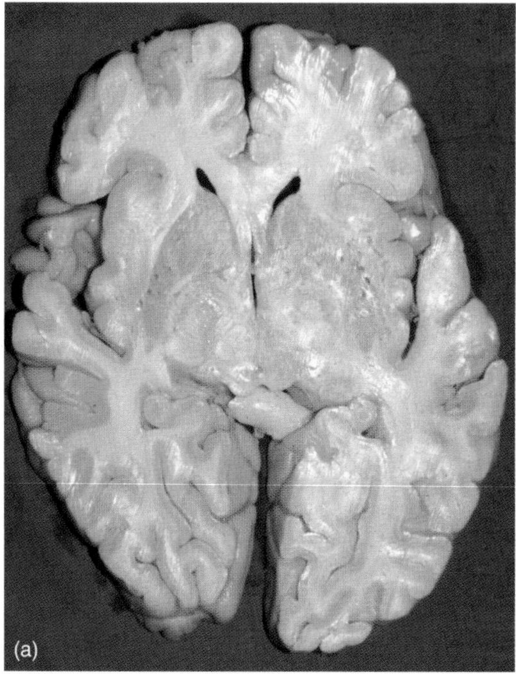

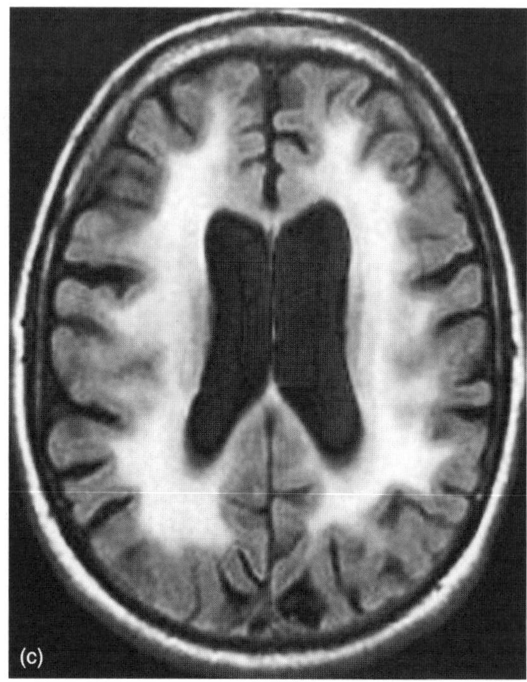

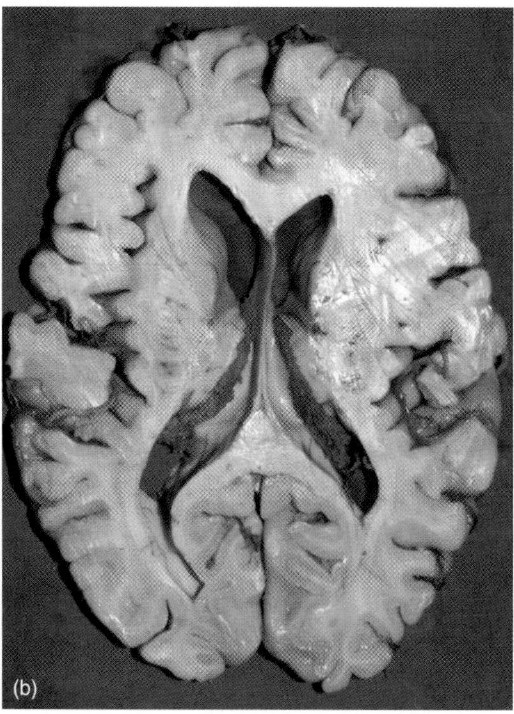

Figure 4.21 Hydrocephalus *ex vacuo*. (a) Normal brain cut in axial plane. (b) Alzheimer's disease. There is considerable atrophy, particularly of the temporal lobes including the hippocampi, and enlargement of the lateral ventricles. The changes are similar in amount and distribution as (c), compared with (a). (c) MRI T1-weighted image. There is frontotemporal atrophy with compensatory symmetrical enlargement of the subarachnoid space and ventricular system.

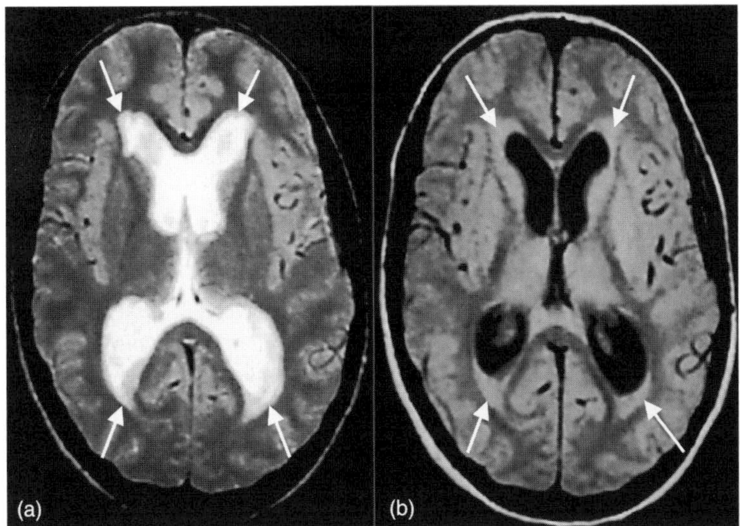

Figure 4.22 Obstructive hydrocephalus. (a) Left panel. MRI T2-weighted image. There is uniform enlargement of the third and lateral ventricles due to midline mass lesion in posterior fossa of 13-year-old patient. (b) Right panel. MRI proton density of same case as (a). Note periventricular change in keeping with interstitial edema.

Table 4.5 Obstructive hydrocephalus

- Site of obstruction can be identified by the enlargement of the ventricular system proximal to the obstruction
- If at an interventricular foramen, one lateral ventricle enlarges
- If in the third ventricle or the aqueduct, both lateral ventricles enlarge
- If at exit foramina of the fourth ventricle, the entire ventricular system enlarges

system enlarges. For example, if the obstruction is at the interventricular foramen (Monro), one lateral ventricle enlarges (Fig. 4.23); if it is in the third ventricle or the aqueduct, both lateral ventricles enlarge; if it is at the exit foramina of the fourth ventricle due to some previous inflammatory process, the entire ventricle system enlarges; if the obstruction is in the subarachnoid space at the level of the tentorium again the entire ventricular system enlarges but on this occasion the hydrocephalus is communicating in type.

Other possible causes of hydrocephalus are *increased production* of CSF, or *decreased absorption.* Increased production of CSF may occur in patients with a papilloma of the choroid plexus but there may also be obstructive elements and shedding of tumor cells or hemorrhage from the tumor may have an irritant effect leading to obliteration of the subarachnoid space. It has been suggested that decreased absorption of CSF may be a sequel to subarachnoid hemorrhage, the arachnoid granulations being partly obliterated by macrophages containing hemosiderin.

Normal pressure hydrocephalus

This is probably a misnomer and is characterized by ventricular enlargement and a clinical syndrome consisting of dementia, disturbance of gait and urinary incontinence or urgency. In 50% of cases there is a preceding cause – subarachnoid hemorrhage, trauma, meningitis or radiation-induced. In the remaining 50% the cause is not known. Routine measurement of the CSF pressure may show it to be normal but if continuous monitoring of ICP is undertaken then episodes of moderate intracranial hypertension can often be demonstrated particularly during sleep. For this reason it has been suggested that a more appropriate term would be *intermittent hydrocephalus.* The patients may be improved by reducing hydrocephalus through a

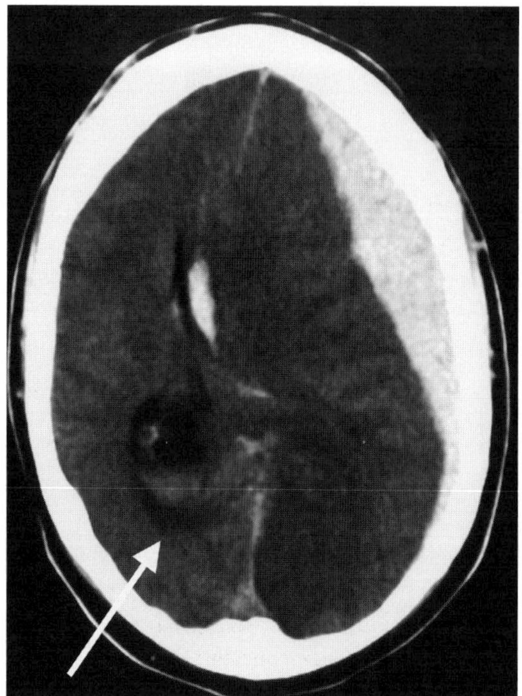

Figure 4.23 Obstructive hydrocephalus. CT scan of a 28-year-old patient with a head injury who developed an acute subdural hematoma. As a result of the mass affect of the hematoma and associated swelling there is a shift of the midline structures and enlargement of the contralateral ventricular system (arrow). The selective hydrocephalus is due to obstruction of the foramen of Monro.

ventriculo-peritoneal shunt, but careful investigation and selection of patients are required particularly in the elderly as some degree of ventricular enlargement associated with cognitive impairment is not uncommon.

Benign intracranial hypertension (pseudo-tumor cerebri)

A controversial subject in which the patients – women more frequently than men – have a high ICP and headache but in whom the ventricular system is not enlarged. It is characterized by increased ICP without evidence of an intracranial mass lesion, obstruction of CSF pathways, infection or hypertensive encephalopathy. Diagnosis is dependent on excluding obstruction to venous outflow or absorption of CSF. Risk factors include obesity, endocrine disturbance and various drugs, which includes oral contraceptives, tetracycline and nalidixic acid. Because the high ICP is evenly distributed throughout the craniospinal axis there are no intracranial pressure gradients and therefore shifts and herniation of the brain do not develop.

CHAPTER 5

VASCULAR AND HYPOXIC DISORDERS

David I Graham

INTRODUCTION

Vascular diseases of the nervous system ('strokes' or cerebrovascular accidents) are common causes of admission to hospital due to the rapid onset of a focal disturbance of brain function of presumed vascular origin, and of more than 24 h duration. The most common causes are *cerebral infarction* and *spontaneous intracranial hemorrhage* (Table 5.1). Although it may be difficult to make the correct diagnosis clinically, modern neuroimaging techniques such as computed tomography (CT) and magnetic resonance imaging (MRI) do so with considerable accuracy. Much useful information about the pathogenesis of cerebrovascular disease and its mortality and its morbidity have been gained from prospective epidemiological studies. In the United Kingdom, as in other westernized countries, cerebrovascular disease constitutes a major health problem accounting for some 10% of all deaths, and is surpassed only by heart disease and cancer. Approximately 30% of all strokes are fatal, approaching 50% after cerebral hemorrhage and an immediate mortality of less than 20% after cerebral infarction.

Table 5.1 Principal types and frequency (%) of cerebrovascular disease

Type	Frequency (%)
Cerebral infarction	**85**
Thrombotic	60
Embolic	25
Intracranial hemorrhage	**15**
Intracerebral	9
Subarachnoid from rupture of saccular aneurysm	5
Bleeding into an infarct (reperfusion injury)	1

Although most common in the elderly, 'strokes' occur in all age groups. The annual incidence in the United Kingdom varies from between 150 and 200 per 100 000 with a prevalence of 600 per 100 000 of which some 30% are severely disabled, and only 10% return to normal activity.

Data from prospective studies suggest that some 85% of 'strokes' are due to infarction (about 60% thrombotic and 25% embolic), leaving some 15% due to hemorrhage (9% from spontaneous intracerebral hemorrhage, and 5% subarachnoid hemorrhage from a ruptured saccular aneurysm).

In spite of much laboratory work, our understanding of the pathophysiology of 'stroke' has not been successfully translated into improved outcome in clinical trials using neuroprotective agents, hence the current emphasis of prevention based on the identification of various *risk factors* which increase the likelihood of 'stroke': the principal risk

Table 5.2 Risk factors for cerebral infarction

- Hypertension
- Cardiac disease
  - Enlargement
  - Coronary heart disease
  - Failure and arrhythmias
  - Rheumatic heart disease
- Diabetes mellitus (increased two-fold)
- Blood lipids, cholesterol, smoking, diet obesity, soft water, hematocrit
- Oral contraceptives
- Disease of neck arteries
- Hereditary factors

Table 5.3 Risk factors and frequency of intracranial hemorrhage

Risk factor	Frequency (%)
Hypertension	70
Cerebral amyloid angiopathy	10
Rupture of saccular aneurysm	5
Arteriovenous malformation	Not known
Neoplasms	5
Mild trauma in association with coagulation disorders and anticoagulants	5
Vasculitis	Not known
Drug abuse, e.g. cocaine	5
Hemorrhagic transformation of infarct	Not known

factors for cerebral infarction are given in Table 5.2. With regard to cerebral infarction, atheroma and hypertension play dominant roles; further important factors include heart disease, diabetes mellitus and open surgery on the heart. Various environmental factors have also been incriminated and include cigarette smoking, diet, obesity, whether the drinking water is hard or soft, coffee drinking, alcohol consumption, stress, physical activity and climate. There is also an increasing appreciation that the close relatives are slightly at greater risk than non-genetically related family members of the 'stroke' patient. On the other hand, factors that predispose to spontaneous intracranial hemorrhage (Table 5.3) are hypertension, the formation of saccular aneurysms on the basal blood vessels comprising the Circle of Willis, hematological abnormalities in which there is thrombocytopenia, mycotic aneurysms, vascular malformations, various primary and secondary tumors, amyloid (congophilic) angiopathy, substance abuse and reperfusion injury which in some instances has been facilitated by fibrinolytic therapy for the treatment of embolic infarction.

BLOOD SUPPLY OF THE BRAIN AND SPINAL CORD

The cerebral hemispheres

The *arterial supply* to the cerebral hemispheres is derived from branches of the *Circle of Willis* at the base of the brain, which is essentially an anastomosis between the *vertebro-basilar* and the internal *carotid systems*. The configuration of the Circle of Willis is subject to considerable variation but the normal circle is illustrated (Fig. 5.1). The *posterior cerebral arteries* are the final branches of the basilar artery that supplies the cortex of the occipital lobes, including the visual cortex, and the medial and inferior surfaces of the temporal lobes excluding the temporal poles (Fig. 5.2). The *middle cerebral arteries* supply the lateral surface of the cerebral hemispheres, except for strips along the upper border – anterior cerebral artery, and the lower border – posterior cerebral artery (Fig. 5.2). Included in this area is the auditory cortex and the insular cortex deep to the Sylvian fissure. The *anterior cerebral arteries* supply the medial surface of the hemisphere as far back as the parieto-occipital sulcus, plus the superior rim of the lateral surface not supplied by the middle cerebral artery (Fig. 5.2). There are anastomoses between these arteries on the surface of the brain. The deep gray and white matter are supplied by *striate arteries* which arise from the Circle of Willis and the proximal portions of the cerebral arteries as perforating branches. All of these blood vessels are essentially end arteries.

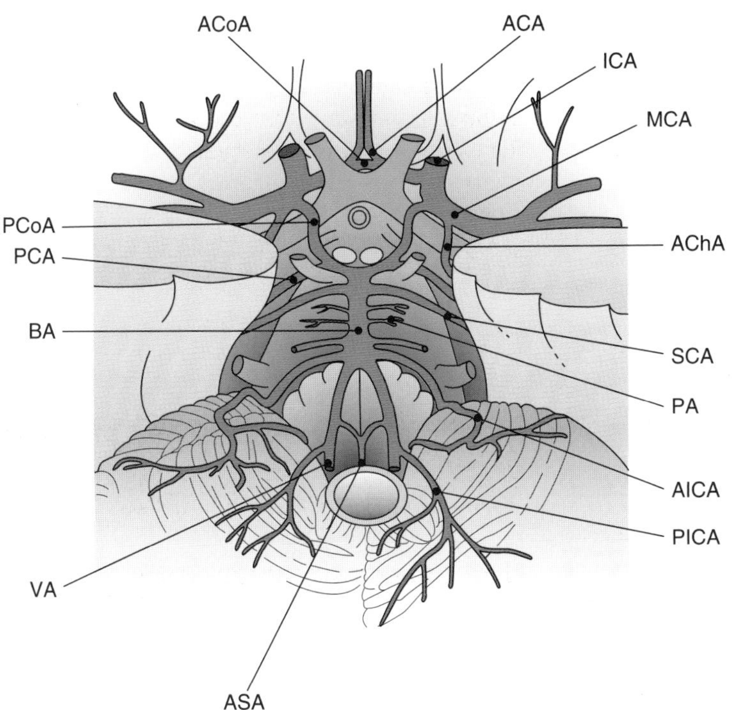

Figure 5.1 Diagram of the Circle of Willis. ACA = anterior cerebral artery; ICA = internal carotid artery; MCA = middle cerebral artery; AChA = anterior choroidal artery; SCA = superior cerebellar artery; PA = pontine arteries; AICA = anterior inferior cerebellar artery; PICA = posterior inferior cerebellar artery; ASA = anterior spinal artery; VA = vertebral artery; BA basilar artery; PCA = posterior cerebral artery; PCoA = posterior communicating artery; ACoA = anterior communicating artery.

There are three main groups of *external cerebral veins* which drain the surface of the hemispheres. These are the superior, the superficial middle and the inferior veins, all linked by two anastomotic veins: the superior (between the superior and the superficial middle) and the inferior (between the superficial middle and the inferior). There are about a dozen *superior cerebral veins* which drain via the bridging veins into the *superior sagittal sinus*. The posterior veins are oblique and enter the sinus against the direction of blood flow. The *superficial middle cerebral veins* run forward in the Sylvian fissure and drain into the *cavernous sinus* on either side of the pituitary fossa. The *inferior veins* are inconspicuous and drain into the nearest venous sinus. The paired *internal cerebral veins* form when the thalamo-striate and the choroidal veins run backwards in the roof of the third ventricle; they then unite to make the *great cerebral vein of Galen* which empties into the *straight sinus*. The great cerebral vein receives many tributaries from the deeper structures of the cerebral hemispheres.

The hind brain

The blood supply of the hind brain is derived chiefly from the vertebro-basilar system (Fig. 5.3). The peripheral branches are not end arteries and their territories overlap. The upper surface and the dorsal angle of the cerebellar hemispheres are supplied by the *superior cerebellar artery*: the artery curves around the brainstem in the ponto-mesencephalic groove and is separated from the posterior cerebral artery by the occulomotor nerves proximally, and the tentorium cerebelli distally. Deep parts of the cerebellum are supplied by the *anterior inferior cerebellar artery*, which is usually the smallest of the three cerebellar arteries. The *posterior inferior cerebellar arteries* arise from the vertebral artery usually some 2 cm below the ponto-medullary junction and supply the dorsolateral sector of the medulla, the inferior surface of the cerebellar hemispheres, and the roof of the fourth ventricle and its choroid plexus. The brainstem derives its blood supply from the paramedian and short perforating branches of the vertebro-basilar system.

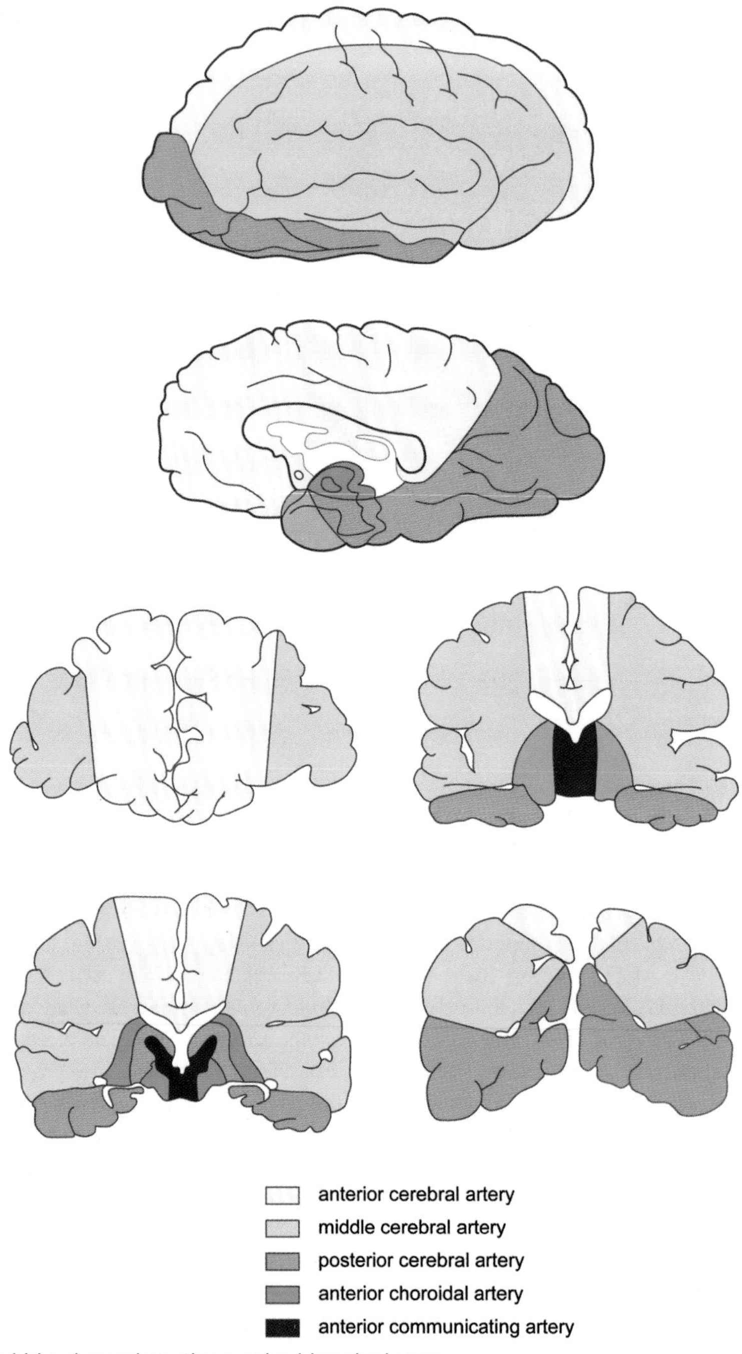

Figure 5.2 Arterial blood supply to the cerebral hemispheres.

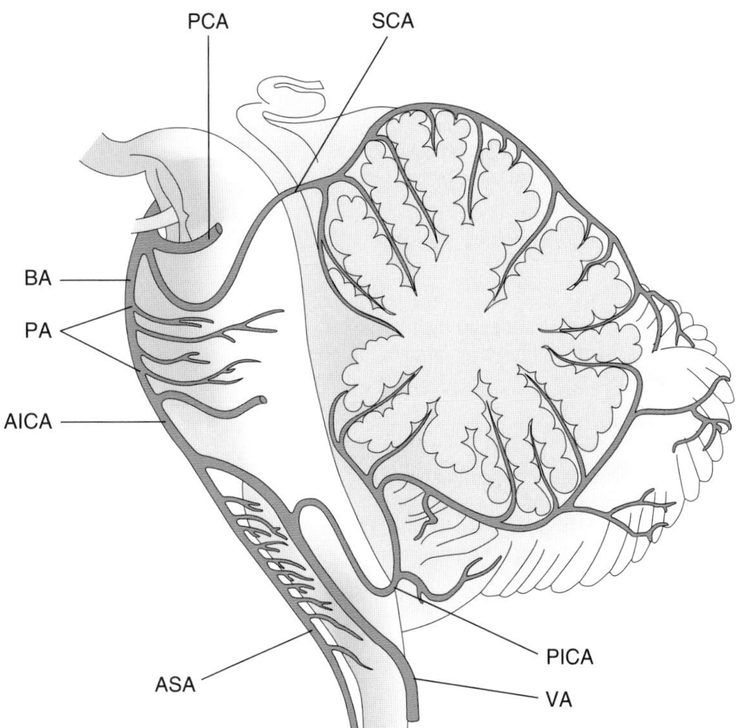

Figure 5.3 Arterial blood supply to the hindbrain. Abbreviations as in Fig. 5.1.

The venous drainage of the brainstem is chiefly a rostral continuation of the spinal veins, and the cerebellum drains into the great cerebral vein of Galen and the straight venous sinus.

The Circle of Willis, the anastomostic channels between the major cerebral arteries on the surface of the cerebral hemispheres and in the cerebellum, and the potential anastomoses via the ophthalmic artery, and between the external and internal carotid arterial systems are of the greatest importance if the blood flow through the internal carotid or the vertebral arteries are compromised in any way. Thus, there is an increased incidence of cerebral infarction if these potential anastomoses are deficient as a result of some anomaly in the Circle of Willis, or of acquired arterial disease such as atheroma.

Spinal cord

The blood supply of the cord is derived from the spinal branches of the vertebral, deep cervical, intercostal and lumbar arteries which all arise from the aorta in a segmental manner (Fig. 5.4). Each spinal artery divides into an anterior and posterior *radicular artery* which run along the ventral and dorsal nerve roots, respectively. The initial arrangement provides each segment of the cord with its own blood supply, but the pattern has undergone considerable phylogenetic change and in Man most of the anterior radicular arteries are small and never reach the cord. Between four and nine anterior radicular arteries, of which one, the artery of *Adamkiewicz* (which usually lies between the vertebral bodies of T8 and L1 on the left) is considerably larger than the others, reaches the anterior sulcus of the cord and contributes to the longitudinal anastomosis of the *anterior spinal artery.* Variations in the anatomy of the anterior radicular arteries are of considerable surgical importance. The anterior spinal artery in the ventral median fissure gives rise to branches which supply the ventral gray and white matter of the cord. The posterior radicular arteries are much more variable in number and size and there are more of them than anterior radicular arteries. They contribute to the freely *anastomosing posterior spinal arteries*, the central

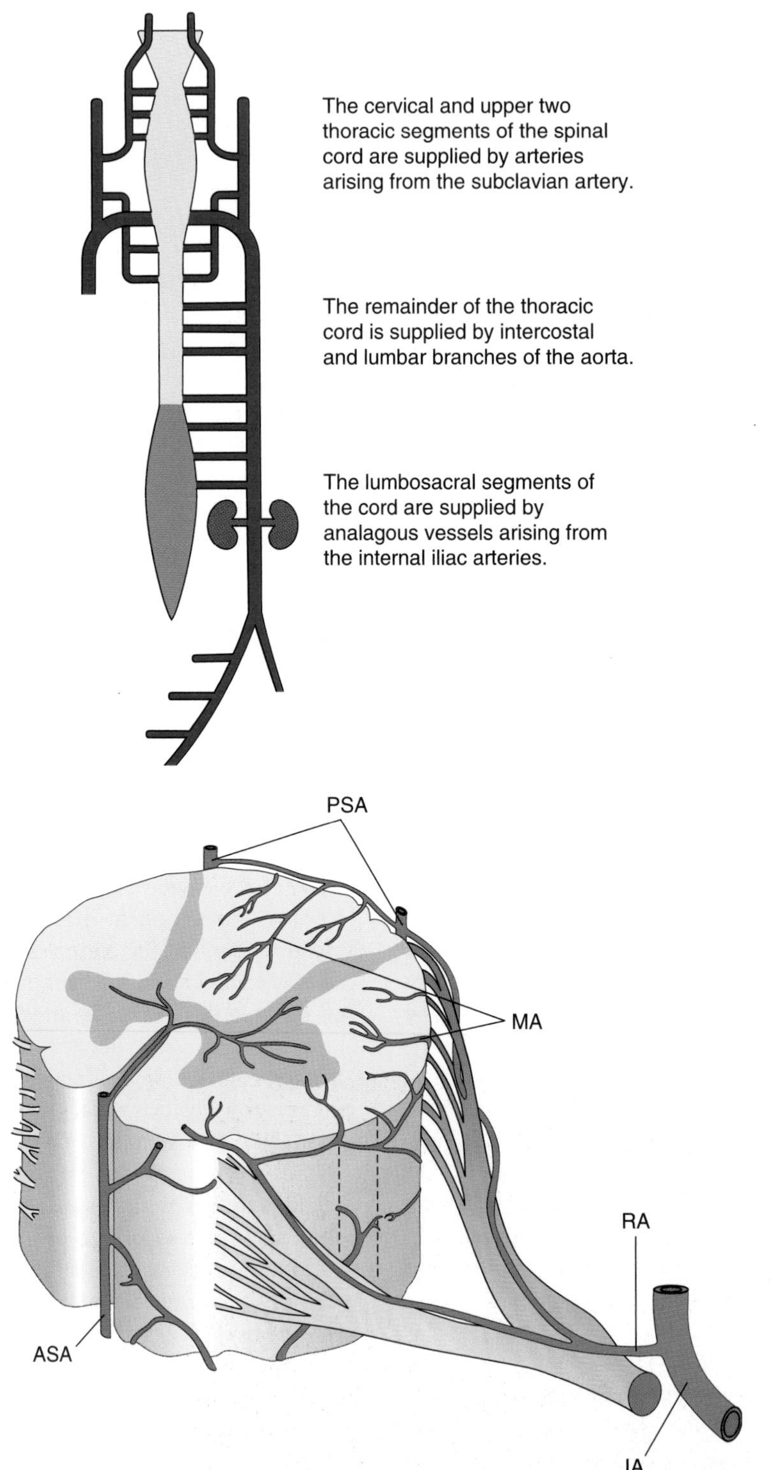

Figure 5.4 Arterial blood supply to the spinal cord. PSA = posterior spinal artery, MA = branches of meningeal arteries, RA = radicular artery, IA = intercostal artery, ASA = anterior spinal artery.

branches of which supply the dorsal columns of the cord. The territories overlap but anastomoses have not been reported within the cord.

The venous drainage of the cord is via six plexiform longitudinal blood vessels, one along each median sulcus and the others on either side of it.

MAINTENANCE OF CEREBRAL BLOOD FLOW AND OXYGEN SUPPLY

The brain is very susceptible to oxygen deprivation. The supply of oxygen depends on the *cerebral blood flow* (CBF) and the oxygen content of the blood. Cerebral blood flow, in turn, depends on the *cerebral perfusion pressure* (CPP), which is the difference between the *mean systemic arterial pressure* and the *intracranial pressure*. Since the most important factor in maintaining an adequate supply of oxygen to the brain is the CBF, there are protective mechanisms to preserve it.

Preservation of CBF, when systemic arterial pressure is low, is brought about by *autoregulation*, which can be defined as the maintenance of a relatively constant blood flow in the face of changes in CPP. As the systemic arterial pressure falls, the cerebrovascular resistance also falls because of autoregulatory dilation of cerebral arterioles, as a result of which CBF remains within normal limits over a wide range of systemic arterial pressures. When cerebral vasodilation is maximum, however, cerebrovascular resistance cannot fall further (the lower limit of *autoregulation*): the critical level of systemic arterial pressure at which autoregulation fails is about 50 mmHg (Fig. 5.5). Thus, when systemic arterial pressure falls below this level, CBF also falls. There is also an upper limit of autoregulation beyond which the autoregulatory vasoconstriction of the cerebral arterioles is inadequate (about 160 mmHg); CBF then increases and dysfunction of the blood–brain barrier develops (*hypertensive encephalopathy*).

Cerebral arterioles also respond to alterations in the blood gases when systemic arterial pressure is within normal limits: an increase of $Paco_2$ or a decrease in Pao_2 produces arteriolar vasodilation and hence a fall in cerebrovascular resistance and an increase in CBF. Thus, if arteriolar vasodilation resulting from hypoxia or, in particular, hypercapnia, exists prior to any reduction in systemic arterial pressure, maximal vasodilation will occur at a higher systemic arterial pressure than in the normocapnic–normoxic state. Hence, CBF will become linearly related to systemic arterial pressure at a relatively high systemic arterial pressure. Patients with pre-existing arteriolar vasodilation are particularly vulnerable to a fall in systemic arterial pressure because the potential autoregulatory preservation of CBF is impaired. Autoregulation

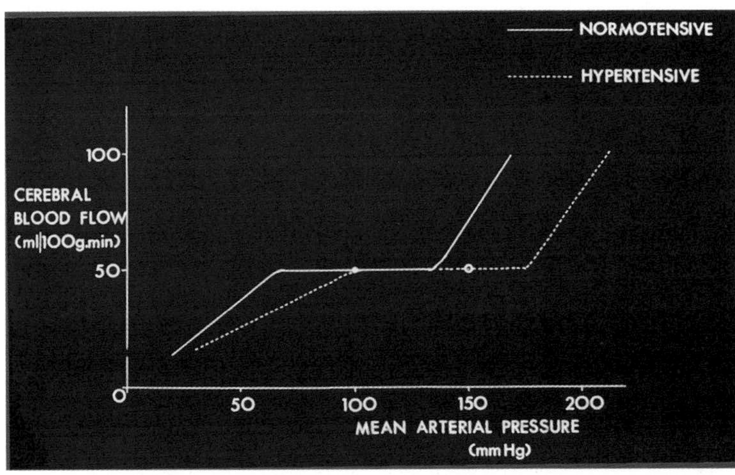

Figure 5.5 Autoregulation of cerebral blood flow. Diagrammatic representation of the relationship between cerebral blood flow (CBF) and mean arterial blood pressure in normotensive and hypertensive subjects. Note the 'shift to the right' of the autoregulatory curve in the hypertensive subjects; ————, normotensive subjects; ---------------- , hypertensive subjects.

may also be deficient if a patient is hypoxemic, for example in the post-anesthetic period, and appears to be lost or at least severely impaired, in a wide range of acute conditions producing brain damage, e.g. acute head injury, hemorrhagic and ischemic 'strokes' or a brief episode of hypoxia. Such patients are particularly susceptible to any episode of acute cardio-respiratory failure and especially after a fall in systemic arterial pressure. In patients with chronic hypertension there is a shift of the autoregulatory curve to the right, with the result that CBF commences to fall at a higher systemic arterial pressure than in normotensive individuals (Fig. 5.5).

Energy is produced in the brain almost entirely from the oxidative metabolism of glucose. The amount of glucose consumed is very high (60 mg/min), and reflects on the inability of the brain to make use of other substrates. Oxidative metabolism of glucose yields energy in the form of high energy phosphate compounds, the most important of which is adenosine triphosphate (ATP). In the normal brain, CBF to a particular part of the brain varies depending on the metabolic needs i.e. the supply of oxygen and glucose are 'coupled'.

In any medical emergency, for example after cardiorespiratory arrest, a severe episode of hypotension, status epilepticus, carbon monoxide or barbiturate intoxication or hypoglycemic coma, the vital factor with regard to the ultimate clinical outcome is whether or not satisfactory resuscitation can be achieved before irreversible brain damage has occurred.

CLINICAL SYNDROMES

Transient ischemic attacks

Transient ischemic attacks (TIAs) are defined as episodes of focal neurological symptoms due to an inadequate blood supply to the brain, these attacks are usually sudden at onset and resolve within 24 h or less without a residual neurological deficit. Their particular importance is that they are often a precursor of cerebral infarction. The great majority of TIAs are due to emboli arising from the heart, or from plaques of atheroma in the aortic arch or the extracranial blood vessels; others are due to a fall in perfusion pressure as a result of a heart disorder or stenosis of a blood vessel. Some 90% of TIAs occur within the arterial distribution of the carotid artery, symptomatology including hemiparesis, hemisensory disturbance, dysphasia or mononucular blindness leaving some 7% occurring in the territory of the vertebro-basilar arterial system presenting with loss of consciousness, bilateral limb motor-sensory dysfunction, binocular blindness, vertigo, tinnitus, diploplia or dysarthria. The natural history of TIAs is that between 5 and 10% will develop infarction in each year of follow-up irrespective of the territory involved, the risk being greatest some 3–6 months after the initial TIA.

'Stroke' due to cerebral infarction

Various clinical syndromes have been described and correlated with either the occlusion of a large blood vessel or one of its branches. The outcome of occlusion depends in part on the collateral blood supply primarily from the Circle of Willis but in addition the external carotid artery may distribute blood to the anterior or middle cerebral arteries through meningeal branches and retrogradely through the ophthalmic artery to the internal carotid artery. Therefore, in clinical practice it is possible to recognize clinical syndromes associated with occlusion of any one of the major arteries supplying the brain. Occlusion of the deep penetrating arteries produces subcortical infarction and is characterized clinically by preservation of cortical function: examples of the clinical syndromes include pure motor hemiplegia, pure sensory–motor, dysarthria–clumsy hand, ataxic hemiparesis and severe dysarthria with facial weakness. Lacunar or subcortical infarction accounts for some 17% of all thrombo-embolic 'strokes'.

A simple and practical classification of infarction has evolved that establishes the diagnosis and is used to predict outcome (Table 5.4).

Hemorrhagic 'stroke'

The clinical effects of intracerebral hemorrhage are due in part to the mass effect and the location of the hematoma. Most present with sudden onset

Table 5.4 Clinical classification of cerebral infarction

Circulation syndrome	Clinical features
Total anterior	Motor and sensory deficit, hemianopia and disturbance of higher cerebral function
Partial anterior	Any two of above or isolated disturbance of cerebral function
Posterior	Signs of brainstem dysfunction or isolated hemianopia
Lucunar	Pure motor stroke, or pure sensory stroke, or pure sensorimotor stroke, or ataxic hemiparesis

of headache followed either by rapid loss of consciousness or gradual deterioration in the conscious level over 24–48 h the associated signs and symptoms depending on whether the hematoma is supratentorial, cerebellar or pontine in location.

Patients with subarachnoid hemorrhage present with sudden onset of severe headache associated with a transient or prolonged loss of consciousness, or epilepsy. Nausea and vomiting commonly occur and symptoms include meningism, neck stiffness, seizures and focal signs in association with coma. As a result of the mass effect of an associated intracerebral hematoma, papilledema or subhyloid or vitreous hemorrhage may been seen by fundoscopy.

Selective vulnerability

Most diseases or disorders of the CNS affect only particular parts of the brain this pattern either being pathognomonic of a particular disease or disorder or providing clues to its pathogenesis. Although, the concept of selective vulnerability has been extended to include a whole range of diseases or disorders, in its most classical form the differing susceptibility of the brain to hypoxia has been known for many years: in general, neurons are the most sensitive, followed by oligodendroglia and astrocytes, whereas the microglia and the blood vessels are the least vulnerable. Although, two major hypotheses *viz.* the vascular theory and the concept of pathoclisis have been advanced to account for the characteristic distribution of hypoxic brain damage, it is now quite clear that there are many contributing factors some of which are anatomical, others vascular, and yet others of a neurochemical–metabolic nature. For example recent work has suggested that a strong correlation exists between the excitatory properties of glutamate and related excitatory amino acids and their ability to induce neuronal damage mediated through various glutamate receptor subtypes principal amongst which are three named after their selective agonists – *N*-methyl-D-aspartate (NMDA), quisqualate and kainate. The receptors for these amino acids play an important role in the selective neuronal loss that occurs after cardiac arrest although the pattern of damage does not correlate precisely with the density of NMDA receptors. More likely, the pattern of selective vulnerability is determined by the localization of calcium binding proteins and their vulnerability to the action of the excitotoxic amino acids.

STRUCTURAL CHANGES RESULTING FROM HYPOXIA AND CEREBROVASCULAR DISEASE

These may be limited to neurons (selective neuronal necrosis and programmed cell death) and may also involve glia and blood vessels (infarction).

Selective neuronal necrosis

Studies in experimental animals and selected human material have shown that there is an identifiable sequence of changes, *the ischemic cell process*, which is the neuropathological common denominator in all types of hypoxia and has been described in detail in Chapter 3. Identification of neuronal changes that are attributable unequivocally to hypoxia may be difficult in the human brain because

Table 5.5 Temporal course and microscopic features of selective neuronal necrosis

Time (h) after hypoxia	Histological changes
1	Microvacuolation (rarely seen in human material)
1–2	Ischemic cell process
1–6	Ischemic cell process, with incrustation formation
15–18	Homogenizing cell change

of histological artefact that results partly from autolysis, partly from slow penetration of fixative, and partly from the short comings in the processing of tissue, these leading to artefacts such as *dark cells, hydropic cells, perineuronal* and *perivascular spaces* and the features of the respirator brain (see Chapter 3). In any histological assessment of the brain, it is of the utmost importance that the pathologist recognizes the ischemic cell process and can distinguish it from these artefacts. The artefacts do not coincide with areas of selective vulnerability, they are most numerous on the surface of the brain, and are not related to the duration of survival after an episode of hypoxia. Thus, any evidence of the ischemic cell process or of a vital reaction in a respirator brain (see Chapter 3) must be interpreted as having preceded the onset of clinical brainstem death. The temporal course and nature of selective neuronal necrosis are given in Table 5.5.

Programmed cell death

For some years it has been suggested that calcium-mediated mechanisms were the final common pathway leading to cell death after injury to the CNS. Recent data have suggested that changes in the level of intracellular calcium leads to apoptosis or necrosis, and that apoptosis is the morphological manifestation of programmed cell death and has typically been associated with the formation of the normal CNS during development as well as its maintenance. Apoptotic neurons, oligodendrocytes and astrocytes have all been observed within injured brain and both *in vivo* and *in vitro* studies have shown that while excitatory amino acids increase intracellular calcium and free radicals, all of which may cause cells to undergo apoptosis, it is also apparent that neurons can undergo apoptosis via many other pathways and that a shift in the balance between pro- and anti-apoptotic factors towards the expression of proteins that promote death, may be one mechanism involved. Thus, there is a balance between survival promoting proteins such as Bcl-2 and Bcl-xL, and death inducing proteins such as Bax, c-Jun the tumor suppresser gene *p53*, and the caspase family of proteases, all of which influence the activation of caspase 8 and 9 and the executioner caspases 2, 3, 6 and 7.

Infarction

Cerebral infarction, i.e. necrosis of neurons, neuroglia and blood vessels, is due to a local arrest or reduction in cerebral blood flow. It can affect an entire arterial territory or, if there is some collateral circulation from adjacent arterial territories, the infarct may be restricted to the central part of the arterial territory (Fig. 5.6a and b).

There are basically three stages in the development of an infarct, depending on its age. Recent infarcts are soft to touch and distinctly swollen (Fig. 5.7): indeed a large infarct may swell to the extent of acting as an intracranial expanding lesion to produce distortion and herniation of the brain and an increase in intracranial pressure. It may be *anemic or hemorrhagic*, depending on whether some blood flow has been restored through the infarct and on whether necrosis of blood vessel walls has occurred, thus, allowing extravasation of blood into the necrotic tissue – *reperfusion injury*. An intensely hemorrhagic infarct may superficially resemble a hematoma but the distinctive feature of a hemorrhagic infarct is the preservation of intrinsic brain architecture within it. In a brain that has undergone recent infarction, the histological appearances are these of coagulative necrosis (Table 5.6). Within gray matter the outlines of dead neurons are recognizable, their cytoplasm is intensely eosinophilic and the nucleus stains poorly with hematoxylin.

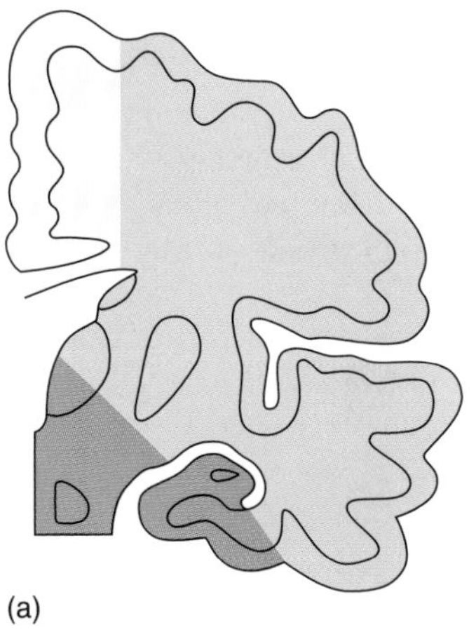

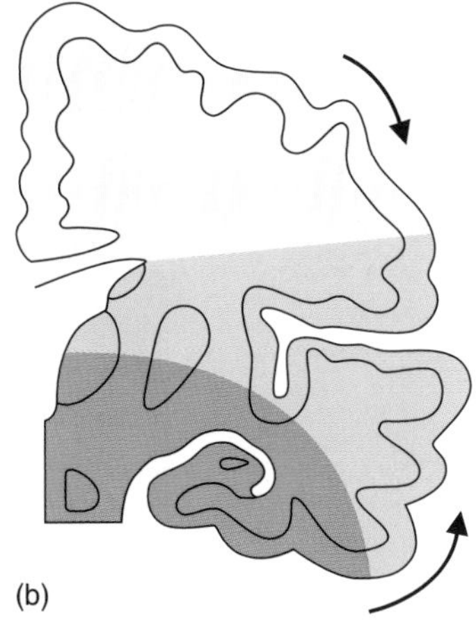

Figure 5.6 Diagrammatic representation of infarcts in the territory supplied by the middle cerebral artery. (a) Infarct involving the entire territory. (b) Infarct restricted to the central territory. Arrows in (b) indicate collateral inflow from the anterior and posterior cerebral arteries.

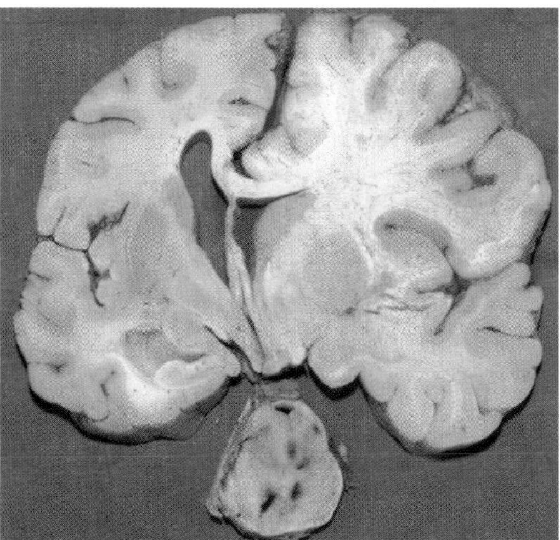

Figure 5.7 Cerebral infarction. There is a large swollen infarct in the territories supplied by the right anterior and middle cerebral arteries. Note the shift of the midline structures to the left and the supracallosal hernia. There was a tentorial hernia and there is secondary hemorrhage into the brainstem.

This picture, which is recognizable within the first 4 to 6 h, is followed by patchy decreasing stainability (Fig. 5.8a). Incrustations are not seen in the central region of a large infarct but occur frequently at its edges. Within 12–20 h the infarct has a sharply demarcated edge (Fig. 5.8b) due to a spongy appearance in the neurophil caused by a combination of the swelling of astrocytic processes and of axons, and loss of staining of myelin. Neutrophil polymorphs may be conspicuous in relation to necrotic walls of blood vessels. Within about 24 h early reactive changes, as shown by proliferation of microglia, astrocytes and capillaries, occur in the normal tissue adjacent to the infarct: reactive microglia also appear early around any surviving blood vessels

Table 5.6 Histological changes and time course of cerebral infarction

Time after infarction	Histological changes
4–6 h	Coagulative necrosis (ischemic cell change)
15–20 h	Defined margin between ischemic and normal brain, spongy neuropil due to swelling of astrocytes, neuronal necrosis, and pallor of myelin staining
24–30 h	Early appearance of polymorphs in meninges and blood vessels at margin of lesion; endothelial enlargement; extravasation of red blood cells
24–36 h	Activation of microglia and astrocytes
36–48 h	Appearance of macrophages and early separation of infarct from normal brain
1–2 weeks	Liquefaction of tissue; gliosis
Months	Cavitation and completion of glial scar; decrease in size and number of astrocytes; atrophy of damaged tissue

Figure 5.8 Recent infarction. (a) In the cerebral cortex, where there is irregular pallor of staining. (b) In the white matter, where there is a sharply defined border between the abnormal (pale) and normal white matter.

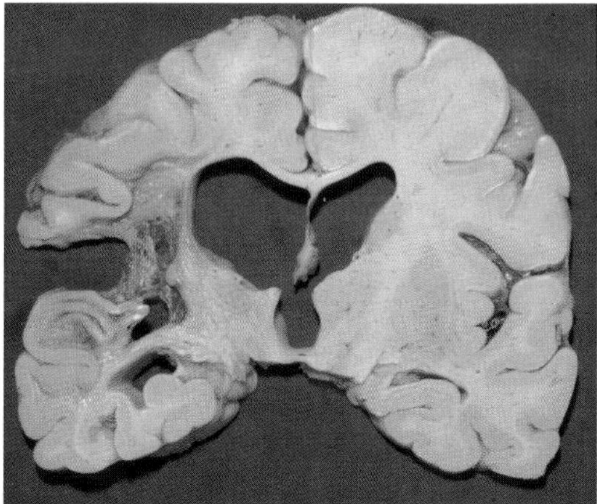

Figure 5.9 Old infarction. The original infarct is represented by shrunken cystic tissue in the central distribution of the left middle cerebral artery. Note the ipsilateral compensatory (*ex vacuo*) hydrocephalus.

within the infarct. Within 1–2 weeks the infarct becomes soft to touch and the swelling resolves: the affected gray matter may already be slightly shrunken and granular. At this stage, in addition to the reactive changes mentioned above, there are sheets of macrophages throughout the infarct (see Fig. 3.33). If the patient survives for several months or more, the dead tissue is removed and the infarct ultimately comes to be represented by a shrunken cystic lesion (Fig. 5.9). The cysts are often traversed by small blood vessels and glial fibers and some macrophages usually persist. If the infarct is in a cerebral hemisphere, shrinkage of the infarct is usually accompanied by enlargement of the adjacent lateral ventricle (hydrocephalus *ex vacuo*). Wallerian-type degeneration will occur in any nerve fibers that have been destroyed. Thus, if the infarct involves the internal capsule, there is progressive degeneration and shrinkage of the corresponding pyramidal tract in the brainstem and in the spinal cord.

Hemorrhage

The appearance of a hematoma is similar regardless of causation. From the edges of recently formed bleeds red blood cells can be seen to spread a short distance into adjacent brain tissue. There is a thin rim of surrounding coagulative necrosis within some 24 h of the onset of the bleed associated with which there is an increasing amount of swelling due to disruption of the blood–brain barrier. Like infarcts there is an inflammatory cell response characterized initially by the appearance of polymophonuclear leukocytes which become prominent between 24 and 48 h. Thereafter, there is a mononuclear cell infiltrate particularly of macrophages which because of phagocytosis within 3–4 days become siderophages from the ingestion of blood-derived pigment. The formation of hemosiderin may be detected by the Perl's stain between 1 and 2 days after the appearance of macrophages. Hemosiderin may be present at the site of the hematoma within both astrocytes and macrophages providing the light brown–yellow coloration that is often present within the walls of a residual cavity. As the hematoma undergoes liquefaction so its wall becomes defined by a glial scar which begins within about 7 days of the bleed.

CAUSES OF CEREBROVASCULAR DISEASE

About three quarters of cases are due to either occlusion (50%), to atheromatous/thrombotic or non-atheromatous disease of the blood vessel wall, embolism (25%) or hemorrhage (20%) (Table 5.7).

Cerebral infarction

Atheroma (atherosclerosis)

This is the most common and important arterial disease in adults in developed countries. Although it may occur to some extent in young adults, it is much more severe and extensive in the middle-aged and elderly. As the plaques gradually enlarge they become confluent and encroach upon the lumen of the blood vessel and may be complicated by calcification and ulceration. The process may progress to complete occlusion of the blood vessel, due either to intramural bleeding into the base of the plaque, or, more often, the formation of thrombus.

The blood vessels most commonly affected are the internal carotid and vertebral arteries, followed by the basilar and middle cerebral arteries and then by the posterior inferior cerebellar arteries. Atheroma of the cerebral arteries is usually associated with atheroma in other parts of the body, including the arteries of the limbs. Correlation between the occurrence of coronary atheroma and that of cerebral atheroma is usually close, although coronary atheroma tends to be more severe. Occasionally, however, the person with marked atheroma in the aorta and coronary arteries may have little or no disease in the cerebral arteries; the reverse may also occur.

Extensive atheroma does not necessarily lead to cerebral infarction because at normal blood pressure the internal cross-sectional area of an artery must be reduced by up to 90% before blood flow is impaired. If, however, there is an episode of hypotension (see below) the flow may be reduced sufficiently to cause ischemic damage.

Table 5.7 Principal causes of cerebrovascular disease

Infarction (50%)
- Atheroma – stenosis/occlusion
- Non-atheromatous disease
- Collagen disease: rheumatoid arthritis, SLE vasculitis; polyarteritis or temporal arteritis; granulomatous vasculitis; Wegener's
- Miscellaneous; sarcoidosis, trauma, infection

Embolism (25%)
- Atheromatous plaque in the intracranial and extracranial arteries, or arch of aorta
- The heart
- Miscellaneous: air, fat and tumor emboli

Diseases of the blood
Venous thrombosis
Reduced cerebral perfusion
Hemorrhage (20%)
- Hypertension
- Saccular aneurysm
- AV malformation
- Neoplasm
- Amyloid vasculopathy
- Coagulation disorder
- Anticoagulant therapy
- Drug abuse
- Trauma

The extracranial cervical arteries

Atheroma of the *internal carotid arteries* in the neck and of the *cervical vertebral arteries* is of considerable importance in the pathogenesis of cerebral infarction. Atheroma is particularly common at the lower end of the internal carotid artery, which may become severely stenosed and, ultimately, lead to thrombotic occlusion. Many individuals with thrombosis of one or even both internal carotid arteries do not necessarily develop a cerebral infarct because of the collateral circulation. Other causes of carotid artery occlusion include embolism, dissecting aneurysm, trauma, blood dyscrasias, aortic arch syndrome and inflammation of the base of the skull. When an internal carotid artery is occluded, reverse flow through the ophthalmic artery connecting the external carotid artery with the upper end of the internal carotid artery is an important source of a collateral circulation.

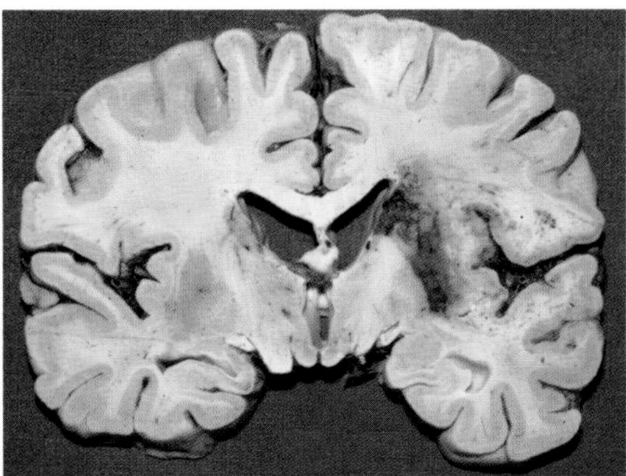

Figure 5.10 'Capsular' infarct that affects the body of the caudate nucleus and the internal capsule. There is hemorrhagic transformation as a result of reperfusion.

Occlusion of an internal carotid artery may be without symptoms or signs, may reveal itself by episodic attacks of transient motor or sensory impairment, or present as a gradual or sudden onset of permanent hemiplegia. If infarction occurs, it may take several forms: massive infarction within the entire territory supplied by the middle cerebral artery (Fig. 5.7, page 93) and sometimes involving the anterior cerebral arterial territory as well; infarction of the cortex around the Sylvian fissure with or without involvement of the basal ganglia and the internal capsule; infarction restricted to the internal capsule – so-called 'capsule infarct' (Fig. 5.10); small infarcts in deep gray and white matter (Fig. 5.11); and infarction within the boundary zone between the territories supplied by the anterior and middle cerebral arteries (Fig. 5.24, page 107).

Stenosis or occlusion of the vertebral arteries affects the vertebro-basilar territory and, if the collateral circulation is inadequate, there is infarction in the brainstem (Fig. 5.12), in the cerebellum (Fig. 5.13) or in the territory of the posterior cerebral artery (Fig. 5.14a and b). Indeed, in patients with a clinical syndrome of infarction in the territory of one posterior inferior cerebellar artery, occlusive arterial disease is often in the vertebral artery and not in the posterior inferior cerebellar artery itself.

Thus, the hemodynamic disturbance leading to cerebral infarction is complex and it is often difficult

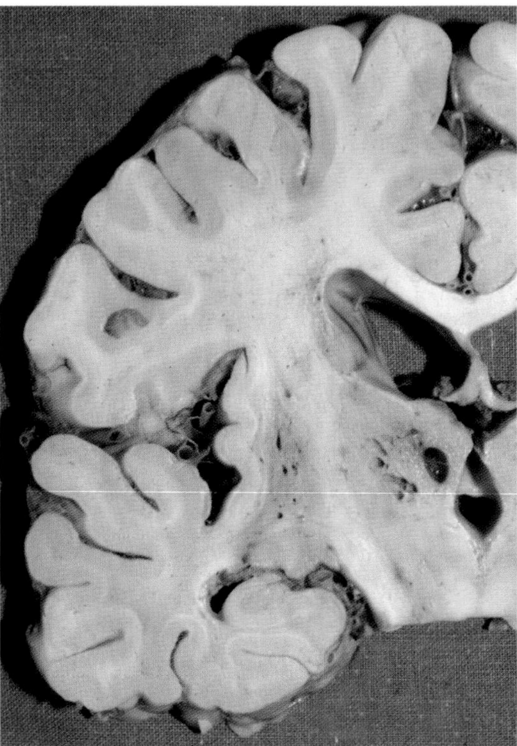

Figure 5.11 Lacunes. There are several small cysts in the basal ganglia.

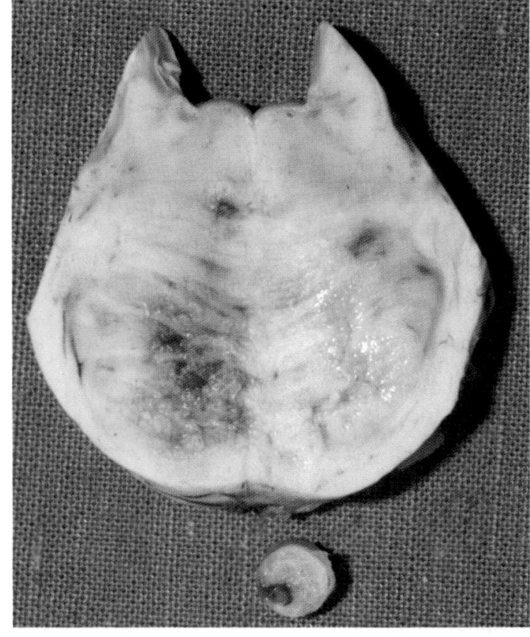

Figure 5.12 Infarction of brainstem due to thrombotic occlusion of the basilar artery.

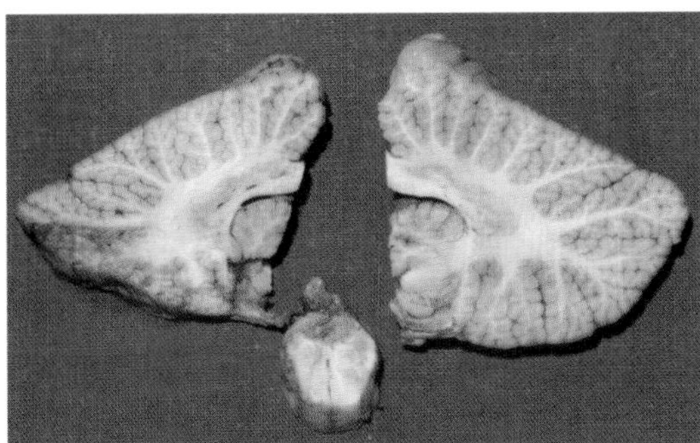

Figure 5.13 Old infarct in distribution of one posterior inferior cerebellar artery. There was also a small infarct in the ipsilateral dorsolateral sector of the medulla.

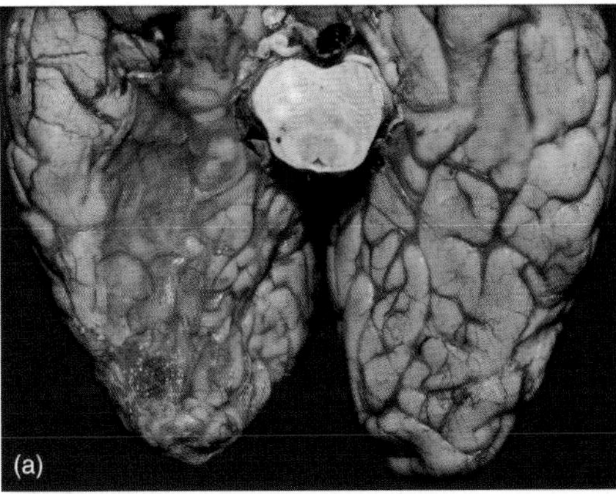

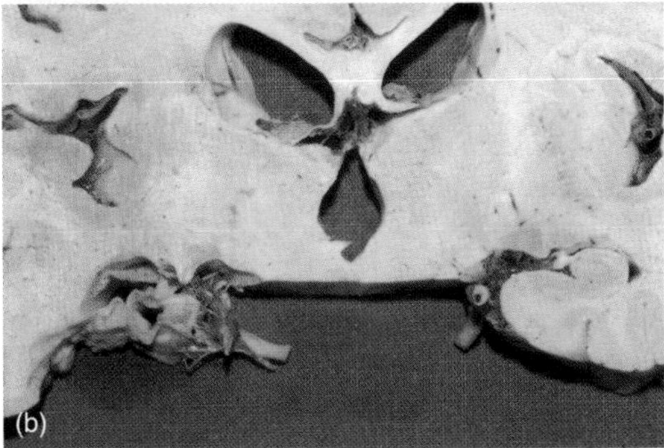

Figure 5.14 Old infarct in distribution of right posterior cerebral artery. Found incidentally at autopsy. (a) There is involvement of the medial and inferior aspects of the right temporal and occipital lobes. (b) Coronal section to demonstrate infarction of structures in the medial part of the temporal lobe. Compare with other side.

to ascribe an infarct to a particular arterial lesion and, especially in the presence of arterial stenosis, cerebral infarction is often the result of a combination of systemic circulatory insufficiency and atheroma of extracranial or intracranial cerebral arteries, or of both.

Obstruction of the subclavian and *brachiocephalic (innominate) arteries* is rarely a cause of cerebral infarction although of some clinical importance as a causative factor in the *subclavian steal syndrome.* In this condition, clinical evidence of cerebral ischemia may be precipitated by exercise of the upper limbs, thus 'stealing' blood from the basilar artery and the Circle of Willis to the subclavian artery distal to the occlusion.

The intracranial arteries

The anatomical distribution of arteries in the brain is remarkably constant and the neurological deficit that results from occlusion of individual blood vessels may be so well defined that clinicians can often say with confidence which artery, or branch of an artery of the carotid and/or vertebral basilar system is involved.

Common causes of occlusion of these blood vessels are embolism (mainly from the heart or internal carotid arteries), thrombosis (formed locally on atheroma or propagated from extracranial cervical arteries), vasospasm in patients with rupture of a saccular aneurysm, arteritis (micro-organisms, collagen diseases, etc.), and mechanical deformation in patients with mass lesions that are producing midline shift and internal herniation. The middle cerebral artery is more often occluded than any other cerebral artery, and it is often secondary to embolism or the cephalad extension of thrombus from the internal carotid artery. Infarction within the distribution of the posterior cerebral arteries is a common incidental finding post mortem in the elderly.

Autopsy studies have established that occlusion of one vertebral artery may be asymptomatic. Whereas thrombus forming on atheroma is the most common cause of a neck extracranial artery occlusion, these blood vessels may also be distorted by osteoarthritis of the cervical spine which, together with atheroma, may be sufficient to cause obstruction as a result of certain temporary movements of the neck, namely hyperextension, intubation for general anesthesia, osteopathic manipulation, etc. Other causes of occlusion include a subluxation of the atlanto-occipital joint in rheumatoid arthritis, and as a birth injury after assisted cephalic breach presentation. Occlusion of the basilar artery is usually due to atheroma. Most of the clinical syndromes associated with cervical vertebro-basilar disease present with ischemia either of the hind brain or the medial portions of the occipital lobe. In some patients there is extensive infarction of the brainstem and the patient dies, whereas others develop the 'locked-in' syndrome in which a conscious mute patient is completely paralyzed apart from eye movements.

The spinal arteries

Occlusion of the *anterior spinal artery* causes infarction of the ventral two thirds of the cord and is more common than occlusion of the *posterior spinal artery*. Occlusion is usually due to thrombosis secondary to trauma, subluxation of the spine, cervical spondylosis, or embolism. Occlusion of the spinal arteries is a common complication of a dissecting aneurysm of the aorta, the pattern of damage being determined by the location of the dissection. The lower thoracic regions of the cord are the most vulnerable due to interference of blood flow through intercostal arteries. Sometimes the entire cord is involved, but on other occasions the damage is limited to the central gray matter. Infarction in either or both of these vascular territories may occur without arterial occlusion, and it is precipitated by changes in spinal blood flow, as may occur after prolonged hypotension, disease of the aorta and of the intercostal or lumbar arteries, embolism after surgery, and in association with coarctation of the aorta.

Embolism

About 25% of ischemic 'strokes' are due to emboli that rise either from atheromatous plaques in the intracranial or extracranial arteries or from the aortic arch, or the heart. There is a very strong association between heart disease and ischemic 'stroke' and about 75% of patients who have had a 'stroke' have features of heart failure, atrial fibrillation or an enlarged heart and in patients with ischemic heart disease there is some two- to five-fold increased incidence of 'stroke'. The embolus may arise from valvular heart disease, arrhythmias, bacterial and non-bacterial endocarditis, atrial myxoma, prosthetic valves, a patent foramen ovale, or cardiomyopathy, and when it occurs as a complication of ischemic heart disease presentation occurs some three weeks after the acute onset of myocardial infarction. Rarely, a thrombotic embolus reaching the heart from the systemic veins may pass through a patent foramen ovale to enter the systemic arterial circulation (*paradoxical embolism*). Brain damage due to embolism may also complicate cardiac surgery and, more recently, open heart surgery with cardiopulmonary by-pass have created new sources of cerebral embolism that include air, fat, particles of silicone and platelet/fibrin emboli from the pump oxygenator.

Fat embolism may develop as a complication of trauma particularly when there are fractures of long bones. Most of the fat will be trapped in the lungs and occasionally emboli will enter the systemic circulation. Death may occur within 3–4 days and the white matter of the brain may be diffusely studded with petechial hemorrhages. Fat globules may be identified in the small arterioles and the walls of small blood vessels are often necrotic. Air embolism may develop during abortion, neurosurgical procedures in the sitting position, catheterization procedures and during sub-atmospheric decompression. Under these circumstances infarction is often found within the arterial boundary zones consequent upon a reduced cardiac output and a reduced blood flow to the brain.

Nitrogen embolism may occur if there is a sudden reduction of atmospheric pressure from an elevated level to normal, as encountered by underwater divers and workers in caissons. Under these circumstances dissolved gases in the blood come out of solution and nitrogen forms small bubbles that cause the 'bends' and 'chokes'. The principal neuropathological findings are multiple foci of ischemic damage particularly in the gray matter of the cerebral hemispheres or in the spinal cord. Lesions have been attributed to a mixture of gases and fat embolism combined with hypotension. With survival, both ascending and descending Wallerian degeneration may be seen.

Emboli arising from tumors of the bronchus, breast, etc., form as metastatic lesions often with a slow and progressive clinical course until such time as they become space-occupying. However presentation may be acute and may mimic a 'stroke-like' illness.

Hypertension

The cerebral circulation in hypertension

The absolute value for cerebral blood flow of 50 mL per 100 g/min is the same in hypertensive and normotensive subjects. In chronic hypertension there is an alteration in the autoregulation curve as a result of which chronically hypertensive patients adapt to remarkably high blood pressures without developing hypertensive encephalopathy implying that the alterations in their blood vessels increase tolerance to high blood pressure. However, hypertensive patients are vulnerable to cerebral ischemia during periods of hypotension. Thus, anti-hypertensive agents may themselves reduce the blood pressure to a level which, though normal, may lead to a fall in the cerebral blood flow (Fig. 5.5). Hypertension is a major risk factor for cerebrovascular disease (Table 5.8).

The acute, usually transient, cerebral syndrome of *hypertensive encephalopathy* may complicate acute glomerulonephritis, toxemia of pregnancy and malignant phase hypertension. The exact pathogenesis remains unclear but it has been attributed to spasm of the cerebral blood vessels and to excessive vasodilation, damage to the blood–brain barrier and cerebral hyperemia. There is also an association between a slowly developing dementia (leukoariosis) and hypertension.

Next to increasing age, hypertension is a major risk factor that predisposes to cerebral infarction and hemorrhage. The risk is equal in males and females and is proportional to the height of the blood pressure (Table 5.8). The risk is mediated through the deposition of large amounts of atheroma in the large cerebral blood vessels and the development of atheromatous plaques in chronic severe hypertension on the penetrating arteries of the internal capsule, basal ganglia and pons. Hypertension also produces changes in the walls of arteries and arterioles, the latter undergoing hyaline arteriosclerosis. Lacunes or small cavities in the basal ganglia (Fig. 5.11, page 96) and in the pons of elderly subjects are associated commonly with high blood pressure: some appear as expanded perivascular spaces, others as small infarcts or resolving hemorrhages. When numerous in gray and white matter the term *état lacunaire* and *état criblé*, respectively, are used. There is also an association between hypertension and multi-infarct dementia (see Chapter 17).

Table 5.8 Hypertension and the brain

- Altered response of cerebral blood vessels to chronic hypertension with a shift of the autoregulatory curve to the right
- Increased amount of atheroma
- Hyaline arteriosclerosis
- Infarction
- Lacunes
- Intracerebral hemorrhage
- Multi-infarct dementia
- Leukoariosis
- Hypertensive encephalopathy

VASCULITIS AND COLLAGEN VASCULAR DISEASES

There are many types of vasculitis that may cause either infarction or hemorrhage (Table 5.9) principal amongst which are the vasculitides and the collagen vascular diseases.

It is likely that these disorders have a common immune basis for their causation insofar as they are all thought to represent an immune complex vasculitis. As a result of a disturbed immune system, antibody–antigen complexes are formed which become lodged within the luminal surface of the blood vessel and activate the complement cascade which in turn causes necrosis and hemorrhage within the blood vessel wall. Although, immune in nature the mechanism of giant cell arteritis/temporal arteritis and granulomatous vasculitis is

Table 5.9 Vasculitis and collagen vascular diseases

Vasculitis
- Associated with connective tissue disease
- Micropolyangiitis
- Allergic angiitis
- Takayasu's arteritis
- Giant cell arteritis/temporal arteritis
- Isolated angiitis of the CNS
- Churg–Strauss angiitis

Collagen vascular diseases
- Systemic lupus erythematosus
- Rheumatoid arthritis
- Granulomatous vasculitis e.g. Wegener's granulomatosis
- Arteritis due to micro-organisms

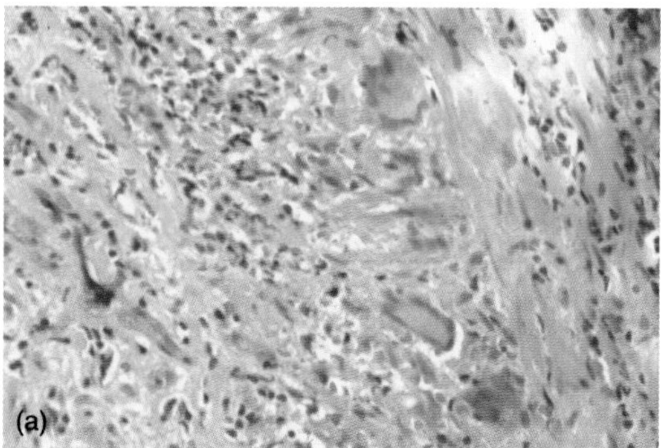

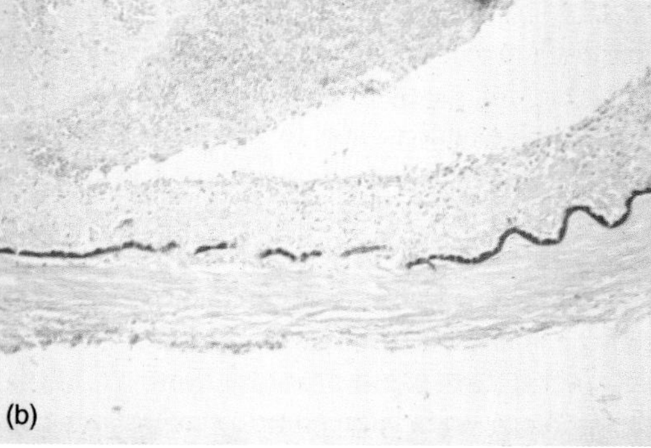

Figure 5.15 Giant cell arteritis. (a) Multinucleated giant cell close to junction between intima and media. There is infiltration of the intima and media by monocytes and some lymphocytes. (b) Irregularly damaged internal elastic lamina in relation to multinucleated cells. (a) H&E, (b) Van Gieson/elastica.

somewhat different in that cellular immune mechanisms predominate.

There is neurological involvement in some 80% of patients with micropolyangiitis (polyarteritis nodosa) as a result of involvement of both small and medium sized arteries. In addition, peripheral nerve involvement is common (mononeuritis multiplex) and Cogan syndrome may be a feature. Diagnosis may be established by renal or peripheral nerve biopsy and imaging may show multiple irregularities and microaneurysm formation. Diagnosis is facilitated by an elevated erythrocyte sedimentation rate (ESR) and C-reactive protein, antinuclear cytoplasmic antibodies, circulating immune complexes and IgM rheumatoid factor in addition to anemia, leukocytosis, and eosinophilia.

Intercurrent illnesses such as infection or neoplasia may trigger an immune complex deposition on the basement membranes of various capillaries and venules. In addition to the systemic symptoms, a rash, fever, arthralgia and multiple organ involvement, some 30% of the patients may also have neurological features that include neuropathy and 'stroke-like' features. Skin biopsy may show a perivenular inflammation in keeping with allergic angiitis (hypersensitivity vasculitis).

Another vasculitis is that of Takayasu's (pulseless) disease in which there is a giant cell arteritis involving the aorta and its major branches. This predominantly affects Asian females in the third and fourth decades. Patients present either with non-specific signs and symptoms or features of myocardial ischemia, peripheral vascular disease or neurological vascular 'stroke-like' symptoms.

Presenting with headache in the elderly, giant cell (temporal) arteritis is an auto-immune disease that may affect any extra- or intracranial blood vessel including the superficial temporal artery. There is a pangranulomatous reaction as shown by the presence of lymphocytes, plasma cells, and occasional neutrophil polymorphs in the walls of arteries of all sizes. Giant cells of either Langhans' or foreign body type are almost always invariably present (Fig. 5.15a and b), either in the media close to the damaged internal elastic lamina or in the adjacent intima. Involvement of the ophthalmic artery, including the ciliary arteries and the central artery of the retina, is particularly important. Because of its accessibility, the temporal artery is the most popular choice for biopsy. Diagnosis is achieved by a high ESR, an elevated C-reactive protein and hepatic alkaline phosphatase together with a positive tissue diagnosis on biopsy. Also within this category are *isolated angiitis of the CNS* in which patients present with headache, seizures, encephalopathy and 'stroke' in the absence of systemic symptoms. A distinctive syndrome of eosinophilia, pulmonary infiltrates, neuropathy and encephalopathy or 'stroke' is that of *Churg Strauss angiitis* and a rare disorder termed *granulomatous vasculitis* (Wegener's granulomatosis), the latter occurring in males aged 20–50 years for which upper or lower respiratory tract granulomata are associated with glomerulonephritis. Neurological involvement includes direct granulomatous invasion of the skull base and 'stroke-like' symptoms.

Clinical evidence of CNS involvement in *systemic lupus erythematosus* is said to occur in some 75% of patients and may predate systemic manifestations. The signs and symptoms may include psychiatric change including dementia, seizures, hemiplegia, cranial or peripheral nerve involvement and 'stroke-like' symptomatology. The pathology is that of small blood vessel disease but rarely including an active vasculitis. Alternative mechanisms for the symptomatology include embolism and coagulopathy (anti-phospholipid antibodies). Diagnosis is achieved by identifying circulating antibodies to nuclear protein, e.g. anti-DNA (ANA), elevated immunoglobulins and prolonged prothrombin time and anti-phospholipid antibodies (60%).

In the pre-antibiotic era acute carotid arteritis sometimes developed in children and young adults with tonsillitis and retropharyngeal inflammation. In some cases of acute purulent meningitis, particularly due to *pneumococci* or *menigococci* there is often histological evidence of acute arteritis of the pial blood vessels, where they are surrounded by inflammatory exudate. In subacute or chronic meningitis, as in *tuberculous meningitis* and in *meningovascular syphilis*, blood vessels become thickened and narrowed due to endarteritis obliterans (Fig. 5.16). Arteritis may also be caused by various fungal and parasitic diseases, such as *aspergillosis*, *mucomycosis*, and *cryptococcosis*.

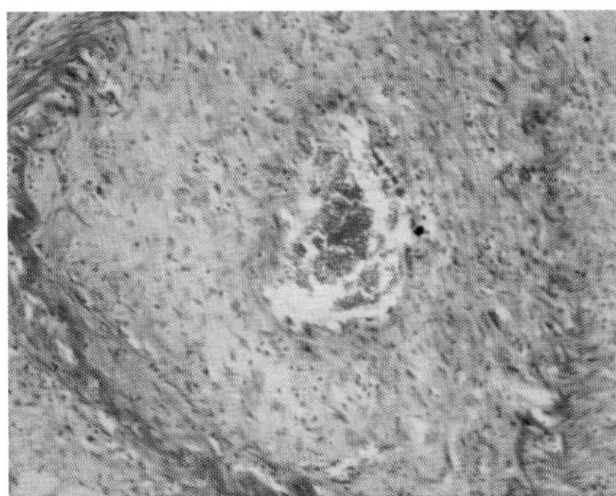

Figure 5.16 Endarteritis obliterans in tuberculous meningitis. The adventitia is thickened and infiltrated by chronic inflammatory cells. The media is normal and there is marked concentric thickening of the intima. H&E.

DISEASES OF THE BLOOD

Patients who present with 'stroke-like' symptoms may be manifesting hematological abnormalities principal amongst which are shown in Table 5.10.

Disseminated intravascular coagulation is a complication of sepsis, malignancy, pregnancy and various immune reactions which result in a consumptive coagulopathy leading to a bleeding tendency with hemorrhage into skin and other organs including the nervous system. Diagnosis is confirmed by a low platelet count along with an increased prothrombin time and elevated fibrin degradation products and reduced fibrinogen levels.

Involvement of the CNS occurs in *sickle cell* disease, this disorder being common in Black populations and sporadically throughout the Mediterranean and Middle East litorals. It is a genetically determined disorder in which abnormal hemoglobin is present in the red blood cells as a result of which sickling occurs if the arterial oxygen saturation is reduced. There may be neurological involvement in both *polycythemia rubra vera* (primary) and *secondary polycythemia* as a result of increased viscosity which reduces CBF and increases the tendency towards thrombosis. The diagnosis is established by elevated hemoglobin and packed

Table 5.10 Diseases of the blood

- Disseminated intravascular coagulation
- Hemoglobinopathies
- Polycythemia
- Thrombocytopenia
- Hypergammaglobinemia
- Antiphospholipid antibodies
- Antithrombin III, protein C and protein S deficiency
- Thrombotic thrombocytopenic purpura

cell volumes. The secondary type occurs in association with respiratory, renal and congenital heart disease.

Abnormality of platelets such as *idiopathic thrombocytopenia* or drug induced, or due to myeloproliferative disorders may be associated with intracranial hemorrhage and *thrombocytosis* in which there is an elevation of the platelet count above 600 000/mm^2 again is part of a myeloproliferative disorder that may also present with 'stroke-like' illnesses particularly thrombotic episodes.

Various immune states including *hypergammaglobulinemia* in which there is an increase in serum gamma globulin arising either as a primary event or secondary to leukemia or myeloma also occurs with neurological involvement in some 20% of cases probably as a result of increased blood viscosity. 'Stroke-like' illness has been associated with *hyperfibrinogenemia* which also increases coagulation and blood viscosity and may occur as a result of infections in association with pregnancy and malignancy.

Relatively recently 'stroke-like' illnesses occurring in association with *antiphospholipid antibodies* and *antithrombin III protein C*, and *protein S deficiency* have been described manifesting as an increased risk of thrombotic 'stroke' including cerebral venous sinus thrombosis. Patients who present with fever, purpura and multi-organ involvement together with neurological features of diffuse encephalopathy or intracranial hemorrhage may have *thrombotic thrombocytopenic purpura*. The main laboratory findings are those of hemolytic anemia, hematuria and thrombocytopenia.

THROMBOSIS OF THE VEINS AND VENOUS SINUSES

Infarction due to venous thrombosis accounts for about 1% of all 'strokes', modern imaging techniques enabling increased recognition. There are two principal types, namely *primary* (non-infectious) and *secondary* (due to pyogenic infection) (Table 5.11).

Some 85% of cases are due to thrombosis of the superior sagittal (Fig. 5.17) and lateral sinuses, some 10% of cases are due to thrombosis of the deep cerebral veins and about 5% of cases are due to thrombosis of the cavernous sinus.

Primary thrombosis of the cortical veins and superior sagittal and cavernous sinuses may complicate pregnancy in the puerperium, in various hematological disorders, with the use of oral contraceptives and with extreme dehydration in children (marasmus). The cerebral cortical vein more than the sagittal sinus occlusion is associated with venous infarction. Secondary thrombosis is most often found as a complication of pyogenic infection. For example, the superior sagittal sinus may become thrombosed if infection spreads from the frontal sinuses or a compound fracture of the skull. Likewise, the lateral and cavernous sinuses may become occluded if infections spread from either the middle ear or the central part of the face, respectively. If the thrombus fragments and is carried into the blood stream, pyemia and systemic abscesses may develop.

MISCELLANEOUS CAUSES OF CEREBRAL INFARCTION

These are various and diverse. For example the brain and spinal cord may be damaged by *X-irradiation*. The immediate response may be an acute inflammatory vasculitis, but more characteristically there is a delayed response in which small blood vessels undergo marked proliferative changes, with hyaline degeneration in their walls and necrosis of surrounding brain tissue.

Table 5.11 Venous thrombosis

Primary (non-infectious)
- Head injury
- Dehydration (marasmus)
- Pregnancy, puerperium
- Contraceptive pill
- Coagulation disorders
- Malignant meningitis

Secondary due to pyogenic infection from
- Face and jaw
- Paranasal sinuses

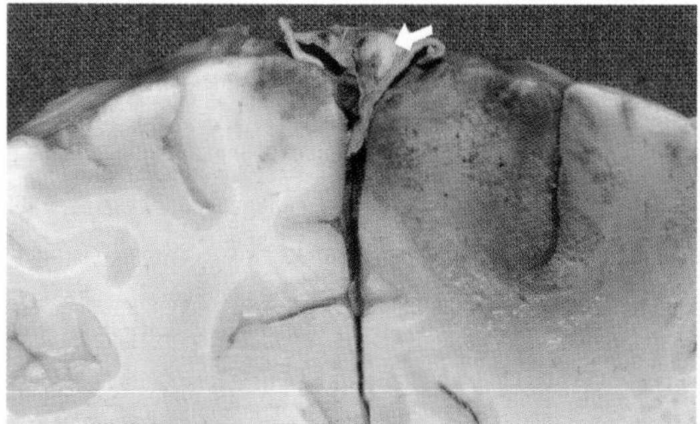

Figure 5.17 Thrombotic occlusion of the superior sagittal sinus (arrow). There is hemorrhagic infarction of the supramedial sectors of the cerebral hemispheres.

Occlusive vascular disease has also been recorded in cases of addiction to *heroin and LSD*, as a complication of *inflammatory bowel disease*, in association with *migraine* and in patients with *inherited disorders of connective tissue.*

Radiological evidence of *vasospasm* of the cerebral arteries is seen commonly in association with subarachnoid hemorrhage due to rupture of a saccular aneurysm (see below) and after severe head injury. In both situations it is an important factor in the genesis of ischemic brain damage. Also in these circumstances vascular complications are common in patients who develop brain shift and internal herniation due to raised intracranial pressure (see Chapter 4). Also a reduced *cerebral perfusion* as a result of cardiac arrest or an episode of hypotension (see below) may cause cerebral infarction.

Dissection of the carotid artery in the neck is the most frequently reported site and occurs most commonly in middle-aged adults: it is either spontaneous or associated with trauma. Spontaneous cervical carotid dissection usually occurs in otherwise healthy subjects, but is associated with *fibromuscular dysplasia* or *Marfan syndrome* in 20% of cases. *Traumatic dissection* may follow direct puncture of the carotid artery for arteriography, or may develop after a neck injury caused by over the shoulder-restraining harness in a road traffic accident: sometimes the trauma is trivial. Traumatic dissection has been associated with most sporting activities, coughing, chiropractic manipulation and vigorous neck turning. Dissection of the intracranial carotid system is rarely due to trauma, and more commonly occurs in association with cystic medial necrosis, fibromuscular dysplasia, atheroma or homocysteinuria.

Fibromuscular dysplasia involves intracranial as well as extracranial blood vessels and appears like a 'string of beads', the patient presenting with infarction as a result of thrombotic occlusion or from an associated saccular aneurysm. Another unusual form of cerebrovascular disease is that due to *cervical rib* which can result in aneurysm formation in the subclavian artery with endothelial damage, thrombus formation and embolization down the arm or retrograde spread of thrombus and embolization to the vertebral and common carotid arteries.

In *Moya Moya disease*, cerebral angiography shows an unusual network of small blood vessels – likened to a 'puff of smoke' at the base of the brain. This condition predominates in the Japanese. Pathologically, there is stenosis or occlusion of the terminal portions of the internal carotid arteries, and the proximal portions of the anterior and middle cerebral arteries. The etiology is unclear. Patients may present with either congenital or acquired forms, the latter occurring in association with previous meningitis, oral contraception or granulomatous disease (e.g. sarcoidosis).

Increasingly, a number of inherited disorders are being recognized as causes of cerebrovascular disease. For example, homocystinuria a recessively inherited disorder is due to the accumulation of homocystine in blood which damages the vessels and induces premature occlusive arterial disease. There is also a group of young patients with *mitochondrial cytopathies* with combined involvement of skeletal muscle and the CNS: these include mitochondrial, encephalomyopathy, lactic acidosis and stroke-like episodes (MELAS). In most patients, the disorder is attributed to a single point mutation in mitochondrial DNA. The pathogenesis of the cerebral infarction is not clear; suggestions include endothelial accumulation of abnormal mitochondria and the effects of the mitochondrial defect on secondary mediated cerebral ischemia.

Cerebral autosomal dominant arteriopathy with subcortical infarcts and leukoencephalopathy (CADASIL) is an inherited non-amyloid arteriopathy that causes multiple infarcts and dementia in patients without hypertension: it is due to a defect in notch 3 located on chromosome 12p13 (Fig. 5.18a and b).

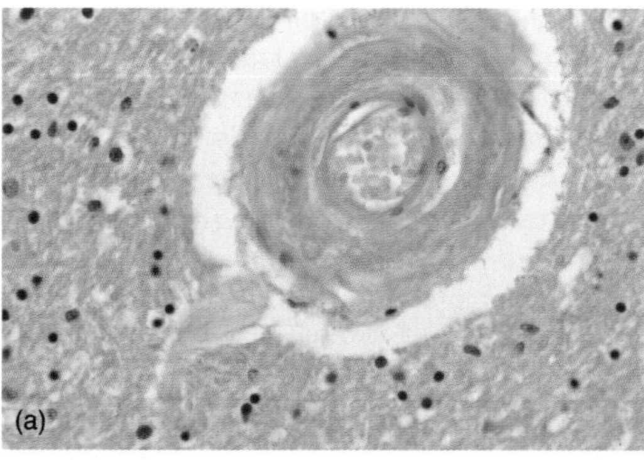

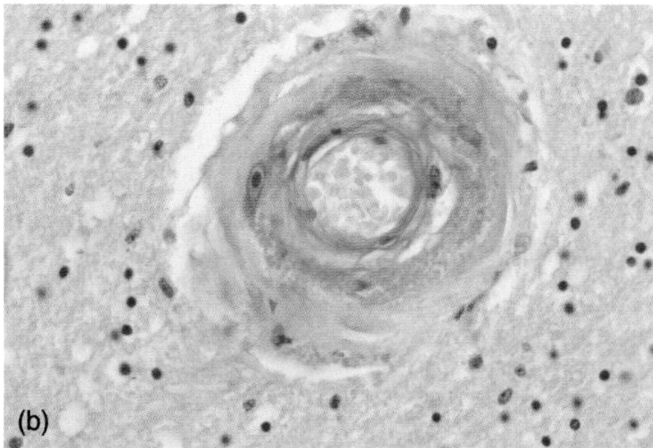

Figure 5.18 CADASIL. The media and adventia are thickened by (a) granular non-amyloid material that is (b) also PAS positive. (a) H&E, (b) PAS.

BRAIN DAMAGE DUE TO CARDIAC ARREST

Brain damage brought about by cardiac arrest is characterized by widespread selective neuronal necrosis which typically has a pattern of selective vulnerability (Table 5.12). Patients may die soon after an episode of cardiac arrest, and there will be no abnormalities identified in the brain. If the patient lives for about 12 h, the brain may again appear entirely normal macroscopically even when it has been properly fixed prior to dissection. The microscopic analysis will show widespread neuronal necrosis in the sites referred to above (Fig. 5.19). In this context little significance should be attached to pallor of nuclear staining, swelling or vacuolation of cytoplasm or loss of Nissl granules, since these can be brought about by autolysis in the brain. Furthermore, many of the patients may have been maintained on artificial ventilation for some hours and during this period autolytic change may proceed in the brain (see Chapter 3). What the

Table 5.12 Pattern of selective vulnerability after cardiac arrest

In cortex
- More severe in parietal and occipital lobes than in the frontal lobes
- More severe in depths of sulci than at crests of gyri
- May be restricted to cortical layers III, V and VI

In hippocampus
- Common in the CA1 and CA4 sectors

In subcortical gray matter
- Common in amygdaloid nuclei
- Variable in basal ganglia
- Common in anterior, dorsomedial and ventrolateral nuclei of thalamus

In cerebellum
- Characteristically, there is diffuse necrosis of Purkinje cells

In brainstem
- Uncommon in adults; more common and severe in young children when there may be necrosis of sensory nuclei

pathologist must identify is incontravertible evidence of classic ischemic cell change with or without incrustations (see Chapter 3). If the patient survives for more than 24–36 h, the pathologist's task is made easier because of more established abnormalities in neurons and the appearance of early reactive changes in astrocytes, microglia and endothelial cells. With the passage of a few days, many of the dead neurons disappear and reactive changes become more intense, including the formation of macrophages. At this stage it may also be possible to identify microscopically, selective damage in the hippocampus (Fig. 5.20a–d) and in the cerebral cortex within sulci, especially in the occipital lobe. A particularly conspicuous histological abnormality is the proliferation of microglia in the cerebellar cortex in relation to the disintegrating dendrites of the Purkinje cells. This is often referred to as microglial shrubwork (Fig. 5.21) and is clear evidence that some Purkinje cells have been destroyed. Indeed, pathologists should hesitate to state that there is a loss of neurons in any part of the brain unless there are corresponding reactive changes. Occasionally, patients who have sustained severe hypoxic brain damage remain alive in a vegetative state for long periods. When this occurs the affected gray matter becomes shrunken and is often cystic. Because the axons and neurons that have been destroyed undergo Wallerian-type degeneration, there is also considerable loss of white matter throughout the brain, leading to symmetrical enlargement of the ventricular system – compensatory hydrocephalus (Fig. 5.22a and b).

There is very little accurate information about the shortest period of cardiac arrest that is likely to produce brain damage in humans. In the context of true circulatory arrest at normal body temperature, complete clinical recovery is unlikely if the period of arrest is more than about 10 min. It is important to realize, however, that adequate cerebral perfusion does not necessarily recommence as soon as the heart rate and arterial blood pressure become recordable, and a poor pre-arrest or post-arrest circulatory state may be as important as the duration of complete arrest in the pathogenesis of brain damage.

BRAIN DAMAGE DUE TO HYPOTENSION

Brain damage due to a generalized reduction in CBF occurs characteristically in association with an episode of severe systemic hypotension. Brain damage may take several forms, but in the commonest type, ischemic damage is concentrated in the boundary zones between the main cerebral and cerebellar arterial territories (Fig. 5.23). If the patient survives only a short time, the brain will appear normal macroscopically. After a few days, however, it is usually possible to see wedge-shaped,

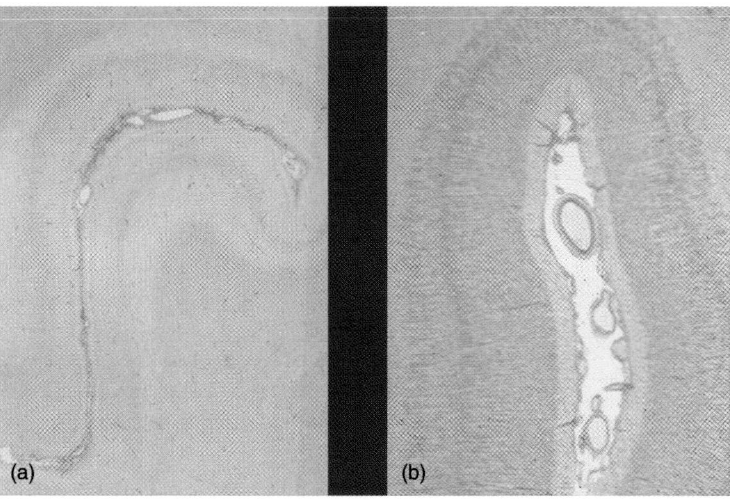

Figure 5.19 Cardiac arrest. Cerebral cortex. (a) There is subtotal laminar necrosis of the III, V and VI cortical layers with selective sparing of the II and IV layers (darker staining) compared with (b) which shows normal cerebral cortex. Left, cresyl violet. Right, H&E.

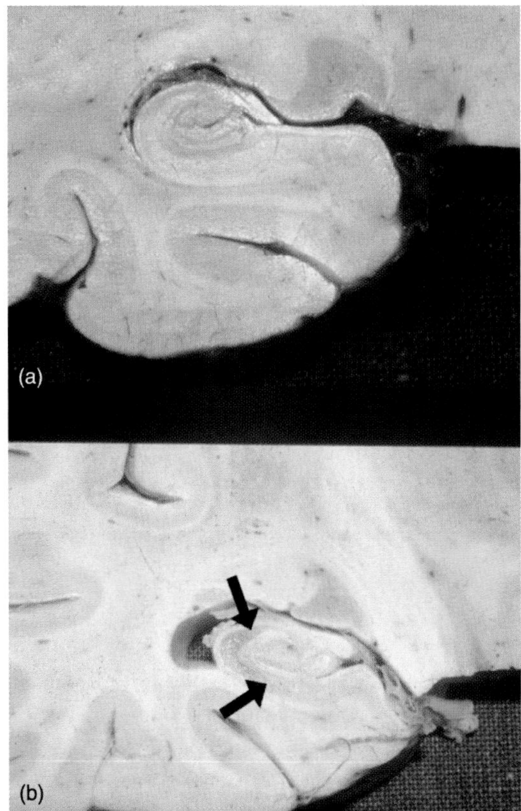

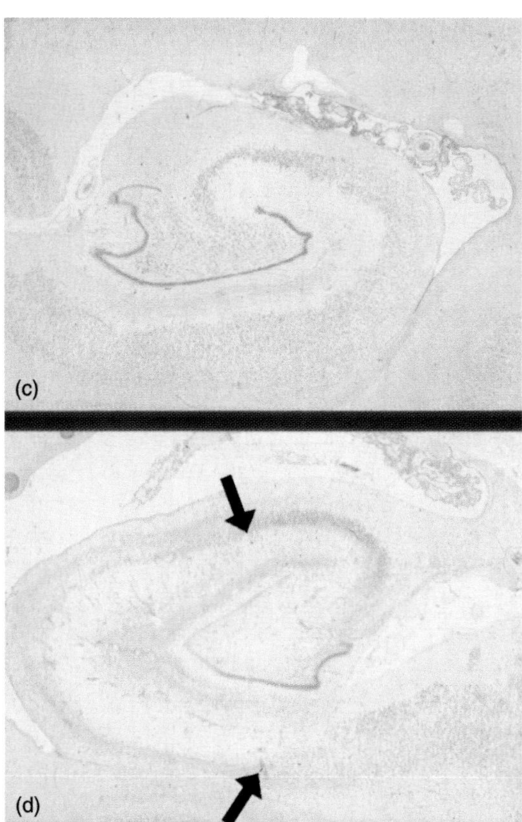

Figure 5.20 Cardiac arrest. Hippocampus. (a) Top: Normal. (b) Bottom: There is necrosis of the Sommer sector (CAl) (between arrows). (c) Top: Normal. (d) Bottom: There is necrosis of the CAl sector (between arrows). (c) and (d) celloidin, cresyl violet.

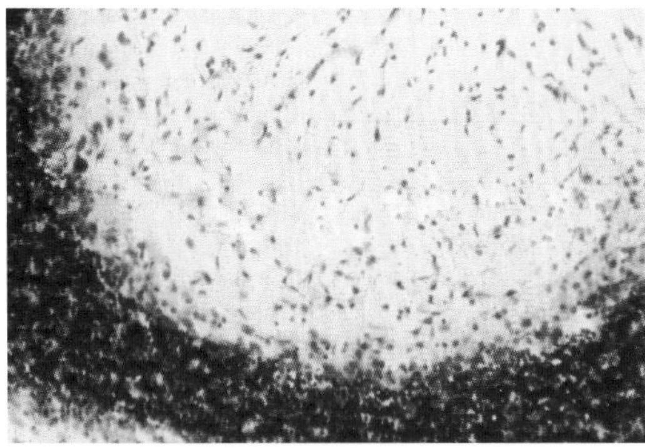

Figure 5.21 Cardiac arrest. Cerebellum. The Purkinje cells have undergone necrosis and as a result there is a reactive astrocytosis and proliferation of microglia in the molecular layer.

often hemorrhagic, infarcts in the arterial boundary zones (Fig. 5.24a and b). These may, however, be small, and may take the form of sharply defined irregular foci of necrosis, mainly in the cortex but sometimes also in the adjacent white matter. Infarcts tend to be largest in the parieto-occipital regions, where the territories of the anterior, middle and posterior cerebral arteries meet. There is variable involvement of the basal ganglia, particularly of the head of the caudate nucleus and in the upper third of the putamen. The hippocampi, despite the extreme vulnerability to hypoxia, are usually not involved.

This type of brain damage appears to be caused by a major and abrupt episode of hypotension followed by rapid return to normal arterial pressure. Because of the precipitate decrease in arterial pressure, autoregulation fails and the regions most remote

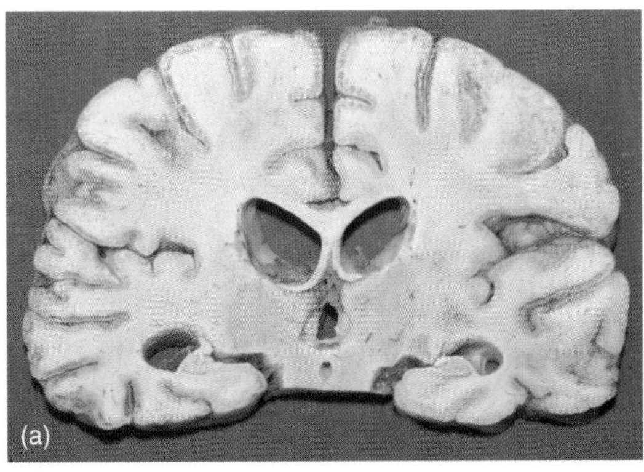

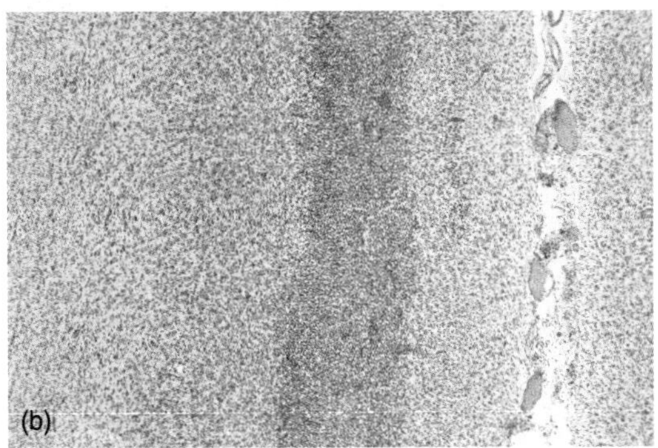

Figure 5.22 Cardiac arrest. (a) The cortex is greatly narrowed and there is enlargement of the ventricles. The hippocampi and the thalami are shown. (b) Laminar necrosis of layer III. H&E.

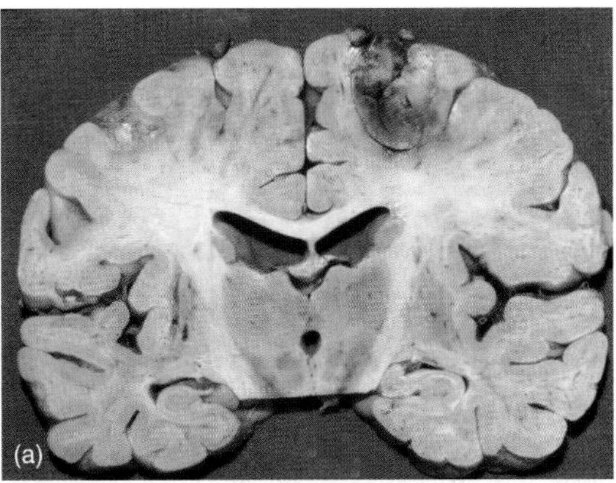

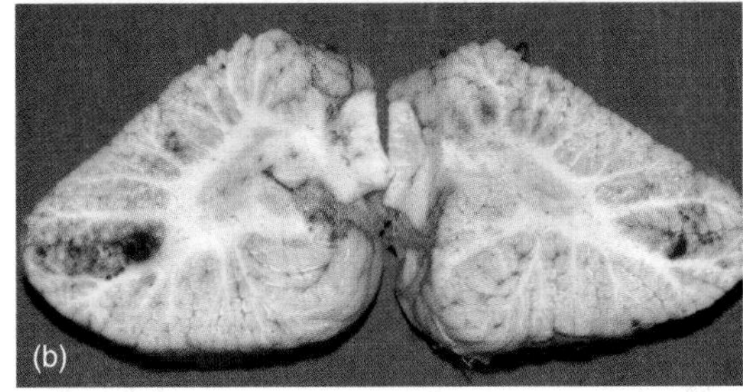

Figure 5.24 Arterial boundary zone infarction. (a) There is asymmetrical hemorrhagic infarction of the sides and depths of the superior frontal sulci in the boundary zones between the anterior and middle cerebral arteries. (b) There is hemorrhagic infarction in the boundary zones between the superior and posterior inferior cerebellar arteries.

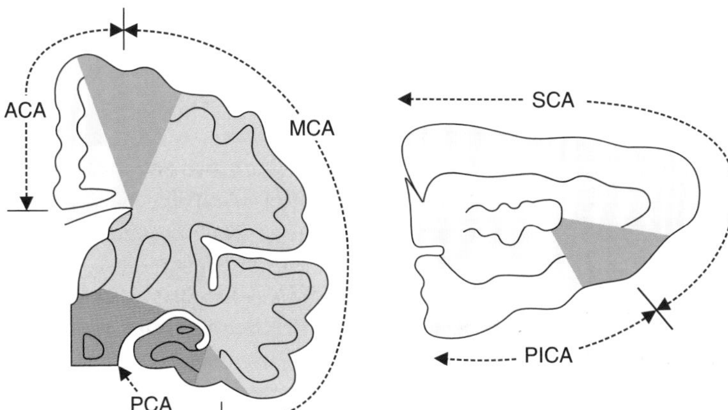

Figure 5.23 Arterial boundary zones (dark blue) in the cerebral and cerebellar hemispheres. They lie between the ACA/MCA, MCA/PCA and SCA/PICA territories. ACA = anterior cerebral artery; MCA = middle cerebral artery; PCA = posterior cerebral artery; SCA = superior cerebellar artery; PICA = posterior inferior cerebellar artery.

from the parent arterial stems, i.e. the boundary zones, are thus subjected to the greatest reduction in cerebral blood flow. Many examples of this pattern of brain damage have been described, but in the great majority there has been a known episode of hypotension or good clinical grounds for suspecting that the patient had experienced at least a transient episode of hypotension, such as brain damage occurring in the course of a major operation under general anesthesia or in association with a myocardial infarct. If the brain damage is particularly severe the hippocampi may be involved, but if the hypotension is less severe and of longer duration, damage to neurons is more widespread, is usually accentuated in the arterial boundary zones and there is again relative sparing of the hippocampi. Structural damage due to a generalized reduction in cerebral perfusion pressure is characteristically bilateral and may occur in the absence of any occlusive arterial disease. One hemisphere may be more severely affected than the other, and this is readily explicable because of the frequency with which there are anatomical variations in the Circle of Willis.

Since hypotension can produce severe brain damage in the absence of any occlusive arterial disease, the significance of any reduction in cardiac output in the patient with pre-existing arterial stenosis in the pathogenesis of hypoxic brain damage should now be clear. It seems likely that such a combination of circumstances more often accounts for the co-existence of cerebral and myocardial infarction than in the widely held view that cerebral infarcts in patients with recent myocardial infarcts are usually embolic in type.

BRAIN DAMAGE DUE TO HYPOGLYCEMIA

Respiratory 'CO_2/O_2' of the brain is almost 1, indicating that oxidation of glucose is the principal source of energy. Hypoglycemia in humans may lead to permanent brain damage in such diverse situations as an excessive amount of insulin given for the treatment of diabetes mellitus or psychosis, in the rare instance of islet cell tumor of the pancreas, and in examples of hypoglycemia in infants.

In cases of short survival, the brain may appear normal macroscopically. If survival is for more than a few weeks, there may be atrophy of the cortex and hippocampi, and enlargement of the ventricular system. Microscopy shows that the brain damage is very similar in type and distribution to that seen after cardiac arrest except that there is usually greater involvement of the superficial layers of the neocortex and often relative sparing of Purkinje cells in the cerebellum.

Experimental work has shown that the blood glucose must fall to about 1 mmol/L for about 60 min before brain damage is produced, although a higher level blood sugar may produce similar damage complicated by hypotension, hypoxemia or epilepsy.

EPILEPSY

Epilepsy is usually considered as the occurrence of two or more seizures and is the consequence of paroxysmal uncontrolled discharge of neurons within the CNS. The clinical manifestations range from a major motor convulsion to a brief period of lack of awareness.

Epidemiology shows that the incidence of epilepsy (new cases/year) is approximately 40–70 in 100 000 in the developed world, and usually presents in childhood or adolescence but may occur for the first time at any age and that some 5% of the population suffer a single seizure at some time. Half a percent of the population have recurrent seizures and it should be stressed that epilepsy is a symptom of numerous disorders and that in the majority of patients the cause remains unclear despite careful history taking, examination and investigation.

The modern classification of epilepsy is based upon the nature of the attack rather than the presence or absence of an underlying cause. Attacks that begin *focally* from a single location within one hemisphere are thus distinguished from those of a *generalized* nature which probably commence in deeper midline structures and project to both hemispheres simultaneously. According to the classification of the International League against Epilepsy there are partial (focal, local) seizures, generalized seizures (convulsive or non-convulsive)

Table 5.13 Causes of epilepsy

Cause	Percent of cases
No cause found	75
Head injury	5
Cerebrovascular disease	5
Central nervous systems infections	5
Congenital disorders	5
Hypoxia, drugs, alcohol and tumors	5

and unclassified seizures. With the increasing use and sophistication of electrophysiological and neuroimaging techniques the accuracy of the clinical diagnosis of symptomatic epilepsy has greatly improved the differential diagnosis including vasovagal attacks, cardiac arrhythmias, migraine, hypoglycemia, episodic confusion, panic attacks, narcolepsy and pseudoseizures. It is only in some 25% of cases that the cause of the epilepsy can be established (Table 5.13) the most frequent underlying conditions being congenital disorders, head injury, cerebrovascular disease and various infections of the CNS with fewer cases being due to drugs and alcohol, hypoxia and neoplasms. Therefore, in some 75% of cases an obvious cause cannot be established although there is often an increase in the various risk factors such as family history, convulsions in childhood or difficult birth delivery. The cause of epilepsy varies with age of onset (Table 5.14), may also be associated with systemic disease and may be precipitated by certain drugs such as anti-depressants and anti-psychotics, and those used in the treatment of tumors.

The etiology of generalized epilepsy is much less clear, there being genetic factors some of which are thought to be due to ligand or voltage gated channelopathies.

Treatment

The majority of patients respond to drug therapy. In intractable cases surgery may be necessary but only if a focal lesion can be identified. Modern investigative techniques include videotelemetry and imaging with MRI, SPECT or PET scanning. Operative techniques include anterior temporal lobectomy with

Table 5.14 Causes of focal seizures with or without generalization by age of onset and in order of frequency

Newborn
- Hypoxia
- Intracranial hemorrhage
- Metabolic
  - Hypocalcemia
  - Hypoglycemia
  - Hyperbilirubinemia
  - Inborn errors of metabolism
- Trauma

Infancy
- Febrile convulsions
- CNS infections
- Head injury
- Congenital disorders
- Inborn errors of metabolism

Childhood
- Head injury
- CNS Infection
- Vascular malformation
- Congenital disorders
- Tumors

Adolescence and early adulthood
- Head injury
- CNS infection
- Tumors
- Vascular malformations
- Drugs and alcohol

Late adulthood
- Drugs and alcohol
- Head injury
- Tumors
- Cerebrovascular disease
- Neurodegenerative disease
- CNS infection

removal of the epileptogenic focus in the hippocampus and the medial part of the temporal lobe: in some 50% the patients become seizure free and in a further 30% gain significant improvement from seizure control. The other operative technique is that of extra-temporal cortical resection which incorporates a frontal, parietal or occipital epileptogenic focus: the results here are less satisfactory than for temporal resection. Other procedures include selective amygdaloid hippocampectomy which is a less extensive resection procedure, section of the corpus callosum which prevents spread and reverberation of seizure activity between the hemispheres: in children with irreversible damage to a hemisphere over 80% of selected patients become seizure free after hemisphorectomy.

Anterior temporal lobectomy specimens

As the lesions causing this type of epilepsy may be small it is very important that each specimen, either a surgically resected temporal lobe or a brain, is cut into thin slices and examined systematically. A number of pathologies may be identified (Table 5.15).

Macroscopic abnormalities may be few at the time of brain cutting although histological examination may reveal changes which could be responsible for the seizures (see above). In general the main types of lesion that have been identified are those of a dysgenetic nature, consequences of trauma that include healed contusions, and neuronal loss and gliosis. The later changes are common, the hippocampus being damaged in some 50–60% of patients, the cerebellum in 45% and the thalamus, amygdaloid and cortex each in 25%. The most common abnormality in the hippocampus is scarring of the medial part of the temporal lobe due to gliosis of the CAI sector (Sommer sector) known as Ammon's horn sclerosis (Fig. 5.25) and laminar damage in layers II and III of the middle and inferior temporal and hippocampal gyri. These features are almost always severe and widespread although, sometimes the sector involvement in the hippocampus may be mild. In addition, there may be dispersion of the dentate granular cell layer. Changes in the cerebellum consist of diffuse loss of Purkinje cells, some loss of granule cells and an associated astrocytosis. The etiology of the neuronal loss and gliosis is not clear. The question as to whether these abnormalities are the cause or the result of the epilepsy remains controversial. Thus, it has been suggested that they may be secondary to hypoxia occurring during birth, when the circulation through the posterior cerebral arteries may be compromised. However, lesions may be found in structures supplied by other arteries, raising the possibility that they may be secondary to the epilepsy and not the cause of it.

Table 5.15 Anterior temporal lobectomy: neuropathology

- Ammon's horn sclerosis, which is by far the most common abnormality
- Hamartomas made up of glia, mixed neuronal glia and vascular lesions
- Lesions made up of astrocytes and/or oligodendrocytes that are probably neoplastic
- Lesions composed of glia and neuronal tissue, which may appear either as hamartomas or gangliogliomas
- Dysembryoplastic neuroepithelial tumors
- Vascular lesions which are angiomatous malformations
- Inflammatory lesions
- A sequel of head injury
- Developmental abnormalities consisting of cysts and cortical malformations such as polymicrogyria

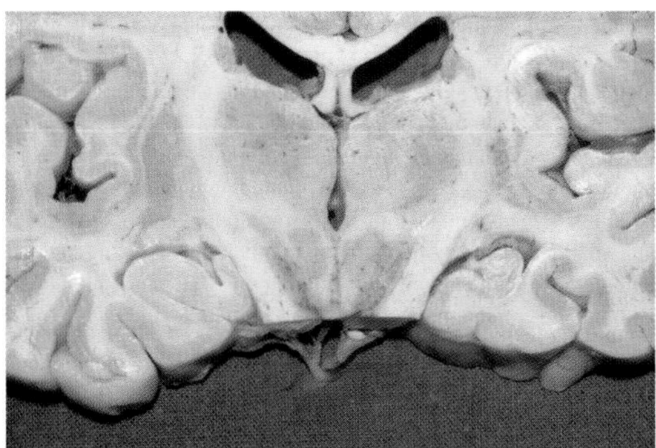

Figure 5.25 Unilateral sclerosis of the right hippocampus. There is associated enlargement of the temporal horn.

The lesions found after cortical resection are similar to the focal abnormalities found in temporal lobectomies, although with much higher proportions of focal cortical dysplasia and Rasmussen syndrome.

Febrile convulsions

These are usually manifested as generalized seizures occurring in some 2–5% of children under the age of 5 years during the course of a febrile illness occurring probably as a result of water and electrolyte disturbance. Follow-up suggests that these seizures are self-limiting without long-term sequelae. There is considerable debate as to whether or not hippocampal sclerosis is a cause or a consequence of febrile seizures in childhood. The great majority of cases develop normally and only a few percent develop chronic epilepsy.

Death in epilepsy

There is an overall increased risk of premature death in patients with epilepsy, the significant excess of deaths being due to accidents, and drowning. Sudden unexpected death in epilepsy (SUDEP) occurs in about 10% and is the major form of death in patients in the 20–40 year age group. It has been defined as 'sudden, unexpected, witnessed or unwitnessed, non-traumatic and non-drowning death in patients with epilepsy with or without evidence of a seizure and excluding documented status epilepticus, in which post mortem examination does not reveal a toxicological or anatomical cause for death'. It has been postulated that death results from cardiac arrhythmia or respiratory failure during or immediately after the seizure. In some two thirds of brains examined it is possible to identify abnormalities which may have either been the cause of the epilepsy or result from epilepsy and include malformations, hippocampal sclerosis, tumors, old infarcts and healed contusions.

Status epilepticus

This refers to seizure activity that is continuous, or intermittent but without intervening recovery, for a prolonged period, commonly set at 60 min for adults and 30 min for infants and children. This state may be life threatening with the development of pyrexia, deepening coma and circulatory collapse. In many cases it is symptomatic of underlying brain disease and may occur with frontal lobe lesions, after head injury, and reducing drug therapy, with alcohol or other sedation, drug intoxication, infections and metabolic disturbances or pregnancy. In fatal cases naked eye abnormalities may be limited to swelling although subsequent microscopy will probably – if survival has been long enough, show widespread irreversible hypoxic damage in vulnerable areas. Post mortem studies in children present a more consistent picture of damage than studies in adults and suggest a higher degree of vulnerability in infants and children up to 3 years of age. Loss of pyramidal neurons in the Sommer sector (CAI) is often almost total and in the cerebellum loss of Purkinje cells may be severe in association with cell loss in the granular layer. There is usually severe neuronal loss in cortical laminae II and III and the thalamus may show severe damage. Comparative studies have shown that there is no definitive difference in the pattern of damage in young children compared with adults; the difference is the greater chance of finding damage in children and its greater severity.

It was at first thought that the acute brain damage seen in children dying after status epilepticus was hypoxic–ischemic in nature complicated by secondary events occurring during or after the seizures. However, there is now strong experimental evidence that local enhancement of excitatory activity and metabolic rate are contributing factors to the hippocampal damage and that there is a complex inter-relationship between both local and systemic factors that include hyperpyrexia, and degrees of hypoxia and arterial hypotension the combinations of which contribute to cortical and cerebellar damage. The final common pathway may be activation of NMDA receptors with enhanced calcium entry and subsequent cell death.

INTRACRANIAL HEMORRHAGE

These may be due to either trauma as a result of head injury or to non-traumatic cases such as a result of asphyxia at birth or cerebrovascular disease. Trauma is the usual cause of bleeding into the extradural and subdural spaces and not uncommonly may be the cause of intracerebral bleeding into the subarachnoid space as a consequence of contusional injury. However, intracerebral hematoma and large amounts of subarachnoid hemorrhage are frequently spontaneous and the subependymal and intraventricular hemorrhages seen in premature infants are strongly associated with perinatal hypoxia.

Intracerebral hemorrhage

Modern imaging techniques have greatly improved the identification of intracerebral hemorrhage with a result that although the number of fatal cases has fallen the incidence has remained the same. The most common causes are shown in Table 5.3, page 84. Many of the hematoma occur in late middle-aged individuals with hypertension and were attributed by Charcot in the middle of the nineteenth century to hemorrhage from miliary aneurysms arising from small perforating cerebral arteries: this has been confirmed by post mortem micro-angiographic studies. They are usually multiple, tend to occur on arteries less than 25 μm in diameter, but may attain a diameter of 2 mm. In contrast, micro-aneurysms are rare in normotensive individuals, although a few can be demonstrated in subjects over the age of 65 years, and are considered to be the origin of spontaneous intracranial hematomas in elderly normotensive individuals.

In 80% of cases with hypertension the hematoma is in the region of the basal ganglia or thalamus – the so-called capsular hemorrhage (Fig. 5.26a). Since the hemorrhages are arterial in origin the hematoma usually enlarges rapidly and causes considerable destruction of brain tissue, and because of the rapidly expanding lesion and distortion with herniation of the brain, death often occurs within 24–48 h as a result of raised intracranial pressure. The hematoma may rupture into the ventricles or through the surface of the brain directly into the subarachnoid space. A few patients may survive the acute episode, presumably because the hematoma is relatively small and because it has developed slowly, thus leaving more time for spatial compensation. The hematoma becomes brown in color and reactive changes in astrocytes, microglia and the small blood vessels appear around it. If the patient survives, the hematoma is ultimately completely absorbed and replaced by clear fluid, thus forming a so-called 'apoplectic cyst' (Fig. 5.26). In the remaining one fifth of cases hypertension-associated cases, the hematoma occurs in the hind brain, either in the pons or in the cerebellum (Figs 5.28 and 5.29).

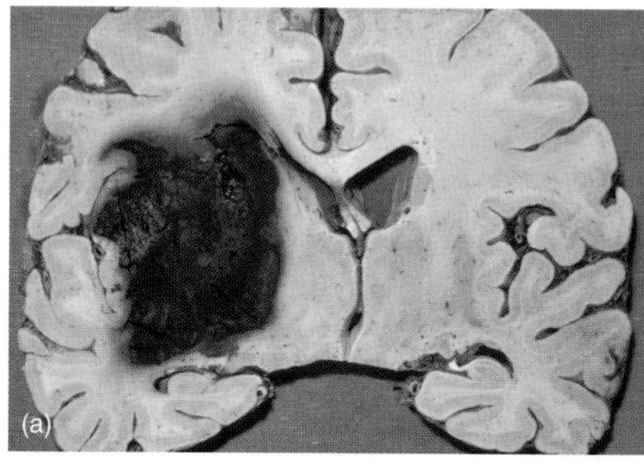

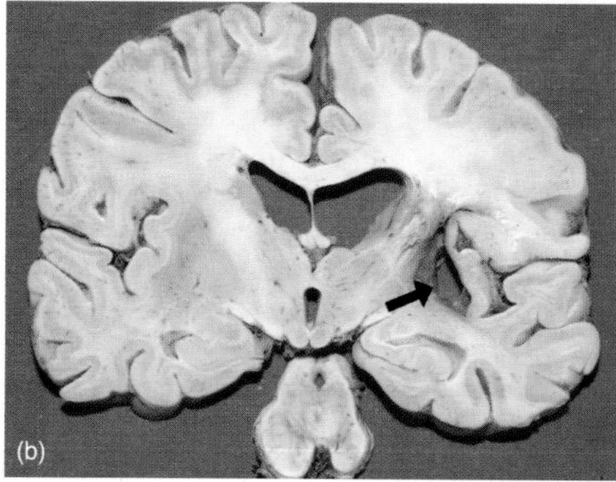

Figure 5.26 Intracerebral 'capsular' hematoma. The patient was hypertensive. (a) Recently formed hematoma. (b) Old intracerebral hematoma. There is an apoplectic cyst (arrow) in the capsule lateral to the lentiform nucleus, the walls of which were orange–brown in color. In the brainstem of the same patient there is ipsilateral descending degeneration in the corticospinal tract.

Primary pontine hemorrhage needs to be distinguished from hemorrhage secondary to raised ICP and internal herniation (see Chapter 4). This is usually not difficult, although a large primary supratentorial hematoma may track downwards into the upper brainstem.

Some 10% of spontaneous intracerebral hematomas occur in association with cerebral amyloid angiopathy. It is frequently lobar, i.e. peripherally located particularly in elderly normotensive patients. There may be more than one bleed and the hemorrhages may be multiple in time and site and because of their superficial location they are commonly associated with hemorrhage into the

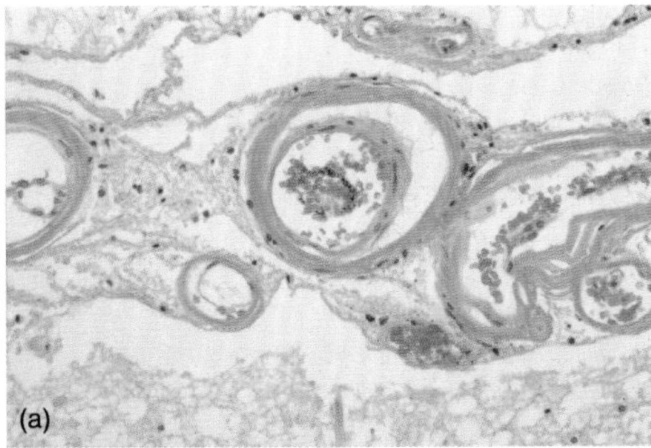

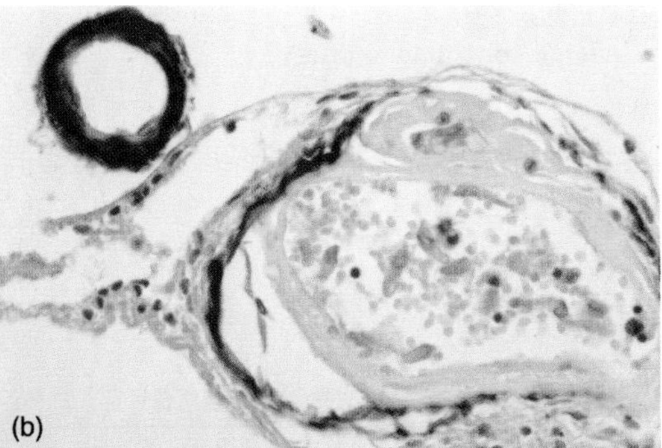

Figure 5.27 Cerebral amyloid angiopathy in non-demented patient. (a) Arterial wall thickened by amorphous material with double barrel appearance. (b) Strongly immunoreactive for β-amyloid. (a) H&E. (b) Immunohistochemistry for β-amyloid.

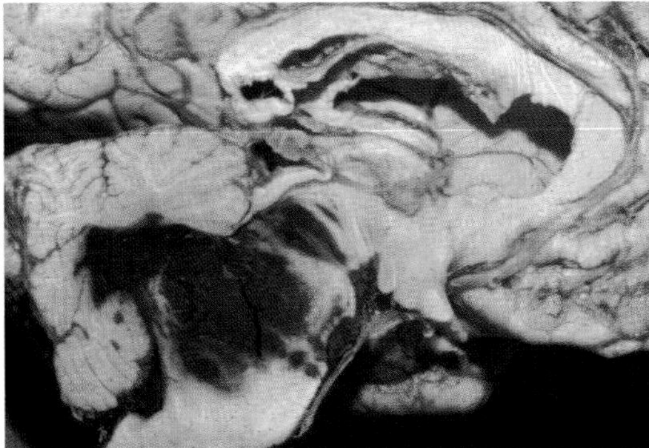

Figure 5.28 Recent hematoma in the pons.

subarachnoid space (Fig. 5.27a and b). It is most commonly associated with the deposition of β-amyloid and less commonly cystatin C and (BRI) protein.

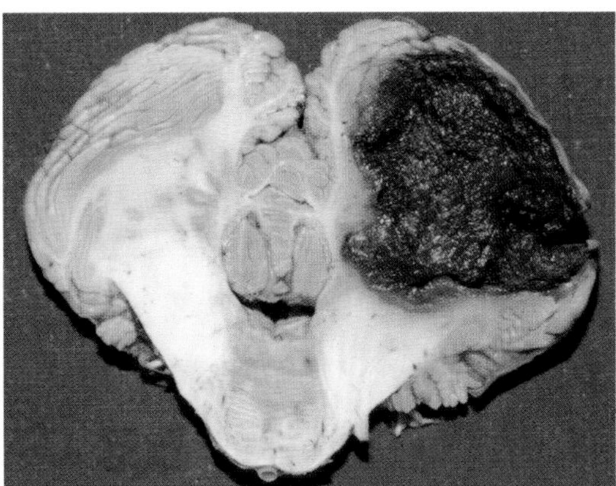

Figure 5.29 Recent hematoma in cerebellum.

Less common causes of hemorrhage are *vasculitis*, particularly in patients with collagen diseases, and rupture of a *mycotic aneurysm*, a *saccular aneurysm* or a *vascular malformation* (see below). In some instances, however, the cause cannot be determined in spite of careful examination of the brain. In such circumstances the hematoma is probably due to rupture of the small hidden angioma. Hemorrhage may occasionally occur in either *primary or secondary brain tumors*: it is most likely to occur in patients with glioblastoma and bleeding into metastatic tumor may be severe, and occurs most often into deposits from the bronchus and malignant melanoma.

Drug abuse is a considerable risk factor for the development of an intracerebral hemorrhage particularly in those who use cocaine, heroin, and sympathomimetics such as amphetamines: at greatest risk are those who are relatively young compared with the general population. The hematomas are commonly lobar in the subcortical white matter and the bleeding usually develops within minutes to a few hours after the use of the drug, the two principal pathogenetic mechanisms being either an acute rise in the blood pressure or arteritis. There is also an association with *alcohol abuse* the hemorrhages again tending to be lobar in site. Some 5% of patients presenting with spontaneous intracerebral hematoma are receiving anticoagulants or have coagulation disorders which either singly or in combination with mild trauma increase the predisposition to hemorrhage. Not only is the

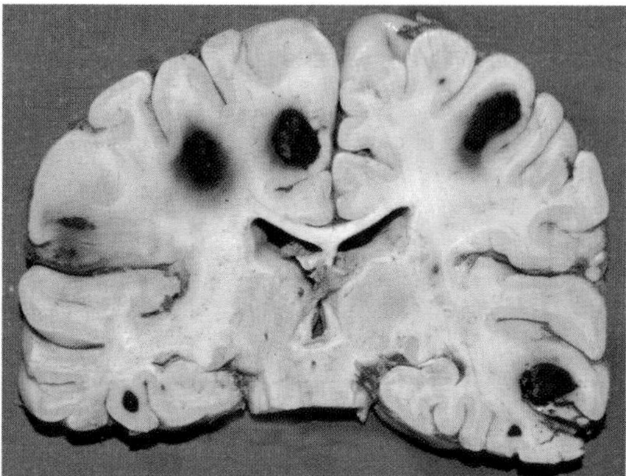

Figure 5.30 Multiple recent intracerebral hematomas in patient with thrombocytopenia due to leukemia.

risk of bleeding increased when conventional anticoagulants are used in the treatment of ischemic 'stroke' when hemorrhagic transformation may occur, but may also be directly caused in the development of hematomas. Thrombolytic therapy may similarly cause ICH and such therapy when used for acute myocardial infarction carries a risk of 0.3–0.8%. This risk is higher when the thrombolytic treatment is given for acute cerebral ischemia the incidence of ICH being 3.5 times higher among patients treated with thrombolytics than in non-treated patients.

Multiple hemorrhages are often seen in the white matter in patients with *thrombocytopenia.* Such patients fall into two main categories: those with and those without leukemia (Fig. 5.30). Thrombocytopenia is also probably the most important factor in the bleeding tendency sometimes seen in alcoholics and in patients with aplastic anemia or disseminated intravascular coagulation.

Petechial hemorrhages (*brain purpura*) may develop under many circumstances: in most instances the hemorrhages being restricted to white matter (Table 5.16).

Hemorrhage into the spinal cord

Bleeding into the spinal cord (*hematomyelia*) is common after trauma and often occurs without any evidence of fracture or subluxation. Spontaneous bleeding is rare, although it may occur in patients

Table 5.16 Causes of petechial hemorrhages

Associated with trauma
- Diffuse brain injury including acute vascular injury
- Fat embolism

Not associated with trauma
- Asphyxia
- Thrombocytopenia
- Disseminated intravascular coagulation
- Hypertensive encephalopathy
- Acute hemorrhagic leukoencephalopathy
- Cerebral malaria
- Endotoxic shock
- Allergic reactions to drugs

with thrombocytopenia or with a spinal vascular malformation. These factors are also considered to feature in those patients who present with bleeding into the extradural spinal space.

Subarachnoid hemorrhage

Bleeding may either occur alone within the subarachnoid space or in association with bleeding elsewhere in the CNS. The most common cause is contusion-laceration after head injury and many samples of CSF obtained by lumbar puncture contain red blood cells (Table 5.17). Some 75% of spontaneous, i.e. non-traumatic bleeding into the subarachnoid space are due to rupture of a *saccular aneurysm* with fewer cases being due to *vascular malformations* with secondary hemorrhage occurring in the association with intracerebral bleeds as a result of *vasculitis, tumor* or a *bleeding diathesis.* Overall spontaneous subarachnoid hemorrhage occurs in approximately 10–15 per 100 000 of the population per year.

Modern imaging techniques, particularly a CT scan, not only confirms the diagnosis of subarachnoid hemorrhage in over 95% of the cases if undertaken within 48 h of the bleed, but also from its location, provides a strong indication as to its cause. CT/MR angiography and digital angiography are undertaken to detect an aneurysm even if under 3 mm in size. In spite of these various techniques angiography may fail to reveal the source of the subarachnoid hemorrhage in some 10% of patients.

Table 5.17 Causes of subarachnoid hemorrhage

Cause	Percent
Trauma	
• Contusion and lacerations	Almost 100
• Part of severe diffuse injury	80
• Lumbar puncture	Not known
Spontaneous (non-traumatic)	
• Rupture of saccular aneurysm	75
• Vascular malformation	5
• Bleeding diathesis	5
• Anticoagulants	Not known
• Tumors	Not known
• Vasculitis	Not known
• Undefined	15

Saccular aneurysms

These occur on the arteries of the base of the brain in between 1 and 2% of the adult population. They are found more commonly in women than in men, are a not uncommon incidental finding at autopsy, and are often referred to as congenital aneurysms, although in fact they are due to a defect in the medial coat at the bifurcation of one of the large cerebral arteries in the subarachnoid space (Figs 5.31 and 5.32). Segmental degeneration of the internal elastic lamina, probably brought about by early atheroma and hypertension, may be prerequisites for the development of an aneurysm. The arterial wall at the bifurcation then commences to bulge. It has been established from serial angiographic studies that the sac may enlarge progressively. Support for the role of hemodynamic stress in the formation of a saccular aneurysm is provided by their recurrent formation on blood vessels supplying arteriovenous malformations. The contribution of hypertension on the development of an aneurysm is unclear, and the relative importance of these factors varies at different ages. Additional risk factors include a family history (×4) and polycystic kidney disease (×4) and although the genetic basis remains unknown procollagen 3 deficiency may play a role in some patients. Multiple aneurysms are found in approximately 25–30% of patients with aneurysmal subarachnoid hemorrhage: in such patients there are usually two or three but sometimes five or more.

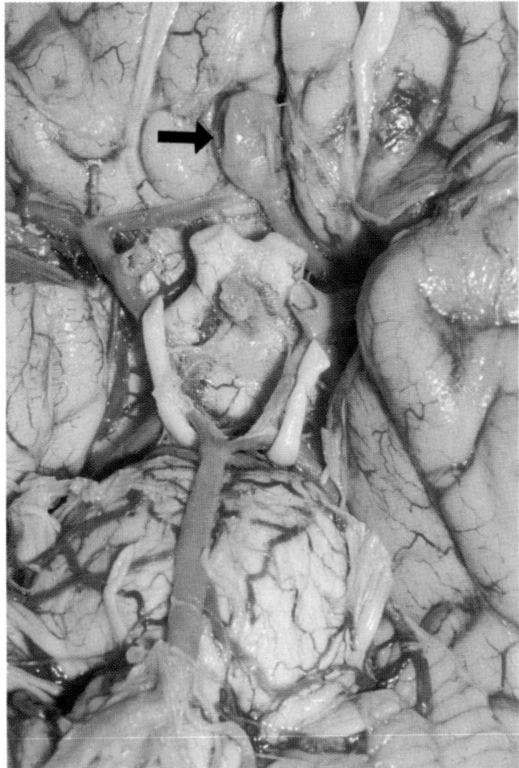

Figure 5.31 Saccular aneurysm arising from anterior communicating artery (arrow). Incidental finding at autopsy.

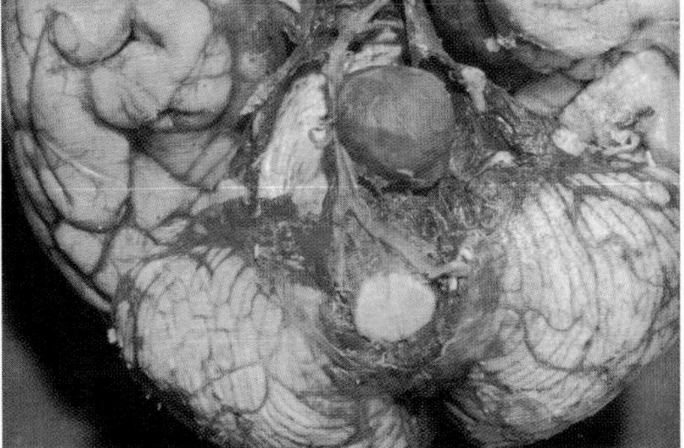

Figure 5.32 Saccular aneurysm arising from the upper end of the basilar artery. The patient died after bleeding into the subarachnoid space of the basal cisterns.

There is said to be an association between multiple aneurysms and coarctation of the aorta, adult type 3 polycystic disease of the kidney and renal artery stenosis, a possible common denominator being hypertension. However, patients with these conditions are not invariably hypertensive and in some instances it is thought that there may be a collagen type 3 deficiency.

The great majority of aneurysms are thin-walled: they range in size from small blisters measuring some 1–2 mm in diameter to large sacs measuring several centimeters across. The latter are usually thick-walled, often contain laminated thrombus, rarely rupture, and may cause focal neurological signs from local pressure on the brain or cranial nerves (Fig. 5.33). Most aneurysms that rupture measure some 5–10 mm in diameter. Risk factors associated with aneurysmal rupture include smoking, hypertension and alcohol excess but other factors also include exhaustion, straining or coitus but in many patients there is no such associated relationship. Saccular aneurysms are found most commonly at certain sites (Table 5.18). About 30% of aneurysms are located at the junction between the internal carotid and the posterior communicating arteries, about 35–40% at the junction between the anterior communicating and the anterior cerebral arteries within the interhemispheric fissure, and about 20–25% at the division of the middle cerebral artery within the Sylvian fissure. The commoner sites of the remaining aneurysms are on the pericallosal artery as it winds around the anterior part of the corpus callosum, at the junction between the internal carotid and middle cerebral arteries, at the upper end of the basilar artery, at the junction between the vertebral and the posterior inferior cerebellar arteries, and at the junction between the internal carotid and ophthalmic arteries immediately beyond the cavernous sinus. Most patients present having had a subarachnoid hemorrhage but a few present with symptoms or signs due to compression of adjacent structures, and in others an aneurysm may be found incidentally.

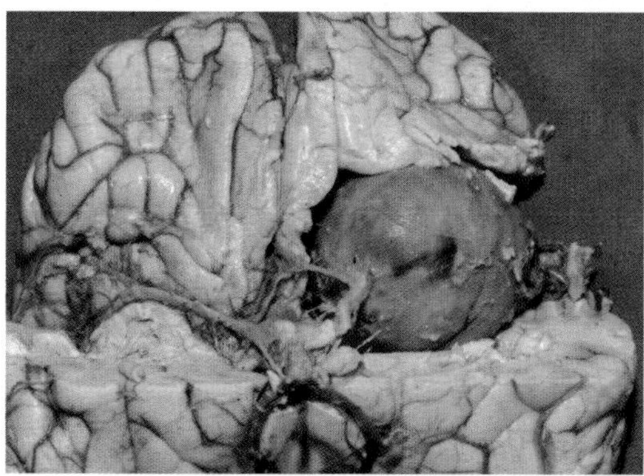

Figure 5.33 'Giant' saccular aneurysm. There is a large unruptured aneurysm on the left middle cerebral artery.

Table 5.18 Sites of saccular aneurysms (less common sites are shown in brackets)

Site	Percent
Anterior communicating artery	35–40
(Pericallosal artery)	
Posterior communicating artery	30
Carotid bifurcation	
(Anterior choroidal artery)	
(Ophthalmic artery)	
Middle cerebral artery at bifurcation or trifurcation	20–25
Basilar artery	10
Posterior inferior cerebellar artery	

Intracranial complications following rupture of saccular aneurysm

These may be early or delayed (Table 5.19).

Early

Reference has already been made to the natural history of a ruptured saccular aneurysm when it was noted that subarachnoid hemorrhage carries a

Table 5.19 Intracranial complications after rupture of saccular aneurysm

Early
- Rebleeding into subarachnoid space
- Intracerebral hematoma with or without extension into ventricles
- Subdural hematoma
- Caroticocavernous fistula
- Acute hydrocephalus

Late
- Cerebral infarction
- Hydrocephalus
- Hemosiderosis of meninges
- Epilepsy

high initial mortality risk which gradually declines with time. Of those who survive the initial bleed, rebleeding and cerebral infarction are the major causes of death.

Rebleeding is a major complication following aneurysmal subarachnoid hemorrhage. In the first 28 days in untreated patients approximately 30% will rebleed of which 70% die. In the following few months the risk gradually falls off but it never drops below 3.5% per year.

When an aneurysm ruptures there is usually subarachnoid hemorrhage (Fig. 5.34). This may be limited to the immediate vicinity of the aneurysm, although frequently there is extensive hemorrhage throughout the subarachnoid space. Recurrent hemorrhage is common in many patients who sustain subarachnoid hemorrhage having a recent clinical history of some headache and neck stiffness which was not recognized at the time as a minor subarachnoid hemorrhage. In fatal cases the basal cisterns and much of the subarachnoid space over the surfaces of the cerebral hemispheres and the cerebellum are filled with recent blood clots. When undertaking a post mortem examination on such a case it is important to try to find the aneurysm prior to fixing the brain, since fixed blood clot is very difficult to remove without destroying the aneurysm. Blood also tracks along the spinal cord, most of it localizing in the subarachnoid space on the posterior surface of the cord. Sometimes quite a large hematoma may develop in the subarachnoid space usually within the Sylvian fissure in association with an aneurysm on the middle cerebral artery, or between the medial surfaces of the frontal lobes in association with an aneurysm on the anterior communicating artery.

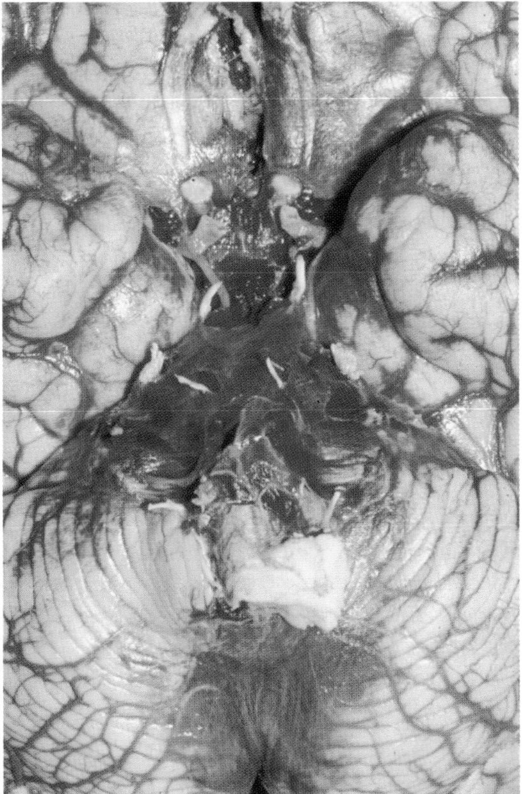

Figure 5.34 Recent subarachnoid hemorrhage due to rupture of a saccular aneurysm on the anterior communicating artery.

Intracerebral hematoma is also a common occurrence when an aneurysm ruptures. There is usually some subarachnoid hemorrhage in addition, but sometimes the fundus of the aneurysm is so deeply embedded in the brain as a result of previous small leaks from the aneurysm, the aneurysm ruptures directly into the brain without there being any obvious subarachnoid hemorrhage. The hematoma lies adjacent to the aneurysm and occurs in the inferomedial part of the frontal lobe(s) in association with anterior communicating artery aneurysms (Fig. 5.35), and in the temporal lobe in association with an aneurysm on a middle cerebral artery

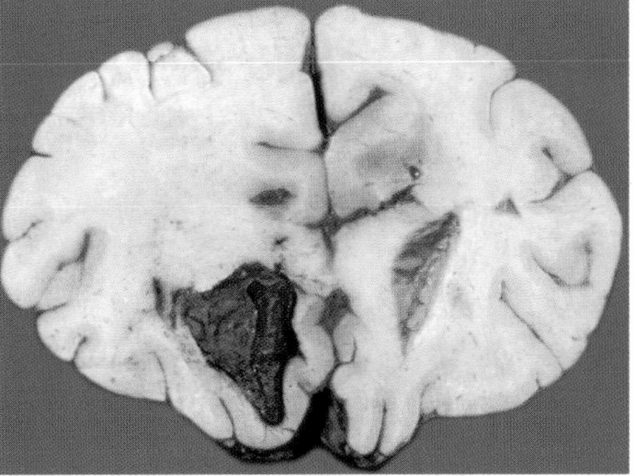

Figure 5.35 Intracerebral hematoma. There is a recently formed hematoma in the infero-medial sector of the left frontal lobe due to rupture of saccular aneurysm arising from the anterior communicating artery.

(Fig. 5.36) or on a posterior communicating artery (Fig. 5.37). The hematoma may rupture into the ventricular system, particularly an aneurysm on the anterior communicating artery or at the bifurcation of the basilar artery. Brain swelling around an intracerebral hematoma may increase its mass effect. Rupture of an aneurysm on the middle cerebral artery may occasionally produce an *acute subdural hematoma*: this is particularly important in medico-legal cases where trauma is suspected. Also, an aneurysm on the internal carotid artery may rupture into the cavernous sinus, causing a *caroticocavernous fistula.*

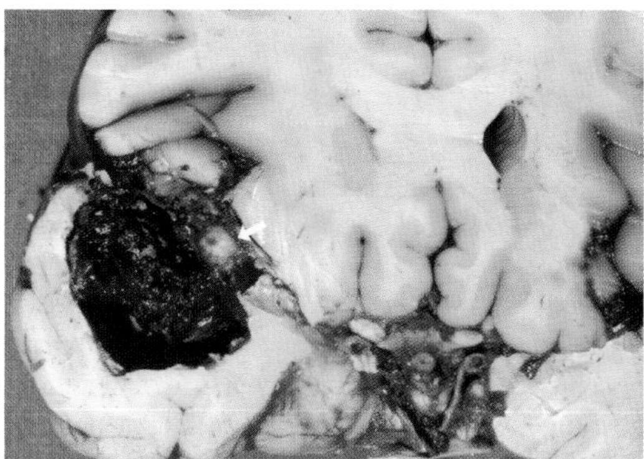

Figure 5.36 Intracerebral hematoma. There is a recently formed hematoma in the temporal lobe closely associated with a saccular aneurysm arising from the middle cerebral artery (arrow). Careful dissection was required to identify the aneurysm.

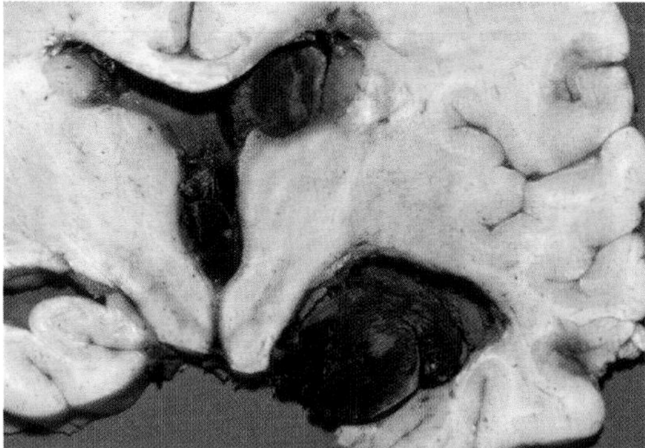

Figure 5.37 Intracerebral hematoma. There is a recently formed hematoma in the medial portion of the right temporal lobe due to rupture of a saccular aneurysm arising from the junction between the posterior communicating and the internal carotid arteries.

Acute hydrocephalus occurs in some 20% of patients usually in the first few days after the ictus. Mechanisms include blood clot within the basal cisterns or obstruction of the arachnoid granulations causing communicating hydrocephalus, or blood within the ventricular system which may cause obstructive hydrocephalus.

Delayed

These include cerebral infarction, hydrocephalus and epilepsy. The development of cerebral ischemia after subarachnoid hemorrhage is a particularly important contributory factor to mortality and morbidity. While it may be the immediate and direct result of the hemorrhage, more often it develops some 4–12 days after the onset either before or after surgery hence the term delayed cerebral ischemia. Approximately 25% of patients develop clinical evidence of delayed ischemia and of these 25% die. About 10% of the survivors remain permanently disabled. Several factors contribute to the development of ischemia one of which is *vasospasm* which is arterial narrowing on angiography. Such narrowing occurs in up to 60% of patients after subarachnoid hemorrhage and it may be either focal or diffuse. The pathogenesis of vasospasm is complex and may in part be due to the action of various vasoconstrictive substances, e.g. serotonin, prostaglandin, either released from the blood vessel wall or from the blood clot within the CSF. As a result of the action of these substances arteriopathic changes may occur. Additional risk factors include *hypovolemia* which may develop as a result of excess renal secretion of sodium rather than a dilutional effect from inappropriate antidiuretic hormone secretion and a reduced cerebral perfusion pressure consequent upon an intracranial hematoma or hydrocephalus which may cause an elevation in the intracranial pressure.

Infarction occurs most commonly in the region of the brain supplied by the artery on which the aneurysm is situated, but it is not infrequently more widespread.

Hydrocephalus develops late, i.e. months or even years after the hemorrhage in some 10% of patients.

If the subarachnoid hemorrhage is not massive and the patient survives, the blood is gradually absorbed and the pia-arachnoid becomes permanently stained brownish/yellow because of residual hemosiderin within macrophages. If there are recurrent episodes of subarachnoid hemorrhage, the outer cortical layers become more deeply pigmented because of the presence of iron containing macrophages: this condition is known as *subpial hemosiderosis*, and is seen more commonly in association with vascular malformations than aneurysms. *Epilepsy* may occur at any stage after subarachnoid hemorrhage especially if a hematoma has caused cortical damage.

A number of operative techniques have been developed for the management of ruptured aneurysm. These include direct clipping of the aneurysm neck or if this is not possible the techniques of wrapping and trapping may be used. Increasingly endovascular techniques using coil embolization, balloon remodeling and balloon occlusion are being used. Factors that determine the prognosis include age, amount of subarachnoid hemorrhage on CT scan, loss of consciousness, clinical condition on admission and the presence of preexisting hypertension or arterial disease. A particular conundrum is the management of unruptured aneurysms, data suggesting that the risk of rupture depends on the size, site and occurrence of a subarachnoid hemorrhage from a previously treated source. There is evidence that for small aneurysms (less than 7 mm in diameter) without a previous history of subarachnoid hemorrhage the annual risk of rupture is 0.1% whereas for aneurysms greater than 10 mm in diameter and at certain sites such as the basilar bifurcation the annual risk of rupture is between 1 and 3.5%. When two or more members of a family have a history of cerebral aneurysms or subarachnoid hemorrhage then other members of that family (over the age of 25 years) have an increased risk of harboring an intracranial aneurysm (about 8% or four times greater than the rest of the population). A similar increased risk occurs with patients with a genetic predisposition although evidence suggests that for small aneurysms the risk is low.

Other types of aneurysm

Atheroma may be the cause of *fusiform* enlargement of a major cerebral artery; such aneurysms rarely rupture. A rare but not unimportant entity is widespread *ectasia* of major cerebral arteries (Fig. 5.38). This may be partly attributable to atheroma, but it seems more likely that there is a generalized inherent defect of the blood vessel wall. When ectasia is severe, a tortuous basilar artery may produce considerable distortion of the ventral surface of the brainstem. It has also been suggested that ectasia of the basilar artery and its increased pulsation in the posterior fossa may be the occasional cause of hydrocephalus. *Mycotic aneurysms* produced by infected emboli may also occur on a cerebral artery. They are found more commonly in adults than in children, and they are said to be multiple in 20% of cases. The aneurysms are most commonly due to *streptococci* and *staphylococci*, and the organisms spread rapidly from the impacted embolus to the blood vessel wall, which then undergoes acute inflammatory changes, necrosis and aneurysmal dilation. Mycotic aneurysms are said to occur in between 3 and 10% of patients with infective endocarditis. Fungal mycotic aneurysms are also encountered, most often in patients with *aspergillosis* or *candidiasis*. They tend to be larger than aneurysms caused by bacteria and are found most commonly on the major arteries at the base of the brain. They are often multiple and the nasal sinus or heart are frequent sources of infection.

Dissection aneurysm of the aorta is the result of extensive hemorrhage into the media weakened by hypertension and idiopathic cystic medial necrosis. The hemorrhage usually commences as a tear in the ascending aorta and extends into the abdominal

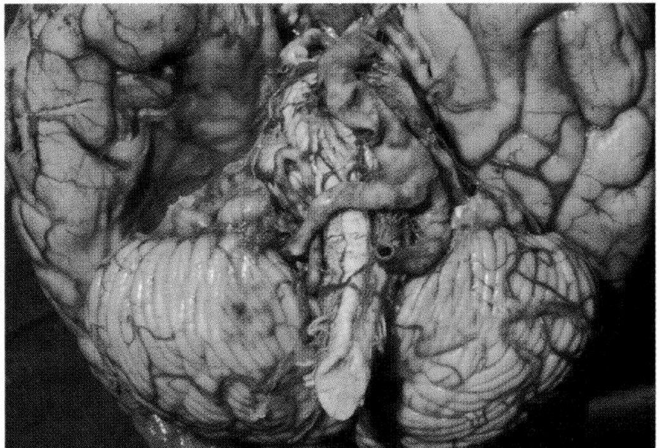

Figure 5.38 Arterial ectasia. The basilar and left vertebral arteries are dilated and tortuous.

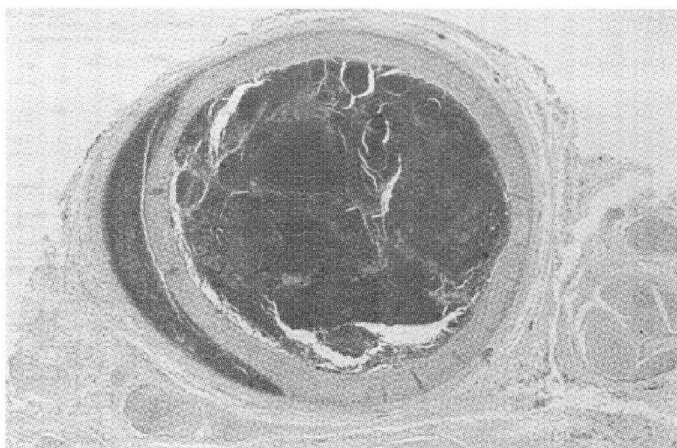

Figure 5.39 Dissecting aneurysm of internal carotid artery after blunt force trauma to the neck.

aorta. The dissection may extend into the extracranial cervical arteries, narrowing their lumens and impairing blood flow to the brain. Dissecting aneurysms of the carotid arteries in the neck and their major intracranial branches may be due to extension from the aorta, develop spontaneously, or be due to neck injury (Fig. 5.39) or follow a carotid puncture or angiography. Dissecting aneurysms of the intracranial arteries are rare, and usually occur in children and young adults: causes include head injury, migraine, arteritis, fibromuscular dysplasia and inflammation. Following dissection, the aneurysm may rupture and cause subarachnoid hemorrhage or produce thrombotic occlusion of the blood vessel, and infarction of the tissue supplied by the affected artery.

Vascular malformation of the brain and spinal cord

These may range in size from capillary angiomas in which there is an area of dilated capillaries to large lesions composed of a plexus of rather thick walled vascular channels - *arteriovenous malformations* (Fig. 5.40). A third type is that of cavernous angioma which is a plum-colored, sponge-like mass composed of a collection of blood-filled spaces. These lesions occur most commonly in young adults and are usually on the surface of the brain or the spinal cord, but they are sometimes restricted to the deeper structures of the brain and do not reach the surface.

Between 40 and 60% of patients with arteriovenous malformation present with hemorrhage often with an intracerebral or intraventricular component. They tend to bleed in younger patients, i.e. between 20 and 40 years and are less likely to have a fatal outcome, and unlike subarachnoid hemorrhage, do

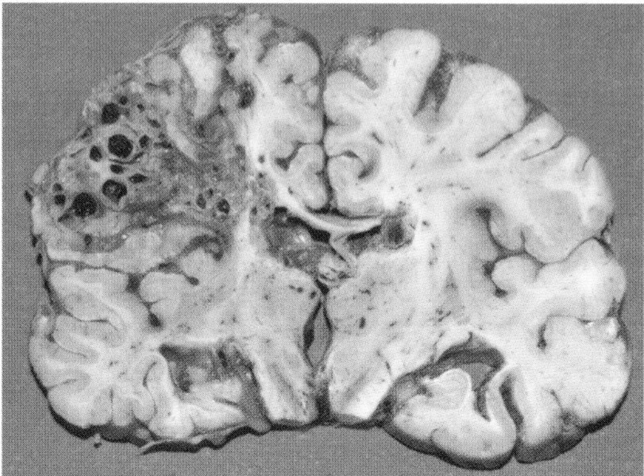

Figure 5.40 Arteriovenous malformation of cerebrum.

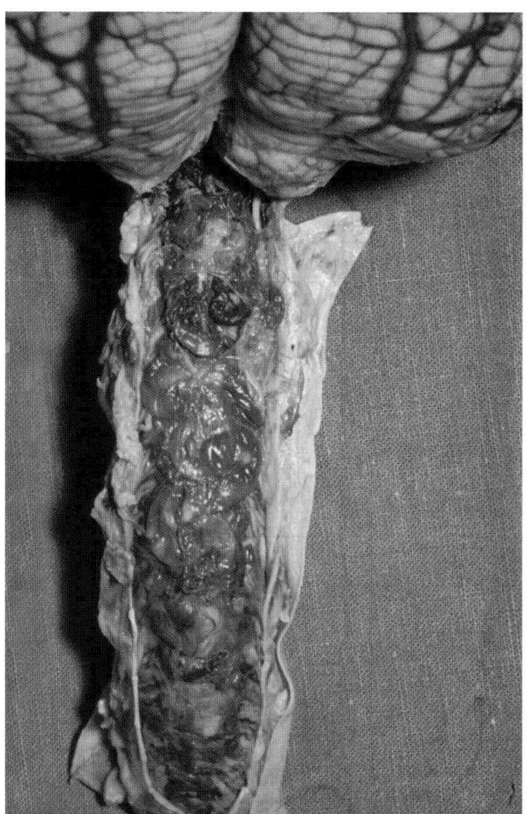

Figure 5.41 Arteriovenous malformation of spinal cord.

not have the complications of vasospasm and delayed ischemia. The annual risk of patients without a history of previous hemorrhage is between 2 and 4% and the mortality from hemorrhage is in contrast to rupture of a saccular aneurysm, relatively low at between 10 and 15%. Patients may also present with epilepsy, neurological deficits, headaches and diagnosis is usually achieved by CT scan, MRI and confirmed by angiography. Management includes incision, stereotactic radiosurgery and embolization.

Cavernous angiomas are said to occur in some 0.5% of the normal population. They may present with hemorrhage, epilepsy or with focal neurological signs and the risk of bleeding is about 1% per year.

Other anteriovenous malformations include aneurysm of the *vein of Galen* in which patients either present in the neonatal period with severe high output cardiac failure due to the associated arteriovenous shunt, in infancy with cranial enlargement due to obstructive hydrocephalus, or in childhood with subarachnoid hemorrhage. In the Sturge–Weber syndrome which is angiomatosis affecting the facial skin, eyes and leptomeninges and dural arteriovenous fistulae, arterial blood drains directly into either a venous sinus, cortical vein or a combination of both: one such example is a caroticocavernous fistula which may follow trauma or rupture of a saccular aneurysm of the carotid artery. Spontaneous closure frequently occurs although embolization with a detachable balloon may be required.

Rupture of a spinal malformation (Fig. 5.41) may lead to subarachnoid or intramedullary hemorrhage. The latter is associated with the rapid onset of severe neurological symptoms, depending on the level of the malformation. The condition known as subacute necrotic myelitis, or *Foix–Alajouanine disease*, which most often occurs in elderly males, consists of small blood vessels within the lumbosacral parts of the spinal cord and in the adjacent subarachnoid space have markedly thickened walls that may be cuffed by lymphocytes. The structural changes that occur are those of small, often multiple, infarcts within the spinal cord, and often a progressive degree of paraparesis.

CHAPTER 6

BACTERIAL INFECTIONS

James A R Nicoll

GENERAL PRINCIPLES OF INFECTION

Many different types of organisms including bacteria, viruses, fungi and others can infect the central nervous system and its coverings. Bacterial infections are dealt with in this chapter and viral, fungal and other infections are dealt with in the following chapter. There are certain features that are relevant to all infections. The brain and spinal cord are relatively well-protected by bone and by the dura from infective agents and consequently blood-borne (hematogenous) spread is more common than direct spread of infection. Direct spread of infection may occur following a skull fracture or as a result of spread of infection from a localized infection in the middle ear, air sinuses or the bone of the skull or spine. A few infective agents, particularly viruses, gain access to the central nervous system (CNS) by spread along peripheral nerves. Once infection becomes established in the CNS local defense mechanisms are relatively ineffective and if micro-organisms gain access to the cerebrospinal fluid (CSF) they can disseminate rapidly throughout the subarachnoid space and the ventricles. Immuno-compromised individuals are susceptible to overwhelming infection, often from organisms that are relatively non-pathogenic in the immunocompetent (i.e. opportunistic infections). Points to note in the autopsy of infection are listed in Table 6.1. Sites of infection are given in Table 6.2, and cytological and biochemical findings in various infections are listed in Table 6.3.

ACUTE BACTERIAL MENINGITIS

In acute bacterial meningitis there is spread of bacteria through the subarachnoid space over the brain surface, within the ventricular system, and over the surface of the spinal cord accompanied by an acute inflammatory exudate (predominantly neutrophil polymorphs). Acute bacterial meningitis is a medical emergency and rapid clinical and laboratory diagnosis is necessary. CSF examination with microscopy for bacteria and characterization of inflammatory cells, biochemistry and culture and/or polymerase chain reaction (PCR) is necessary. Appropriate antibiotic therapy, if given sufficiently early, can be life-saving and prevent permanent disability. Increasingly, immunization against the common causative organisms of bacterial meningitis is becoming available for prevention of the disease.

Epidemiology and clinical features

Clinical presentation of meningitis in adults and children includes headache, vomiting, pyrexia, neck

Table 6.1 The autopsy in infection of the central nervous system and its coverings

Initial examination
- Assess clinical history and review existing microbiological information.
- Discuss sampling procedures and specimen handling with microbiologists.
- Assess risk of the procedure to the staff involved (e.g. HIV, TB).

Macroscopic examination
- Search for systemic evidence of sepsis.
- Search for localized focus of infection (middle ears, air sinuses, bone of skull and spine).

Examination of the central nervous system
- Is there pus in the extradural, subdural or subarachnoid compartments?
- Assess brain swelling and effects of raised intracranial pressure (e.g. internal herniations and brainstem compression).
- Are there focal abscesses?
- Is there a necrotizing encephalitis?

Sampling for microbiology
- Sample CSF with a sterile needle and syringe through the skin via a cisternal puncture before opening the scalp or from the lateral ventricles through the corpus callosum after removing the calvaria and opening the dura.
- In suspected meningitis, after removing the calvaria and opening the dura, lift the frontal lobes and swab the base of the brain – even if there is no visible pus.
- Swab visible pus at any location.
- In suspected encephalitis without macroscopic lesions, take samples of cerebral gray and white matter from several different locations, including medial temporal cortex (herpes simplex virus).

Table 6.2 Sites of infection

Bone	Osteitis, osteomyelitis
Extradural space	Epidural (extradural) abscess
Dura	Pachymeningitis
Subdural space	Subdural empyema
Subarachnoid space	Meningitis (strictly speaking, leptomeningitis)
Intracerebral	Cerebral abscess, encephalitis
Intraventricular	Ventriculitis

stiffness, photophobia and a skin rash. Seizures and focal neurological signs, including cranial nerve palsies, may also occur. Imaging is not helpful in the acute stage of infection but may show meningeal enhancement in later stages. Without effective antibiotic therapy there is rapid progression to coma and mortality is high.

The common causative organisms of acute bacterial meningitis are commensals of the upper respiratory tract mucosal epithelium. In the developing countries meningitis occurs in epidemics but in developed countries meningitis is usually sporadic. In most cases bacteria reach the meninges by hematogenous spread. In such cases there is therefore always a bacteremia and sometimes a septicemia, which is particularly common in epidemics of meningococcal meningitis.

Meningococci (*Neisseria meningitidis*) are spread by droplet infection from carriers who harbor the bacteria in the nasopharynx. Meningococcal infection can cause death as a result of septicemia before there is any evidence of meningitis. An important feature of meningococcal septicemia is a hemorrhagic rash and a common terminal event in rapidly fatal cases is adrenal hemorrhage and circulatory collapse (Waterhouse–Friderichsen syndrome).

The commonest cause of bacterial meningitis in adults is *Streptococcus pneumoniae* (pneumococcus). The elderly, the immunocompromised and patients who have had a splenectomy are particularly susceptible to pneumococcal infection. Clinical progression of the disease is rapid and is associated

Table 6.3 CSF findings in infections of the CNS

Infection	Cytology	Protein	Glucose
Acute bacterial meningitis (early)	Polymorph neutrophils	Raised	Decreased
Acute bacterial meningitis (late)	Polymorph neutrophils, lymphocytes and macrophages	Raised	Decreased
TB meningitis	Lymphocytes and macrophages (polymorph neutrophils early in the disease)	Raised	Decreased
Neurosyphilis	Sparse lymphocytes	Raised	Normal
Viral meningitis	Lymphocytes	Normal	Normal
Fungal meningitis	Polymorph neutrophils, lymphocytes and macrophages	Raised	Decreased
Neoplastic meningitis	Neoplastic cells, scanty lymphocytes and macrophages	Raised	Decreased
Viral encephalitis	Lymphocytes	Normal	Normal
Brain abscess, subdural empyema, epidural abscess	Sparse cells, variable in type	Raised	Normal

with septicemia, the organisms originating in the respiratory tree.

In neonates initial non-specific symptoms such as irritability, vomiting and poor feeding progress rapidly to coma. There may be nuchal rigidly, a bulging fontanelle and evidence of septic shock. The causative organism is usually *Escherichia coli* or *group B Streptococcus*, although other bacteria can also cause neonatal meningitis. The route of entry is usually oral, from infected amniotic fluid, the maternal genital tract during childbirth or from the skin of carers following birth. The organism usually reaches the CNS by hematogenous spread. However, organisms may gain direct access to the meninges in neonates with open spina bifida defects. The causative organisms and the main routes of spread are given in Tables 6.4 and 6.5.

Patients who have survived an episode of acute bacterial meningitis may have a number of sequelae which result in disability. These include adhesions in the subarachnoid space resulting in obstructive hydrocephalus, cranial nerve palsies due to vascular involvement, epilepsy and cognitive dysfunction.

Macroscopic appearances

The brain is swollen and there is vascular congestion. There may be evidence of transtentorial and cerebellar tonsillar herniation accompanied by brainstem compression. A purulent exudate may be seen beneath the leptomeninges in the subarachnoid space and may be present over the convexities of the cerebral hemispheres (Fig. 6.1). The inflammatory exudate has a particular tendency to collect at the base of the cerebrum and over the cerebellum (Figs 6.2 and 6.3). If antibiotic treatment was given even just a few hours prior to death pus may not be detectable macroscopically, even if the meningitis was the cause of death. The ventricular system may be compressed as a consequence of brain swelling or may be dilated if accumulation of pus within the ventricular system (ventriculitis) has impeded the CSF flow (obstructive hydrocephalus) (Fig. 6.4). It should be noted that age-related collagenous thickening and opacification of the leptomeninges has a parasagittal distribution and should not be confused with the macroscopic appearances of meningitis.

Table 6.4 Routes of spread of bacteria to cause meningitis

- Hematogenous
- Spread from the skull (chronic osteitis, sinusitis, middle ear infection)
- Fracture of the skull base provides a route of entry of bacteria from air sinuses to the subarachnoid space
- Penetrating head injuries with a compound fracture of the skull provide a route of access for bacteria from the external environment
- Iatrogenic. Occasional accidental introduction of bacteria directly into the CSF due to invasive procedures such as lumbar puncture, ventricular CSF shunts and neurosurgery

Table 6.5 Common causative organisms in acute bacterial meningitis

- *Neisseria meningitidis* (particularly in young adults)
- *Haemophilus influenzae* (particularly in children)
- *Streptococcus pneumoniae* (particularly in the elderly)
- *Escherichia coli* and group B streptococci (neonates)

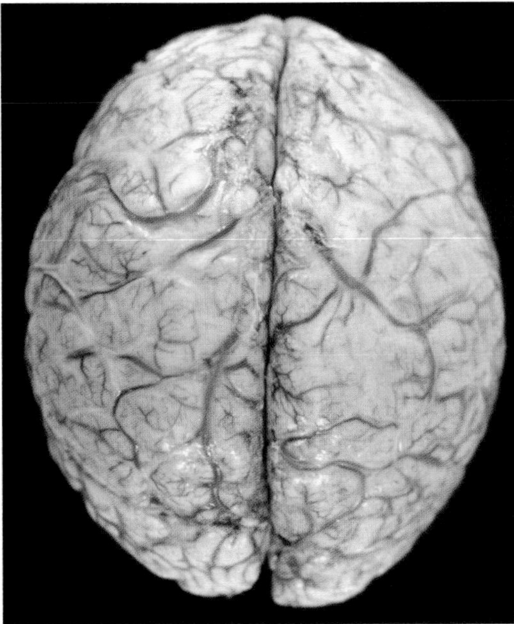

Figure 6.1 Acute bacterial meningitis. Opaque purulent exudate beneath the leptomeninges in the subarachnoid space over the convexities of the cerebral hemispheres.

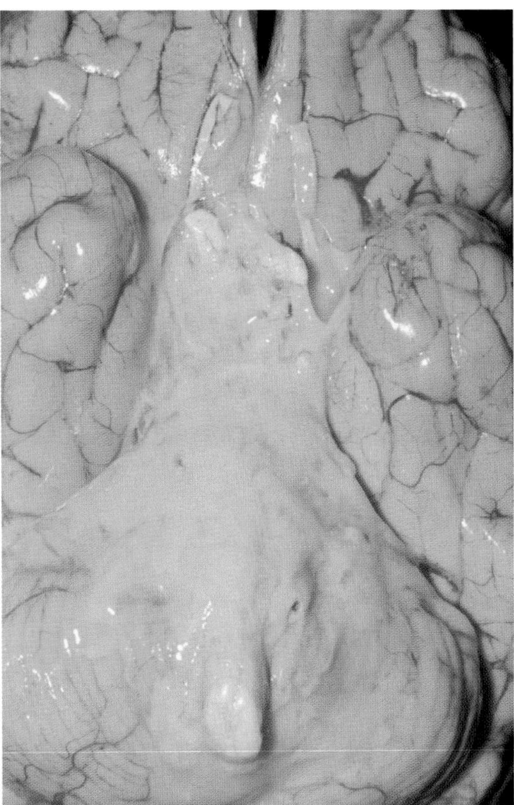

Figure 6.2 Acute bacterial meningitis. Inflammatory exudate tends at the base of the cerebrum and over the cerebellum.

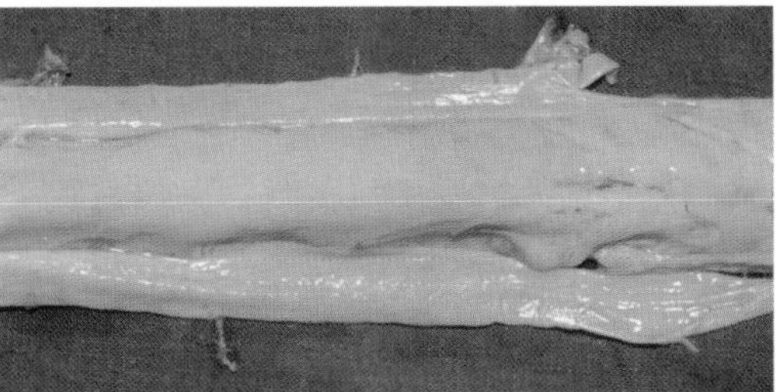

Figure 6.3 Acute bacterial meningitis. Pus within the subarachnoid space over the surface of the spinal cord.

Dissection of the brain may reveal small infarcts due to thrombosis of penetrating arteries or evidence of venous thrombosis.

Microscopic appearances

Microscopic examination shows an inflammatory exudate consisting predominantly of neutrophil

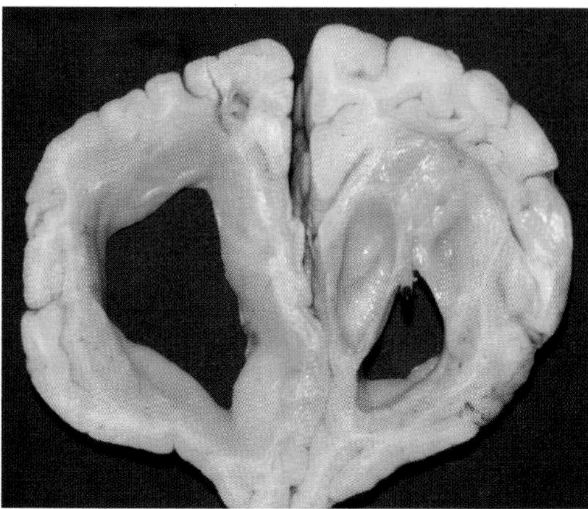

Figure 6.4 Acute bacterial meningitis. Accumulation of pus within the ventricular system can impede the CSF flow and cause an obstructive hydrocephalus. This is an example of acute bacterial meningitis in an infant.

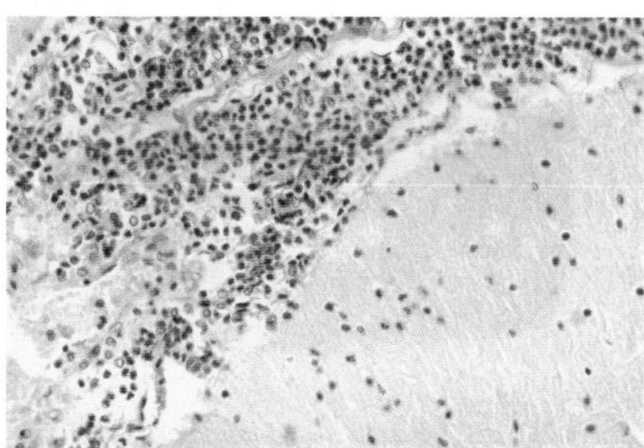

Figure 6.5 Acute bacterial meningitis. There is an acute inflammatory exudate (above left) consisting predominantly of neutrophil polymorphs in the subarachnoid space overlying the brain surface (below right). H&E.

polymorphs in the subarachnoid space (Fig. 6.5). As noted on macroscopic examination, the exudate tends to be more marked over the base of the cerebral hemispheres and over the cerebellum. If the infection persisted during life for more than a few days there may also be lymphocytes, plasma cells and macrophages. The walls of blood vessels crossing the subarachnoid space may be involved in the inflammatory process (vasculitis) (Fig. 6.6) but the underlying brain parenchyma is usually not involved. Thrombosis of small blood vessels affected by inflammation is common and may result in small superficial infarcts. Gram-stained sections may reveal the causative bacteria; however, if antibiotics were given even if only shortly prior to death, then bacteria are not likely to be detectable histologically.

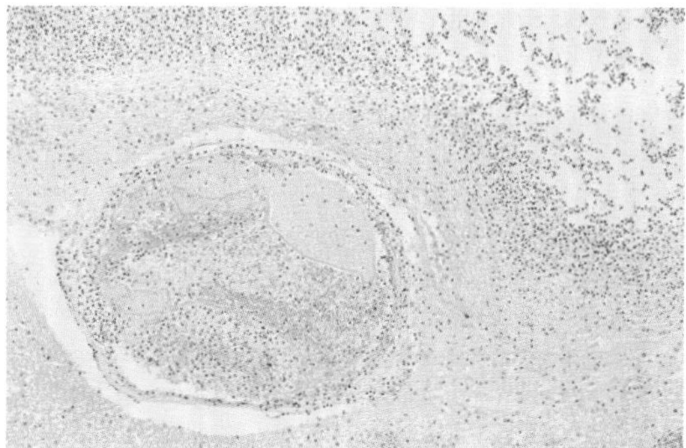

Figure 6.6 Acute bacterial meningitis. Involvement of blood vessels crossing the subarachnoid space by the acute inflammatory process (i.e. vasculitis) may result in small superficial infarcts or ischemic damage to cranial nerves. H&E.

BRAIN ABSCESS

A brain abscess is a focal infection of the brain by bacteria with an associated acute inflammatory reaction. Common organisms are listed in Table 6.6. It is essentially similar to an abscess elsewhere in the body but is the cause of serious problems

Table 6.6 Brain abscess

- Common organisms in brain abscess
  - *Streptococcus milleri*
  - Other streptococci
  - Staphylococci (*S. aureus* is particularly associated with post-traumatic abscess and spinal lesions)
  - Bacteroides
  - Coliforms
  - *Nocardia*
- Infections are often mixed
- It is important to note that brain abscesses may be due to a number of other organisms, particularly in the immunosuppressed, including mycobacteria (see Table 6.7), *Toxoplasma gondii* and fungi (see Chapter 7)

associated with an intracranial expanding lesion, including focal brain damage and raised intracranial pressure. Clinical presentation includes headache, pyrexia, focal neurological signs and seizures. Imaging reveals focal lesions the features of which depend on the maturity of the abscess. An organizing abscess can appear as a ring-enhancing lesion with a differential diagnosis of a glioblastoma. A biopsy may be required to clarify the diagnosis and has the additional benefit of obtaining organisms for microbiological culture and determination of antibiotic sensitivities. Mortality and morbidity are high. Neurological sequelae are common in survivors and include epilepsy, focal neurological signs and cognitive impairment.

The route of infection is either hematogenous or by direct spread. Hematogenous spread occurs from a focus of infection in the lungs or heart, in particular the valves (bacterial endocarditis). Children with congenital heart disease and a right to left shunt are vulnerable because organisms in the blood can bypass the filter of the pulmonary circulation. Intravenous drug abusers are at risk because of introduction of organisms directly into the bloodstream from contaminated needles. Other risk factors for brain abscess include head injury, neurosurgery and immunodeficiency. Direct spread of infection may occur from a focus of infection in the middle ear (chronic suppurative otitis media) or air sinuses. The presence of multiple brain abscesses usually indicates hematogenous spread of organisms (Fig. 6.7). However, direct spread usually results in a single abscess close to the focus of infection such as in the case of a temporal lobe abscess resulting from infection in the middle ear (Fig. 6.8).

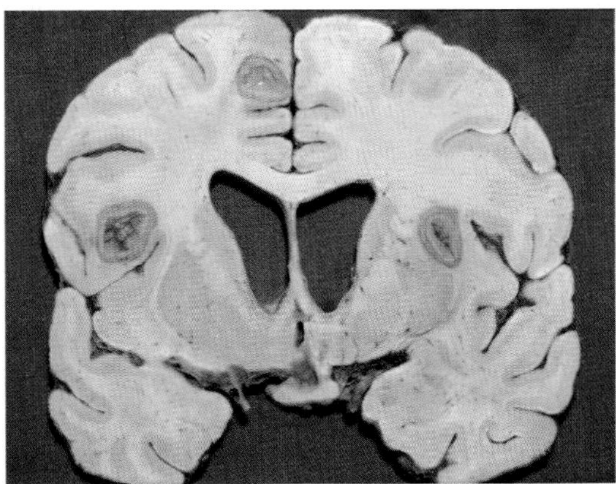

Figure 6.7 Brain abscess. Multiple cerebral abscesses are usually the result of hematogenous spread of infection, in this case from a focus of infection in the lung.

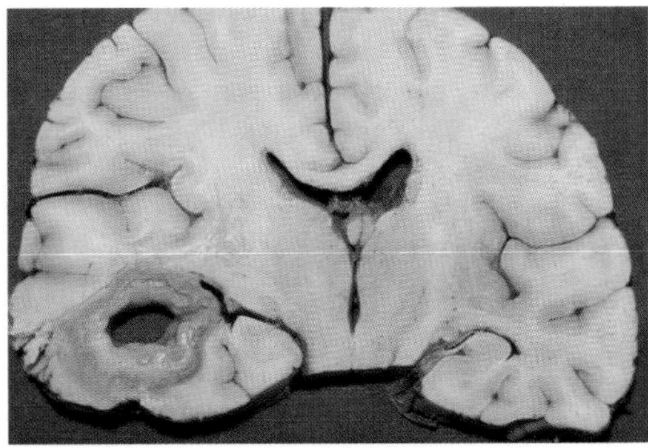

Figure 6.8 Brain abscess. Direct spread of infection to the brain usually results in a single abscess, in this case in the temporal lobe as a result of spread of infection from the middle ear.

Stages in the evolution of a brain abscess

1. Focal cerebritis (1–2 days). An ill-defined area of edema with a polymorph infiltrate and bacteria but without necrosis.
2. Acute brain abscess (2–7 days) (Fig. 6.9). Focal necrosis containing acute inflammatory debris (pus) mixed with bacteria. The surrounding brain tissue is edematous with a developing astrocytic and microglial reaction.

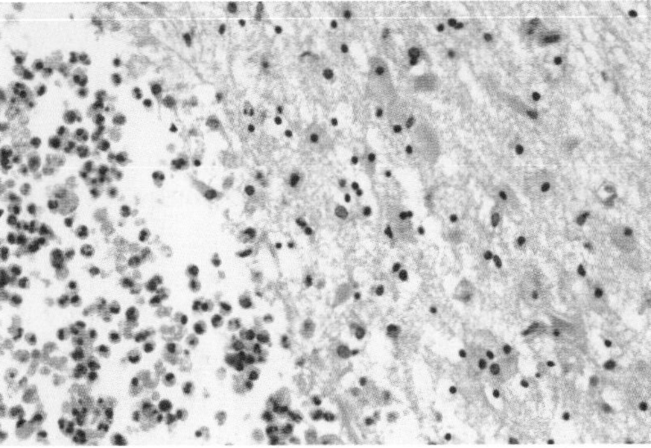

Figure 6.9 Brain abscess. In an acute abscess, within the first few days of infection there is focal necrosis containing acute inflammatory debris (lower left) mixed with bacteria. The surrounding brain tissue (above right) is edematous with a reactive gliosis. H&E.

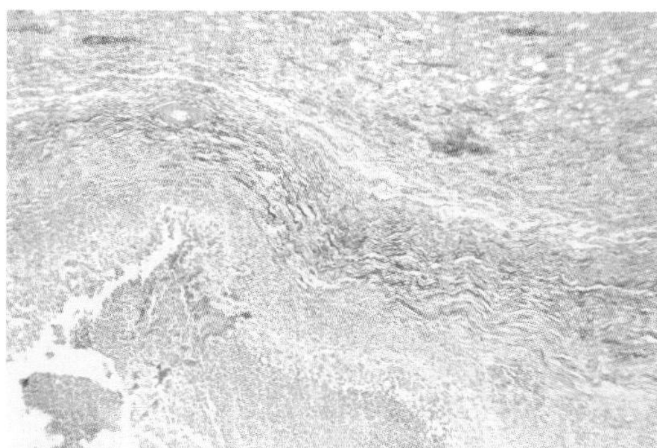

Figure 6.10 Brain abscess. In a chronic abscess, several weeks after the initial infection a collagenous capsule (red) separates the abscess cavity (below) from the surrounding reactive brain tissue (above). Van Gieson.

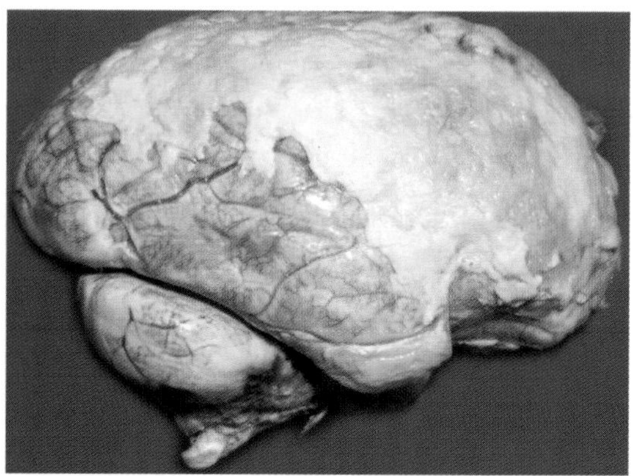

Figure 6.11 Subdural empyema. When an acute inflammatory exudate gains access to the subdural space it spreads extensively over the brain surface between the leptomeninges and the dura.

3. Chronic abscess (1–2 weeks onwards) (Fig. 6.10). Encapsulation of the abscess takes place progressively with the formation of granulation tissue which matures into a fibrous wall. The central zone of necrotic debris, neutrophil polymorphs and bacteria is surrounded by a capsule containing collagen and proliferating fibroblasts, with new blood vessel formation, hyperplastic and hypertrophic glial cells (astrocytes and microglia) and a chronic inflammatory infiltrate of lymphocytes, plasma cells and macrophages. Surrounding the capsule the brain tissue is edematous and gliotic.

EPIDURAL ABSCESS AND SUBDURAL EMPYEMA

Epidural abscess and subdural empyema are acute bacterial infections related to the outer and inner surfaces of the dura, respectively. Pachymeningitis is the appropriate term when the dura itself is involved by the infection.

Epidural (extradural) abscess occurs most commonly in the spine. The abscess extends over several vertebral levels and results in compression of spinal roots or the spinal cord. Infection may be due to direct spread from a local infection such as vertebral osteomyelitis or due to hematogenous spread from elsewhere (e.g. a cutaneous abscess). Infection may also be iatrogenic or result from trauma. An underlying debilitating condition such as diabetes, renal failure, corticosteroid therapy, neoplastic disease or intravenous drug abuse is frequently present. *Staphylococcus aureus, Streptococci* and coliforms are the commonest causative organisms. Histology shows necrotic acute inflammatory debris which evolves into granulation tissue. Intracranial epidural abscesses result from direct spread of infection from a focus of chronic osteitis in the skull, chronic suppurative otitis media, mastoiditis or sinusitis. Epidural abscesses within the cranial cavity tend to be small because the dura is firmly attached to the skull.

Subdural empyema results when infection gains access to the subdural space in which it can spread widely (Fig. 6.11). Subdural empyema is most commonly intracranial where it presents with the clinical effects of an intracranial mass lesion. The routes of infection are generally similar to those for epidural abscess (see above). *Streptococci* and *Staphylococci* are common causative organisms. Clinical presentation of intracranial subdural empyema includes headache, pyrexia, nausea and vomiting, impaired consciousness, seizures and focal neurological signs. Spinal subdural empyema is relatively uncommon and presents with localized pain or the effects of spinal cord compression. At autopsy large collections of pus may be present in the subdural space. Subdural pus can be wiped off the leptomeningeal surface of the brain in contrast to pus in the subarachnoid space (acute bacterial meningitis) which is retained in position by the leptomeninges.

TUBERCULOSIS

Involvement of the central nervous system by *Mycobacterium tuberculosis* is by spread of infection from elsewhere in the body. In developed countries tuberculosis (TB) is now relatively uncommon as a consequence of immunization programs and high standards of living. However, it still occurs, particularly in the economically deprived, vagrants, the immunosuppressed and immigrants from countries with a high prevalence of TB, and remains a major problem in many of the developing countries. TB affects the CNS in three principal ways: tuberculous meningitis, tuberculous abscess (tuberculoma) and spinal osteomyelitis.

Tuberculous meningitis

Tuberculous meningitis is usually caused by hematogenous dissemination of organisms from a site of infection elsewhere in the body, such as the lungs or the gastrointestinal tract. Tuberculous meningitis may be a manifestation of miliary TB or secondary to rupture into the CSF of a small tuberculous focus in the choroid plexus or on the surface of the brain. Occasionally TB gains access to the CNS as a result of suppurative infection penetrating through the dura from a tuberculous lesion in the vertebral column.

The clinical presentation of tuberculous meningitis is subacute with a history of several weeks of nausea, vomiting, malaise and headache with seizures, cranial nerve palsies and other focal neurological deficits. Examination of the CSF is required to make the diagnosis. There is usually a lymphocytosis with a diminished glucose concentration and an increased protein concentration. Traditionally, definitive diagnosis required either identification of alcohol and acid-fast bacilli on Ziehl–Neelsen stained preparations or by culture which takes several weeks. However, now *M. tuberculosis* can be detected in the CSF rapidly by the use of PCR.

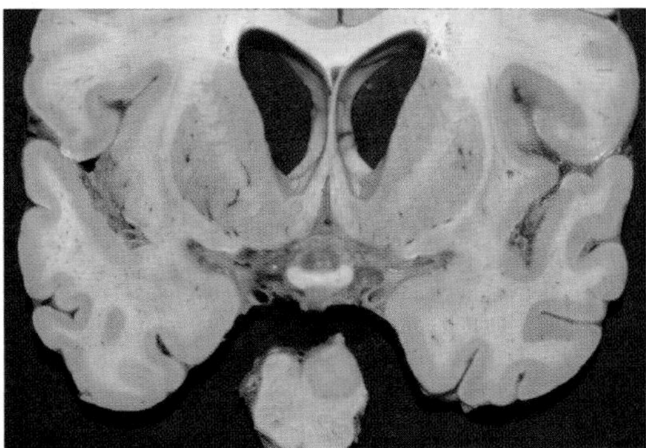

Figure 6.12 Tuberculous meningitis and tuberculoma. A gelatinous or caseous exudate extends over the brain surface in the subarachnoid space (tuberculous meningitis) with a particular tendency for the exudate to accumulate at the base of the brain. Note the tuberculoma, which is a circumscribed tuberculous abscess in the dorsolateral sector of the medulla.

Tuberculous meningitis is a subacute meningitis. Macroscopic examination shows a gelatinous or caseous exudate which is most abundant on the surface of the base of the brain (Fig. 6.12), within sulci and around the spinal cord. Small tubercles (1–2 mm in diameter) may be identified in the meninges. The ventricles may be dilated, reflecting hydrocephalus due to exudate obstructing the flow of CSF. The ventricular lining and the choroid plexus may also be involved.

On histological examination, the subarachnoid space and ventricles contain a chronic inflammatory infiltrate including lymphocytes, plasma cells and macrophages (Fig. 6.13 and Table 6.7). There may be granulomas with central caseous necrosis and surrounding epithelioid cells and multinucleated giant cells. In longstanding infection there may be organization of the exudate with proliferation of fibroblasts and formation of collagen. There may be involvement of superficial blood vessels by the inflammatory process (vasculitis) and arteritis with narrowing of the vessel lumen and intravascular thrombosis. These vascular changes may give rise to small superficial cortical infarcts and ischemic damage to cranial nerves. There may be small associated superficial cortical tuberculomas. Immunosuppressed patients with tuberculous meningitis are less likely to have a typical granulomatous

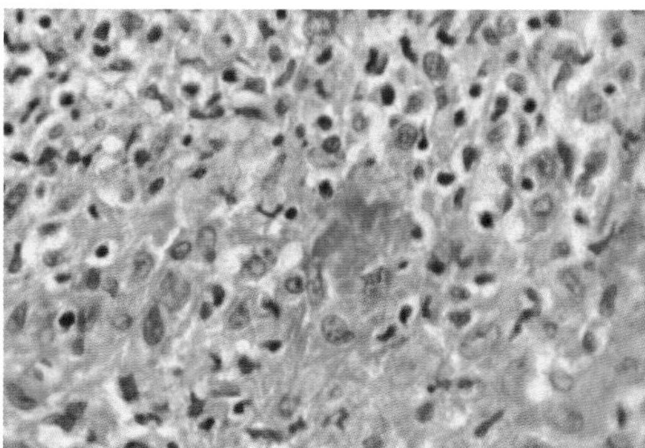

Figure 6.13 Tuberculous meningitis. The subarachnoid space contains a chronic inflammatory infiltrate including macrophages, lymphocytes and plasma cells. H&E.

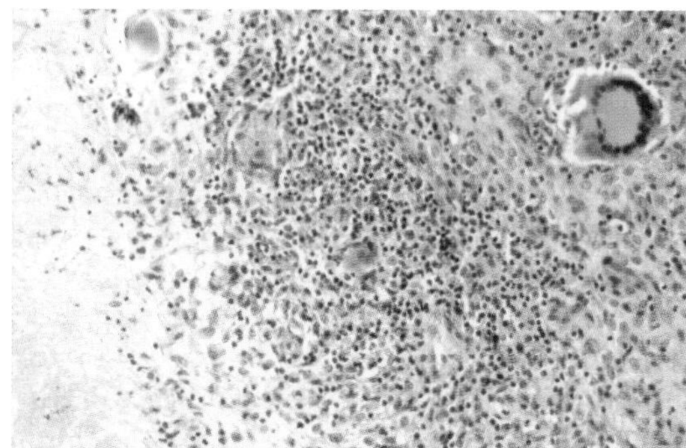

Figure 6.14 Tuberculoma. A localized mass of chronic inflammation including macrophages, lymphocytes, plasma cells and multinucleated giant cells. There may be a central zone of caseous necrosis. H&E.

Table 6.7 Differential diagnosis of granulomatous inflammation (meningitis or abscess)

- Tuberculosis (examine Ziehl–Neelsen stain)
- Fungi (examine PAS and Grocott stains)
- Neurosarcoidosis (after exclusion of an infective cause and a search for systemic evidence of sarcoid)
- Discuss with microbiologists: send fresh tissue for culture and/or PCR

inflammatory reaction. Mycobacteria may be detectable on Ziehl–Neelsen stained sections but this is unlikely in patients who have been treated with anti-tuberculous chemotherapy. Organisms are more likely to be visible in tuberculous meningitis occurring in immunosuppressed patients.

Tuberculoma

A tuberculoma is a chronic tuberculous abscess. Clinical presentation is subacute with focal neurological signs and symptoms, seizures and evidence of raised intracranial pressure. There may be systemic evidence of TB. Tuberculomas are very common lesions in developing countries where TB is rife. In some countries tuberculomas are the commonest form of intracranial mass lesions. Macroscopically, tuberculomas are circumscribed, encapsulated caseous masses (Fig. 6.12), usually in the cerebrum or cerebellum. Histologically, they are composed of a central zone of caseous necrosis surrounded by a collagenous capsule containing lymphocytes, macrophages, multinucleated giant cells and fibroblasts (Fig. 6.14). Longstanding lesions are likely to be calcified. There is a gliotic reaction in the surrounding brain.

Spinal tuberculous osteomyelitis

The spine is commonly involved in tuberculosis. Clinical presentation is subacute with back pain and malaise. Collapse of vertebral bodies affected by the inflammatory process may cause spinal cord compression. The inflammation may involve not only the vertebral bodies but also the intervertebral discs and extend into the epidural space to form an epidural abscess.

SYPHILIS

Syphilis is very uncommon in developed countries, although it may occur in the immunosuppressed, particularly in the context of AIDS. In primary syphilis there is proliferation of the spirochete *Treponema pallidum* at the site of entry to the body causing a chancre which subsequently heals. In secondary syphilis there is hematogenous spread of organisms which gain access to the CNS. There may be transient meningoencephalitis at this stage with an increase in lymphocytes and protein in the CSF. Neurosyphilis takes two principal forms: tertiary neurosyphilis and parenchymatous neurosyphilis. Tertiary syphilis occurs 7–10 years after the primary infection whereas parenchymatous neurosyphilis occurs later, as long as 20 years after the primary infection.

Tertiary neurosyphilis

Tertiary neurosyphilis may present as meningovascular syphilis or as a gumma.

Meningovascular syphilis takes the form of a subacute meningitis with lymphocytes and plasma cells in the subarachnoid space and a periarteritis. Extension of the inflammatory process into cranial and spinal nerves and the periarteritis may cause focal neurological signs such as optic atrophy or cranial nerve palsies.

Gummas occur in the meninges, particularly over the convexity of the cerebral hemispheres or over the cerebellum. They are usually attached to both the dura and the brain, in which they become embedded, but occasionally they are confined to the dura. Within the abnormal tissue there is necrosis, periarteritis and infiltration by lymphocytes and plasma cells.

Parenchymatous neurosyphilis

Parenchymatous neurosyphilis takes two forms: paretic dementia and tabes dorsalis. Both forms can co-exist.

Paretic dementia is a subacute encephalitis associated with a progressive cognitive decline. Histologically there is perivascular cuffing of blood vessels by lymphocytes and plasma cells within the CNS and in the subarachnoid space. In the cerebral cortex there is neuronal loss, reactive astrocytosis and proliferation of rod-shaped microglia. There is progressive cerebral atrophy with widening of sulci and dilation of the ventricles.

Tabes dorsalis is selective degeneration of the dorsal spinal roots and dorsal columns in the spinal cord (Fig. 6.15). It may be associated with chronic inflammation in the spinal leptomeninges and dorsal root ganglia. The lumbosacral nerve roots tend to be the most severely affected. Clinically, there is pain and paraesthesia with subsequent loss of pain and proprioceptive sensation leading to trauma and ulceration of the lower limbs.

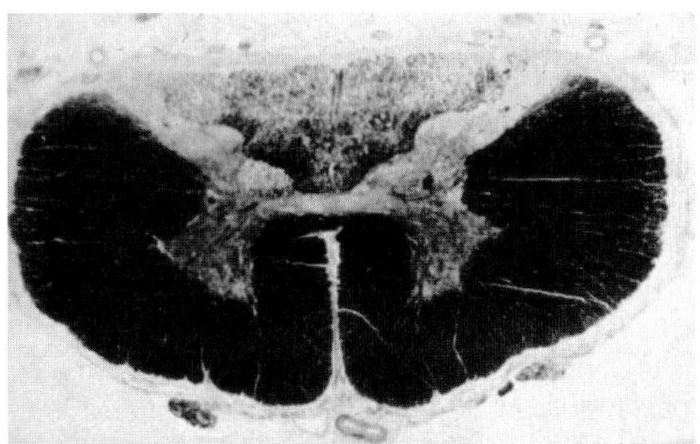

Figure 6.15 Syphilis. In tabes dorsalis there is selective degeneration of the dorsal spinal roots and dorsal columns in the spinal cord. There may be an associated chronic inflammatory infiltrate in the leptomeninges and dorsal root ganglia.

OTHER CAUSES OF CHRONIC MENINGITIS

Neurosarcoidosis is the term given to involvement of the CNS by sarcoidosis. Neurosarcoidosis is usually accompanied by widespread systemic disease but it may sometimes apparently be confined to the CNS. The chronic granulomatous inflammation typical of sarcoidosis may affect the leptomeninges, particularly at the base of the brain in the region of the hypothalamus, the optic nerves and infundibulum. The leptomeninges overlying the cerebellum may also be affected. Classically the granulomas of sarcoidosis are non-caseating. The inflammatory process may involve the cranial nerves leading to cranial nerve palsies. Diagnosis of neurosarcoidosis requires thorough exclusion of a specific and potentially treatable infective cause for the inflammation, and a search for clinical evidence of systemic involvement by sarcoidosis.

Neoplastic meningitis occurs when there is involvement of the subarachnoid space by tumour cells and can present with the clinical features of a subacute meningitis. Cranial nerve palsies are common. The neoplastic cells may be derived from a CNS tumour such as a glial tumor or a primitive neuroectodermal tumour. Alternatively, the cells may represent metastatic spread from neoplastic disease elsewhere in the body including carcinoma, melanoma and leukaemia/lymphoma. The diagnosis of neoplastic disease can be made by cytological examination of the CSF. Immunocytochemistry may be helpful in identifying the type of tumor in patients who have no other clinical evidence of malignant disease. Cytological investigation is therefore an essential part of the investigation of patients with subacute meningitis. In some patients with clinically suspected neoplastic disease several repeated attempts at sampling the CSF are required before neoplastic cells are identified. A meningeal biopsy is sometimes performed.

Lyme disease is due to infection with the spirochete *Borrelia burgdorferi* which is transmitted by bites from animal-borne ticks. Part of the multisystem manifestation of Lyme disease is a chronic meningoencephalitis.

Whipple's disease very rarely involves the CNS. There is infiltration of the basal ganglia and brainstem and the overlying leptomeninges by macrophages containing the Gram positive bacillus *Tropheryma whippelii.* Diagnosis can be confirmed by brain biopsy, or biopsy of the small intestine, and recognition of the characteristic organisms in macrophages and by PCR.

Chemical meningitis can result from intrathecal administration of drugs, contrast medium in neuroradiological studies, and following neurosurgery on cysts containing irritant material such as craniopharyngiomas, dermoid and epidermoid cysts.

CHAPTER 7

VIRAL AND OTHER INFECTIONS

James A R Nicoll

VIRAL INFECTIONS

Most viral infections of the central nervous system (CNS) are severe and have a high morbidity and mortality unless appropriate specific antiviral therapy is available, and is administered before brain damage has occurred. Fortunately, the CNS appears to be relatively protected from viral infections. Many of the viruses which do affect the CNS are common causes of systemic infection, such as herpes viruses and enteroviruses, and involvement of the CNS is relatively uncommon. When it does occur it is a medical emergency which requires rapid diagnosis and treatment in order to avoid irreversible brain damage. The diagnosis may be achieved by identification of viral DNA in the cerebrospinal fluid (CSF) by using polymerase chain reaction (PCR) analysis. Serological studies, identifying the antibodies generated by the host response to the virus in samples of serum and CSF, are also important. In the past, brain biopsy played an important role in the diagnosis of viral infections of the CNS, but this is now rarely performed and pathologists will more often encounter viral infections at autopsy. If a post mortem examination is to be performed on a patient with a suspected viral infection then liaison with the virologist is essential to ensure that appropriate samples are obtained. Fresh brain tissue, sampled bearing in mind the anatomical targets of the different viruses, is important, together with specimens of CSF and serum.

Viruses affect the nervous system in diverse ways. Some viruses affect specific cell types. For example, rabies virus and enteroviruses affect neurons. Other viruses affect both neurons and glial cells (e.g. herpes viruses and arboviruses). JC virus specifically infects oligodendrocytes to cause demyelination in progressive multifocal leukoencephalopathy.

Some viruses have characteristic anatomical patterns of involvement of the nervous system (Table 7.1). For example, herpes simplex virus type 1 (HSV-1) causes encephalitis which selectively involves the medial temporal lobes, cingulate gyrus and insular cortex. Cytomegalovirus encephalitis tends to involve the walls of the ventricles. Some enteroviruses specifically target lower motor neurons in the spinal cord and brainstem (poliomyelitis).

Table 7.1 Regions of the central nervous system affected by various viral infections

- Meningitis – infection restricted to the subarachnoid space and leptomeninges
- Encephalitis – involvement of the brain
- Meningoencephalitis – involvement of the meninges and brain
- Ventriculitis – involvement of walls of the ventricles
- Encephalomyelitis – involvement of brain and spinal cord
- Poliomyelitis – involvement of the gray matter of the spinal cord
- Radiculitis – involvement of nerve roots

Varicella zoster virus and herpes simplex virus become latent in sensory ganglia.

Viruses can have a variety of effects on cells, including cell lysis, latency, transformation, cell fusion and modification of the antigen composition of the infected cell. To be susceptible to infection by a particular virus the host cell must have specific receptors on its plasma membrane.

Different age groups are susceptible to different infections. Immunosuppressed patients are vulnerable to overwhelming infection with viruses that in immunocompetent people fail to cause disease of the nervous system or have only restricted involvement.

Routes of infection

Most viruses gain entry to the body through the mucous membranes of the respiratory or gastrointestinal tract. Infection through the skin also occurs, but usually via a bite or an abrasion or, iatrogenically, via a needle. Most viruses that affect the CNS replicate at an extraneural site such as submucosal lymphoid tissue in the intestine, in the muscle, or in subcutaneous tissue where virus has entered through the skin. The virus travels to the CNS most commonly by blood spread, following a viremia, when virus passes through the blood–CSF barrier into the subarachnoid space, or through the blood–brain barrier into the CNS parenchyma. Transport of viruses along peripheral nerves is an important route of entry to the CNS for some viruses, such as rabies virus, herpes simplex virus and varicella zoster virus. It has also been postulated that viruses may gain access to the CNS from the nasal mucosa via the olfactory bulbs and tracts. Once a virus has reached the subarachnoid space it can be easily disseminated via the CSF pathways. Cell-to-cell spread with transmission along axons is probably an important mechanism of spread of virus within the CNS. Viral involvement of the nervous system usually takes the form of an acute infection such as aseptic meningitis or encephalitis. Some viruses cause subacute or chronic infections, such as JC virus in progressive multifocal leukoencephalopathy and measles virus in subacute sclerosing panencephalitis.

Immunization programs for some viruses have dramatically reduced the prevalence of the associated diseases (e.g. poliomyelitis). Effective treatments are available for some viruses (herpes simplex virus and HIV) but for many viruses there is not yet any effective antiviral therapy.

Viral meningitis

Viral meningitis is usually a mild and self-limiting disease. It occurs particularly in children and is most frequently caused by one of the enteroviruses, including coxsackie virus and echovirus, and poliovirus in vulnerable populations. Infections occur most commonly in the summer. Since viral meningitis is infrequently fatal its pathology is rarely encountered. Histological examination (Fig. 7.1) reveals infiltration of the subarachnoid space by lymphocytes, plasma cells and macrophages. There may be mild cuffing of blood vessels in the superficial layers of the cortex by the inflammatory infiltrate.

Herpes virus infections

The herpes viruses are very common DNA viruses which are almost ubiquitous in many populations. The herpes viruses that affect the CNS include herpes simplex virus (HSV-1 and HSV-2), varicella zoster (VZV), cytomegalovirus (CMV), Epstein–Barr

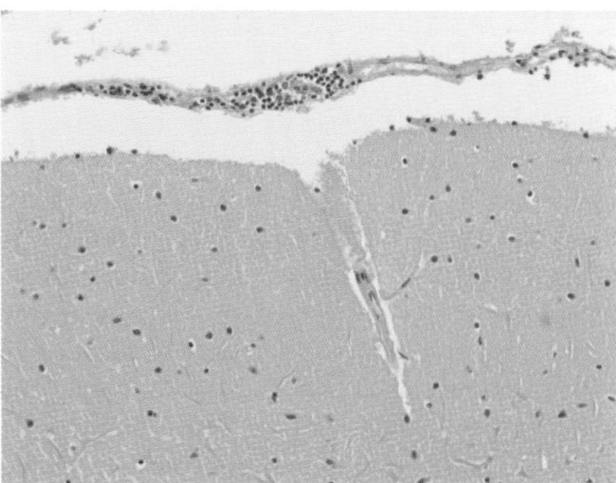

Figure 7.1 Viral meningitis. There is a scanty infiltrate of lymphocytes in the subarachnoid space. H&E.

virus (EBV) and human herpes virus 6. The B virus of monkeys can also affect the nervous system in humans. The herpes viruses exhibit the property of remaining latent within the body after primary infection. Latent virus persists, usually in peripheral sensory ganglia, throughout life and in some people reactivates to cause secondary or recurrent infection.

Herpes simplex virus

Primary infection

HSV-1 and HSV-2 both cause initial infection of the mucous membranes as a result of contact with infected secretions from reactivated virus (cold sores) from another person. HSV-1 is spread predominantly by oral contact and HSV-2 by genital contact. Primary infection is usually asymptomatic.

Establishment of latency in peripheral nerve ganglia

The virus replicates locally at the site of primary infection and is then transported by retrograde axonal transport along sensory nerves to the relevant sensory ganglion. After primary infection of the lips or mouth HSV-1 usually establishes latency in the trigeminal ganglion. Following infection of the genital tract HSV-2 usually establishes latency in the sacral dorsal root ganglia. In the latent state viral DNA and a specific form of mRNA (latency associated transcripts) are detectable in the nuclei of ganglionic neurons. There is no production of viral proteins during the latent phase.

Reactivation of virus

The virus becomes reactivated episodically and is transported along peripheral sensory axons to cause a recurrent superficial infection of the skin or mucosa close to the site of the primary infection (cold sores). The precise reason for reactivation of virus is unclear but triggers include stress, immunosuppression, local trauma and ultraviolet irradiation.

Entry of HSV into the CNS

The route by which HSV enters the brain to cause encephalitis is unclear. Possibilities that have been suggested include (1) spread of reactivated virus along the central projections from the sensory ganglia to reach the CNS, (2) reactivation of virus that had established latency in the brain during primary infection, (3) viremia and (4) along olfactory pathways from the nasal mucosa.

HSV-1 encephalitis

HSV-1 is the commonest cause of viral encephalitis (Table 7.2) in western Europe and the commonest non-epidemic viral encephalitis in the United States. HSV-1 encephalitis is an acute disease which presents with non-specific features of headache, pyrexia and drowsiness, progressing to coma. There may be focal neurological signs or seizures. If the disease process is sufficiently developed, imaging may show the characteristic anatomical distribution of pathology with signal changes in the temporal lobes. A definite diagnosis is based on detection of viral DNA in the CSF by PCR using specific primers. By comparing virus antibody titers in paired CSF and serum samples taken during the acute phase of the disease and 2 weeks later a retrospective diagnosis can be made by detection of a specific intrathecal immune response. However, specific antiviral therapy (such as acyclovir) has dramatically reduced the mortality and morbidity and it should therefore be given immediately on clinical suspicion of the disease. The quality of survival depends on treatment being instituted before brain damage has occurred. Untreated, the disease is rapidly progressive over a few days and is almost always fatal.

Macroscopic examination of the brain (Fig. 7.2) reveals the highly characteristic anatomical pattern of involvement of the temporal lobe (particularly the medial part), insular cortex and cingulate gyrus. The pattern of involvement is somewhat variable and may be asymmetric. The brain is swollen with hemorrhagic necrosis of the affected areas. If the patient survives an acute infection the necrotic tissue in the temporal lobes, the insula and the cingulate gyrus characteristically becomes shrunken and cystic. In immunosuppressed patients the encephalitic process may be more widely disseminated throughout the brain.

Histological examination of the brain of a patient who has died early in the course of the disease

Table 7.2 General features of viral encephalitis

Infiltration by inflammatory cells
- Lymphocytes, plasma cells and monocytes are located predominantly in the perivascular spaces (perivascular cuffing) in the brain and in the subarachnoid space
- Lymphocytes and plasma cells extend from perivascular spaces into brain parenchyma, particularly in regions where necrosis has occurred
- Sparse neutrophil polymorphs may be present in the early stages of infection

Abnormalities in neurons
- Viral inclusions
- Acute necrosis of infected neurons
- Neuronophagia
- Ischemic cell change

Viral inclusion bodies
- Can occur in neurons, astrocytes and oligodendrocytes
- Most are intranuclear
- Appear eosinophilic on hematoxylin and eosin stained sections
- Reflect accumulation of viral particles within the nucleus, displacing the nuclear chromatin to the periphery of the nucleus
- Occur, for example, in: herpes simplex encephalitis, CMV encephalitis ('owl's eye inclusions'), SSPE, rabies (Negri body)

Reactive changes in microglia
- Diffuse hyperplasia
- Hypertrophy and activation (express CD68 and MHC class II)
- Formation of rod cells with elongated nuclei
- Microglial nodules – small clusters of microglia mainly in the gray matter
- Numerous lipid-laden macrophages where necrosis has occurred

Reactive changes in astrocytes
- Diffuse hyperplasia
- Reactive astrocyte morphology in involved regions of the nervous system
- Progression to chronic fibrillary astrocytosis in affected areas in patients who have survived an acute infection

Ischemia and necrosis
- Features of global cerebral hypoxia–ischemia due to brain swelling and raised intracranial pressure
- Prominent necrosis with some viral infections (especially HSV-1), producing histological features of infarction combined with those of chronic inflammation

reveals a diffuse meningoencephalitis with lymphocytes and plasma cells throughout the subarachnoid space and perivascular cuffing by inflammatory cells throughout the CNS (Figs 7.3 and 7.4). There is hyperplasia of microglia and astrocytes. The disease process is characteristically localized to the temporal lobes, the insulae and the cingulate gyri where the inflammatory changes are particularly intense and often accompanied by necrosis (necrotizing encephalitis). Intranuclear viral inclusions (Fig. 7.5) are often detectable in neurons and less frequently within glial cells. Immunohistochemistry with specific HSV-1 antibodies is useful in establishing the diagnosis. Immunohistochemistry reveals viral antigen not only within the inclusions but also more widely within the cytoplasm of neurons and glial cells in affected areas (Fig. 7.6). Viral antigen is detectable up to 3 weeks after onset of the disease. Electron microscopy (Fig. 7.7) can be used to identify viral particles with the targetoid morphology characteristic of herpes virus but this is not specific for HSV-1. Viral DNA

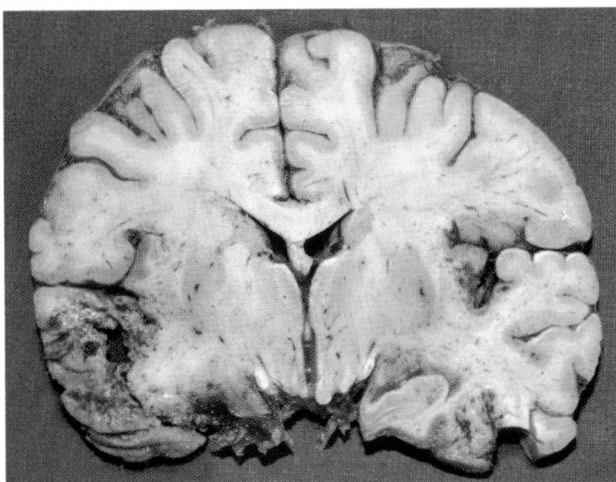

Figure 7.2 Acute herpes encephalitis. The brain is swollen and there is hemorrhagic necrosis affecting the gray matter of the temporal lobes and the insulae bilaterally.

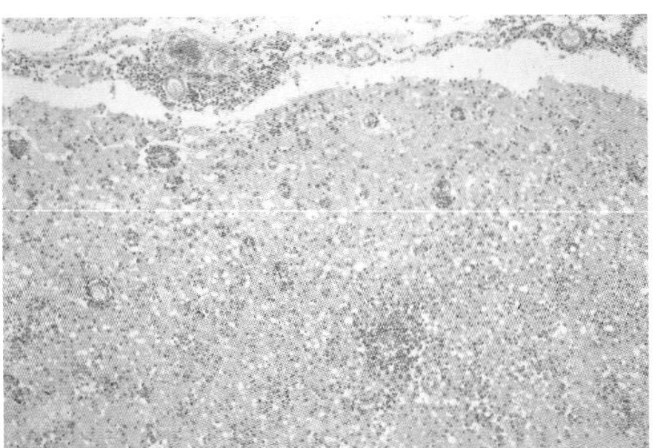

Figure 7.3 Acute herpes simplex encephalitis. There is a necrotizing meningoencephalitis with lymphocytes within the cerebral cortex and subarachnoid space. H&E.

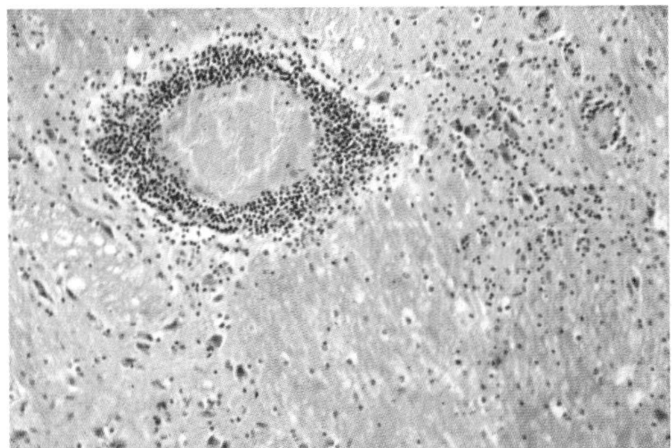

Figure 7.4 Acute herpes simplex encephalitis. There is perivascular cuffing of lymphocytes predominantly within gray matter. H&E.

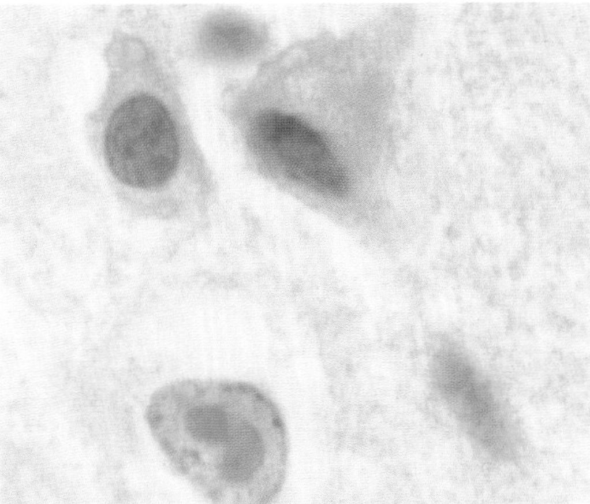

Figure 7.5 Acute herpes simplex encephalitis. Eosinophilic intranuclear inclusion in a neuron (bottom). The inclusions represent intranuclear accumulations of proliferating viral particles. H&E.

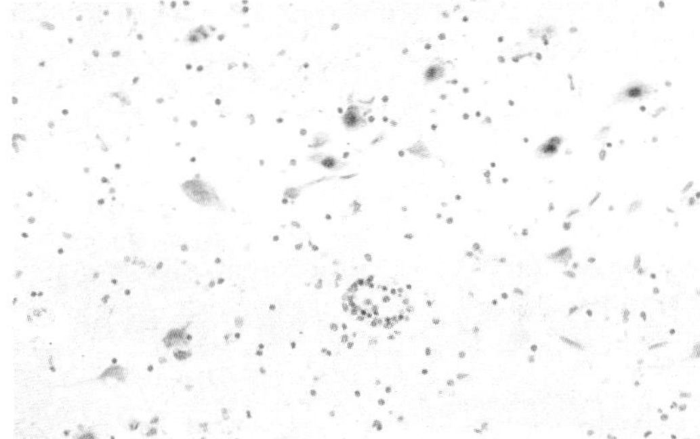

Figure 7.6 Acute herpes simplex encephalitis. Viral antigen is detectable within the nuclei and cytoplasm of neurons and glial cells. Immunohistochemistry for HSV-1.

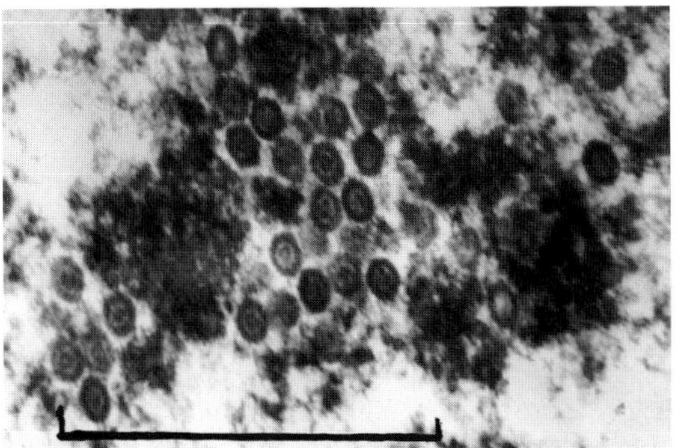

Figure 7.7 Acute herpes simplex encephalitis. Ultrastructurally, herpes virus particles have a characteristic spherical targetoid appearance. This appearance is not specific for herpes simplex virus but is shared by other herpes viruses. Electron microscopy.

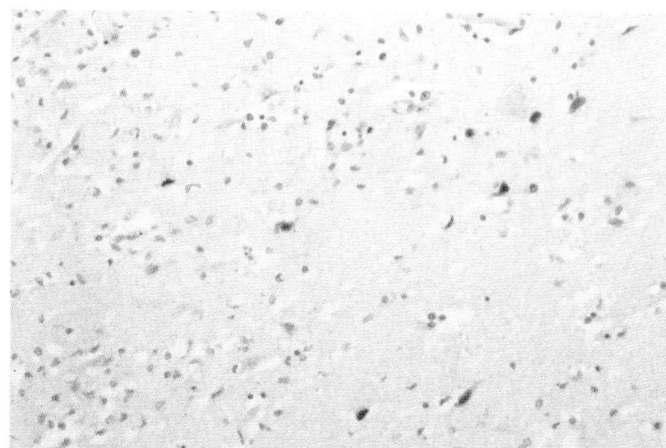

Figure 7.8 Acute herpes simplex encephalitis. Viral DNA has a similar distribution to viral proteins detected by immunohistochemistry. *In situ* hybridization for HSV-1.

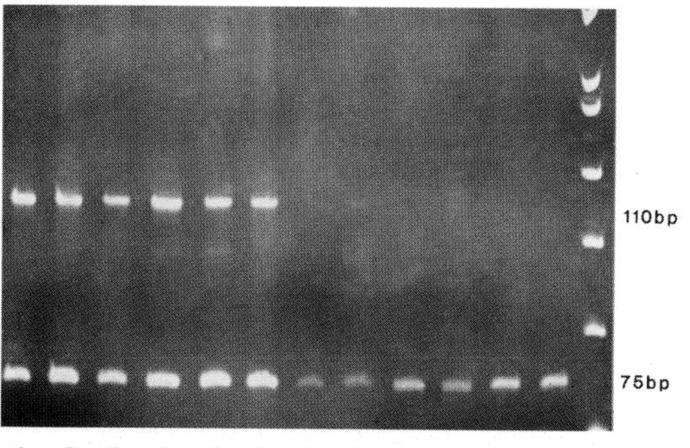

Figure 7.9 Acute herpes simplex encephalitis. Polymerase chain reaction (PCR) using appropriate primers specific for HSV-1 DNA, viral DNA (110 b.p.) can be amplified from affected brain tissue (lanes 1–6) but not uninfected controls (lanes 7–12). The 75 b.p. DNA fragment is from primers which amplify a host sequence, confirming presence of DNA in the samples.

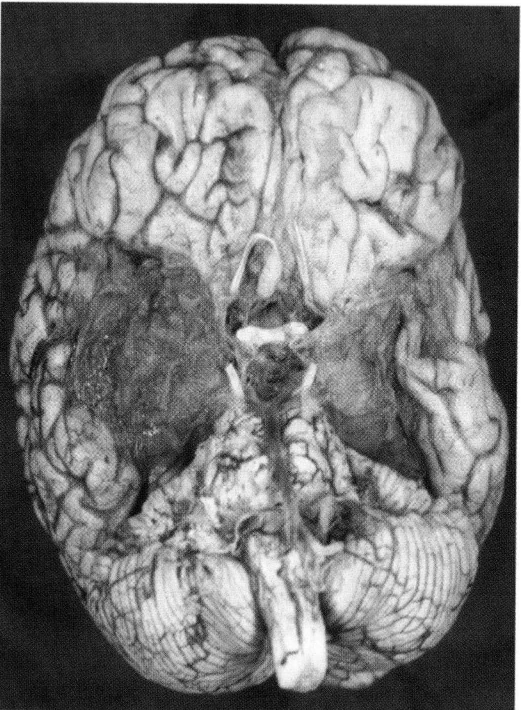

Figure 7.10 Long-term survival after acute herpes simplex encephalitis. The medial temporal lobes, which were severely affected by the acute infection, are reduced to areas of cystic degeneration.

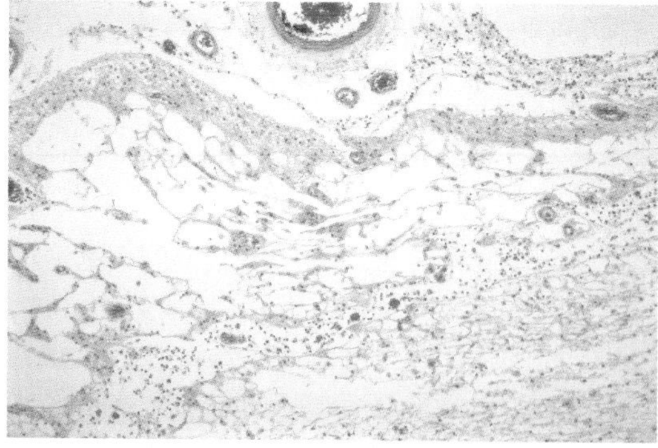

Figure 7.11 Long-term survival after acute herpes simplex encephalitis. There is cystic degeneration and gliosis of affected areas of cerebral cortex. H&E.

can be detected in biopsy or autopsy tissue by *in situ* hybridization or PCR (Figs 7.8 and 7.9).

Long-term survivors of an episode of acute herpes simplex encephalitis in which severe brain damage occurred show cystic degeneration of the affected areas, most notably the medial parts of the temporal lobes (Fig. 7.10). Histologically, there is severe neuronal loss with reactive proliferation of astrocytes and microglia (Fig. 7.11). In patients who die more than 3 weeks after the acute infection viral particles and viral proteins are no longer detectable in the CNS. However, HSV DNA may remain detectable but it is not clear whether this represents simply residual fragments of viral DNA or HSV becoming latent in the brain.

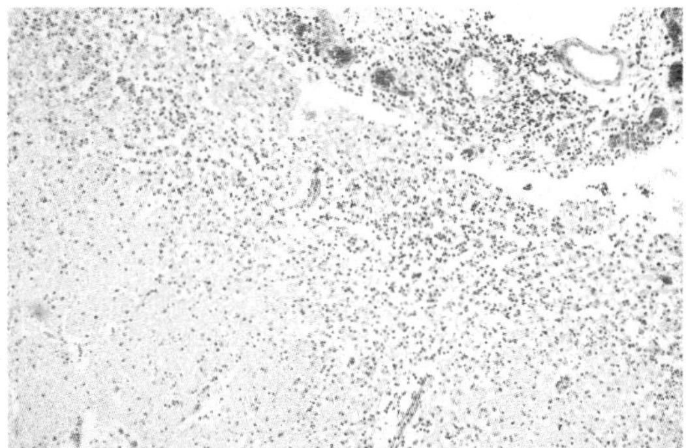

Figure 7.12 Acute neonatal encephalitis. Infection with HSV-2 produces a widespread necrotizing meningoencephalitis with infiltration of the brain and leptomeninges by lymphocytes. H&E.

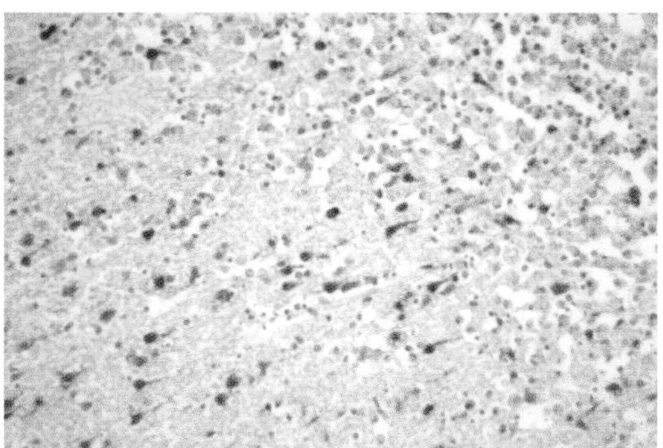

Figure 7.13 Acute neonatal encephalitis. Immunohistochemistry with an antibody specific for HSV-2 demonstrates viral antigen within the nuclei and cytoplasm of neurons and glial cells.

HSV-2 encephalitis

HSV-2 encephalitis occurs in neonates usually following delivery through an infected maternal genital tract. HSV-1 can also cause infection in neonates, although it is much less common, and is presumed to be acquired post-natally. Neonatal HSV infection is often a severe widely disseminated infection involving the brain, liver, adrenal glands, skin, eyes and mouth. The brain is affected by a widespread encephalitis involving the cerebrum, cerebellum and brainstem. The histological appearances are those of a necrotizing meningoencephalitis with infiltration of the leptomeninges and brain by lymphocytes (Fig. 7.12). Nuclear inclusions are often visible and use of specific antibodies or analysis of DNA can distinguish between HSV-1 and HSV-2 infection (Fig. 7.13).

Varicella zoster virus

Varicella zoster virus (VZV) is probably acquired by the respiratory route. Primary infection with VZV produces the systemic disease chickenpox (varicella) which is associated with a viremia. VZV becomes latent in dorsal root ganglia or trigeminal ganglia, presumably being transported to the ganglion cells by retrograde axonal transport. The virus is periodically reactivated and is transported in an anterograde manner down the nerve to cause the characteristic vesicular rash in the area of skin supplied by the ganglion. In its commonest form zoster occurs in a dermatome supplied by one posterior root ganglion, most often in the thoracic region. Alternatively, the ophthalmic division of the trigeminal nerve is commonly affected. Less frequently, cervical or lumbar dermatomes or other branches of the trigeminal nerve may be affected. Recurrent zoster (shingles) is common, particularly in the elderly and in the immunosuppressed. Post-herpetic neuralgia is pain affecting the distribution of the involved nerve and is presumably due to damage to the nerve and the sensory ganglion cells.

Reactivation of virus is associated with swelling of the affected ganglion. Microscopically, there is a lymphocytic infiltrate and there may be neuronophagia.

Maternal infection with VZV during the first trimester is a cause of maldevelopment of the CNS (Table 7.3). Infection in the neonatal period can cause a severe systemic illness. VZV is a rare cause of encephalitis, myelitis, radiculitis, cerebellitis and CNS vasculitis. Such infections are most likely to occur in the immunosuppressed. The inflammatory process may extend into the posterior nerve root and adjacent dorsal sector of the spinal cord and subarachnoid space.

Cytomegalovirus

Primary infection with cytomegalovirus (CMV) is usually asymptomatic but it may present with

Table 7.3 Congenital brain damage resulting from maternal infection

- Cytomegalovirus
- Varicella zoster virus
- Rubella
- HIV
- Syphilis
- *Toxoplasma*

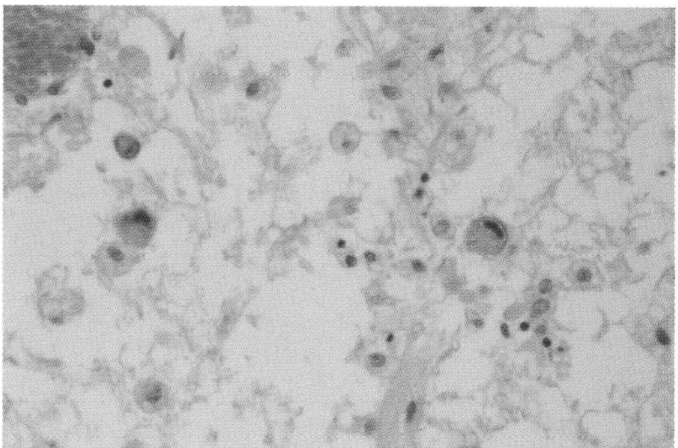

Figure 7.14 Cytomegalovirus encephalitis. Characteristic 'owl's eye' inclusions are present in cells lining the ventricles.

an infectious mononucleosis-type syndrome. In immunocompromised individuals CMV can cause serious disease of the CNS including an encephalitis, myeloradiculitis and retinitis. CMV encephalitis occurs particularly in the context of AIDS and characteristically affects the periventricular regions (ventriculitis). Here, it is associated with a localized lymphocytic infiltrate and the presence of characteristic CMV inclusions ('owls-eye' inclusions) in affected cells which may be neurons or glia (Fig. 7.14). Immunohistochemistry can demonstrate viral proteins and confirm the diagnosis (Fig. 7.15). Viral DNA is detectable by *in situ* hybridization or PCR.

Primary infection with CMV in a pregnant woman can result in transplacental spread of the virus and infection of the fetus. This may result in a severe systemic disease in the fetus associated with a multifocal necrotizing encephalitis and calcification. Surviving children have severe disability associated with seizures, learning difficulties, and hearing and visual loss.

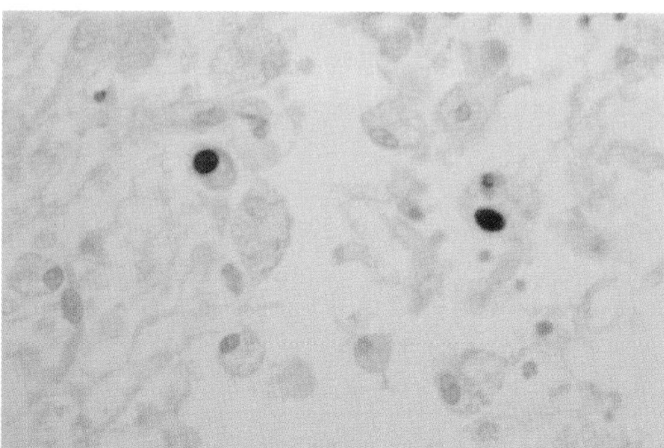

Figure 7.15 Cytomegalovirus encephalitis. Immunohistochemistry for CMV demonstrates the viral antigen, confirming the diagnosis.

Poliomyelitis

Historically, poliomyelitis was a common cause of disability. The disease typically results in asymmetric weakness and wasting of an upper or lower limb. Most cases of poliomyelitis were caused by polio viruses (Types 1, 2 and 3) which are small RNA enteroviruses. It occurred in an endemic form which primarily affected young children, causing 'infantile paralysis'. It also occurred in epidemics with a seasonal incidence, being particularly common in late summer during which adults were also affected. Transmission of the virus is probably by the fecal–oral route. The virus probably replicates in the mucosa of the throat and ileum, spreads to regional lymph nodes, followed by a viremia during which the virus reaches the CNS. Polio affects motor neurons in the anterior horns of the spinal cord and in the motor nuclei of the brainstem and causes paralysis. The prevalence of poliomyelitis was dramatically reduced with the availability of immunization and is now almost completely abolished, not only from developed countries, but also from the developing countries.

The virus selectively attacks motor neurons in the anterior horns of the spinal cord, particularly in the lumbar and cervical enlargements. The motor nuclei in the brainstem are also often affected ('bulbar polio') when there may be early involvement of the respiratory center. In patients who died in the acute stage of the disease, focal hemorrhage was described macroscopically in the anterior horns of the spinal cord and in the motor nuclei of the brainstem. Microscopic examination showed a lymphocytic meningoencephalomyelitis more widespread than the clinical symptoms suggest. However, the anterior horns in the brainstem motor nuclei were particularly severely affected with clusters of microglia around injured neurons (neuronophagia).

In patients with residual paralysis who die long after the acute stage of the disease, the most striking structural abnormality is atrophy of the anterior horns of the spinal cord. There is loss of neurons in the affected segments, which is often asymmetrical, and there is associated gliosis. There is atrophy of the corresponding anterior nerve roots and of the corresponding skeletal muscle. Examination of muscle shows neurogenic atrophy with evidence of denervation and reinnervation.

Post-polio syndrome is the term given to progressively increasing weakness and muscle atrophy in survivors of poliomyelitis many years later. The cause of post-polio syndrome is not well understood but may reflect age-related failure of residual neurons.

Arbovirus infections

Arboviruses are RNA viruses which are transmitted from host to host by blood-sucking insects (arthropod-borne viruses). They give rise to a wide variety of diseases, including several types of encephalitis which are named after the geographical regions in which they occur. The different geographical regions tend to have distinct combinations of arthropod vector and type of arbovirus. Many have a seasonal variation which presumably reflects the life cycle of the relevant arthropod. Infections occur mostly in the summer and early autumn. The vector becomes infected when it is feeding on the blood of an infected host in the viremic stage. After a bite from an infected arthropod the virus causes a viremia during which time the CNS may become infected.

Types of mosquito-borne arbovirus encephalitis include Saint Louis encephalitis, eastern and western equine encephalitis (of the Americas), Japanese encephalitis, Murray Valley encephalitis and West Nile virus. West Nile virus is of particular note because it has spread across North America in recent years. Types of tick-borne arbovirus encephalitis include Russian spring–summer encephalitis and central European encephalitis.

Following an incubation period which varies from several days to a few weeks presentation is with pyrexia and non-specific neurological symptoms, progressing to coma. Macroscopically, there may be vascular congestion and brain swelling with petechial hemorrhages. The clinical features of the various types of arbovirus infection range from aseptic meningitis to a rapidly progressive encephalitis. Some of these diseases resemble poliomyelitis. Microscopically, there is a meningoencephalitis with infiltration, particularly of gray matter, by perivascular cuffs of lymphocytes and plasma cells. There is proliferation of microglia and neuronal necrosis. There are not specific viral inclusions and diagnosis requires specific virological studies.

Rabies

Rabies is endemic in animals in many parts of the world including central and eastern Europe, India and parts of North and South America. Rabies is usually transmitted to humans by the bite of a rabid dog. In developed countries vaccination has reduced rabies in domestic dogs but wild animals remain an important source of the disease, including foxes, skunks, jackals and bats.

The bite of an infected animal injects virus into the skeletal muscle in which the virus replicates and reaches the CNS by traveling along peripheral nerves by retrograde axonal transport. The incubation period of the disease varies greatly and is related to the distance of the bite from the CNS, varying from a few days to several months. Once the virus reaches the CNS there is an acute neurological disease which lasts a few days and may assume a restless form or a paralytic form. The restless form corresponds to the furious rabies of dogs and includes aggressive behavior and hypersensitivity. In the paralytic type there is limb paralysis.

Macroscopically, the brain may appear normal or slightly congested. Microscopic examination shows the features of a viral encephalitis predominantly affecting the gray matter. In addition to perivascular cuffing by lymphocytes, plasma cells and macrophages, there is widespread microglial hyperplasia and neuronophagia. The pathognomic histological feature of rabies is the Negri body which is a sharply defined round or oval eosinophilic intracytoplasmic inclusion 1–7 μm in diameter. Negri bodies tend to be prominent in the hippocampus, cerebellar Purkinje cells and brainstem nuclei. Immunohistochemistry for rabies antigens shows that virus is present in the Negri bodies and also occurs widely in various cell types throughout the CNS. Microglial nodules are prominent. In the paralytic form of rabies there is selectively severe involvement of the spinal cord, particularly in the lower thoracic and lumbar region.

Encephalitis lethargica

Encephalitis lethargica was a pandemic encephalitis which appeared suddenly in 1916, spread rapidly around the world and had disappeared by 1926. The cause of encephalitis lethargica has not been clearly established but it may have been related to the influenza virus. Encephalitis lethargica was characterized by a somnolent stage from which the patient could be wakened easily but then would quickly relapse again into sleep. In patients who died in the acute stage the features of an acute viral encephalitis were observed. Parkinsonism was a prominent feature in survivors.

Persistent virus infections

Rather than result in an acute infection some viruses, when involving the CNS, run a protracted course over a period of months or years.

Subacute sclerosing panencephalitis

Subacute sclerosing panencephalitis (SSPE) is a persistent virus infection of the nervous system caused by the measles virus. Measles virus is a single-stranded RNA virus of the paramyxovirus family. It is a very rare disease which affects young people between the ages of 5 and 20 years. The clinical course of the disease is progressive and is fatal within months or a few years. SSPE tends to occur in children who have had an initial infection with measles virus at less than 2 years of age. The manifestation of SSPE follows several years later.

SSPE appears to be associated with replication of a mutant virus, with failure to produce the viral M protein, and associated with loss of ability of infected cells to produce complete viral particles. There are high levels of antibody to measles virus circulating in the blood and CSF which may as a consequence select for a mutant virus. Persisting passive immunity from maternal antibodies in children exposed to measles virus very early in life may play a role in the pathogenesis. Introduction of measles vaccination has had the effect of substantially reducing the risk of SSPE.

The initial stage of the disease is characterized by personality change and intellectual deterioration. Subsequently, periodic involuntary movements develop which tend to occur at regular intervals, every 5–10 s. There is a progressive deterioration with ataxia, spasticity, dementia, decerebration and seizures, leading to coma and death. CSF examination shows a raised protein and lymphocytes, plasma cells and monocytes.

Macroscopically, the brain appears normal or, particularly if the disease has run a protracted course, there may be generalized cerebral atrophy. The features of hypoxic brain damage, as a consequence of seizures, may be superimposed.

Microscopically (Fig. 7.16), there is a chronic encephalitis with a prominent inflammatory infiltrate in cases where the disease has progressed rapidly. The subarachnoid space and perivascular spaces in gray and white matter are infiltrated with lymphocytes and plasma cells. In cases that have pursued a longer course there is less inflammation, but a prominent proliferation of astrocytes and microglia. Large well-defined intranuclear inclusion bodies are present in neurons and oligodendrocytes. Neuronophagia is common. Neurofibrillary tangles may be present. Cerebral white matter is gliotic with rarefaction of myelinated fibres.

In addition to causing SSPE, measles virus can affect the nervous system in a number of other ways. It can cause aseptic meningitis, measles inclusion body encephalitis in the immunosuppressed (Figs 7.17 and 7.18) and trigger acute disseminated encephalomyelitis (ADEM) (see page 195).

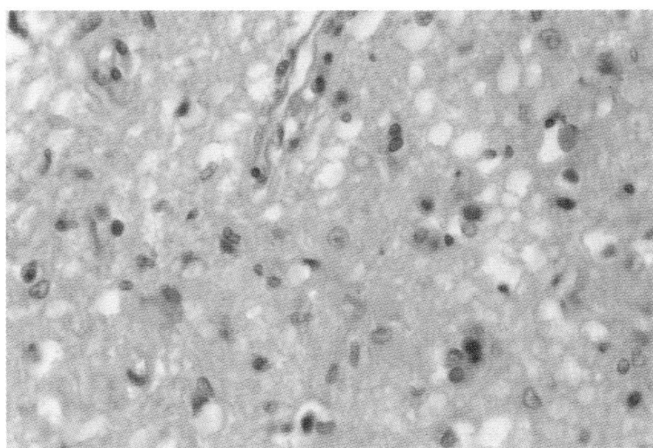

Figure 7.16 Subacute sclerosing panencephalitis. The cerebral cortex is hypercellular due to proliferation of glial cells including astrocytes and microglia. Eosinophilic intranuclear viral inclusions may be seen.

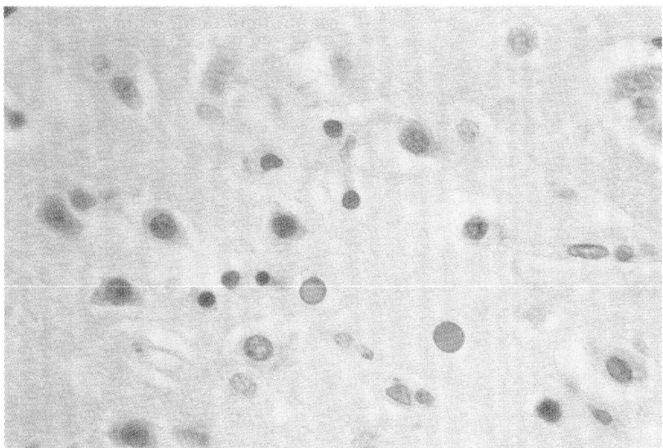

Figure 7.17 Measles encephalitis. In immunosuppressed patients, including those with AIDS, measles virus may cause an acute encephalitis. Intranuclear viral inclusions are identified in the gray matter. H&E.

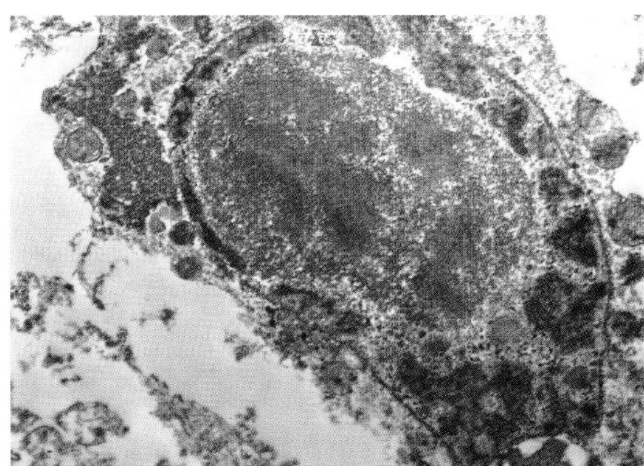

Figure 7.18 Measles encephalitis. The intranuclear inclusions are composed of accumulation of measles virus particles which have a spaghetti-like morphology. Electron microscopy ×60 000.

Progressive multifocal leukoencephalopathy

Progressive multifocal leukoencephalopathy (PML) occurs almost exclusively in patients immunosuppressed due to leukemia, lymphoma, or iatrogenic immunosuppression such as following renal transplantation. PML also occurs relatively commonly in AIDS and is due to the JC virus, a polyoma virus which is almost ubiquitous and is usually apparently asymptomatic. It appears to reside in a latent state and is reactivated as a consequence of immunodeficiency. Clinical presentation is with focal neurological deficits, ataxia, personality change and seizures. The course of the disease is progressive over several months leading to dementia and death. Imaging shows the characteristic patchy abnormalities in the white matter. On macroscopic examination there are multiple small gray foci distributed widely but asymmetrically through the brain, mainly in the cerebral white matter (Fig. 7.19). These foci can coalesce to form large gray areas in which there may be necrosis. The basal ganglia, brainstem and cerebellum are less commonly involved.

Histological examination shows multiple foci of demyelination (Fig. 7.20) associated with which are large bizarre reactive astrocytes (Fig. 7.21), lipid-laden macrophages and abnormal oligodendrocytes. The oligodendroglia have a particularly characteristic

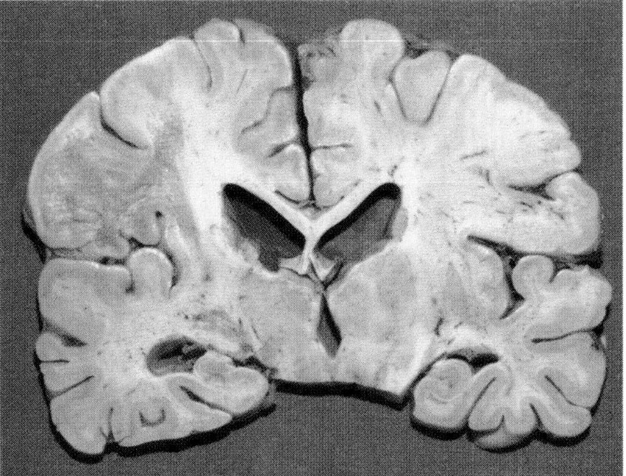

Figure 7.19 Progressive multifocal leukoencephalopathy. There is extensive degeneration of white matter, mainly in the left cerebral hemisphere.

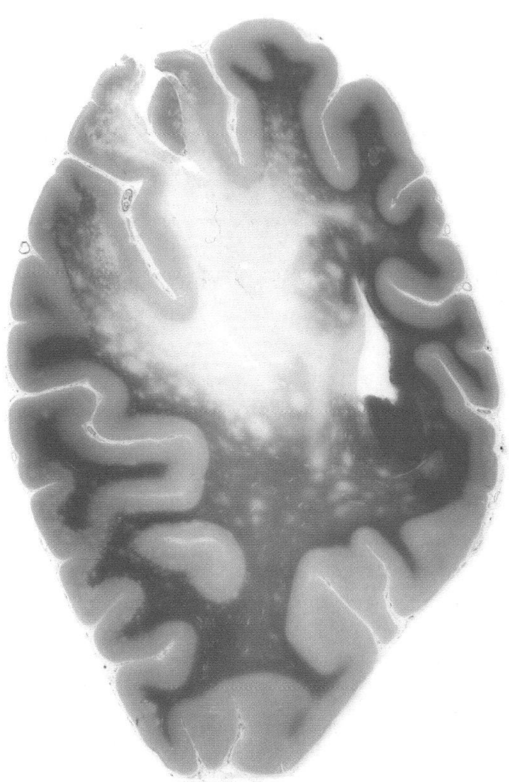

Figure 7.20 Progressive multifocal leuko-encephalopathy. There are multiple small foci of demyelination around a larger confluent area of demyelination. Luxol fast blue/cresyl violet.

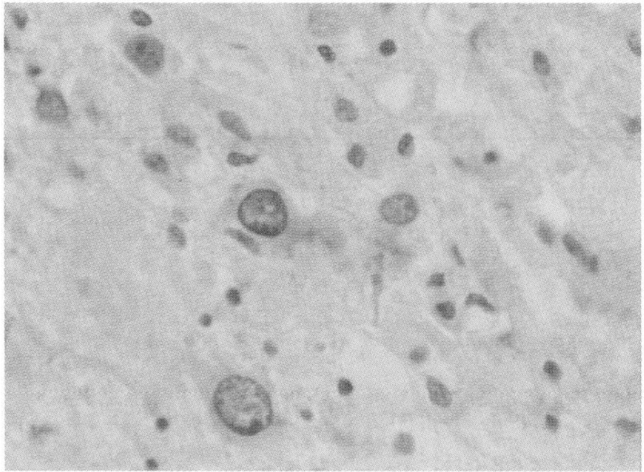

Figure 7.21 Progressive multifocal leuko-encephalopathy. Larger bizarre reactive astrocytes are a characteristic feature. H&E.

appearance (Fig. 7.22), with nuclei that are swollen by inclusions which are purple in sections stained with hematoxylin and eosin. These oligodendrocyte nuclei are filled with polyoma virus particles

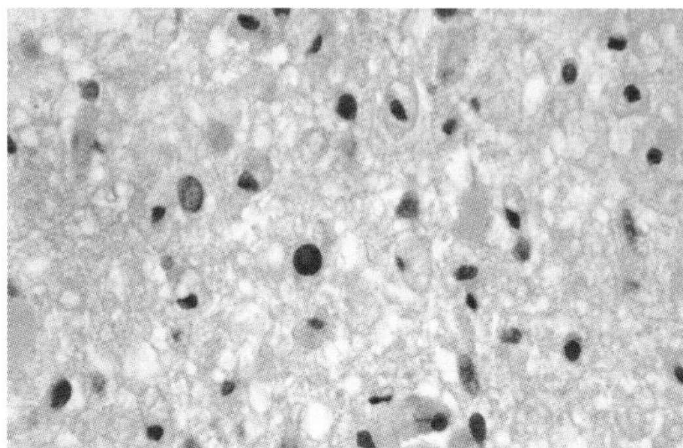

Figure 7.22 Progressive multifocal leukoen-cephalopathy. The oligodendrocytes have a highly characteristic appearance, with purple-staining nuclei that are swollen by accumulation of viral particles. H&E.

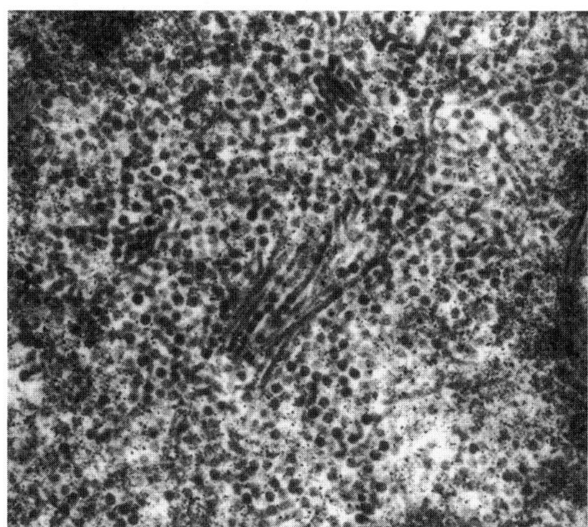

Figure 7.23 Progressive multifocal leukoen-cephalopathy. Electron microscopy shows the nuclei of affected oligodendroglial cells are filled with viral particles with the characteristic small spherical morphology of polyoma virus. Electron microscopy ×5000.

on electron microscopy (Fig. 7.23) and viral nucleic acid can be detected by *in situ* hybridization. The oligodendrocyte inclusions are particularly numerous at the periphery of foci of demyelination and in the immediately adjacent brain. Within the smaller foci of demyelination there is relative sparing of axons, but in the large lesions very few axons remain and there may be frank necrosis.

HTLV1-associated myelopathy

HTLV1-associated myelopathy (HAM), also known as tropical spastic paraparesis, is infection by a retrovirus (HTLV1) mainly affecting the spinal cord. HTLV1 is predominantly sexually transmitted and is endemic in some parts of the world including the Caribbean, South America and Africa. Pathologically, there is myelitis with infiltration of lymphocytes and macrophages in the leptomeninges and the spinal cord. This is associated with demyelination, long tract degeneration and gliosis. Viral nucleic acids can be identified in the spinal cord.

Human immunodeficiency virus

Human immunodeficiency virus (HIV) is an RNA-containing retrovirus. Infection with HIV is present throughout the world, although there are dramatic differences in prevalence. In sub-Saharan Africa, where up to 30% of the population may be infected, HIV has devastated whole communities (Table 7.4). In developed countries transmission has been limited by public awareness campaigns, promotion of the use of condoms, needle-exchange programs for drug addicts, post-exposure prophylaxis for needle stick injuries, screening of blood for transfusion and anti-retroviral therapy of infected individuals. Major means of transmission of HIV infection include sexual transmission, intravenous drug abuse, vertical transmission from mother to child, and occupational exposure in health care workers by needle stick injury. Infection by blood transfusion is now rare.

HIV infects T lymphocytes and macrophages after binding to CD4 receptors on the cell surface. Subsequent depletion of these cells is responsible for the reduced ability of an infected individual to resist infection (Table 7.5). Infection with HIV can be identified by demonstration of HIV specific antibodies in blood and by detection of HIV nucleic acid by PCR. Without treatment, HIV positive individuals may remain asymptomatic for many years before progressing to acquired immunodeficiency syndrome (AIDS). In developed countries during the 1980s and early 1990s, prior to the availability of anti-retroviral therapy, CNS lesions in HIV positive patients were biopsied in order to obtain a diagnosis. The commonest forms of pathology identified as causing focal lesions were *Toxoplasma* and PML. Once this was recognized, such lesions tended to be treated with anti *Toxoplasma* therapy without resort to biopsy, specific therapy for PML being unavailable. With the advent of highly active anti-retroviral therapy (HAART) in the mid 1990s the course of disease in HIV positive patients has altered dramatically. HAART can render HIV undetectable in the blood and dramatically reduces the prevalence of opportunistic infections and neoplasms. In under-developed countries where HAART is unavailable progression from HIV positivity to AIDS, with its associated complications, remains unaltered.

Table 7.4 Effects of HIV upon the CNS

- HIV encephalopathy due to direct infection of the CNS by HIV
- Opportunistic infections due to immunosuppression (see Table 7.5)
- Neoplasms (CNS lymphoma)

Table 7.5 Opportunistic infections in AIDS

Fungal infections
- *Cryptococcus neoformans* (meningitis) (Fig. 7.27)
- *Aspergillus fumigatus* (abscesses) (Fig. 7.28)
- Coccidioides (meningitis and abscesses)
- Histoplasmosis
- Candidiasis (Fig. 7.29)
- Mucormycosis (Fig. 7.30)

Viral infections
- Cytomegalovirus (ventriculitis and retinitis) (Figs 7.14 and 7.15)
- Herpes simplex virus (encephalitis) (Figs 7.2–7.13)
- Progressive multifocal leukoencephalopathy (Fig. 7.19–7.21)
- Measles inclusion body encephalitis (Figs 7.17 and 7.18)

Parasitic infection
- Toxoplasmosis (large necrotic abscesses) (Figs 7.31–7.35)

Bacterial infections
- *Mycobacterium avium* intracellulare
- *Mycobacterium tuberculosis* (Chapter 6, Figs 6.12–6.14)
- Neurosyphilis

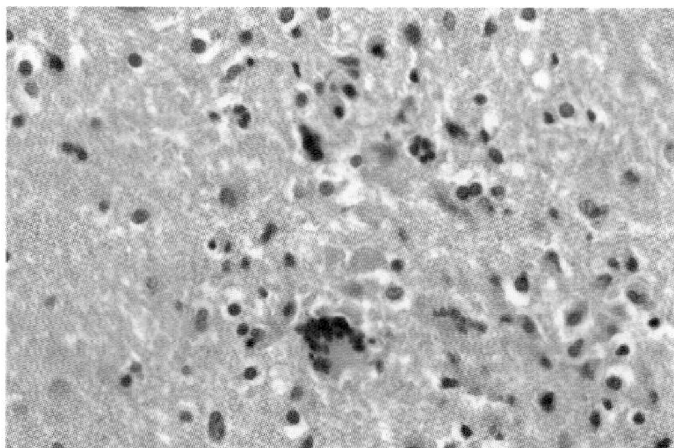

Figure 7.24 HIV encephalopathy. Small multinucleated cells, often in a perivascular location, are a characteristic feature. H&E.

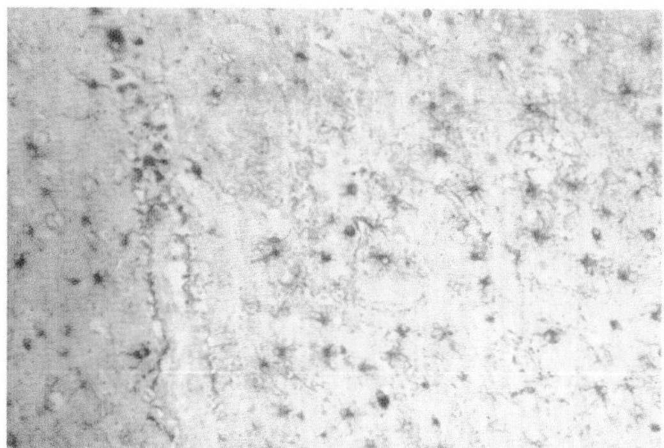

Figure 7.25 HIV encephalopathy. There may be a leukoencephalopathy with white matter rarefaction and gliosis. Immunohistochemistry for GFAP.

HIV encephalopathy

Clinical recognition of HIV-associated dementia correlates poorly with the presence of histological features of HIV encephalopathy and its precise substrate is unclear. HIV encephalopathy shows a variable pattern comprising the following features:

1. Small multinucleated cells, often in a perivascular location, in which HIV antigen can be demonstrated (Fig. 7.24).
2. Leukoencephalopathy with white matter rarefaction and gliosis (Fig. 7.25).
3. Widespread inflammatory changes, with microglial nodules and sparse perivascular lymphocytes (Fig. 7.26).

Macroscopically, the brain may appear normal or may show generalized atrophy. The mechanism by which HIV enters the brain remains uncertain. However, it seems likely to be due to infected circulating monocytes crossing the blood–brain barrier into the brain. Macrophage/microglial infection with HIV results in activation and secretion of cytokines and other neurotoxic substances. HIV appears not to infect neurons in the brain, but some viral proteins (e.g. GP120) may be directly neurotoxic.

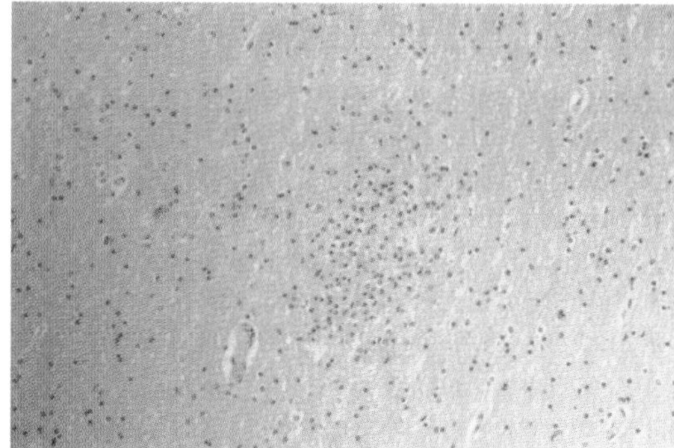

Figure 7.26 HIV encephalopathy. Scattered microglial nodules are often encountered and are presumed to be the consequence of an opportunistic viral infection, although the specific virus responsible may not always be identified. H&E.

Vacuolar myelopathy

Vacuolar myelopathy is common in patients with AIDS. It results in spastic paraparesis and incontinence. The pathology resembles subacute combined degeneration of the spinal cord with vacuolation of white matter in the dorsal and lateral columns.

FUNGAL INFECTIONS

Fungi are ubiquitous in the environment but cause CNS disease in humans relatively rarely. Some fungi may produce disease in humans in the absence of any obvious predisposing factors but more often fungal infections are 'opportunistic', occurring in patients in whom the natural defenses of the body are lowered. Immunosuppression occurs in chronic debilitating diseases such as diabetes mellitus or alcoholism, with lymphoma/leukemia or other disseminated malignant processes, iatrogenically by the prolonged use of antibiotics, corticosteroids, cytotoxic drugs or immunosuppressive agents, and in AIDS. Intravenous drug abusers are also vulnerable. Fungal infections of the CNS are invariably secondary to infection elsewhere in the body but lesions at the portal of entry may be small and readily overlooked, with the result that the brain may appear to be the only organ involved. Fungi usually reach the CNS by the bloodstream and the primary focus is most often in the lung. Less commonly, fungi spread directly to the brain from a focus of infection in the sinuses.

Fungal infections usually take the form of either intraparenchymal abscesses or a basal meningitis. In the acute phase of a fungal infection the inflammatory infiltrate is composed predominantly of neutrophil polymorphs, whereas lymphocytes and macrophages predominate in chronic infections. Some fungal infections are associated with a granulomatous inflammation which may include multinucleated giant cells. Faced with a biopsy or autopsy specimen in which there is acute inflammation or a mixed acute and chronic inflammation, or in which an unusual infection of the CNS is suspected, material must be taken for culture, and sections stained with PAS and methenamine silver (Grocott) to identify fungi. Fungi may have the morphology of yeasts or hyphae. To some extent the morphology of the organisms in histological sections can indicate the type of fungus. For example, fine caliber septate hyphae which branch at an acute angle are likely to be *Aspergillus*. Larger non-septate hyphae which are irregular in caliber and branch at right angles are likely to be *Mucor*. However, definitive identification of the organism requires microbiological culture and increasingly, specific antibodies and PCR are used.

Cryptococcus neoformans

Cryptococcus neoformans is a pathogenic yeast and infection with it is not restricted to individuals with impaired resistance to infection. It is thought that an important reservoir of the infection is pigeon manure. The organism gains access to the body through the respiratory tract but pulmonary cryptococcosis is less commonly encountered clinically than infection of the CNS. The commonest clinical presentation is as a subacute meningitis and *Cryptococcus* is the commonest fungal cause of meningitis. Unless the diagnosis is made early in the disease, it is usually fatal. Cryptococcal abscesses are less common (Fig. 7.27). Cryptococci may be identified in the CSF but in dried films they may be mistaken for lymphocytes unless their capsules are sought by the appropriate techniques.

Macroscopically, there is usually an exudate and sometimes small nodules 2–3 mm in diameter in the subarachnoid space, particularly in the interpenduncular fossa and within cerebral sulci. On section, the typical abnormality is the presence of numerous small cysts measuring up to 2–3 mm in diameter in the superficial layers of the cortex. On histological examination encapsulated cryptococci are scattered throughout the subarachnoid space, either singly or as small collections. Cryptococci stain with PAS and methenamine silver and the capsule stains with alcian blue. The size, shape and staining reactions closely resemble those of corpora amylacea, with which cryptococci can be confused. The cysts in the superficial layers of the cortex usually contain masses of cryptococci. Reactive inflammatory changes are often mild, but occasionally there may be a granulomatous reaction similar in many respects to tuberculous meningitis because of the presence of multinucleate giant cells.

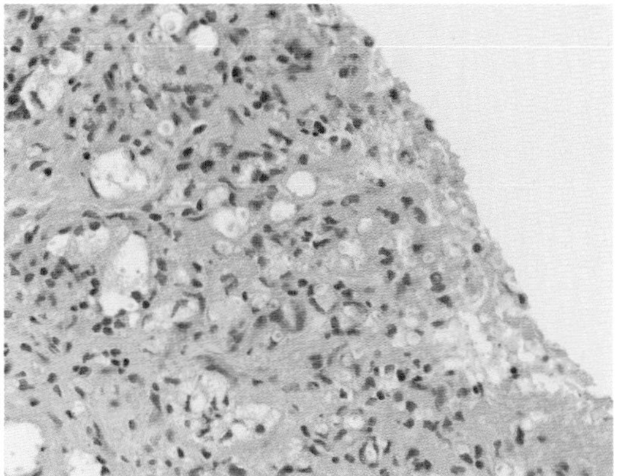

Figure 7.27 Cryptococci are small encapsulated organisms which cause meningitis or, more rarely, intraparenchymal abscess as in this figure. H&E. (Courtesy of Dr I. Mazanti, Southampton.)

Coccidioidomycosis

This fungus (*Coccidioides immitis*) is restricted to regions with a semi-arid climate and occurs particularly in the south-western USA, Mexico and South America. The fungus usually causes only mild transient febrile illness but in a small proportion of cases granulomatous lesions appear in the lungs. The fungus may then be carried to the brain by the bloodstream where it produces a granulomatous meningitis. Occasionally, granulomas may occur within the brain. Histologically, the lesions closely resemble those of tuberculosis but many of the giant cells contain the fungus which appears as spherules about 10–16 μm in diameter filled with endospores.

Blastomycosis

Blastomyces dermatidis is a fungus that exists as a filamentous growth and as a yeast. It is the causal agent of blastomycosis which occurs particularly in the USA, Canada and Mexico. Blastomyces may also produce a pulmonary granulomatous meningitis in which the yeasts occur free or within macrophages. Involvement of the vertebrae is not uncommon and the resulting extradural granulomas may cause spinal cord compression.

Histoplasmosis

Infections by *Histoplasma capsulatum* are common in the USA, South America and southern Africa. Infection probably usually takes place by inhalation. Hematogenous spread to the brain produces a diffuse granulomatous meningitis characterized by a thick yellow exudate in the subarachnoid space with occasional discrete grayish/white opacities resembling tubercules adjacent to blood vessels. On histological examination there are macrophages, lymphocytes and plasma cells, and small granulomas. Granulomas may also occur within the brain.

Aspergillosis

Aspergillus fumigatus generally produces abscesses of varying size which are often multiple in the brain, and early in the disease process the lesions may resemble hemorrhagic infarcts. With time they become well defined abscesses. Histological examination shows varying degrees of infarction, including necrosis of the walls of blood vessels, and a cellular infiltrate consisting of lymphocytes, plasma cells, neutrophil polymorphs and macrophages. *Aspergillus* often provokes a granulomatous reaction characterized by the presence of multinucleate giant cells. *Aspergillus* has fine-caliber septate hyphae which branch at an acute angle (Fig. 7.28).

Candidiasis

Candida albicans is a yeast which is a normal commensal of the skin and intestine. *Candida* commonly infects the oral or vaginal mucosa. It can cause a meningitis and intraparenchymal microabcesses. With appropriate stains, *Candida* appears as yeast forms with pseudohyphae which may virtually replace necrotic blood vessel walls (Fig. 7.29 and Fig. 14.60, page 289).

Mucormycosis

Mucormycosis has a particular propensity to infect uncontrolled diabetic patients in whom the infection tends to start in paranasal air sinuses or in the adjacent skin. It produces a rapidly progressive necrotizing infection and spreads though the bone of the base of the skull and the cavernous sinuses to involve the adjacent brain where it produces an

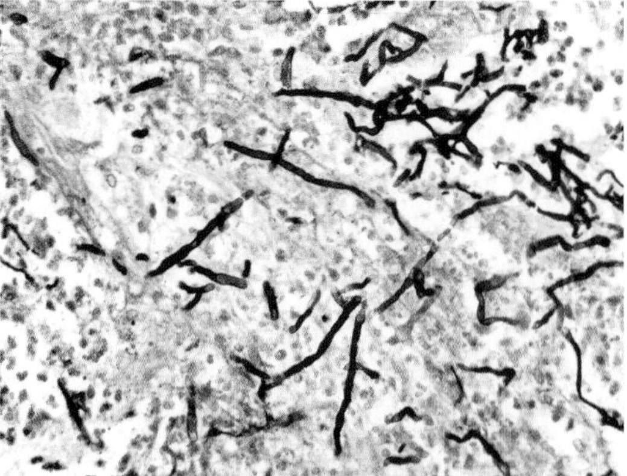

Figure 7.28 *Aspergillus* has a characteristic appearance. The fungal hyphae are of uniformly fine caliber, are septate, and branch at an acute angle. Methenamine silver.

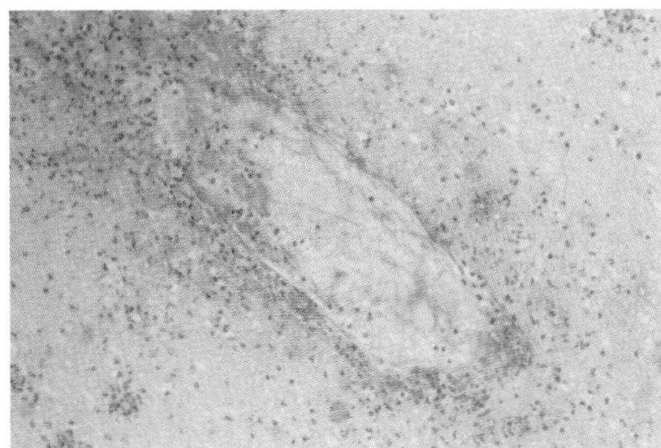

Figure 7.29 *Candida* commonly involves the walls of blood vessels within the brain parenchyma, leading to necrosis, as seen here. H&E.

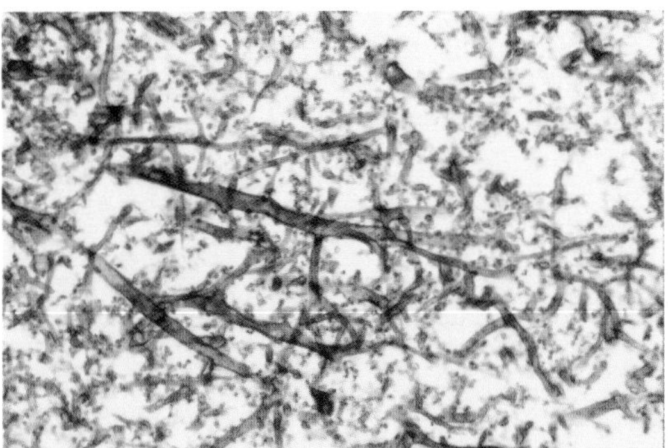

Figure 7.30 Mucormycosis. The hyphae of *Mucor* are large and irregular in caliber, non-septate, and branch at right angles. Methenamine silver.

acute necrotizing meningitis and, on occasion, abscess formation. The orbit may be involved. On microscopic examination there is necrosis of the walls of blood vessels and tissue, and there are large non-septate hyphae which are irregular in calibre and branch at right angles (Fig. 7.30). Granulomatous inflammation is not a common feature.

PROTOZOAL INFECTIONS

Toxoplasmosis

This is a common protozoal infection of humans caused by *Toxoplasma gondii*, a coccidian parasite.

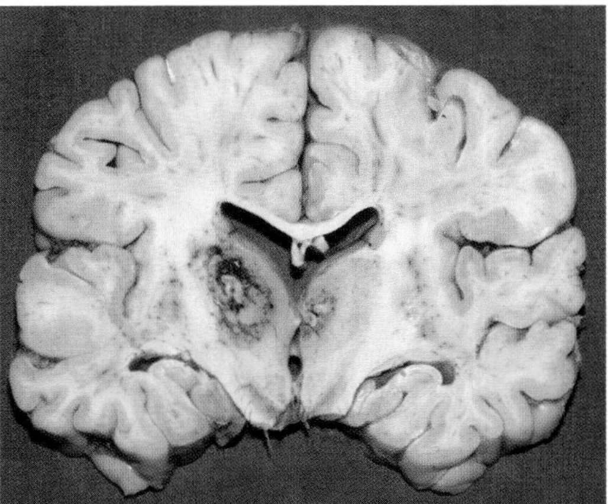

Figure 7.31 Cerebral toxoplasmosis occurs mainly in the immunosuppressed and causes intraparenchymal abscesses.

Toxoplasma gondii is widespread in nature but its principal life occurs in cats, and infection in humans is probably most often acquired by contamination with cat feces, and as a result of consuming infected undercooked meat. Infection in immunocompetent individuals is usually asymptomatic although there may be a lymphadenopathy.

Toxoplasma infection of the brain may be congenital, following transplacental transfer in a pregnant woman sustaining a primary infection. Congenital toxoplasmosis is associated with severe abnormalities which include multifocal necrosis, with calcification, hydrocephalus and chorioretinitis.

In adults, cerebral toxoplasmosis occurs in the context of immunosuppression, usual due to AIDS, and is probably due to reactivation of dormant infection. In the immunosuppressed, *Toxoplasma* causes multifocal necrotizing lesions in the brain (Fig. 7.31). Histologically, the lesions are abscesses consisting of a necrotic central focus surrounded by a mixed acute and chronic inflammatory reaction (Fig. 7.32). The inflammatory infiltrate may be relatively sparse in severely immunosuppressed patients. The organisms can be identified in the rim of cellular reaction surrounding the necrotic zone (Fig. 7.33). They take the form of small round or oval basophilic tachyzoites which are 2–4 μm in diameter lying distributed singly within the tissue or clustered together inside cysts (bradyzoites) which measure 20–100 μm in diameter.

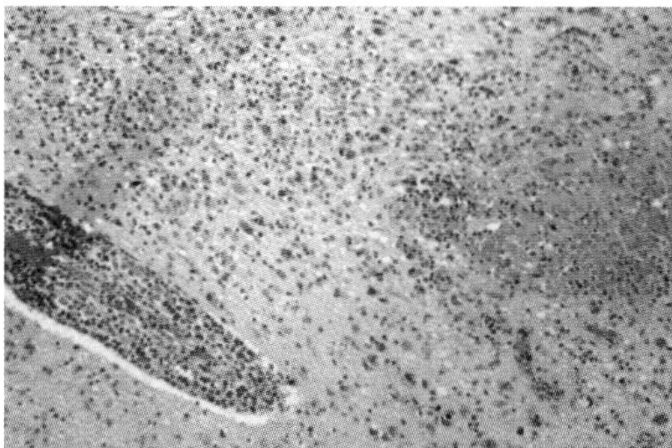

Figure 7.32 *Toxoplasma* abscesses have a central zone of necrosis, with a mixed inflammatory infiltrate. In severely immunosuppressed patients the inflammatory infiltrate may be relatively sparse. H&E.

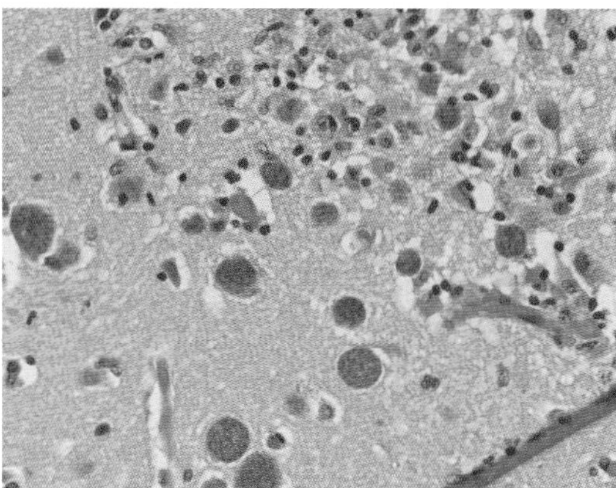

Figure 7.33 *Toxoplasma* cysts can be identified, with a careful search, in H&E stained sections at the periphery of the abscess. (Courtesy of Dr N. Cohen, Southampton).

The organisms are much easier to see in sections immunostained with a specific *Toxoplasma* antibody which confirms the diagnosis (Figs 7.34 and 7.35).

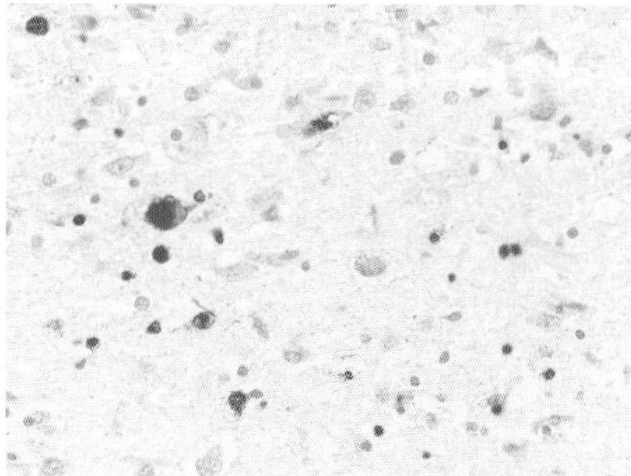

Figure 7.34 Immunohistochemistry with a specific antibody for *Toxoplasma* makes the organisms more readily identifiable and confirms the diagnosis. The organisms may be clustered together inside cysts (bradyzoites) or distributed singly within the tissue (tachyzoites). (Courtesy of Dr N. Cohen, Southampton.)

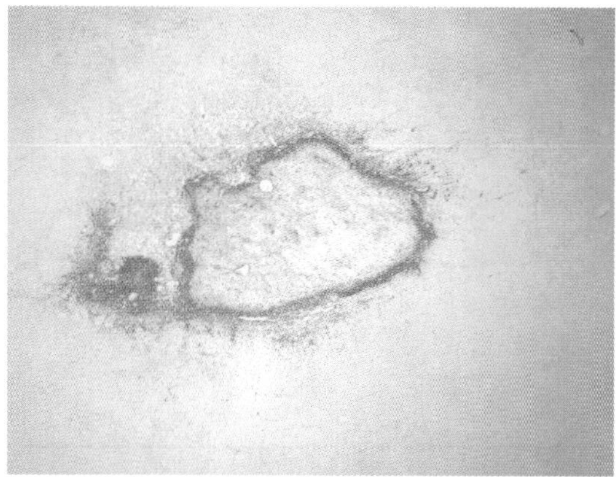

Figure 7.35 A low-power view of a *Toxoplasma* cyst demonstrates the distribution of the organisms in a ring at the margin of the zone of necrosis. Immunohistochemistry for *Toxoplasma*. (Courtesy of Dr N. Cohen, Southampton.)

AMEBIASIS

Primary amebic meningoencephalitis

This rare disease is caused by free-living amebae which are ubiquitous in the environment, particularly in soil and fresh water. Cases have been described from many parts of the world, including the United Kingdom. The ameba most frequently implicated is *Naegleria fowleri*, and the infection is acquired by swimming in warm lakes or pools contaminated with the amebae. The amebae spread by the olfactory passages to produce acute meningitis. The disease is acute, rapidly progressive and usually fatal. Pathologically, in fatal cases there is a purulent meningitis, and the olfactory bulbs and tracts may be hemorrhagic. Microscopic examination shows a fibrinopurulent exudate containing macrophages and neutrophil polymorphs. The inflammatory cells may extend for a short distance along perivascular spaces into the cerebral cortex, where there may be a necrotizing vasculitis. Amebae are usually present in large numbers, particularly around the blood vessels. Amebae can be found in the CSF obtained by lumbar puncture during life.

Granulomatous amebic encephalitis

This disease is usually due to *Acanthameba* and takes the form of a subacute or chronic infection. There is a chronic granulomatous inflammatory infiltrate which involves the meninges and has a perivascular distribution within the brain. The granulomas may have central necrosis and contain multinucleate giant cells. The *Acanthamebae* (15–40 μm) have vacuolated cytoplasm, a central nucleus and may be encysted.

Amebic abscess

This is caused by *Entameba histolytica*, a parasite that commonly causes colitis in tropical and subtropical regions. In most cases of amebic abscess in the brain, there is a primary infection in the liver, intestine or lungs. Cerebral abscess is rare and tends to be a late complication of amebiasis and is secondary to hematogenous dissemination of the ameba. Pathologically, amebic abscesses are usually solitary, and the wall of the cavity is poorly defined. Histological examination shows an inner zone of necrotic tissue and a broader outer zone of diffuse infiltration by lymphocytes, plasma cells and macrophages. Amebae are present in the abscess wall and are large (25 μm) with a relatively small, usually eccentric pale-stained nucleus, closely resembling lipid-laden macrophages.

MALARIA

Cerebral malaria is common in tropical and subtropical regions and is almost always due to infection with *Plasmodium falciparum*, transmitted by the bite of the *Anopheles* mosquito. It usually occurs in people lacking immunity to malaria, including infants and foreign visitors. Unless diagnosed early and appropriate treatment is instituted, the mortality rate is high. In fatal cases the most characteristic features are cerebral edema and the presence of numerous petechial hemorrhages through-out the brain. On histological examination (see Fig. 14.58, page 289) small blood vessels are plugged with red blood cells within which the plasmodia may be identified, and malaria pigment is seen in relation to capillaries. There may also be ball and ring hemorrhages. To what extent the structural abnormalities are related to disseminated intravascular coagulation, to acute hemorrhagic leukoencephalopathy, or to the presence of the parasites remains unclear.

TRYPANOSOMIASIS

African trypanosomiasis (sleeping sickness)

Infection of humans with *Trypanosoma brucei* results from the bite of the tsetse fly. T. brucei *rhodesiense*, a disease of East Africa, usually follows a fairly acute course and a pancarditis is often more conspicuous than an encephalitis. T. brucei *gambiense* is the cause of classic sleeping sickness, a disease found in central and West Africa, and characterized by subacute encephalitis. In a patient dying as a result of sleeping sickness, the brain may be swollen, macroscopically normal, or atrophic if the course of the disease has been protracted. Some treated patients develop acute hemorrhagic encephalitis. The histological features are those of a non-specific lymphoplasmacytic meningoencephalitis, the encephalitis being much more severe than the meningitis. The most striking feature is cuffing of blood vessels by lymphocytes and plasma cells and, in the more severe cases, these cells extend into the adjacent parenchyma. The inflammatory reaction is particularly severe in the deep white matter, the basal ganglia, the brainstem and the deep structures in the cerebellum, and tends to be mild in the cerebral and cerebellar cortex. In the more florid cases there are often collections of lymphocytes, plasma cells and microglia in the brain not directly related to blood vessels, and there is usually diffuse microglial hyperplasia in gray matter. So-called morular cells, plasma cells filled with immunoglobulin, are a characteristic but not diagnostic feature of the disease. Trypanosomes are not identifiable in the brain. The pancarditis takes the form of diffuse infiltration of the pericardium and endocardium with lymphocytes and plasma cells, and focal collections of such cells within the myocardium.

American trypanosomiasis (Chagas' disease)

This disease occurs mainly in South America, particularly in Brazil. *Trypanosoma cruzi* is transmitted by house bugs and is usually acquired in childhood. The disease may be acute, particularly in children, and is associated with encephalitis or myocarditis. The disease may also be chronic, both in children and in adults, and is associated with involvement of the autonomic nervous system causing megaesophagus, megacolon and cardiomyopathy. Encephalitis is more common in acute than in chronic cases and takes the form of numerous small inflammatory foci consisting of lymphocytes, plasma cells and microglia throughout the brain. They are more commonly seen in white matter than in gray matter. The parasites may be seen within glial cells.

OTHER INFECTIONS

Various other parasites including cestodes, trematodes and nematodes may affect the brain. The more common ones are described below.

Cysticercosis

This is caused by the pork tapeworm, *Taenia solium*, a cestode. In many parts of the world cysticercosis is very common. When humans are infected, usually as a result of eating undercooked pork, the adult worm lives in the small intestine but if ova reach the stomach, the embryos penetrate the wall of the intestine and are then disseminated throughout the body by the blood stream. Involvement of the muscle, brain and eyes is common. As the larvae develop, cysts measuring up to about 1 cm in diameter form. They are frequently multiple within the brain and are often asymptomatic. Less frequently, thin-walled racemose cysts form grape-like clusters in the basal cisterns or ventricles. Viable larvae invoke little inflammation, but when the organisms die there is a surrounding mixed inflammatory infiltrate which progresses to fibrosis and calcification.

Hydatid disease (echinococcosis)

Hydatid disease is caused by the larvae of *Echinococcus granulosus*, which is also a cestode. The adult worm occurs in the dog and sheep, and humans may be infected by ingesting food contaminated with ova. Hydatid cysts occur most often in the liver, and in many patients with a cerebral hydatid cyst there is also a cyst in the liver. The cerebral cysts are usually single, spherical and unilocular and can ultimately reach a size of several centimetres in diameter. They comprise a laminated translucent chitinous outer layer with an inner germinal layer to which ova are attached.

Schistosomiasis

The CNS is one of the rarer sites of infection by *Schistosoma* which is a trematode whose host is a snail. Granulomas resulting from infection in the brain are usually caused by *S. japonicum* but granulomas may also occur in the vertebral canal caused by *S. haematobium* or *S. mansoni*.

CHAPTER 8

TRAUMA

David I Graham

INTRODUCTION

Within the United Kingdom, trauma is responsible for more deaths in all age groups under the age of 45 years than any other single cause, and head injury is the single most important factor in death due to trauma. Between one third and one half of all deaths due to trauma are due to head injury. In the UK, with a population of approximately 60 million, about 1500 patients per 100 000 report to accident and emergency (A&E) departments and some 300 patients per 100 000 are admitted to hospital because of a head injury. Of those admitted to hospital, some 30% are dead in 6 months, 60% are severely disabled, 20% are moderately disabled, 3% are vegetative and some 30% make a good recovery. There is an accumulating population of disabled survivors from head injury, one family in 300 having a member with such a disability.

Injury to the spinal column is less common, there being in the UK some 1.3–2.7 patients per 100 000 of the population who sustain severe paralysis as a result of trauma. In some 50% of patients hospitalized for paraplegia or quadriplegia, trauma is the cause. In non-military practice about 45% of all new cases of spinal injury result from road accidents, 30% are due to falls and the remainder are due to sporting injuries and occasionally to gunshot wounds.

There are various processes that singly or in combination may damage the CNS after trauma. What distinguishes mild, moderate and severe categories of traumatic injuries is not so much the nature of the pathology as its amount and distribution. Therefore, there is likely to be a clinical and neuroradiological continuum from mild to severe damage, the structural basis of which might be inferred from postmortem studies of patients who have died with varying degrees of disability after trauma.

BLUNT HEAD INJURY

Any classification of brain damage after blunt injury must take into account the full spectrum of clinical presentation and outcome, from the patient who remains in coma from the moment of injury until death, to the patient who is apparently normal after the initial injury, but who as the result of a complication subsequently relapses into fatal coma. Given that some structural damage is likely in all forms of head injury an important determinant of outcome is the pre-injury condition of the brain. For any given level of injury, a good recovery is more likely in a healthy individual whose brain is normal than an individual who either because of pre-existing developmental or acquired disorders, had an abnormal brain. For example, the outcome even after relatively minor head injury in a patient who has already experienced a 'stroke' or head injury is likely to be that much worse than if such premorbid conditions are not present.

Earlier classifications based on clinico-pathological correlations in patients after head injury helped to identify potentially preventable complications and in particular those who 'talked and died' or 'talked and deteriorated'. The fact that the patient had talked only to deteriorate or subsequently die was (and still is) taken as evidence that the initial structural damage was not great, although the head injury had initiated a progressive sequence of events that led subsequently to a fatal outcome or persisting disability. Injury to the brain was therefore considered to be either *primary* (induced by mechanical forces) which occurred at the moment of injury or *secondary* (not mechanically induced) and which developed on an already mechanically injured brain. Such secondary damage could be due to complications either initiated via or independent of the primary damage. These secondary processes therefore are not unique to the head-injured patient, being commonly found in other types of intracranial disease.

It is now established that the principal mechanisms of damage after trauma are either *contact* or *acceleration/deceleration* (Table 8.1). Lesions caused by contact result either from something striking the head or vice versa and consist of local effects such as laceration of the scalp, fracture of the skull, with or without an associated extradural hematoma, surface contusions and lacerations, and intracerebral hemorrhage. In contrast, acceleration/deceleration damage results from head movements in the instant after injury and lead to intracranial and intracerebral pressure gradients as well as shear, tensile and compressive strains. Such inertial forces are responsible for two of the most important types of damage encountered in blunt head injury, *viz.* acute subdural hematoma resulting from the tearing of subdural bridging veins, and widespread damage to axons. Yet another classification has been derived based on the increase in clinical and neurological appreciation that the brain damage after trauma is either focal or diffuse and that such a classification is a useful means of grouping patients based on the appearances seen on a computed tomography (CT) scan (Table 8.2). The replication of these pathologies under controlled laboratory conditions has not only served to explain the patterns of brain damage occurring in humans, but also provided key information on the mechanisms and time course of various pathologies that are responsible for the brain damage after blunt head injury. Such information is critical in both the prevention of blunt head injury and in the identification and measurement of at least potentially avoidable factors contributing to brain damage after head injury.

Table 8.1 Mechanisms of damage after blunt head injury

Contact	Acceleration/deceleration
Lacerations of scalp	Tearing of bridging veins with formation of subdural hematoma
Fracture(s) of skull with or without an associated extradural hematoma	Diffuse traumatic axonal injury, tissue tears, and associated intracerebral hematoma(s)
Surface contusion and lacerations, and associated intracerebral hematoma(s)	Acute traumatic vascular injury

Glasgow database

With the full co-operation of the appropriate legal authorities and the forensic pathologists in the west of Scotland, a comprehensive database of brain damage in fatal head injuries has been established

Table 8.2 Classification of damage after blunt head injury

Focal	Diffuse-multifocal
Injury to scalp	Ischemic damage
Fracture(s) of skull	Axonal injury
Surface contusions and lacerations	Vascular injury
Intracranial hematoma(s)	Brain swelling
Raised intracranial pressure and associated vascular changes	Meningitis

Table 8.3 Classification and frequency of the principal types of lesions after fatal blunt head injury

Classification	Frequency (%)
Focal lesions	
• Fracture of the skull	75
• Surface contusions and lacerations	95
• Intracranial hematoma(s)	60
• Associated with raised	
• intracranial pressure	75
Diffuse (multifocal) lesions	
• β-APP immunohistochemistry	95
• Brain swelling	53
• Vascular damage	<5
• Ischemic damage	55
• Meningitis	4

in the 35-year period since 1968 consisting of a consecutive series of over 1500 fatal blunt injuries (Table 8.3). In most cases the brains were suspended in 4% formol saline for at least 3 weeks before being dissected in a standard fashion. The cerebral hemispheres were sliced in the coronal plane, the cerebellum at right angles to the folia and the brainstem horizontally. Comprehensive histological studies were undertaken in the majority of cases.

Current concepts of the pathophysiology of blunt head injury

Blunt head injury can be viewed as a clinical syndrome resulting from a combination of events mainly to neural and/or vascular components as a result of mechanical distortion of the head and brain (Fig. 8.1). Brain injury involves processes that are initiated at the time of head injury but may require hours or days to develop. The principal mechanisms of cellular dysfunction are the direct effects of trauma – deformation of membranes, dysfunction due to neurochemical, neurotransmitter and receptor changes, calcium-mediated damage, damage due to oxygen radicals and lipid peroxidation, and changes in association with inflammation

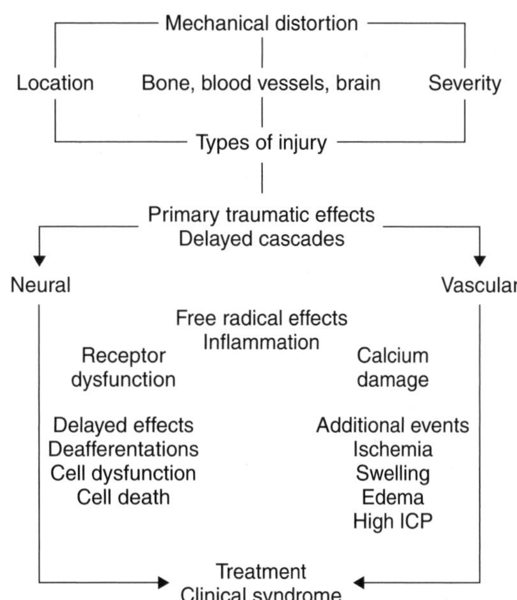

Figure 8.1 Principal features of traumatic injury to the head and brain

Table 8.4 Principal mechanisms of cellular injury after blunt head injury

Initial traumatic events
Deformation of membranes
Neurochemical, neurotransmitter and receptor changes
• Catecholamine neurotransmitters
• Monoamine neurotransmitters
• Excitatory amino acids
• Endogenous opioid peptides
• Platelet activating factor
• Various ions *viz.* Mg^{2+}, Ca^{2+}
Calcium-mediated damage
• Receptor mediated
• Voltage dependent
• Traumatic membrane defect
• Coupled receptor/channel
Oxygen-derived free radicals and lipid peroxidation
Inflammatory and cellular responses

(Table 8.4). These pathways singly or in combination result in either cellular necrosis or programmed cell death some of the cells showing features of apoptosis.

FOCAL LESIONS

Principal amongst these are fracture of the skull, surface contusions and lacerations, intracranial hematoma and brain damage associated with raised intracranial pressure.

Fracture of the skull

The different types are listed (Table 8.5). The more severe the head injury, the greater the frequency of the fracture of the skull. For example, the frequency is 3% in those who attend A&E departments, 65% in patients admitted to a neurosurgical unit and 80% in fatal cases. A fracture of the skull may be limited to the vertex, to the base of the skull, or may affect both. In 62% the fracture affects the vault of the skull with an extension into the base in 17%. A depressed fracture occurs in some 11% of patients and if either compound or penetrating may act as a potential source for intracranial infection. Fractures at the base of the skull may pass through the middle ear or the anterior cranial fossa producing CSF otorrhea or rhinorrhea, respectively, and they are potential sources for later infection.

There is a strong association between the presence of a fracture of the skull with the development of an intracranial hematoma, particularly if the patient had a depressed level of consciousness after the injury. For example, it has been determined that only 1 in 6000 patients attending A&E who did not have any of these features subsequently developed an intracranial hematoma, whereas the risk becomes 1 in 4 if these clinical features had been present.

Surface contusions and lacerations

These are the hallmarks of brain damage due to a head injury (Table 8.6). They vary in amount and are usually asymmetrical. Most contusions are found over the lateral surface of the hemispheres (Fig. 8.2), on the under surfaces of the frontal and temporal lobes (Fig. 8.3), in the cortex above and below the Sylvian fissures (Fig. 8.4) and less commonly on the under surface of the cerebellar hemispheres, and they are rarely seen in the occipital lobes. Different types are described (Table 8.7).

Contusions are invariably associated with some bleeding into the subarachnoid space. If more severe they may extend into white matter comprising a mixture of hemorrhage and necrosis, at the margins of which is an area of swelling (Fig. 8.5a and b). An actual hematoma may develop within the affected

Table 8.5 Types of skull fracture

- Linear or fissure
- Depressed if fragments of the inner table are displaced inwards by at least the thickness of the diploe
- Compound if depressed fracture is associated with laceration of scalp and penetrating if there is also a tear in the dura
- Hinge if fracture extends across the base of the skull
- Coup at site of injury
- Contrecoup describes a fracture located a distance from the point of injury
- Growing fractures occur in infancy and are due to interposition of soft tissue and meninges between edges of fracture that may prevent healing.

Table 8.6 Surface contusions and lacerations

- Found in 96% of fatal adult head injuries
- Healed contusions are found incidentally in 2.5% of adult autopsies post mortem
- Pia-arachnoid intact with contusions, but torn with lacerations
- At vertex related to fractures, and inferiorly correspond to irregular bony contours of base of skull
- Characteristically affect crests of gyri
- Appear as punctate hemorrhages or streaks of hemorrhage at right angles to the cortical surface
- In early infancy contusions appear as tears in the subcortical white matter and in the inner layers of the cortex of the frontal and temporal lobes

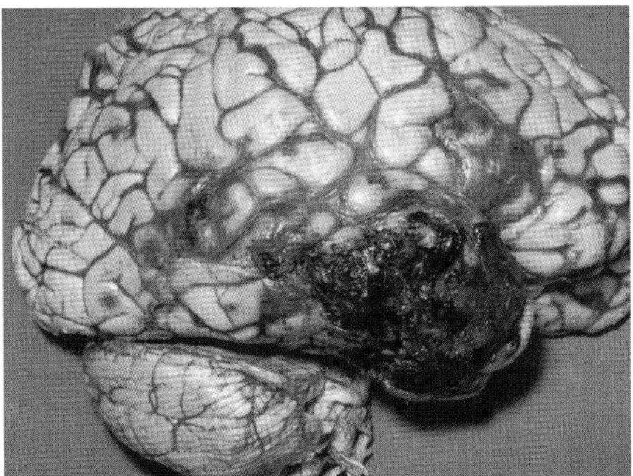

Figure 8.2 Cerebral contusions. There are recent hemorrhagic contusions on the lateral aspect of the right cerebral hemisphere.

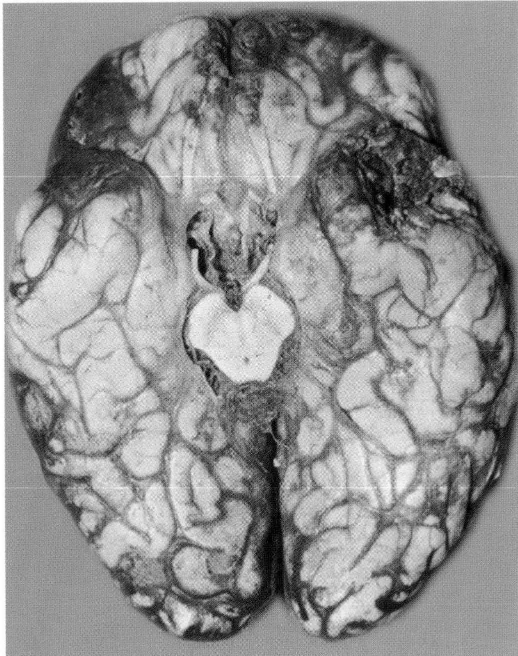

Figure 8.3 Cerebral contusions. There are recent hemorrhagic contusions on the inferior surfaces of the frontal and temporal lobes.

gyrus and if laceration of the pia-arachnoid has taken place, then there may be bleeding into the subdural space. The combination of extensive contusion and an associated subdural hematoma is often referred to as a 'burst lobe'.

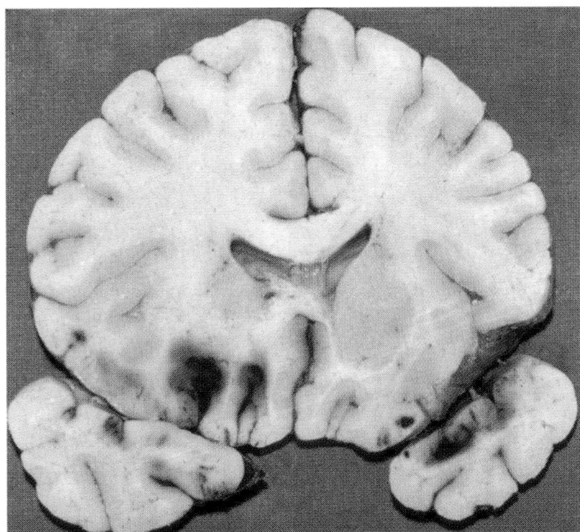

Figure 8.4 Cerebral contusions. There are recent hemorrhagic contusions above and below the Sylvian fissures.

Table 8.7 Types of contusion and laceration

- Fracture contusions occur at sites of a fracture
- Coup contusions occur at the site of impact in the absence of a fracture
- Contrecoup contusions occur in brain away from the point of impact
- Herniation contusions occur where the parahippocampal gyri and the cerebellar tonsils make contact against the edge of the tentorium and the foramen magnum respectively at the time of injury
- Gliding (parasagittal) contusions describe focal hemorrhage in the cerebral cortex and subjacent white matter at the superior margins of the cerebral hemispheres: they are usually bilateral, asymmetrical and are related to diffuse brain damage

In patients who die almost immediately after a head injury, contusion is composed essentially of perivascular hemorrhage (Fig. 8.6a and b) which may also extend into the white matter. Adjacent tissue undergoes necrosis as shown by the presence of ischemic cell change. There are then reactive changes in the form of proliferation of capillaries, astrocytes and microglia: often there is also associated edema (see Fig. 8.5b). The dead tissue is ultimately removed and the contusion comes

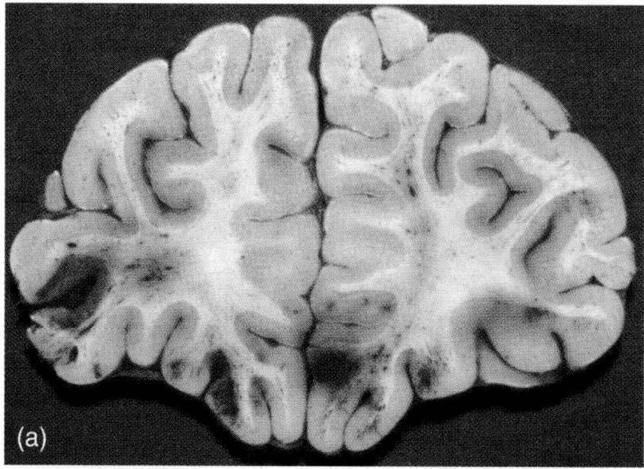

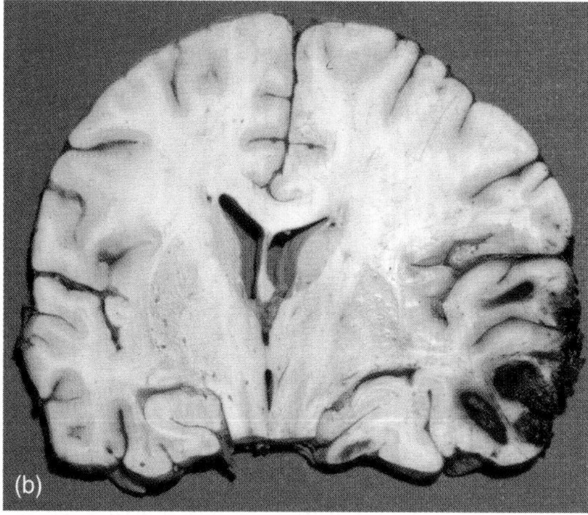

Figure 8.5 Cerebral contusions. There are recent hemorrhagic contusions, *viz.* (a) on the inferior aspects of the frontal lobes, and (b) on the lateral aspect of right temporal lobe. There is also associated swelling with midline shift and internal herniae.

to be represented by a shrunken and gliosed rather fenestrated scar, often remaining pigmented from residual hemosiderin containing macrophages – siderophages (Fig. 8.7a and b). An old contusion tends to be triangular in shape, its broad base being at the crest of a gyrus and its apex in the digitate white matter.

Intracranial hematoma

This is present in about 66% of blunt head injuries and is the most common cause of deterioration and death in patients who have experienced a lucid interval after head injury. Most are evacuated surgically. Regardless of the severity of the head injury there is always the possibility that an intracranial hematoma may complicate the injury. The bleeding usually begins at the instant of injury and by the time of admission to hospital some 3–4 h later there is a hematoma in between 30 and 60% of patients. Serial CT scans have also shown that some hematomas do not develop until 2 or more days after the injury: these are referred to as delayed hematomas. Neuroradiological investigations have also shown that intracranial hematomas are often present before they produce clinical deterioration, associated swelling of the brain and shifts and herniation being probably largely responsible. There are several types of traumatic intracranial hematoma and they are usually classified according to the anatomical compartment in which they develop (Table 8.8).

Extradural (epidural) hematoma

This consists of an ovoid mass of clotted blood that lies between the bone at the vault or the base of the skull and the dura (Table 8.9). As the source of the bleeding is usually arterial the hematoma enlarges fairly rapidly, gradually stripping the dura from the scalp to form a circumscribed ovoid mass that progressively indents and flattens the adjacent brain (Figs 8.8 and 8.9a and b). In some cases bleeding is from venous sinuses. In many cases there is very little associated underlying brain damage. Small hematomas may become completely organized, although larger ones may undergo partial organization, becoming cystic and filled with dark viscous fluid. After about 2 weeks the hematoma becomes smaller and in the majority of patients have completely resolved by 4–6 weeks after the injury. Occasionally, they may calcify. If untreated, large hematomas may cause midline shift leading to the formation of internal herniae, and compression of the midbrain.

In fire-related deaths where the head has been exposed to intense heat there may be fissure fractures of the skull and heat hematomas in the extradural space. These hematomas have a pink spongy appearance which are said to be characteristic of heat injury and different from the dark

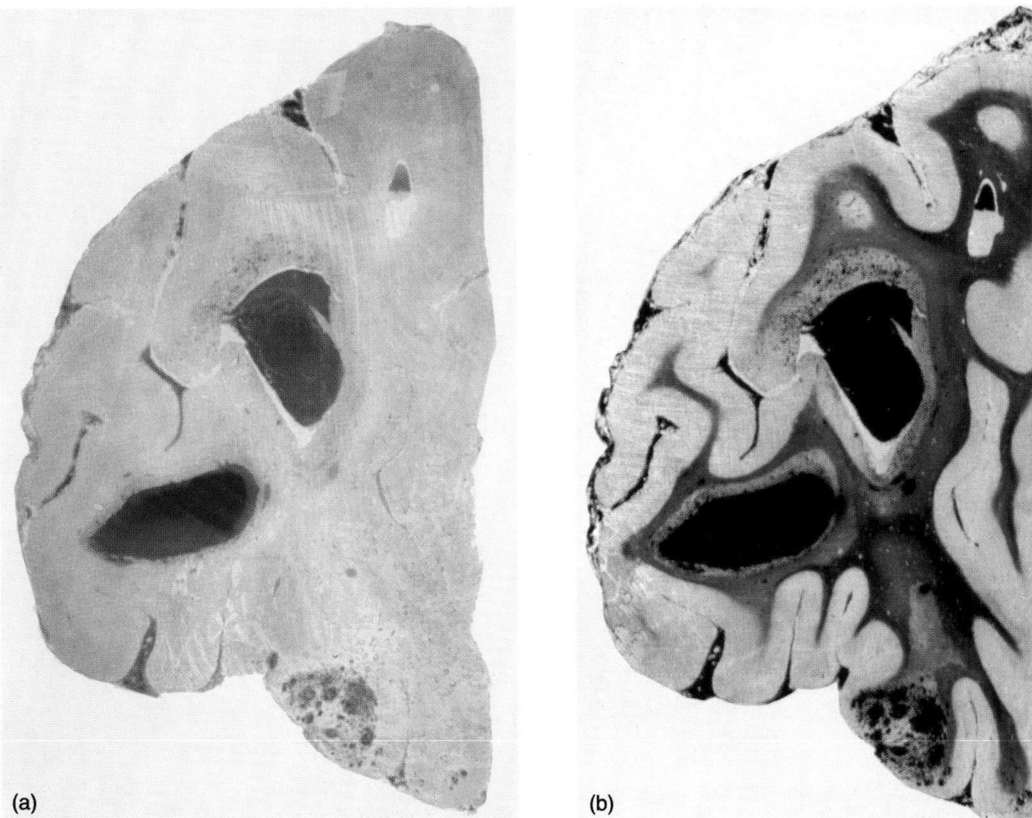

Figure 8.6 Cerebral contusions of frontal lobe. (a) There is subarachnoid and intracerebral hemorrhage. (b) There is pallor of staining in the adjacent tissue. Celloidin: (a) cresyl violet, (b) myelin stain.

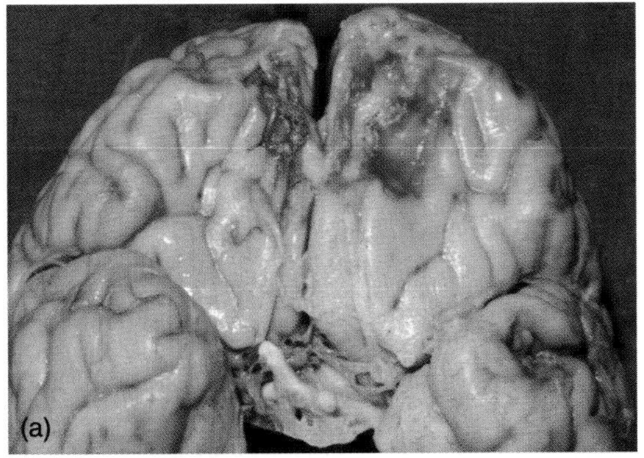

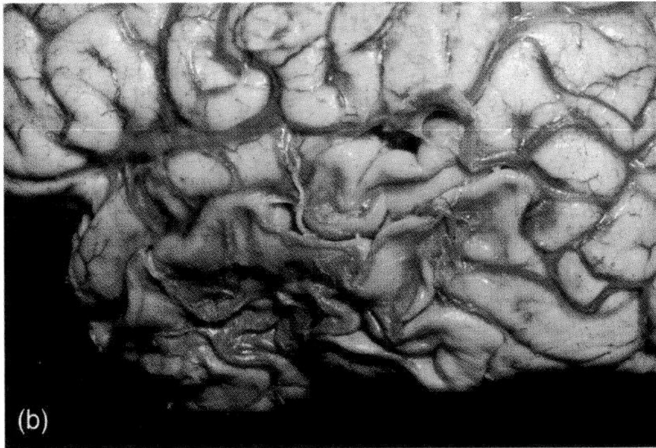

Figure 8.7 Cerebral contusions. There are old shrunken contusions, *viz.* (a) on the inferior surfaces of the frontal lobes (cf. Fig. 8.2), and (b) on the lateral aspect of the left temporal lobe.

red appearance of the blood in the conventional extradural hematoma: they also follow closely the distribution of the charring on the outer surface of the skull.

Intradural hematoma

Principal amongst these is the acute subdural hematoma (Table 8.10). Small amounts of bleeding

Table 8.8 Types and frequency of intracranial hematoma

Type	Frequency (%)	
Extradural	10	} 66
Intradural	56	
• Subdural	13	
• Subarachnoid	3	
• Discrete intracerebral or intracerebellar hematomas not in continuity with the surface of the brain	15	
• 'Burst' lobe: an intracranial or intracerebellar hematoma in continuity with a related subdural hematoma	25	

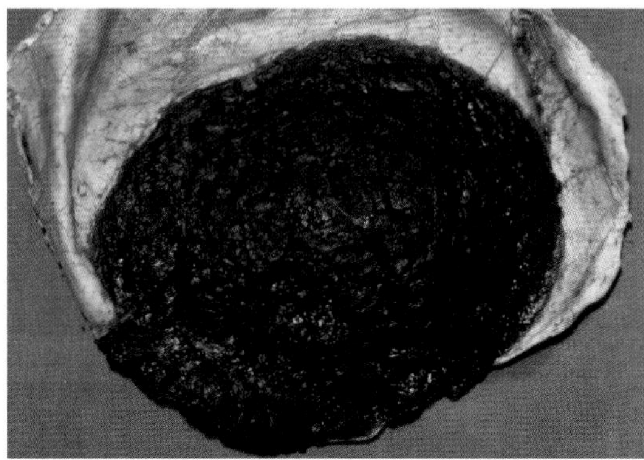

Figure 8.8 Extradural (epidural) hematoma. There is a sharply defined hematoma in the extradural space.

Table 8.9 Extradural (epidural) hematoma

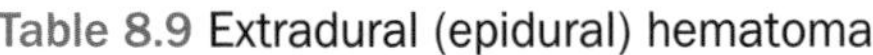

- Present in 5–15% of fatal head injuries
- In 85% of adults there is an associated fracture: in children a fracture is commonly absent
- In 70% of cases there is a fracture in the squamous part of the temporal bone; related to the middle meningeal artery in remaining cases they are frontal or parietal or even occur in the posterior fossa
- The hematoma reliably indicates the site of the fracture
- They are most common in young adults and are rarer in children and in the elderly
- In 5–10% of cases they co-exist with an intradural hematoma

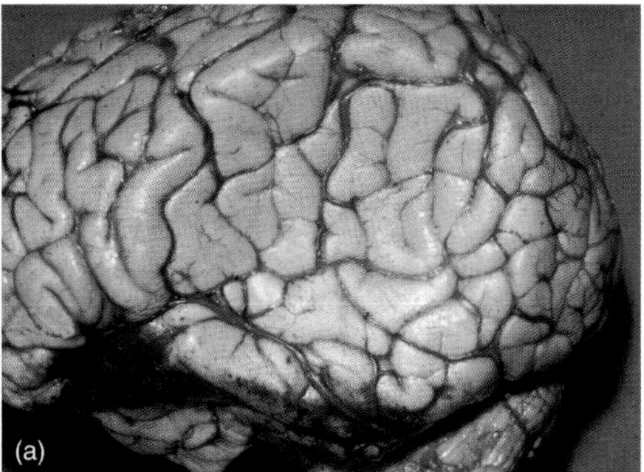

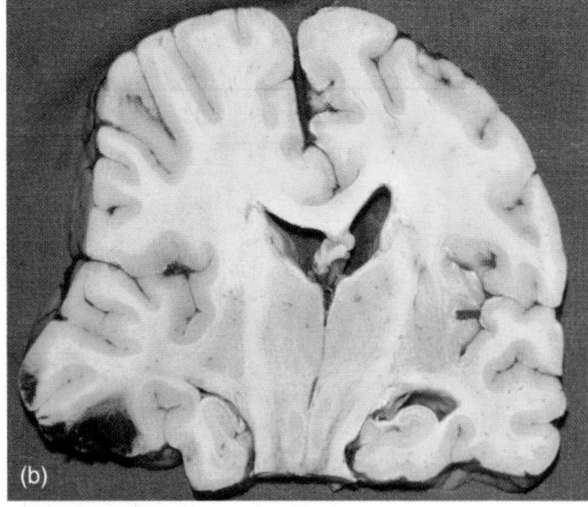

Figure 8.9 Extradural (epidural) hematoma. (a) Concave indentation of lateral aspect of left cerebral hemisphere. (b) Same as case (a). Note midline shift and internal herniation. There is a small recent hemorrhagic contusion.

within the subdural space are common in fatal head injury. Because this blood can spread freely throughout the subdural space it tends to cover the entire hemisphere with the result that a subdural hematoma is usually larger than an extradural hematoma. In the great majority of cases, subdural hematomas are due to rupture of veins that bridge the subdural space where they connect the upper surface of the cerebral hemisphere to the sagittal sinus, occasionally they are arterial in origin. The majority of acute subdural hematomas are associated with underlying brain damage and therefore the mortality and morbidity are greater in subdural

Table 8.10 Acute subdural hematoma

- Present in 13–20% of fatal head injuries
- In 70% of cases injury is produced by a fall or an assault
- About 70% of cases have a fracture of the skull, but in about 50% of these cases the fracture is contralateral to the side of the hematoma
- The peak incidence of intradural hematoma is in the fifth and sixth decades
- Only 2–3% of traumatic hematomas are in the posterior fossa where intradural hematomas are as common as extradural
- Present in a proportion of victims of child abuse
- There is an association between an acute subdural hematoma and swelling of an ipsilateral cerebral hemisphere: such swelling often persists after the hematoma has been evacuated
- In over 60% of cases there is infarction of the related cerebral hemisphere

than in extradural hematomas. This is particularly true in cases with a 'burst' frontal or temporal lobe.

The current literature classifies subdural hematoma as acute when it is composed of clotted blood (usually within the first 48 h after injury), subacute where there is a mixture of clotted and fluid blood (developing between 2 and 14 days after injury) and when the hematoma is fluid (developing more than 14 days after injury). With increasing survival the hematoma undergoes a sequence of changes (Table 8.11). Chronic subdural hematoma occurs weeks or months after what may appear to have been a trivial head injury (Fig. 8.10). The hematoma becomes encapsulated and slowly increases in size: they are more common in older than in younger patients and in alcoholics, and there is an association with long-term anticoagulation therapy and patients with coagulation defects such as hemophilia. The hematoma slowly increases in size, probably as a result of repeated small hemorrhages that are due

Table 8.11 Histological changes in subdural hematoma with increasing survival

Time after injury	Hematoma	Dural side	Arachnoidal side
Acute	Fresh red blood cells (RBCs)	Fibrin and a few fibroblasts	Fibrin
Subacute	Loss of definition of RBCs outline Hemosiderin formation	Fibroblast layer 2–5 cells thick	Fibrin
1–2 weeks	Leaking of RBCs Angiofibroblastic invasion of clot that is breaking up	Fibroblast layer equal to 25–50% thickness of dura	Fibroblastic membrane
Chronic, 3–4 weeks	Vascular channels well developed. Liquefied clot	Fibroblastic layer equal to thickness of dura. Siderophages throughout membrane	Well-formed membrane
1–3 months	Hyalinization of the membranes. There are dilated capillaries and secondary hemorrhages		
>3 months	Not possible to give accurate estimation of the age of the hematoma. The neomembranes fuse and there are scattered siderophages: they eventually become collagenized to look like dura. Occasionally calcification or ossification occur		

Modified from JM Hardman The pathology of traumatic brain injury. In: Thompson RA, Green JR (eds) *Advances in neurology*, vol. 22. New York: Raven Press, 1979: 15–50.

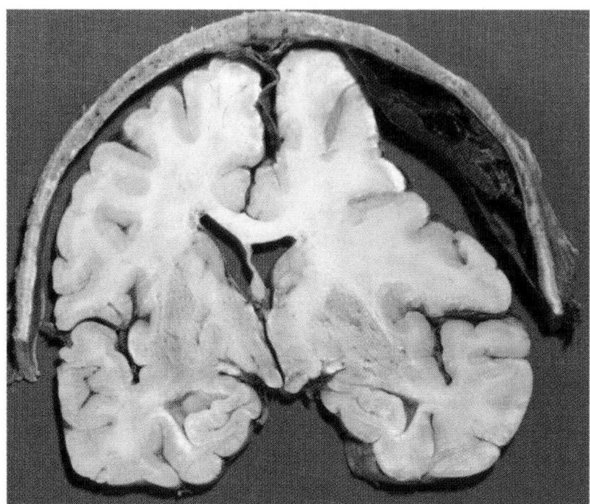

Figure 8.10 Chronic subdural hematoma. Mass effect with midline shift and internal herniae.

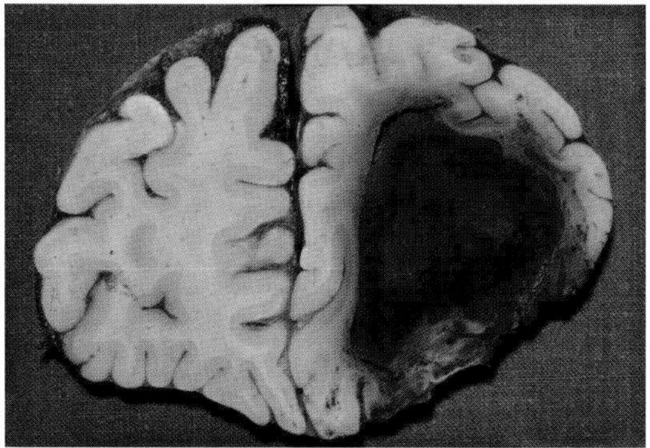

Figure 8.11 Traumatic intracerebral hematoma. There is a large hematoma in the right frontal lobe.

in part to the production of fibrin degradation products in the fluid and in part to the formation of new friable blood vessels in the capsule with a widely patent blood–brain barrier that allows the passage of red cells in and out of the hematoma.

Subdural hematoma is found in a proportion of cases of child abuse and in the 'battered baby' syndrome. Diagnosis is confirmed by needling the fontanelle that yields yellow fluid with a high protein content – *subdural hygroma.*

Intracerebral hematoma

These were present in 16% of the Glasgow series. They occur in two principal forms. One is a hematoma in a frontal (Fig. 8.11) or a temporal lobe (Fig. 8.12) in relation to contusions (Fig. 8.9): and

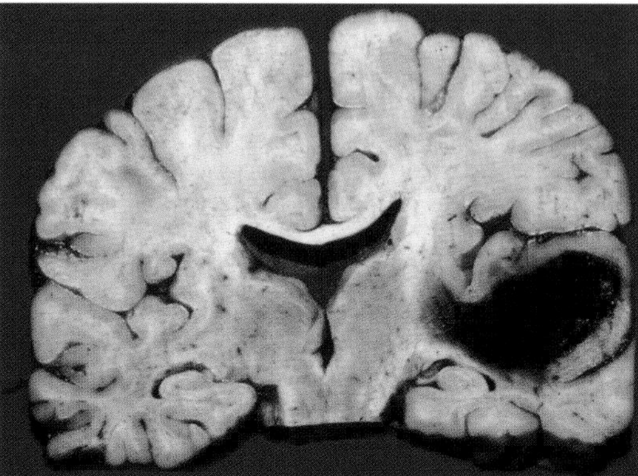

Figure 8.12 Traumatic intracerebral hematoma. There is a recent hematoma in the right temporal lobe that on dissection was in continuity with recent contusions.

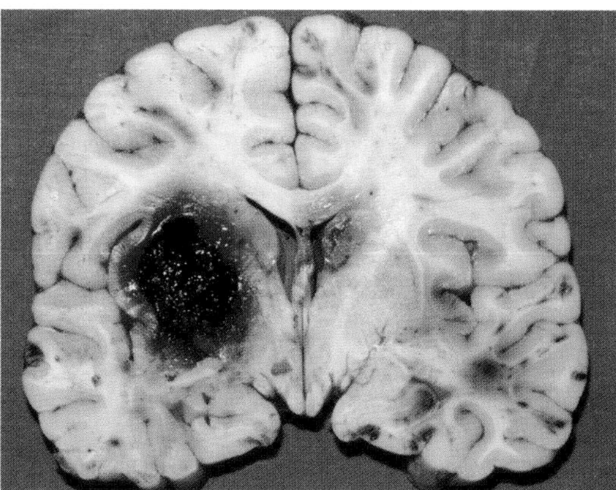

Figure 8.13 Traumatic intracerebral hematoma. There are bilateral 'basal ganglia' hematomas. There are also small 'gliding' contusions and a hemorrhagic lesion in the corpus callosum.

the second often referred to as '*basal ganglia hematomas*' are more common than was previously suspected clinically, and may be multiple, and are usually indicative of a severe head injury (Fig. 8.13).

'Burst lobe'

This is the co-existing of subdural hematoma, cerebral contusion and intracerebral hematoma, and is usually indicative of severe brain damage. The frontal and temporal lobes are most often affected. A burst lobe was identified in 23% of the Glasgow series.

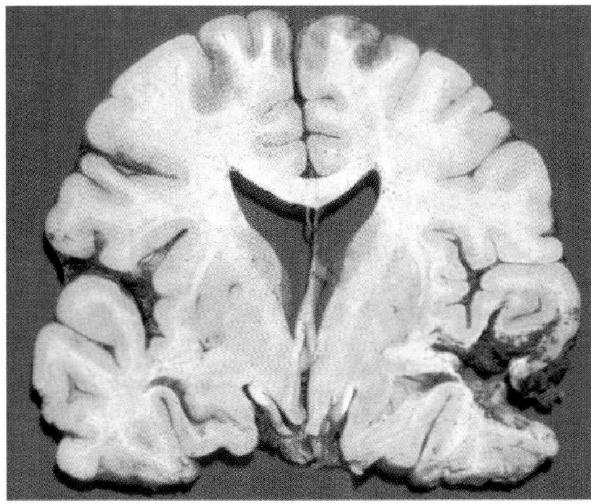

Figure 8.14 Ischemic brain damage. There is focally hemorrhagic infarction of the dorsomedial sectors of each hemisphere. Note contusion of right temporal lobe.

Brain damage due to raised intracranial pressure

This has already been detailed (see Chapter 4). Whether due to contusions with associated swelling or an intracranial hematoma several characteristic features develop (see page 68). The structural criterion of pressure necrosis in one or both parahippocampal gyri (Fig. 4.3, page 69) allows the pathologist to state with some certainty that the intracranial pressure (ICP) has been high during life and is a feature of some 75% of patients who after blunt head injury die in a neurosurgical intensive care unit. The further development of internal herniae is likely to mechanically deform blood vessels sufficient to cause vascular complications (see pages 70–71) which are a common finding in the brains of patients who die after head injury from the effect of a mass lesion. The end result is vascular damage in the brainstem often in the form of centrally replaced hemorrhages in the midbrain and pons. These vascular complications are thought to be due to downward traction on the central perforating branches of the basilar artery causing either their rupture or bleeding into areas of ischemic necrosis.

Death from secondary damage to the brainstem may be the result of one or more intracranial pathologies, such as contusion/laceration, brain swelling and intracranial hematoma.

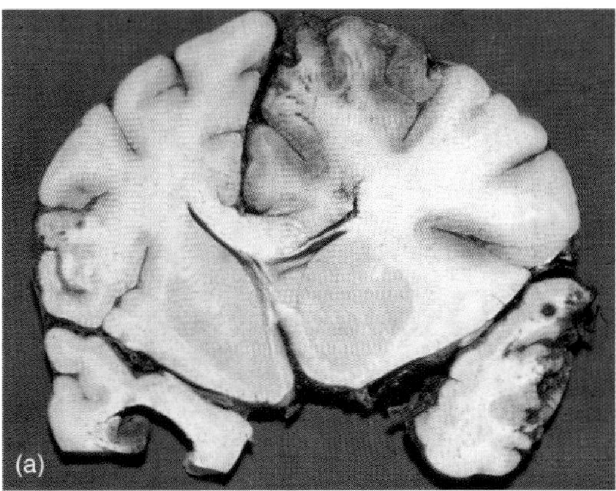

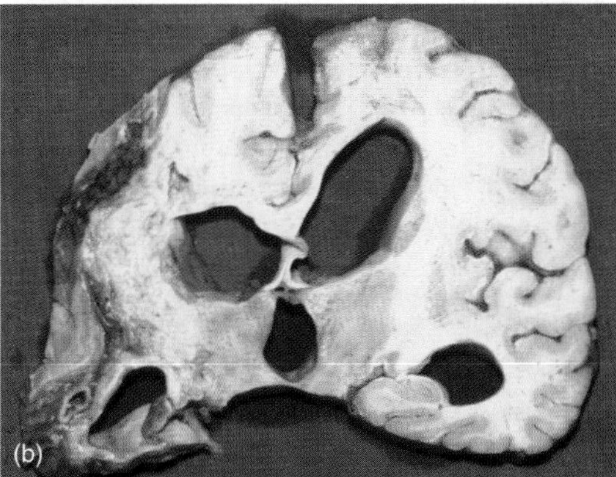

Figure 8.15 Ischemic brain damage. (a) Partly 'hemorrhagic' and anemic infarction in the territories of the right anterior and middle cerebral arteries, respectively. (b) Ischemic brain damage. There are longstanding infarcts in the distributions of the left middle and posterior cerebral arteries. Patient vegetative after head injury that required evacuation of a large left-sided acute subdural hematoma.

Ischemic brain damage

This is a frequent finding in patients who die as a result of a blunt head injury. Much of it occurs adjacent to contusions and hematomas, and is secondary to shift and herniation of the brain, in association with raised ICP (see Chapter 4) such as infarction in the brainstem and in the territories of the internal carotid arteries and of the posterior cerebral arteries. Analysis of the Glasgow database has shown that several decades ago there was ischemic damage in the arterial boundary zone in

20% of cases, and diffuse hypoxic brain damage in 35%. The infarction in arterial boundary zones is sometimes hemorrhagic, when it can be identified macroscopically. In other cases it can only be demonstrated microscopically and it has already been emphasized in Chapter 5 that severe diffuse hypoxic brain damage may defy recognition macroscopically even when it has been present for a few days. With the passage of time, however, reactive changes occur and affected areas become gliosed and shrunken (Figs 8.14 and 8.15).

The pathogenesis of ischemic brain damage resulting from a head injury is not yet established but the available evidence suggests that it occurs soon after injury, and correlations have been established between the presence of hypoxic brain damage and an episode of systemic hypoxia (defined as a systolic blood pressure of less than 80 mmHg for at least 15 min, or a $Pa\text{O}_2$ of 50 mmHg or less at some time after the injury) or high ICP. The basic cause of ischemic damage in arterial boundary zones is a transient period of greatly reduced cerebral blood flow, whereas diffuse hypoxic brain damage is frequently brought about by an episode of cardiorespiratory arrest or status epilepticus. These are well known events in a patient with an acute head injury.

It is important that pathologists are aware of the frequent occurrence of ischemic brain damage in blunt head injury since, as with diffuse traumatic axonal injury, it may only be recognized histologically. Whereas, in some cases it may be possible to identify pure or relatively pure examples of diffuse traumatic axonal injury in cases of which there have been complications of raised intracranial pressure, sometimes because of the widespread distribution of the lesion, the superimposition of one on the other may make it impossible to identify and separate out the two. Further, it is important that pathologists are aware of the frequent occurrence of ischemic brain damage in blunt head injury since, as with diffuse traumatic axonal injury, it may only be recognizable histologically.

Other types of focal injury

In accidents causing hyperextension of the head on the neck, traumatic separation of the pons on the medulla is a well recognized cause of death. In many cases there is an associated ring fracture at the base of the skull or dislocation and/or fracture of the first cervical vertebra. While complete tears are immediately fatal, patients with small or incomplete tears at the pontomedullary junction may survive for some time following injury.

Any of the cranial nerves may be damaged at the time of injury.

Damage can also occur in the hypothalamus and pituitary gland. Occasionally the pituitary stalk is torn, but more frequently the stalk is intact although there is infarction in the anterior lobe of the pituitary. A number of potential mechanisms have been put forward to explain this type of damage including a fracture at the base of the skull that extends into the sella turcica, elevation of the ICP leading to distortion and compression of the pituitary stalk and hypotensive shock, analogous to the situation occurring in post-partum necrosis of the pituitary.

Damage to blood vessels may also occur. It is now possible to identity various vascular lesions by angiography, including *dissection* with occlusion of the internal carotid or vertebral arteries, a *traumatic pseudo-aneurysm*, a *traumatic arteriovenous fistula*, *venous thrombosis*, and the presence and amount of any *vasospasm*.

Multiple petechial hemorrhages are not uncommonly found when patients die from severe head injury. While many of these may be part of diffuse traumatic axonal injury (see below) there are many other causes that include *fat embolism, septicemia*, and a host of *vascular* and *hematological abnormalities* that constitute some of the medical complications of head injury.

DIFFUSE (MULTIFOCAL) LESIONS

This term describes a number of pathologies some of which are a consequence of acceleration/ deceleration applied to either white matter or blood vessels or both and yet others that are secondary to ischemia. While it is true that these pathologies are widely distributed and in some instances are

Table 8.12 Pattern and frequency of hemorrhages and tissue tears in severe cases of diffuse traumatic axonal injury

Location of hemorrhage	Frequency (%)
Dorsolateral sector(s) of upper brainstem	95
Corpus callosum	92
Choroid plexus of IIIrd ventricle	90
Parasagittal (gliding) contusions	88
Hippocampus	88
Periventricular (IIIrd)	83
Interventricular septum	80
Cingulate gyrus	61
Thalamus	56
Basal ganglia	17

diffuse the overall generic term diffuse brain injury is something of a misnomer, as in the majority of cases the pathology is multifocal.

Diffuse traumatic axonal injury

This is one of the most important types of brain damage resulting from a blunt head injury and is the most common cause of coma in the absence of an intracranial hematoma. This type of brain damage has many synonyms and was first described under the heading of *diffuse degeneration of white matter.* There is now international recognition for the term *diffuse traumatic axonal injury* (TAI). In severe cases and in patients surviving for only a few days hemorrhagic lesions are found with a characteristic distribution in midline structures (Table 8.12) which may be seen at the time of brain cutting (Fig. 8.16). These focal hemorrhagic lesions are in contrast to the widespread damage to axons in the specimens. Indeed in some cases the brain may appear fully normal macroscopically and, of course, widespread damage to axons that characterizes this condition can only be identified microscopically. The histological appearances of the lesions depend on the length of survival after injury (Table 8.13). If the patient survives for only a few hours or days the lesions are usually hemorrhagic (Fig. 8.17a and b), but over time these result in shrunken often cystic scars (Fig. 8.18a and b). The changes in the white matter are particularly important. Although, they may be recognized in both H&E and silver-stained preparations as eosinophilic or argyrophilic swellings respectively (Fig. 8.19a and b), the sensitivity of immunohistochemistry using an antibody to the precursor protein of β-amyloid (β-APP) is increasingly becoming apparent. For example, it is now possible to identify axonal β-APP accumulation between 1 and 2 h after injury and early bulb formation at 3 h (Fig. 8.20a and b). The amount of immunostaining increases between 16 and 24 h after which it appears to plateau. Therefore, the amount of axonal injury as demonstrated by immunostaining appears to increase between 3 and 24 h and there are always

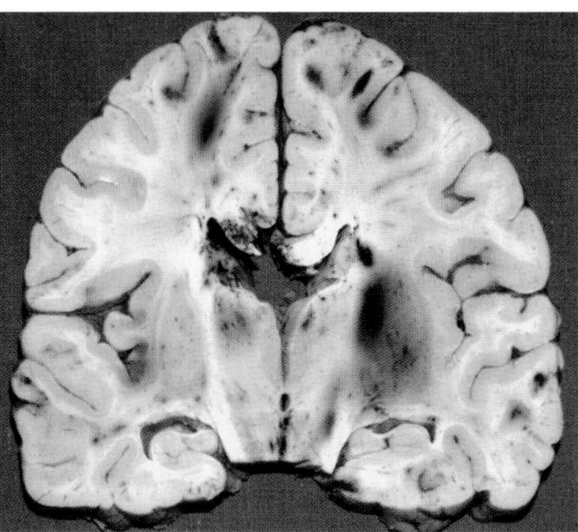

Figure 8.16 Diffuse traumatic axonal injury. There is a hemorrhage lesion in the corpus callosum to the left of the midline. The interventricular septum has been torn. There are also 'gliding' contusions and small hemorrhages in the basal ganglia. Note the absence of surface contusions.

Table 8.13 Diffuse traumatic axonal injury: histological appearances and their time course

Hours
- Hemorrhages and tissue tears
- Axonal swellings
- Axonal bulbs

Days/weeks
- Astrocytosis
- Clusters of microglia (macrophages)

Months/years
- Wallerian degeneration

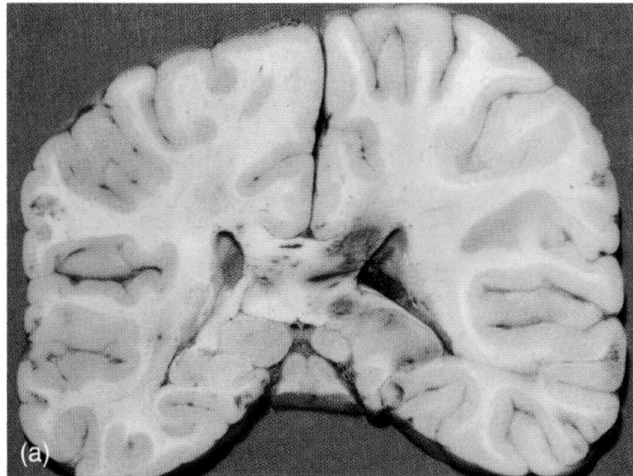

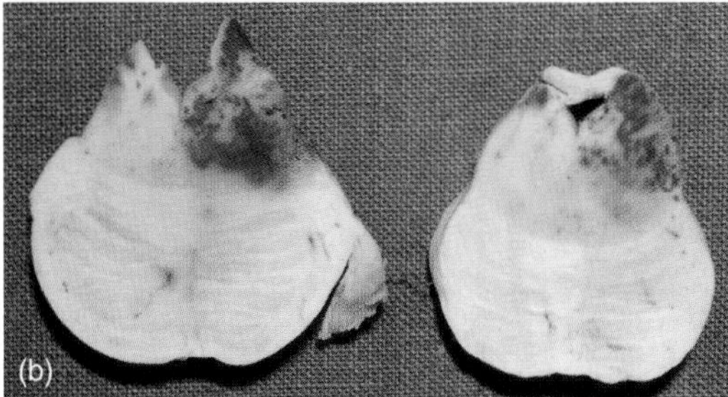

Figure 8.17 Diffuse traumatic axonal injury: short survival. (a) There is a hemorrhagic lesion in the splenium of the corpus callosum. (b) There is a hemorrhagic lesion in the dorsolateral sector(s) of the rostral brainstem.

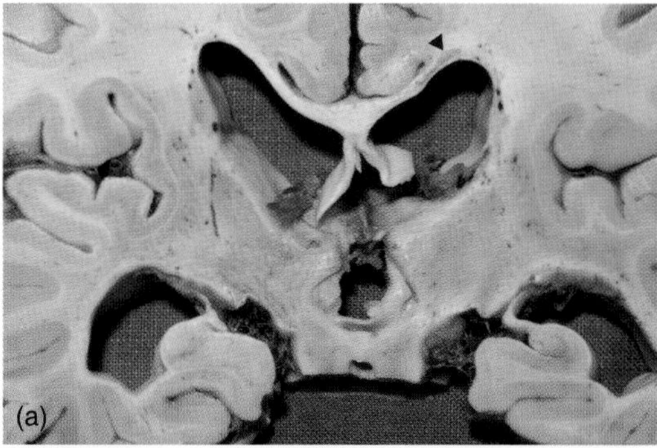

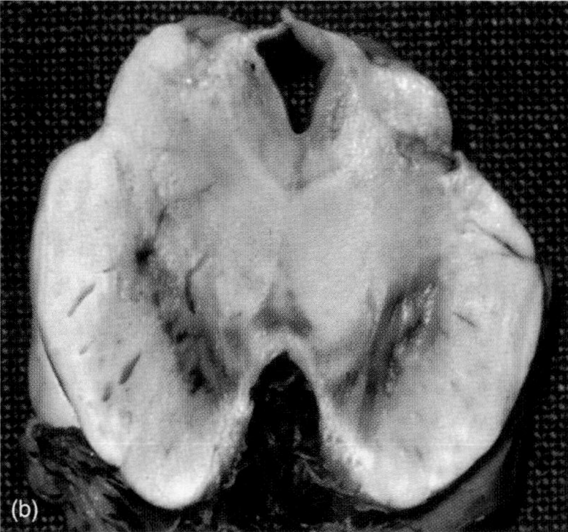

Figure 8.18 Diffuse traumatic axonal injury: long survival. (a) There is a small scar (arrowhead) in the corpus callosum and enlargement of the lateral ventricles. (b) There is a slightly discolored and granular lesion in the dorsolateral sector of the pons.

more axonal swellings than bulbs. If survival extends to a number of weeks then bulbs become less prominent, being difficult to see after 2 months. By 48–72 h there is an astrocytosis and within a few weeks there is a response in microglia and macrophage formation (Fig. 8.21). With a survival of months or years previous axonal damage can be recognized by the identification of the breakdown products of myelin (Fig. 8.22). Therefore, in those patients who survive severely disabled or in a vegetative state, abnormalities in the brain may be limited to small healed superficial contusions and extensive degeneration in the white matter. Coronal sections of such specimens reveal characteristic features of relatively intact gray matter and a greatly reduced amount of central white matter and compensatory enlargement of the ventricular system (Fig. 8.23). In most cases it is still possible to identify, by using the Perl's technique for hemosiderin, the tell-tale focal lesions in the corpus callosum and in the rostral brainstem (Fig. 8.24a and b).

A grading system has been developed that reflects the clinical spectrum of TAI in which a proportion of cases with grade 1 may present with a partial or complete lucid interval whereas all of the patients with grade 3 TAI are in a coma from the time of injury (Table 8.14). The distinct clinicopathological nature of this group of patients is further demonstrated by a statistically significantly lower incidence of fracture to the skull, cerebral contusions, intracerebral hematomas and evidence of a high ICP as compared to patients without this type of brain damage. There is also a high incidence

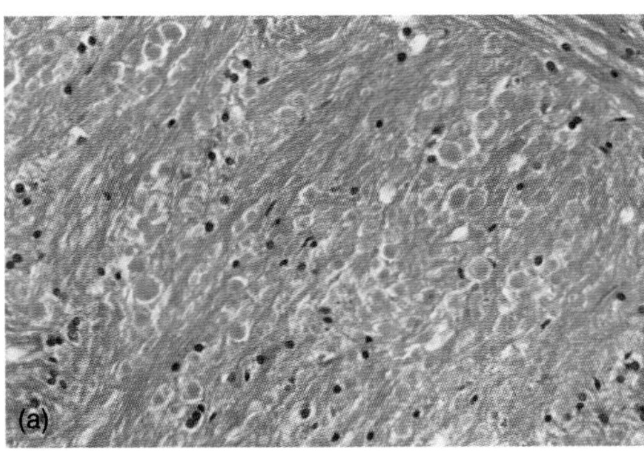

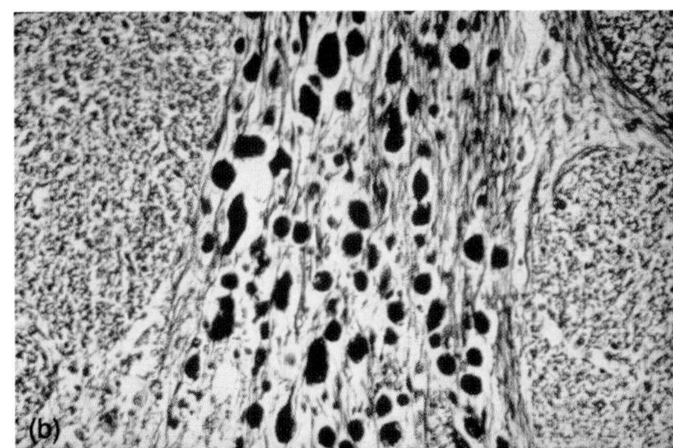

Figure 8.19 Diffuse traumatic axonal injury. In the early stages there are axonal swellings in the white matter. (a) H&E, (b) Silver impregnation.

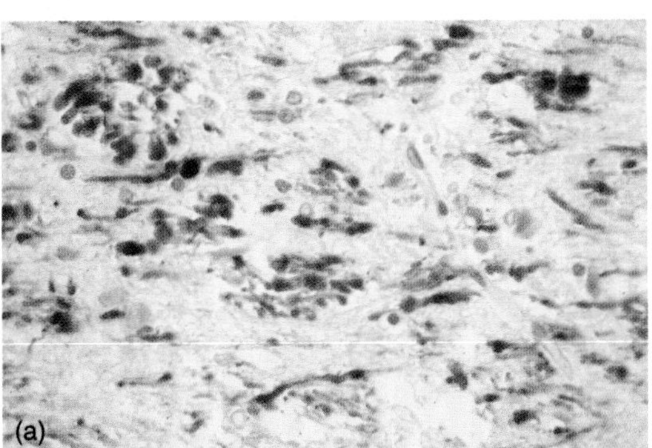

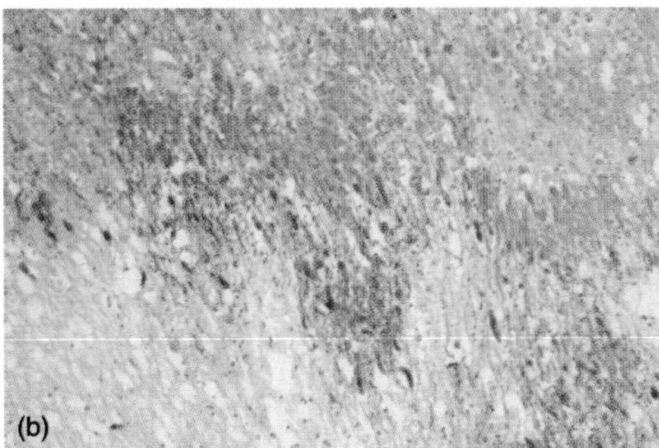

Figure 8.20 Diffuse traumatic axonal injury. (a) Irregularities in the outline of axons are readily identified. These changes are widely distributed although accentuated in the midline structures and are not limited to areas of infarction or hemorrhage. (b) Abnormal axons are frequently seen in 'Z'-shaped patterns in relation to infarcts. (a) and (b) Immunohistochemistry β-APP.

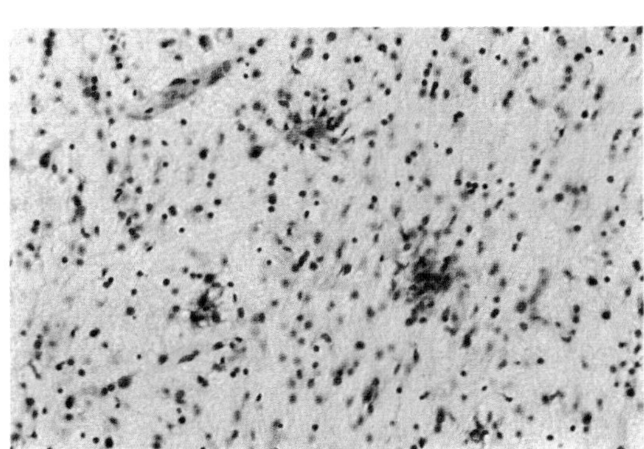

Figure 8.21 Diffuse traumatic axonal injury. There are clusters of microglia/macrophages in the white matter. Cresyl violet.

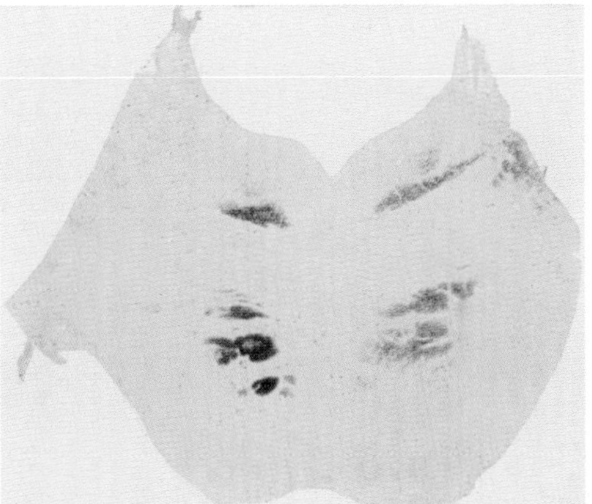

Figure 8.22 Diffuse traumatic axonal injury. There is asymmetrical Wallerian-type degeneration in the corticospinal tracts and in the medial lemnisci. Marchi preparation.

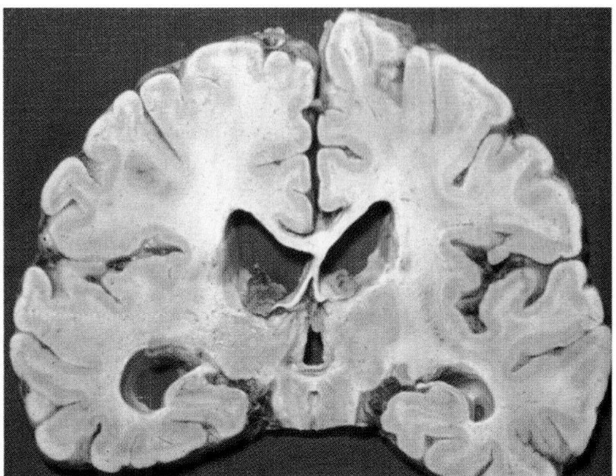

Figure 8.23 Diffuse traumatic axonal injury: patient surviving 21 months in vegetative state. There is a reduction in white matter which is rather granular and gray–white in color, and ventricular enlargement. Note absence of surface contusions.

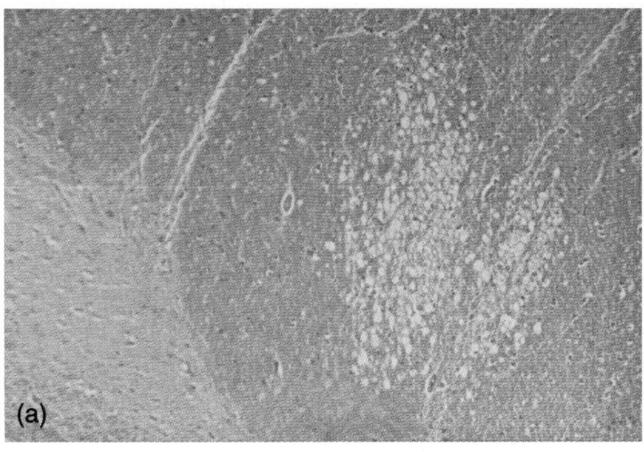

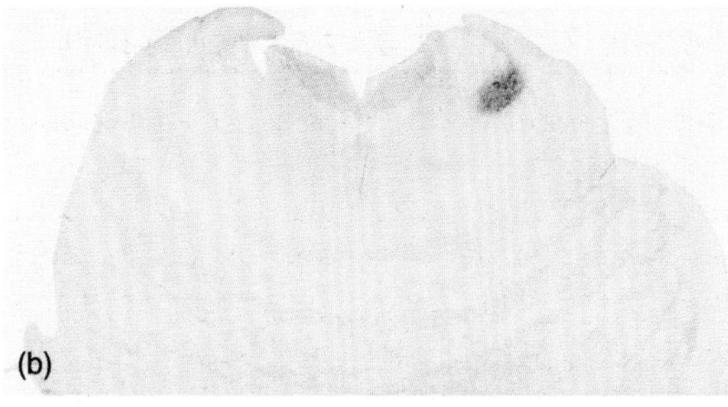

Figure 8.24 Diffuse traumatic axonal injury. (a) In short survivors there may be rarified areas ('tears') in the corpus callosum. (b) In long survivors focal 'tears' may be more easily identified by identifying hemosiderin at sites of previous hemorrhage. (a) H&E stain, (b) Perl's.

Table 8.14 Grading of traumatic axonal injury

Grade	Features
1	Scattered axonal bulbs throughout white matter
2	Also a focal lesion (usually hemorrhagic) in the corpus callosum
3	In addition there is a lesion in the dorsolateral sector(s) or the rostral brainstem

of head injury due to road traffic accidents, although TAI has been described following an assault and after a fall from a height.

The distribution of β-APP immunoreactivity has been examined in multiple brain areas. A common site of axonal injury was in the brainstem occurring in over 95% of cases. The internal capsule and thalamus were positive in 80% of cases and evidence of axonal injury was present in the corpus callosum and parasagittal white in 70%. When interpreting presumed traumatic axonal injury it is essential to establish if the distribution of any of the changes can be accounted for by the presence of hemorrhage or a vascular complication of raised intracranial pressure and internal herniation. Indeed, there are many instances when the amount of β-APP immunostaining that can be attributed to the secondary effects of deformation, shift and internal herniae is so great that it is not possible to comment upon the presence, let alone the amount of any traumatic axonal pathology. Under these circumstances it is advisable to obtain as much clinical information as possible before attempting clinico-pathological correlation. For example, a specimen in which there are large numbers of β-APP immunostained axons is unlikely to be part of the TAI complex if the clinical records indicate that the patient had 'talked' prior to death.

A diagnosis of TAI may be suspected clinically, radiologically, or even at the time of brain cutting, but the diagnosis can only be determined with certainty by the histological examination of the brain. Therefore, how many blocks and from which brain areas are required to establish the diagnosis? The recommended practice is to take 17 blocks as a matter of routine including the left and right parasagittal white matter, the watershed areas, the insular cortex and extreme capsules, the thalamus including internal capsules, the cerebellar peduncles, the corpus callosum at three levels, (anterior, mid and splenium) the midbrain, upper pons and medulla. Fewer blocks, even if taken from brain areas that are known to be particularly vulnerable to shearing injury, are likely to provide an under-estimate of the amount and distribution of TAI. In many cases there is considerable asymmetry of the findings. Further, there may be an anterior–posterior gradient in the corpus callosum and there are instances when axonal damage attributable to TAI can be found only above the tentorium, the brainstem apparently appearing normal.

It has been suggested that a wavy linear pattern of β-APP immunostaining (Fig. 8.20b) is more likely due to infarction than multifocal axonal immunostaining, which is considered to be more typical of TAI. However, it should be remembered that the TAI complex embraces the likelihood of both axonal and vascular damage and so both patterns, that is wavy linear bands and multiple foci of staining may be a feature of TAI. Furthermore, increasing experience with β-APP immunohistochemistry has heightened awareness of pitfalls in the diagnosis of TAI, as swellings and bulbs may be seen in a number of disorders (Table 8.15). Clearly, many disorders need to be considered before concluding that they are necessarily due to head injury. Other factors that need to be considered include the length of time for which a patient may be brainstem dead, i.e. the amount of time for which there has not been any cerebral perfusion and during which time autolysis would be taking place between the intervals of death, autopsy and fixation. Antigen retrieval techniques, *viz.* microwaving, have helped to identify axonal injury under these circumstances, but difficulties in interpretation may arise if in spite of all these possible methods immunohistochemistry fails to identify any evidence of axonal injury in a patient diagnosed clinically and radiologically as having a diffuse brain injury.

Table 8.15 Non-traumatic causes of axonal pathology

- Hematomas
- Infarcts
- Associated with vascular complication of raised intracranial pressure
- AIDS
- Acute demyelination
- Acute cerebritis
- Hypoglycemia
- Carbon monoxide poisoning
- Aging process

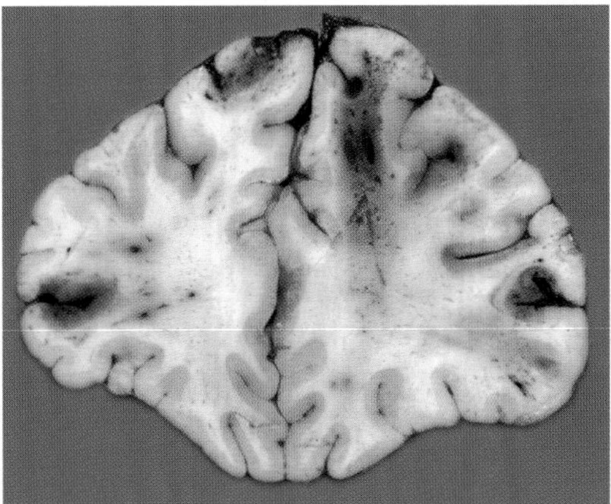

Figure 8.25 Diffuse traumatic axonal injury. There are multiple petechial hemorrhages in the white matter of the frontal lobes.

Diffuse traumatic vascular injury

There is a form of acute brain injury after trauma that is characterized by a series of multiple small hemorrhages that are particularly conspicuous in the white matter of the frontal and temporal lobes, (Fig. 8.25), in and adjacent to the thalamus and in the brainstem: small hemorrhages may also be seen in parasagittal white matter, and in the corpus callosum. This pattern of damage is seen in patients who die either instantly or at the scene of the accident, although a number may survive for up to 24 h. It is thought to represent a severe form of brain injury in which, as a result of acceleration/

deceleration, tearing has occurred in small blood vessels. The relationship between this entity and that of TAI has yet to be established.

Cerebral edema and brain swelling

Vasogenic cerebral edema (see Chapter 4) occurs around contusions and hematomas and may contribute to the effective size of the expanding lesion. Acute congestive brain swelling (see Chapter 4) also occurs after head injury in the form of diffuse swelling in one or both cerebral hemispheres. Development may be very rapid but occasionally appears to be delayed by 24–48 h.

Diffuse swelling of the entire cerebral hemispheres occurs in about 30% of patients with an acute traumatic intracranial hematoma, and is particularly common after evacuation of an acute subdural hematoma (see Fig. 4.13, page 74). Diffuse swelling of both cerebral hemispheres occurs in young children (Fig. 4.14, page 74). The original injury may have been apparently trivial or severe but the pathogenesis of either type of brain swelling in head injury is not known, but because of the rapidity with which it can appear it seems likely that there must be some vasomotor paralysis and loss of autoregulation (see Chapter 4).

Traumatic subarachnoid hemorrhage

Death is usually rapid and at autopsy a large amount of fresh blood is present within the basal cisterns and around the brainstem, and the cranial nerve roots. In many instances death may be attributed to raised ICP and tonsillar herniation leading to respiratory arrest. Small amounts of traumatic hemorrhage are common in survivors. In cases in which large amounts of hemorrhage are present the possibility of injury to a vertebral artery or one of its branches needs to be considered.

Fat embolism

Some patients who sustain a head injury also have multiple injuries including limb and other fractures. Therefore, they are at risk of developing systemic fat embolism. Indeed fulminating fat embolism is a well recognized, if uncommon, cause of a rapid progressive neurological deterioration in a patient without an acute intracranial expanding lesion. In some instances the classical appearance of petechial hemorrhages may be absent despite the presence of extensive fat embolism. In patients with multiple injuries, therefore, the brain has to be screened routinely for fat embolism.

Meningitis

Meningitis is a well-recognized complication of head injury and is usually due to the spread of micro-organisms through an open fracture of the calvaria or through a sometimes unrecognized fracture at the base of the skull bringing the subarachnoid space into continuity with major air sinuses. The latter is often associated with a CSF rhinorrhea or otorrhea or an aerocele. If there is a small defect in the dura at the base of the skull meningitis may be delayed for many months or even years. A small traumatic fistula may also be the cause of recurrent episodes of meningitis. In a small number of cases infection may complicate the insertion of an ICP monitoring device. Shunt-associated infections may present in various ways. Infected ventriculoatrial shunts may present as meningitis, ventriculitis or shunt nephritis.

Dementia pugilistica

It is well recognized that large numbers of concussive or subconcussive blows, such as may be incurred by various sportsmen, and in particular by boxers, sometimes induces the development of neurological signs and progressive dementia that may develop years after the last injury. It affects amateur as well as professional boxers and it is most likely to develop in boxers with long careers who have been dazed, if not knocked out, on many occasions. Studies have revealed a characteristic pattern of damage, the principal features of which are abnormalities in the septum pellucidum with fenestration of its leaves and enlargement of the ventricles (Fig. 8.26a). In some cases there is thinning of the adjacent fornices of the corpus callosum, scarring with neuronal loss in the cerebellum, degeneration in the substantia nigra with a loss of pigmented neurons (Fig. 8.26b), the presence of

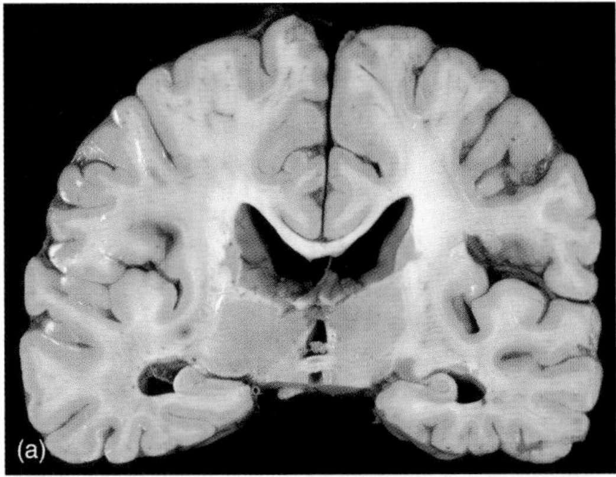

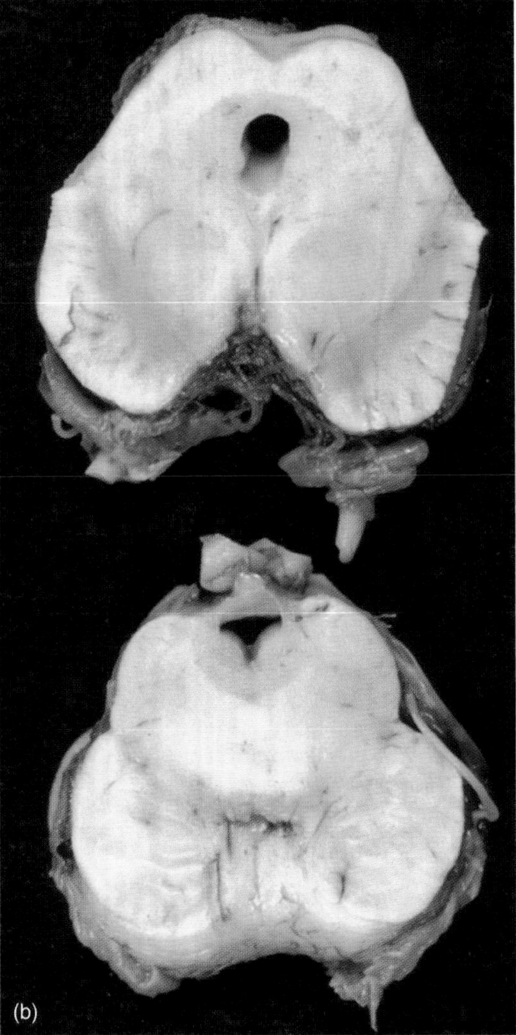

Figure 8.26 Boxers. (a) There is degeneration of the columns of the fornix, and ventricular enlargement. (b) There is pallor of the substantia nigra.

numerous neurofibrillary tangles diffusely throughout the cerebral cortex and in the brainstem, and the recent demonstration of variable amounts of diffuse β-A4 (Aβ) staining plaques.

The autopsy

It should be clear from the foregoing account there are many subtle changes of brain damage in blunt head injury. Only too often, death is certified as being due to a fracture of the skull and cerebral contusions and neither may be the reason for the patient even being in coma. The great majority of patients with a fracture of the skull make an uneventful recovery, and patients with quite severe cerebral contusions may make an excellent recovery if no other type of brain damage is present.

The pathologist must be present when the skull is open so that it can be clearly established whether an intracranial hematoma is extradural or intradural. The volume of the hematoma should be measured, since hematomas of less than 35 mL are unlikely to have been important intracranial expanding lesions unless there is also brain swelling. The pathologist should also assess the tightness of the dura, since this is a useful method of determining whether or not intracranial pressure has been high during life. Some comments relating to the autopsy in children and infants will be found in Chapter 14.

In many severe head injuries the cause of the fatal outcome is immediately apparent, e.g. if there is an intracranial hematoma, evidence of a high intracranial pressure and secondary hemorrhage in the brainstem. Even in these patients there may be other types of brain damage. On the other hand, the pathologist may find a brain of entirely normal appearance when the clinical history clearly indicates that the patient has died as a result of a blunt head injury. Circumstances sometimes dictate that the unfixed brain is sliced rather than being retained after a period of fixation before dissection. Slices of unfixed brain may make it difficult to identify focal lesions in the corpus callosum or rostral brainstem. Furthermore, ventricular size and displacement caused, for example, by swelling, is almost impossible to assess. Even if the brain is sliced and fixed, it must be screened for diffuse traumatic axonal injury, ischemic brain damage and fat embolism. The presence or absence of the last of these can easily be established by taking two or three blocks for frozen section. To establish the presence of diffuse traumatic axonal injury or ischemic brain damage, tissue from the arterial boundary zones, the parasaggital white matter, the corpus callosum, and the hippocampi, the cerebellum and several levels of the brainstem must be examined histologically.

If a patient has survived in coma or vegetative state for some weeks or months after head injury, the most likely cause is diffuse traumatic axonal injury or ischemic brain damage, since most patients who sustain secondary damage in the brainstem rarely survive for more than a few weeks. The situation should be clarified by histological survey but, if the patient has survived for more than two months after injury, the importance of looking for long-tract degeneration has to be emphasized.

Missile head injury

This can be defined as depressed, penetrating or perforating. In a *depressed* injury the missile does not enter the cranial cavity but produces the depressed fracture of the skull. In a *penetrating* injury, the object enters the cranial cavity but does not pass through it. In a *perforating* injury, the object, usually a bullet, traverses the cranial cavity and leaves through an exit wound.

Missile injuries produce focal damage to the brain in the form of lacerations at the site of injury, hemorrhage into the regions of the brain destroyed by the penetration of the object, and varying degrees of swelling around it (Fig. 8.27). Since the damage is focal, there may be no disturbance of consciousness unless some vital structure is damaged by the missile. In a severe missile injury, such as that produced by a bullet, radial displacement forces from the bullet tract may cause remote contusions affecting the undersurfaces of the frontal and the temporal lobes and the cerebellum. Contrecoup fractures (see page 156) may also occur in the orbital plates.

In penetrating and perforating injuries there is a high risk of infection, *abscess* being more common than meningitis (Fig. 8.28), and a higher incidence of post-traumatic epilepsy that is brought about by blunt head injury. Occasionally there may be direct damage to the brainstem in deep penetrating injuries.

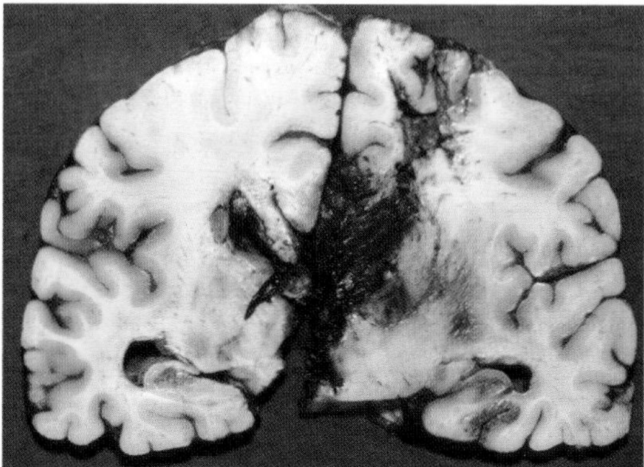

Figure 8.27 Missile head injury. There is a hemorrhagic track that passes downwards and medially from the dorsomedial sector of the right cerebral hemisphere through the ipsilateral corpus callosum and medial thalamus into the third ventricle.

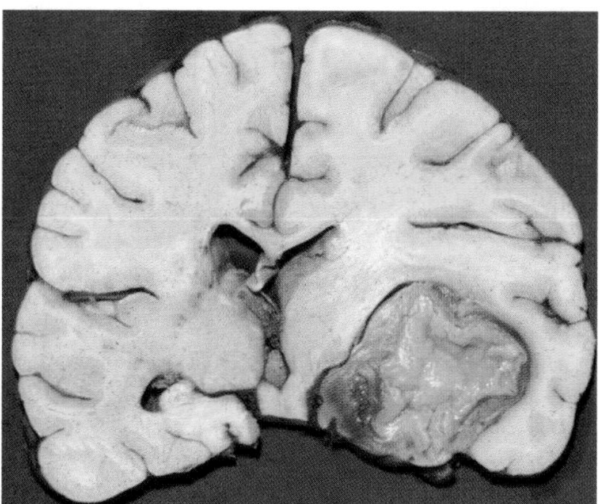

Figure 8.28 Cerebral abscess. There was an air-gun pellet in this acute hemorrhagic abscess.

HEAD INJURY IN INFANCY AND CHILDHOOD

There may be trauma to the brain, and to the spinal cord (see below) during birth. For example, a cephalohematoma is present in some 2.5% of all births. Fractures of the skull are unusual, and are found only in association with prolonged labor and forceps delivery. Subdural hemorrhage at full term is usually due to either a tear in the falx cerebri or in the tentorium cerebelli during a precipitate or breech delivery. In premature babies bleeding is likely to occur during breach presentation, high forceps delivery or excessive distortion of skull bones during birth. Subarachnoid hemorrhage is common and may be due to rupture of blood vessels within the subarachnoid space or in the cerebral hemispheres, with direct extension to the ventricles, or to a tear in the falx or the tentorium.

Head injuries are common in the pediatric age group and most are minor and of little consequence. However, head injury is the single most common cause of death and new disabilities in childhood and the third leading cause of death in children aged less than 12 months, with an overall mortality in cases with a Glasgow Coma Scale (GCS) of less than 8 of between 9 and 52%.

There is evidence to suggest that child abuse accounts for almost 25% of all children admitted to hospital under the age of 2 years, and is second only to car accidents as the cause of the death. Between the ages of 2 and 4 years, falls are the most common cause of head injury and in older children bicycling and car accidents are the most common causes of injury.

Fracture of the skull during the first year of life is not uncommon as the skull is relatively thin and breaks easily after impact. Most skull fractures are linear and are not associated with underlying brain damage, although intracranial bleeding may result. Particular complications include the development of a *subepicranial hygroma*, where a fracture is associated with a dural tear and allows CSF to dissect beneath the periosteum, and a *growing skull fracture* which results from herniation of contused and swollen brain through the torn dura mater thereby separating the bones along the line of the fracture. The fracture tends to 'grow' during the period of rapid growth of the brain.

Extradural hematoma in infancy rarely results from injury to the middle meningeal artery: venous bleeding from the bone is the usual cause. Chronic subdural hematomas occur most commonly at 6 months of age and are rare under 1 year of age.

Child abuse is the major cause of head injury in infants but its true incidence is unknown. Such cases were widely recognized under the term '*battered child*' and the '*shaken baby syndrome*' was used in infants with acute subdural hematoma and subarachnoid hemorrhage, retinal hemorrhages and periosteal new bone formation, at epiphysgeal regions of long bones and was attributed to the to and fro shaking of a child's body producing a whiplash motion of the child's head on the neck. The term 'shaken baby' has been questioned, as inertial force generated by shaking alone is believed to be insufficient to account for the intracranial pathology compared with those caused by impact. These doubts have given rise to the new term of '*shaking impact syndrome*' in which the injuries are attributed to both inertial and impact forces.

There is some evidence that between the ages of 2 and 5 years the still maturing brain responds differently to head injury, than in the older child. For example, there is said to be a smaller risk of developing a traumatic intracranial hematoma in children less than 5 years old than in adults. Thereafter, the frequency and nature of the intracranial pathologies is similar in childhood and adulthood, with the possible exception of diffuse cerebral swelling which has been found to be more common in childhood than in adulthood. This is demonstrated in CT by small ventricles, compression of the basal cisterns but the principal pathological features are the enlargement of the cerebral hemispheres and the obliteration of the CSF spaces. The bilateral hemispheric swelling has been attributed to cerebral hyperemia with an increase in cerebral blood volume.

There have been continuing uncertainties about the nature, the distribution and the pathology in accidental and non-accidental injury in infants and children. Recent clinico-pathological studies have indicated that diffuse traumatic axonal injury of the type seen in adults may only be seen in children older than 12 months. In infants less than 12 months hypoxia/ischemia is the principal finding, any axonal pathology being invariably limited to the craniocervical junction. Therefore, contrary to some literature, diffuse traumatic axonal injury is not a feature of non-accidental head injury in infants and the structural damage that results from hypoxia/ischemia is thought to be consequent upon respiratory distress and/or apnea due to axonal injury at a craniocervical junction.

SPINAL INJURY

This may be classified as either *closed or missile.* The former results from subluxations and fracture dislocations of the vertebral column, and in civilian practice, almost 50% of all new cases of spinal injury result from motor car or motor cycle accidents, with 30% being due to falls and the remainder due to sporting injuries. The vertebrae may return to normal position when the fracture dislocation is said to be *stable.* If the vertebrae are still capable of moving the fracture is *unstable* and any undue movement to the injured patient may intensify damage to the spinal cord. Some two thirds of the patients are less than 40 years of age and some 90% are male.

The cervical spine at the level of C5/6 vertebrae and the thoracic spine are injured most commonly in road traffic accidents, whereas the lumbar spine is damaged most commonly in crush injuries of the type seen in mining accidents or after falls.

There are various mechanisms that result in injury to the spinal cord and include a combination of flexion, rotation, extension and compression. An extension injury is usually due to a hyperextension of the mid-cervical vertebrae which causes separation and dislocation of intervertebral discs, local hemorrhage and possible rupture of the longitudinal ligament. If there is excessive flexion in the cervical spine there is compression of the vertebral bodies, part of which can be displayed posteriorly causing damage to the spinal cord. The spinal canal may be narrowed by fracture dislocation due to rotation, compression fractures when fragments of bone may be displaced backwards, or if the spinal column is angulated acutely with stretching and compression of the dura. In conjunction with cervical spondylosis or ankylosing spondylosis severe damage to the cord may result. Injury to the cord may also result from missiles such as bullets and associated bony fragments which may lodge in the cord or in the case of high velocity missiles may cause severe damage to the cord by pressure changes resulting from shock waves. In civilian practice the cord may be injured by a stab wound, especially if a knife enters the spinal canal anterolaterally.

Pathology of spinal cord trauma

In cases of mild injury where there is only temporary neurological dysfunction, the term *concussion* is used as it is presumed that structural abnormalities are minimal, indeed the external surface of the cord may be normal. In more severe injuries there is *contusion* of the cord, the extent and severity of which will vary from case to case and in many there is extradural, subdural or subarachnoid hemorrhage. The lesion is characterized by hemorrhagic necrosis at the site of trauma, transverse sections revealing an essentially fusiform shaped mass – *traumatic hematomyelia* – which tapers to end in one or more segments above and below the site of injury (Fig. 8.29a, b and c). Histologically, there is swelling, necrosis and petechial hemorrhage formation and axonal swellings and bulb formation may be seen. Myelin sheaths become swollen and disintegrate. Within a few days of injury there is infiltration by polymorphonuclear leukocytes. Gradually, the swelling subsides, small amounts of hemorrhage are absorbed and the necrotic tissue is gradually removed by macrophages. Eventually, a cavity is formed, the margins of which are delineated by an astrocytosis in which iron pigment may be found. In severe cases affected segments are replaced by what is predominantly an astrocytic scar. If the injury involves root entry zones then regenerating axons and Schwann cells may invade the cord and although effective axonal regeneration does not occur the appearance in some cases is similar to that of an amputation neuroma. A late consequence of injury is the development of degeneration in both ascending and descending fiber tracts (see below). Sometimes a longitudinally disposed cavity – *post-traumatic syringomyelia* may track upwards to the medulla or downwards from the damaged section.

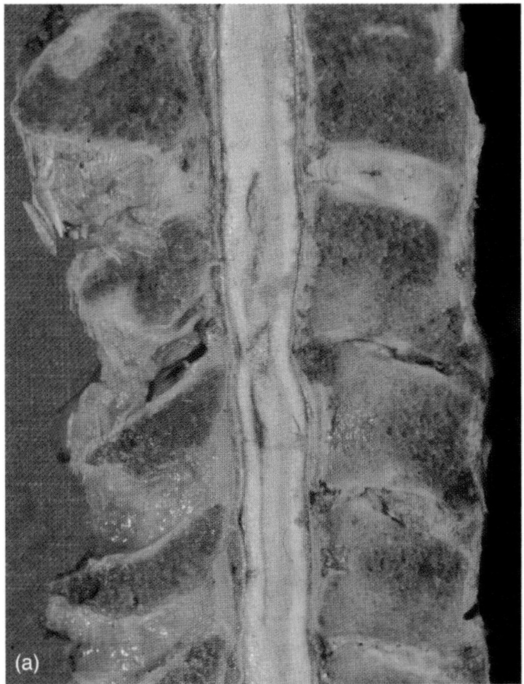

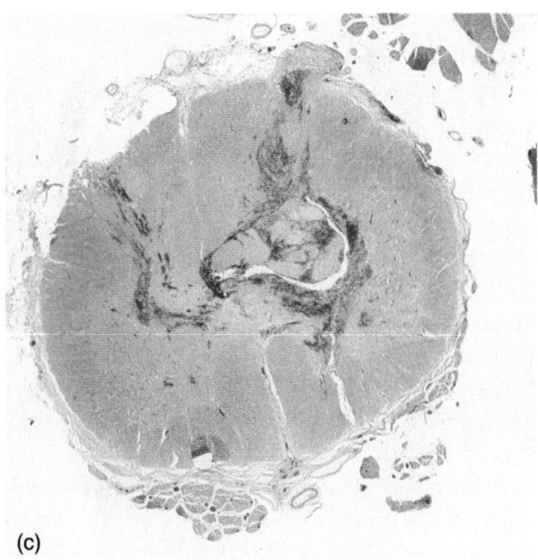

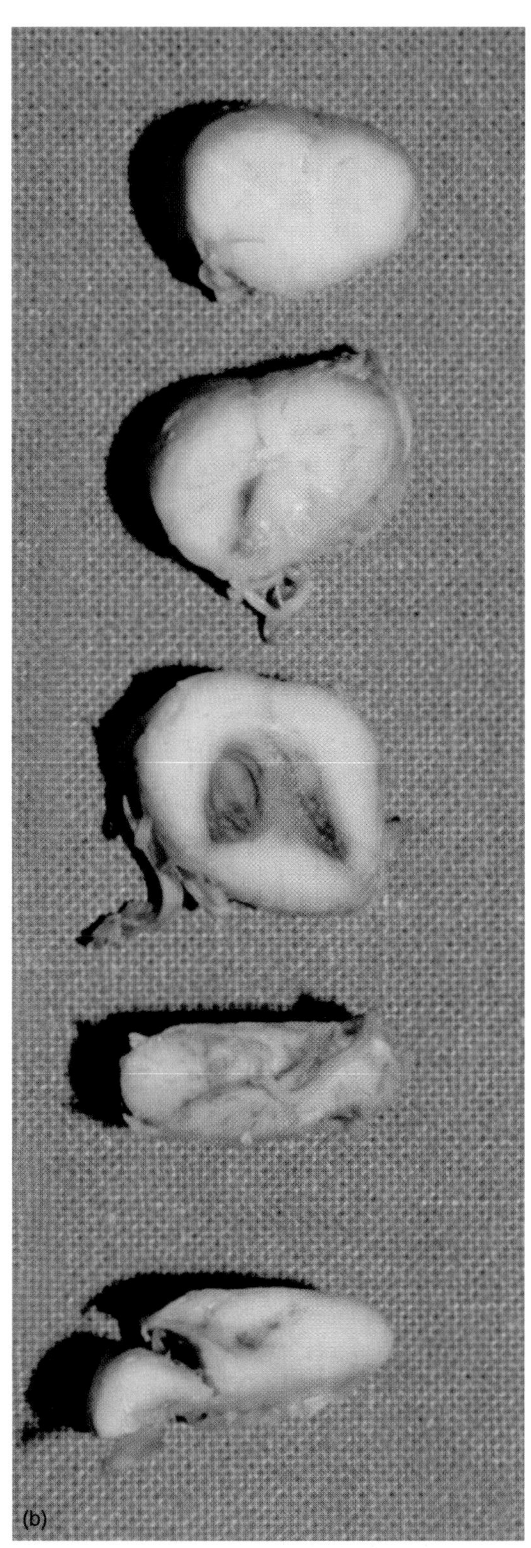

Figure 8.29 Spinal injury. (a) There is a traumatic hematomyelia in relation to a fracture of the cervical spine. (b) A hemorrhagic hematomyelia in transverse segments of the cord in relation to fracture dislocation. The damage is greatest in the middle segment from which it tapers both proximally and distally. (c) Histological section showing centrally placed site of traumatic hematomyelia. H&E.

Postmortem procedures are difficult in this type of case and it is essential to move a block of the vertebral column extending for at least two or three vertebrae above and below the level of the injury. This block should then be fixed. Thereafter, a laminectomy can be done and the spinal cord removed from the vertebral canal, and the specimen can be cut with a band saw in the midline sagittal plane to demonstrate the damaged vertebrae and spinal cord (Fig. 8.29a). In longstanding cases of traumatic paraplegia, the damaged segment of the cord may be densely adherent to bone as a result of the formation of scar tissue.

Other lesions affecting the spinal cord

This is an appropriate place to summarize such lesions since the majority produce a *transverse lesion* which has many features in common with those produced by trauma, namely varying degrees of paraparesis, ranging from a mild weakness in the legs to paraplegia, and varying degrees of degeneration of long-tracks above and below the level of damage to the spinal cord.

Compression of the spinal cord

The causes of spinal compression are many and varied (Table 8.16) and there are different causes in the young, middle-aged, and elderly. The clinical effects depend to a considerable extent on the rate of development of the compressive lesion: these may progress over many months, whereas some of the more rapidly expanding lesions can produce paraplegia within days. The damage to the spinal cord is often partial, leading to the syndrome of hemisection (*Brown–Séquard syndrome*), namely spastic weakness and loss of vibration and joint sense on the same side of the lesion because of involvement of the ipsilateral crossed corticospinal tract and posterior column, whereas involvement of the crossed spinothalamic tract results in disturbance of pain and temperature sense on the opposite side. If the lesion becomes large enough, it will interfere with the blood supply to the cord of the level of the compression and, if surgery is delayed, irreparable structural damage may develop.

Table 8.16 Principal causes of compression of the spinal cord

Lesions in vertebral column
- Prolapsed intervertebral disc
- Cervical spondylosis
- Kyphoscoliosis
- Fracture–dislocation
- Metastatic tumor

Spinal extradural lesions
- Metastatic carcinoma
- Lymphoma
- Myeloma
- Abscess

Intradural extramedullary lesions
- Meningioma
- Schwannoma

Intramedullary lesions
- Astrocytoma
- Ependymoma
- Cyst formation

Many of the causes of compression of the spinal cord are dealt with in more detail in the appropriate chapters. The lesion may arise in the *vertebral column* such as a prolapsed intervertebral disc (see below), whereas in patients with a severe kyphoscoliosis, increasing angulation of the vertebral column may interfere with the blood supply to the spinal cord at that level. The majority of lesions causing compression of the spinal cord, however, arise in the *spinal extradural space*, metastatic carcinoma and lymphoma, including myeloma being the most common. Other lesions are a subacute pyogenic abscess that is usually caused by staphylococci or coliform bacilli, extension of a tuberculous infection in the vertebral body into the extradural space, vascular malformation and tumors of mesenchymal origin. Spontaneous extradural hemorrhage is a recognized clinical entity but its pathogenesis is not clear. The most common *intradural extramedullary lesions* are meningioma and schwannoma. *Intramedullary* tumors within the spinal cord may have similar effects.

Structural abnormalities within the spinal cord will depend on the severity of the compression and, as indicated above, they amount to frank infarction. A peculiar histological feature seen in the spinal cord related to less severe compression is coarse vacuolation of white matter, the cause of which is not known.

Transverse myelitis

This is a clinical rather than a pathological term and is used to describe a transverse lesion in the spinal cord in the absence of a compressive lesion. Causes include infarction, demyelination, caisson disease, infection or hemorrhage (spontaneous hematomyelia).

Following partial or total interruption of the cord in addition to the local damage an inevitable consequence is the development of ascending and descending Wallerian degeneration in the interrupted tracts of the spinal cord. The distribution of the degenerative processes and their time course can be studied by one of two main staining techniques that are used to demonstrate the loss of myelin. First, there is the Marchi technique which is used to demonstrate recent breakdown of myelin within the preceding 2–3 months: the unsaturated fatty acids formed during this process are stained black, while normal myelin remains unstained. Additional histological techniques that yield useful information about myelin breakdown include Sudan IV, Sudan black or oil red O in a frozen section. Myelin sheaths break up into ellipsoids and gradually the products of degeneration are taken up by macrophages, a process that may be seen after 6–8 weeks. Gradually the amount of Marchi-positive material diminishes, but it may remain in affected tracts for many months or even several years (but most laboratories now use immunohistochemistry to identify the number and distribution of microglia and macrophages for such purposes). The degenerative process is accompanied by an astrocytosis which gradually increases over several weeks and it may still be evident some 6–12 months later. The second technique is one used for determining the long-term consequences of the myelin degeneration by identifying the demyelinated areas by their failure to stain with conventional stains, e.g. Luxol fast blue.

Ascending degeneration

The pattern following a transverse lesion is well seen in the lower thoracic spine (Fig. 8.30). In the section taken a few segments above the lesion, degeneration is seen in the posterior columns with the exception of the small area dorsal to the gray commissure where there are chiefly commissurial fibers and the spinothalamic and spinocerebellar tracts. In the cervical region the degeneration of the posterior columns is virtually confined to the gracile tracts. Because the cuneate tract is composed of ascending fibers that have joined the cord above the level of the lesion, normal fibers will be found in the spinocerebellar tracts and in the cuneate tracts up to their nuclei in the medulla. The long-term consequences of this degeneration are well seen with pallor of staining due to loss of myelin in the posterior columns.

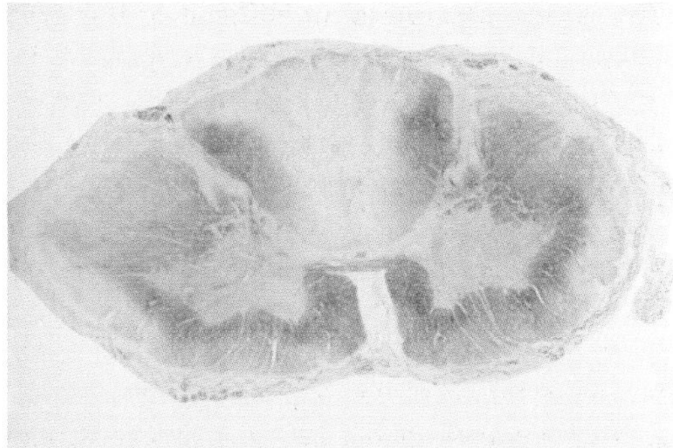

Figure 8.30 Ascending degeneration in spinal cord. There is loss of myelin in the gracile and spinocerebellar tracts. The cuneate tracts are normal because of the inflow of nerve fibres above the lesion in the lumbar spinal cord.

Descending degeneration

In a section taken distal to a transverse section of the cord, marked degeneration is seen in the crossed (lateral) and uncrossed (anterior pyramidal) tracts (Fig. 8.31). A different path of degeneration is seen following a lesion either in the brainstem or in one internal capsule which results in degeneration of the corticospinal tract. In these situations there is degeneration of the crossed pyramidal tract on the opposite side and of the uncrossed pyramidal tract on the same side. As the uncrossed pyramidal tract does not usually extend below the upper thoracic segments, its degeneration will not be seen in sections of the lower thoracic cord.

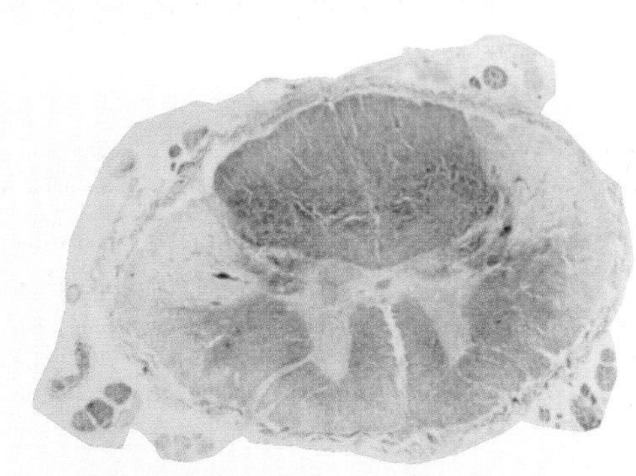

Figure 8.31 Descending degeneration in spinal cord. There is loss of myelin in the corticospinal tracts below a lesion in the cervical spinal cord. Myelin stain.

Prolapsed intervertebral disc

This is a common occurrence. The central part of an intervertebral disc consists of soft fibrocartilage *the nucleus pulposus*, and this is surrounded by a ring of much firmer fibrocartilage *the annulus fibrosus*. As age advances the nucleus pulposus becomes progressively dehydrated and the annulus wider. The annulus is thicker anteriorly, and this presumably accounts for the fact that most disc protrusions occur posteriorly.

A disc may prolapse acutely in an apparently normal spine as a result of sudden physical stress, but more frequently, it occurs secondary to degenerative disease. Most protrusions occur in the lumbar region, the discs most commonly affected being L5/S1 and L4/5. An acute disc prolapse may also occur in the cervical region. Most protrusions are posterolateral (Fig. 8.32a), affecting the related spinal nerve root. The rarer central protrusions are of greater importance since they compress the cauda equina (Fig. 8.32b), the result of which may be paraparesis and sphincter dysfunction.

MRI is the investigation of first choice. If the lumbar disc prolapse is posterolateral then many cases settle spontaneously with conservative treatment, indications for surgery being unremitting leg pain, recurrent attacks or neurological deficits. Surgical techniques include microdiscectomy with over 80% of patients obtaining a good result after surgery. In contrast central disc protrusion usually requires urgent treatment often by laminectomy.

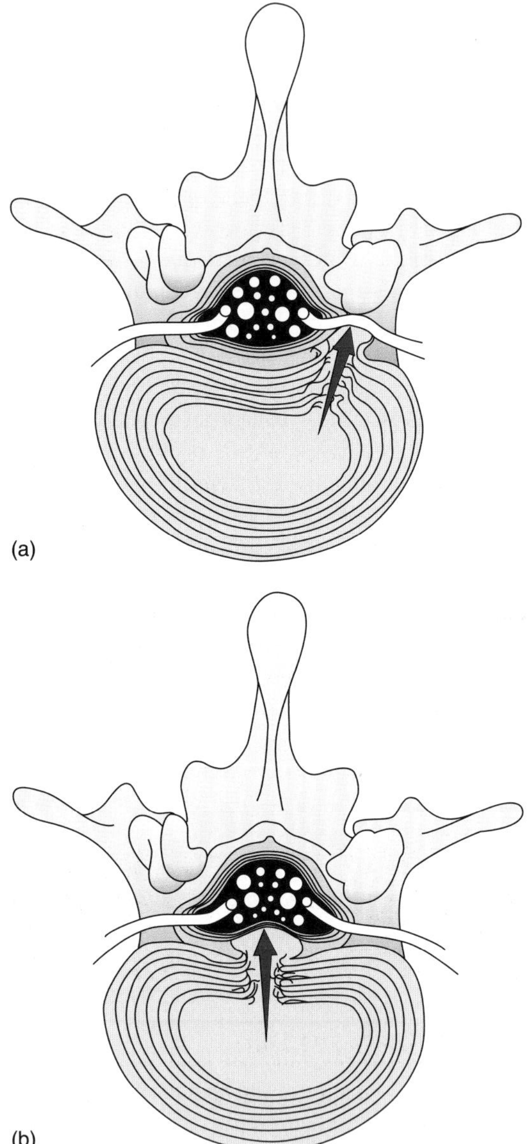

Figure 8.32 Prolapsed intervertebral disc. (a) Posterolateral protusion compressing a nerve. (b) Central protrusion compressing cauda equina.

Cervical spondylosis

This results from degeneration of intervertebral discs in cervical regions. The disc spaces are narrowed and transverse bars develop in the vertebral canal as a result of posterior protrusion of the annulus. There is also a reactive osteophytosis affecting the neurocentral joints and the intervertebral foramina and thickening of the intervertebral ligaments leading to compression of nerve roots and fibrosis of dural root sleeves. As the spondylosis progresses there may, in addition to compression of nerve roots, be interference to the blood supply of the spinal cord, where the vertebral canal is most narrow. There is considerable controversy about the importance of cervical spondylosis, since it has been demonstrated radiologically in some 50% of adults over the age of 50 and in some 75% over 65. It may be, therefore, that secondary ischemic damage in the spinal cord – *cervical myelopathy* – occurs only in individuals with congenital narrowing of the vertebral canal. The structural changes in the spinal cord are a combination of focal infarction and subtotal degeneration of the lateral parts of the posterior columns secondary to damage to axons in the cervical posterior nerve roots. Congenital narrowing of the vertebral canal in the lumbar region – *lumbar stenosis* – may lead to compression of nerves in the cauda equina.

OTHER BONY ABNORMALITIES THAT MAY AFFECT THE SPINAL CORD

Basilar invagination

This is the term applied to abnormal protrusion of the tip of the odontoid process. It may be a developmental malformation but can also occur secondary to osteomalacia or rheumatoid arthritis. As invagination progresses, the odontoid compresses the upper end of the cervical cord and the lower medulla.

Tuberculosis

Where tuberculosis is common, the vertebral column is not infrequently affected, usually in the mid-thoracic region. The cord may be compressed by granulation tissue within the extradural spinal space or as a result of angulation (kyphosis) of the spine.

Paget's disease

When Paget's disease affects the vertebral column there is often some degree of kyphosis, but of greater importance is the generalized reduction in the size of the vertebral canal leading to compression of the spinal cord.

SELECTIVE LESIONS IN NEUROSURGERY

There are several disease processes where clinical improvement can be achieved by stereotactic surgery in addition to the aspiration or biopsy of small deeply seated tumors, cysts or abscesses. The techniques have been developed for lesion-making, in thalamic nuclei for the treatment of tremor relief, pain especially intractable head or neck pain in malignancy, in psychosurgery, for the treatment of obsessive and compulsive illness and intractable depression, and stimulation for movement disorders, such as dystonia and tremor. Other procedures include aspiration and irradiation by the implantation of radioactive seeds, e.g. the treatment of craniopharyngioma, glioma or metastases or external stereotactic irradiation, for the treatment of deeply seated arterio-venous malformations. Such techniques have been developed by the advent of CT and MRI compatible stereotactic systems using frames, and more recently by the development of image-guided frameless stereotaxy which aids accurate positioning of burr holes and bone flaps and the planning of the safest approach to certain tumors, the placement of depth electrodes, defining the extent of resected tissue, the treatment of arterio-venous malformations, abscesses and the location of intra-orbital lesions.

One of the first techniques to be introduced was lesion-making for psychosurgery and the development of *prefrontal leukotomy* (Fig. 8.33). The number of cases requiring such surgery has diminished with the introduction of improvements in drug

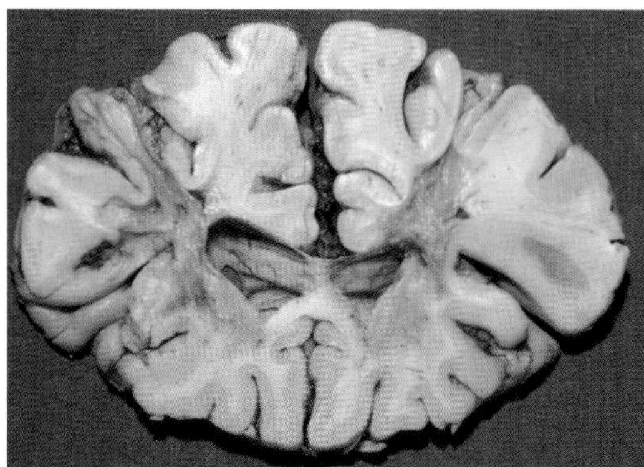

Figure 8.33 Prefrontal leukotomy. There is considerable longstanding destruction of white matter in the frontal lobes.

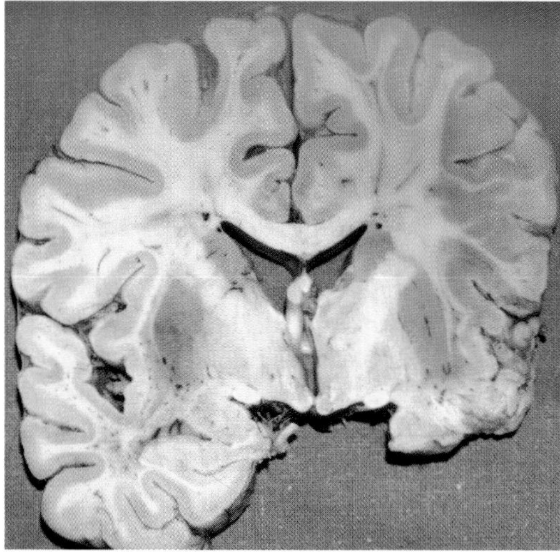

Figure 8.34 Partial temporal lobectomy. Patient presented with intractable seizures due to a neuronal migration disorder in right cerebral hemisphere.

treatment but stereotactic surgery is still used as a method of lesion-making in selective patients where drug treatment has failed; such surgery includes subcaudate tractomy, limbic leukotomy (Fig. 8.34), anterior internal capsulotomy and amygdalotomy. Another technique is that of cordotomy which is aimed at destroying the spinothalamic fibers in the spinal cord, sometimes undertaken in patients with intractable pain.

There is some evidence that the surgical introduction of grafts and cells into the brains of adult rats can re-establish damaged connections in the host brain and restore functions lost or damaged as a result of a preceding lesion. These techniques have opened up the possibility that at least some types of neurons in the CNS may possibly be replaced by new implants of neuronal tissue. Such grafting techniques have particular relevance to the neurodegenerative disorders of Parkinson's disease and Huntington's disease. Although, the possibility that dopaminergic neurons could be grafted to patients with Parkinson's disease has been discussed since the first reports of successful dopamine neuron grafting in rodents, there still remain many unanswered questions. In an attempt to overcome immunological rejection, and to avoid the ethical implications of using human fetal tissue, alternative sources of catacholamine-containing donor tissue have been sought by genetic engineering. There have already been a number of clinical trials with autografts of adrenal medulla to the striatum in Parkinson's disease. These studies have shown that the grafting of human dopamine neurons in patients with Parkinson's disease is not only feasible, but when used in association with various factors, the graft is likely to survive and may result in some functional recovery.

TRAUMA BY NON-MECHANICAL FORCES

Included in this category are the effects of radiotherapy and other forms of radiation.

Radiotherapy

Radiotherapy is the mainstay of treatment in malignant brain tumors. The most important complications in the CNS result from the effects of ionizing radiation, and the concept that the human brain is resistant to the effect of therapeutic irradiation is no longer held. The type, frequency and extent of post-radiotherapy complications depend on many factors, which include the total dose of radiation, the number of fractions, the dose per fraction, the total treatment time, the volume of tissue irradiated, the elimination of 'hot spots' by use of multiple fields and the use of other treatments such as steroids and radiosensitizers for antineoplastic chemotherapy.

The main effect of irradiation on a tumor is to produce necrosis. This is particularly true for radiosensitive tumors such as germinoma or lymphoma (see Chapter 15), where large fluid-filled cysts lined with glial tissue can be found after treatment. In less radiosensitive tumors, including glioma, extensive central necrosis may be produced although peripheral tumor may remain. Tumor radiation may also lead to a change in tumor cytology. Typically, multinucleate giant cells with irregular hyerchromatic nuclei are found: the number of mitotic figures is reduced. Pathological effects of radiation on the tumor blood vessels include thickening, hyalinization, and occlusion of blood vessels with proliferation of collagen in perivascular regions.

Radiation can cause injury to scalp and bone although megavoltage irradiation is relatively skin sparing, the exit dose to the skin must be considered. Skin erythema and hair loss are common. Hair loss may be patchy or extensive and may be permanent. A combination of irradiation in certain chemotherapeutic regimens may exacerbate skin reactions and increase the risk of permanent hair loss. Necrosis of bone flaps is a potential risk but is not often a clinical problem, but impaired wound healing does occur. Treatment of various intracranial tumors is particularly valuable and also plays an important part in the management of some benign tumors such as pituitary adenoma and craniopharyngioma. In some tumors that disseminate throughout the CSF pathways, e.g. medulloblastoma, whole neural axis irradiation minimizes the risk of distant occurrence.

Treatment of intracranial tumors using radiotherapy utilizes *megavoltage* X-rays, an electron beam from a *linear accelerator, accelerated particles from a cyclotron*, or gamma rays from *cobalt*. More modern techniques have been developed to minimize irradiation to adjacent normal brain. These are delivered through standard techniques. Such methods include: *conformal therapy*, where the beams are shaped to conform with the shape of the tumor; *stereotactic radiosurgery* where a beam from a linear accelerator is focused on a selected target; *interstitial techniques* whereby tumor is treated from within by the implantation of multiple radioactive seeds; *beam-intensity modulated radiotherapy* which allows the delivery of high doses of radiation to very localized regions adjacent to vital structures such as the skull base; and *proton therapy*.

Effects of irradiation upon normal brain

These have been studied according to the time of their manifestations: *acute reactions* occur during the course of irradiation; *early delayed reactions* appear a few weeks to 2–3 months later; and *delayed reactions* appear from a few months to many years after irradiation. Acute reactions are usually minor with conventional doses and fractionation, particularly when steroids are used. They cause symptoms and signs of raised intracranial pressure. The reaction is dose related and is probably due to increased edema, that usually responds to an increase in the dose of steroids. Early delayed reactions are usually transient and disappear without treatment. Clinical features include lethargy, somnolence and an intensification of pre-existing symptoms and signs. Transient somnolence and lethargy have been reported in 80% of children given 25 Gy whole-brain radiotherapy as a prophylactic treatment for acute lymphoblastic leukemia; it has also been reported in adults given 1.8 Gy daily fractions to a dose of 60 Gy. Very occasionally early delayed reactions may lead to the patient's death, neuropathological examination then revealing multiple small foci of demyelination with perivascular infiltration by lymphocytes and plasma cells. In some instances there is evidence of damage to blood vessels. The early delayed reaction probably results from injury to oligodendrocytes, the latent interval of clinical recovery being consistent with the time required for myelin replacement.

Late delayed reactions are caused either by diffuse damage to white matter accompanied by ventricular enlargement – a *leukoencephalopathy* – or as a space-occupying gliovascular reaction known as *radionecrosis*. These features tend to occur from about one to many years after treatment, and may be delayed by up to 30 years. There are many reports of radionecrosis after irradiation of intracranial or extracranial tumors, such as nasopharyngeal carcinoma, parotid carcinoma, or basal cell carcinoma

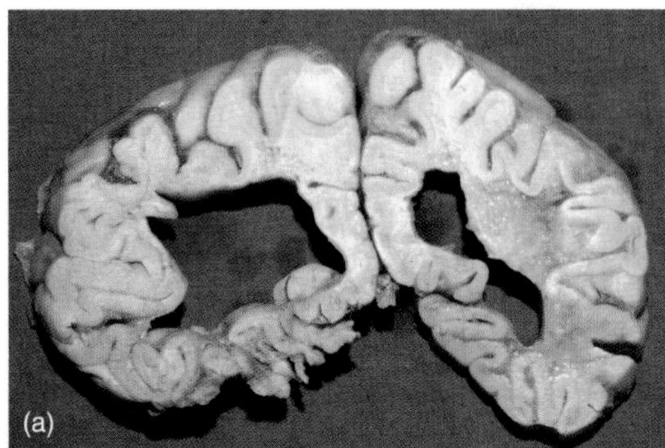

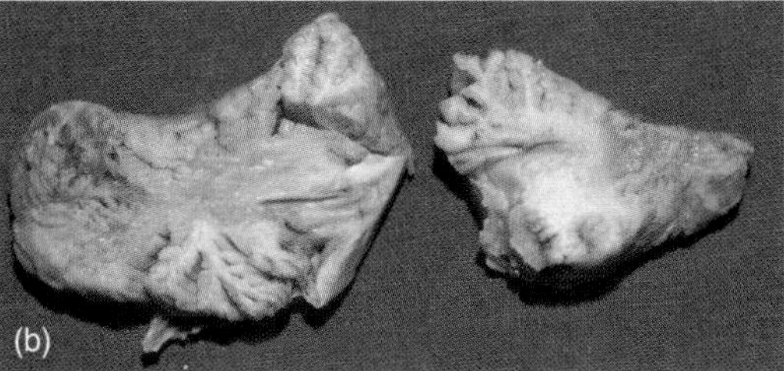

Figure 8.35 Delayed radiation necrosis. (a) There is necrosis, mainly in the white matter, of the occipital lobes. (b) Necrosis is present in the white matter of the cerebellar hemispheres.

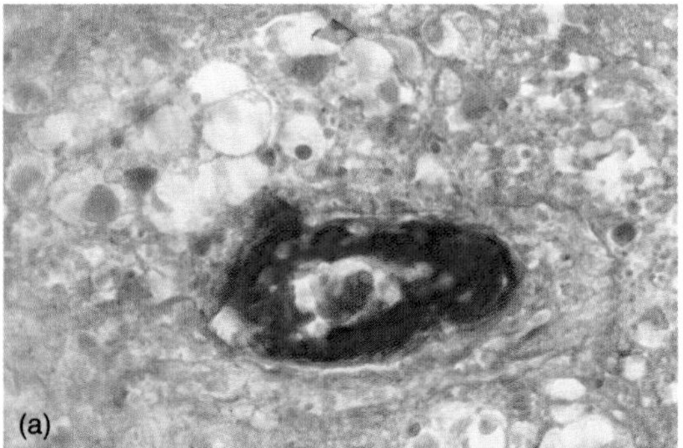

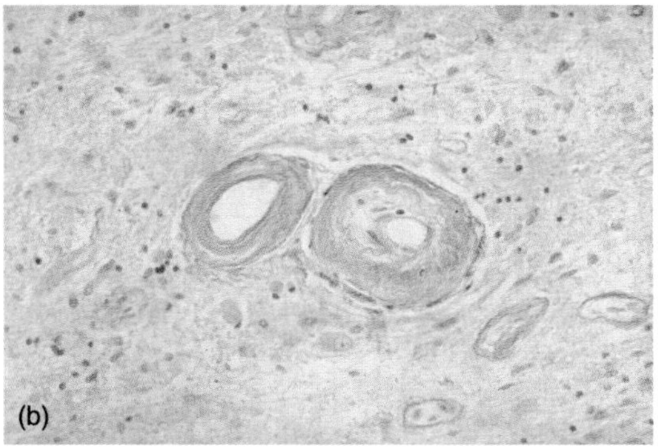

Figure 8.36 Radiation necrosis. (a) Small blood vessel showing fibrinoid necrosis. (b) There is hyalinization and endothelial proliferation in small blood vessels. (a) Martius scarlet blue, (b) H&E.

of the scalp. The macroscopic appearances of radionecrosis are similar to those of a malignant glioma. White matter is expanded and replaced by focally cystic, waxy, pale yellow tissue in which there may be petechial hemorrhage (Fig. 8.35a and b). In longstanding cases the affected tissue becomes granular and is apt to crumble. Anatomical definition is blurred, but in the main gray matter is spared. Histologically, the process is characterized by appearances that range from coagulative necrosis around which there is no or minimal reactive change, to foci of demyelination, loss of axons and infiltration by lipid-containing macrophages, lymphocytes and plasma cells. The most important change, however, is fibrinoid necrosis (Fig. 8.36a) and hyalinization of the walls of blood vessels (Fig. 8.36b) and proliferation of endothelium, which may be sufficient to cause an obliterative endarteritis and thrombotic occlusion of small blood vessels. Additional features include the formation of telangiectatic blood vessels, the proliferation of perivascular fibroblasts, and the formation in some areas of large amounts of relatively acellular collagen, an associated astrocytosis often with bizarre multinucleated cells (Fig. 8.37) and foci of calcification. Similar changes may be seen in the spinal cord: referred to as *radiation myelopathy* (Fig. 8.38), a complication that is said to occur in between 1 and 2% of patients who have received radiation in the corresponding region. Changes in the cerebellum, however, are of a different nature, the main feature consisting of the formation of small cysts in the Purkinje cell layer of the cortex, with some loss of both Purkinje cells and granule cells with subsequent atrophy of folia, demyelination and gliosis (Fig. 8.39). Eventually the Purkinje cells are replaced by a series of confluent cystic spaces associated with which there is exudation of fibrin which spreads readily along the molecular layer, hyaline thickening on the walls of blood vessels, and focal calcification.

The pathogenesis of radionecrosis remains uncertain; vascular change, a direct effect of radiation

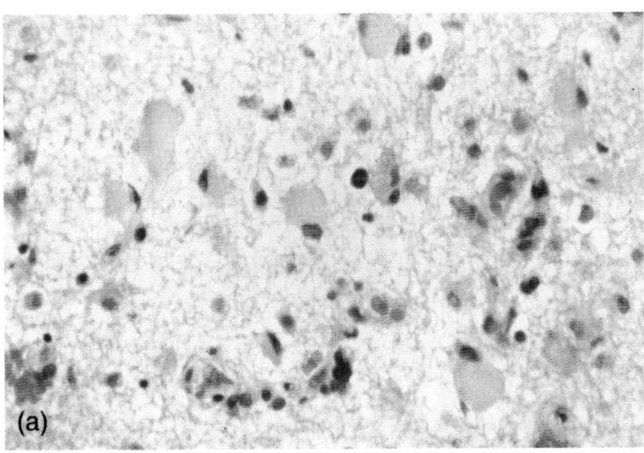

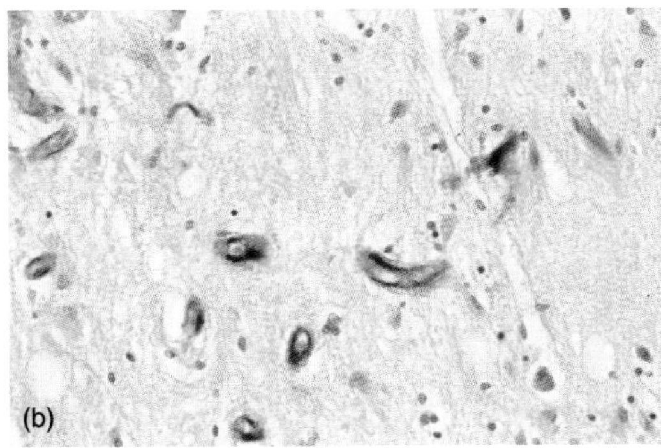

Figure 8.37 Radiation necrosis. (a) Astrocytosis including bizarre-shaped astrocytes some of which are multinucleated. (b) Foci of calcification. (a) H&E, (b) Von Kossa.

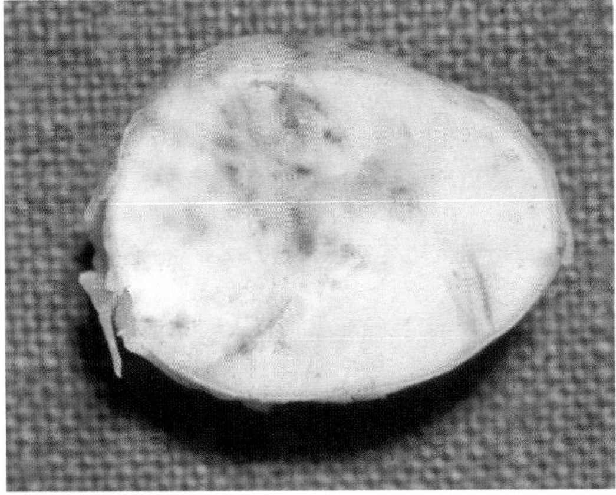

Figure 8.38 Radiation necrosis in spinal cord.

on the glia, and immunological mechanisms have all been proposed. The risks of developing radionecrosis are not clearly defined, although there is a general consensus that daily fractions of 1.8–2 Gy to a total dose of 65–70 Gy would normally be well

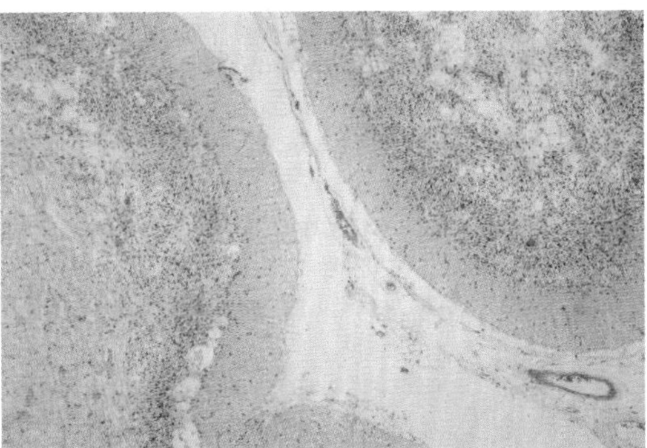

Figure 8.39 Radiation necrosis. There is a lacy pattern of vacuoles between the Purkinje cells and the granular neurons. Also there is associated atrophy of the folia, demyelination of the white matter and gliosis. H&E.

tolerated, and occasional cases of radionecrosis will occur. In general the incidence and necrosis is progressively greater with high irradiation doses: below 54 Gy this complication is rarely seen, between 57 and 65 Gy it may develop in up to 3% of patients, and above 65 Gy the incidence may be as high as 18–20%.

A *diffuse leukoencephalopathy*, which may be necrotizing, is also associated with radiotherapy. Most of the reported cases have been treated simultaneously with various chemotherapeutic agents, and it is likely that this disease is primarily a complication of drug treatment. Intellectual deficits may follow irradiation in both children and adults, and various studies in children have suggested that low doses of about 25 Gy are due to little or no intellectual disturbance, though mild pschomotor dysfunction and general slowing down may be seen. Complications of radiotherapy are greater in the developing brain, and radiotherapy to the CNS is usually delayed as long as possible in young children. Additional complications include *hypothalamopituitary dysfunction*, especially of growth hormone regulation. Other complications include blindness, which is thought to be secondary to demyelination in the visual pathways and occasionally radiation-induced damage to both large *extracranial* and *intracranial arteries* has been described.

An interesting phenomenon is the induction of *brain tumors* as an uncommon complication of cerebral irradiation. Commonest examples are meningeal fibrosarcomas, which have generally been complications for radiation of pituitary adenomas. Such complications have also been noted following low dose irradiation for acute lymphoblastic leukemia. Meningiomas can also be induced either by a dose of irradiation for the treatment of intracranial tumors or following low-dose treatment of benign scalp disorders, such as ringworm. An increasing number of children are surviving after radiotherapy for intracranial tumors. There have, as a result, been increasing numbers of reports of further neuroectodermal tumors developing in these children. Doses of radiation have been very wide, ranging from 1.5 to 60 Gy and the latency period has been 5–25 years. Mostly these tumors are anaplastic astrocytoma or glioblastoma and appear within the first three decades of life.

Other types of radiation

These include *laser* and *ultraviolet radiation* both of which are capable of causing tissue necrosis in the CNS, the former having been introduced for targeted therapy of deep-seated intracerebral tumors.

Electromagnetic trauma, including injury by *lightning*, has been described. Changes including coagulative necrosis, hemorrhages and brain swelling. Damage to the spinal cord may also occur in the form of atrophy of the dorsal and lateral columns.

CHAPTER 9

DEMYELINATING DISEASES

James A R Nicoll

MYELIN AND DEMYELINATION

Myelin

The myelin sheath in the central nervous system is composed of multiple layers of oligodendrocyte cell membrane wrapped around the axon. The myelin sheath of a single axon is divided by nodes of Ranvier into short segments (internodal segments). A single oligodendrocyte provides an internodal segment of myelin to several axons in its vicinity. The function of myelin is to provide electrical insulation of the cell membrane of the axon so that the ion fluxes across the axon membrane, resulting in the action potential, take place only at the nodes of Ranvier. As a consequence, the action potential jumps from node to node (saltatory conduction) providing rapid transmission of the electrical impulse along the axon.

Demyelination

Demyelination can be defined as selective loss of the myelin sheath of a nerve fiber with preservation of the axon. This definition excludes disorders of myelin formation during development (leukodystrophy, see Chapter 12). It is also distinct from loss of entire myelinated fibers (i.e. loss of both the axon and the myelin sheath) which occurs in infarction and in white matter atrophy. A consequence of demyelination, with loss of the myelin sheath wrapping an axon, is that saltatory conduction no longer takes place, resulting in complete conduction failure or slowing of conduction of the action potential along the axon. Table 9.1 lists the main disorders that occur as a result of demyelination.

Table 9.1 Demyelinating diseases

Primary demyelinating diseases
- Multiple sclerosis
- Acute disseminated encephalomyelitis
- Acute hemorrhagic leukoencephalopathy

Other disorders in which demyelination may occur

Viral
- Progressive multifocal leukoencephalopathy (JC virus)
- HTLV-1 associated myelopathy

Metabolic/nutritional
- Central pontine myelinolysis
- Marchiafava–Bignami disease
- Mitochondrial disease
- Subacute combined degeneration of the spinal cord (vitamin B_{12} deficiency)

Toxic
- Methotrexate
- Carbon monoxide
- Solvent abuse

DETECTING DEMYELINATION

Neuroimaging

As magnetic resonance imaging (MRI) is sensitive to alterations in tissue water content, it provides a sensitive method of detecting the loss of the lipid associated with demyelination. Patients who present with clinical signs suggestive of multiple sclerosis (MS) often already have other clinically silent lesions which are detectable by MRI.

Visual evoked responses

The slowing of conduction caused by demyelination forms the basis of a diagnostic electrophysiological test. Visual evoked responses involve flashing patterns of light before the eyes while monitoring the response in the visual cortex using electrodes on the occipital scalp. If there is demyelination in part of the optic pathway, as is common in MS, the conduction time (latency) is increased.

Macroscopic

As myelin is composed predominantly of cell membrane it has a high lipid content and, consequently, the regions of the central nervous system containing the highest density of myelinated fibers appear white to the naked eye (i.e. the white matter). Areas of demyelination within the white matter lose their white appearance and become gray in color.

Microscopic

Histologically, myelin is demonstrated by Luxol fast blue (LFB) or by immunohistochemistry for myelin proteins e.g. myelin basic protein, myelin oligodendrocyte glycoprotein (MOG) or myelin-associated glycoprotein (MAG). It is important to realize that lack of staining for myelin alone is not diagnostic of selective demyelination. It is necessary to demonstrate preservation of axons within the area of myelin loss using a silver stain such as Palmgren or neurofilament immunohistochemistry in order to distinguish demyelination from, for example, infarction.

EXPERIMENTAL MODELS

Experimental allergic encephalomyelitis (EAE) is an animal model which involves peripheral injection of brain extract or myelin proteins. Immune-mediated demyelination occurs in the central nervous system 8–10 days later. Most models are monophasic and resemble acute disseminated encephalomyelitis (ADEM). The relevance of EAE to MS is unclear but it does demonstrate that an appropriately triggered immune system can cause selective demyelination.

MULTIPLE SCLEROSIS

Multiple sclerosis (MS) is by far the commonest demyelinating disease affecting the CNS. In MS well-circumscribed foci of demyelination (plaques) are distributed throughout the CNS. A defining feature of MS is that the episodes of demyelination are disseminated in space and time, i.e. foci of demyelination arise in different anatomical regions of the CNS at different times. There is great variation in the location of the plaques in MS and all areas of the CNS may be affected including the cerebral white matter, the optic nerves, the brainstem, the cerebellum and the spinal cord. Although more difficult to detect, plaques can also occur in the gray matter.

In MS there is loss of apparently normal myelin sheaths with relative preservation of axons and, consequently, individual axons have lost their myelin sheaths (i.e. there is demyelination). There are two qualifications in this definition. Firstly, that the myelin sheaths have been normally formed during development, thereby excluding the leukodystrophies. Secondly, that the preservation of axons compared with myelin is relative. It is becoming increasingly recognized, however, that some axonal loss may occur, particularly in the chronic stage of the disease.

Demyelination in MS is mediated by the immune system. The reason for the attack on myelin is not yet known, but it is presumed to be a consequence of the interaction of genetic and environmental factors. Despite an intensive search there is no convincing evidence that an infective organism is responsible for the demyelination, although exposure to a common virus during adolescence in genetically susceptible individuals has been postulated as a trigger for demyelination later in life. Inflammation is a prominent feature of the early stage of demyelination.

Etiology

The etiology of MS is outlined in Table 9.2.

Genetic factors

Multiple sclerosis does not appear to be inherited as a single gene trait. However, there is evidence that genetic factors are involved. There is a 15–20-fold increased risk of MS in first-degree relatives of patients with MS. The concordance rate for MS is many times higher in monozygotic twins than dizygotic twins. There is an association of MS with certain human leukocyte antigen (HLA) types. This evidence suggests that genetically determined variation in the control of the immune response may be relevant in the pathogenesis of MS. In addition to susceptibility to developing MS, it is likely that some of the variation in clinical course of patients with MS is genetically determined. Current evidence suggests that patients with the *APOE* $\epsilon 4$ allele are more likely to develop progressive disease.

Environmental factors

The prevalence of MS varies considerably around the world, being virtually absent at the equator and increasing with distance to the north or south. The prevalence is highest at high latitudes including in northern Europe, North America, south-east Australia and New Zealand. One of the highest recorded prevalence rates for MS anywhere (approximately 1 in 500) was from a community-based study in north-east Scotland. The reason for this intriguing distribution is unclear but suggestions include exposure to sunlight being a protective factor. Migration studies have shown that migration before around 15 years of age from a high to a low incidence area reduces the likelihood of developing MS (e.g. northern Europe to Israel). Conversely, migration before about 15 years of age from a low to a high incidence area probably increases the risk of developing MS. Migration after the age of 19 years does not affect the risk of developing MS. Although the geographic variation in the prevalence of MS may to some extent reflect the genetic susceptibility of different populations, the migration studies point to the influence of environmental factors. A possible explanation for these observations is that exposure to a childhood viral infection may act as a trigger for the disease later in life.

Viruses

There is no convincing evidence that an infective agent causes MS. MS has not been transmitted to experimental animals by inoculation of affected brain tissue. Evidence has been sought for the involvement of many viruses in MS including measles, vaccinia, rubella, herpes simplex virus, human herpes virus 6, HTLV-1, JC virus and canine distemper virus, but specific viral proteins or nucleic acid have not been consistently demonstrated.

Immunological factors

MS appears to be an autoimmune disorder in the sense that the attack on myelin is mediated by the immune system. Cells of the immune system (lymphocytes, plasma cells and activated microglia and macrophages) are present in the acute phase of demyelination. Anti-myelin antibodies are present in the peripheral blood of patients with MS but these seem not to be specific in that they may also be present in patients without MS. There is also decreased activity of circulating suppressor T cells during an attack. The genetic association with

Table 9.2 Etiology of MS

Although the cause of MS is not yet known the various pieces of evidence can be drawn together to form a working hypothesis as follows:

Immune-mediated demyelination is triggered in genetically susceptible individuals by a common infective organism acquired in childhood.

certain HLA antigen types supports a key role for the immune system in MS.

Clinical features

The presenting signs and symptoms of MS are usually those of focal lesions in the CNS (Table 9.3). Painful inflammation of the optic nerve associated with blurred vision (optic neuritis) is a common presentation. Peak onset is in the age range 20–40 years and onset is very uncommon in childhood or after 60 years of age. MS is more common in women than in men with a ratio of about 3 to 2. It is a chronic disease with a very variable and unpredictable clinical course (Table 9.4). Typically, the early years are characterized by relapses, with onset of focal neurology over a matter of hours or days, followed by remission with recovery of function over days and weeks. In later years there is often progressive deterioration leading to irreversible disability. However, occasionally, patients may have a single episode, for example of optic neuritis, without further symptoms. At the other end of the spectrum is a disease course characterized by rapid and relentless progression leading to death within months (acute MS).

There is a correlation between the anatomical location of the plaques and the consequent clinical signs and symptoms. For example, involvement of the optic pathways leads to visual impairment. Disordered control of eye movements results from brainstem lesions. Cerebellar plaques cause ataxia and disordered control of speech. Involvement of long ascending and descending tracts causes focal sensory disturbance and loss of motor control. Demyelination may occur at multiple levels in the spinal cord and this contributes to paraplegia and loss of bladder control. Extensive cerebral lesions may be associated with impaired cognitive function.

Most patients with MS survive for many years or decades and die from an unrelated disease. However, severely disabled patients may die from infective complications of immobility such as bronchopneumonia or septicemia resulting from a urinary tract infection or pressure sores.

Table 9.3 A clinical diagnosis of multiple sclerosis

1. Clinical evidence of focal neurological deficits disseminated in space and time
2. Identification by magnetic resonance scans of multiple well-circumscribed lesions within the white matter
3. Visual evoked responses providing electrophysiological evidence of slowing of conduction of action potentials along demyelinated axons
4. Oligoclonal bands in CSF indicating an active immune response within the CNS

Table 9.4 Variants of MS

- Classic or chronic MS (Charcot type) – relapses and remissions in early years often followed by progressive disability in later years
- Acute MS (Marburg type) – rapidly progressive disease which is fatal within months
- Neuromyelitis optica (Devic type) – simultaneous demyelination in the optic nerves and spinal cord. There may or may not be progression to chronic MS
- Concentric sclerosis (Balo type) – a very uncommon pattern of pathology in which plaques are large and have concentric rings of alternating demyelination and myelin preservation

Pathology

Plaques in MS appear macroscopically as well-circumscribed areas of gray discoloration within white matter (Figs 9.1–9.4). On external examination plaques may be seen involving the pial surface of the optic nerves and chiasm, the midbrain, pons, medulla and spinal cord. On dissection of the brain, plaques are typically numerous and scattered throughout the cerebral white matter, brainstem, cerebellar white matter and spinal cord (Figs 9.1– 9.4). They are very variable in size but most often in the range 2–10 mm in diameter. The distribution of plaques may seem almost random although some locations are more frequently involved. Plaques involve the walls of the lateral ventricles (periventricular plaques) (Figs 9.1, 9.5 and 9.6), the deep cerebral white matter, the interface between the cortex and white matter and the optic nerves and chiasm (Fig. 9.7). Plaques can occur

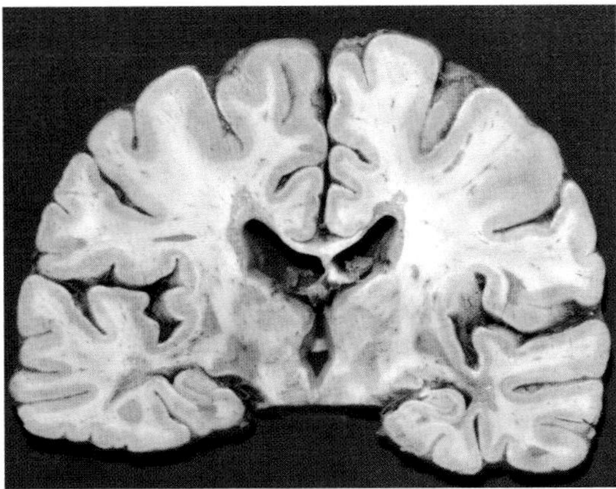

Figure 9.1 Multiple sclerosis. Coronal section of cerebrum. There are multiple well-demarcated gray foci of demyelination (plaques) scattered widely throughout the white matter. They are particularly prominent around the lateral ventricles.

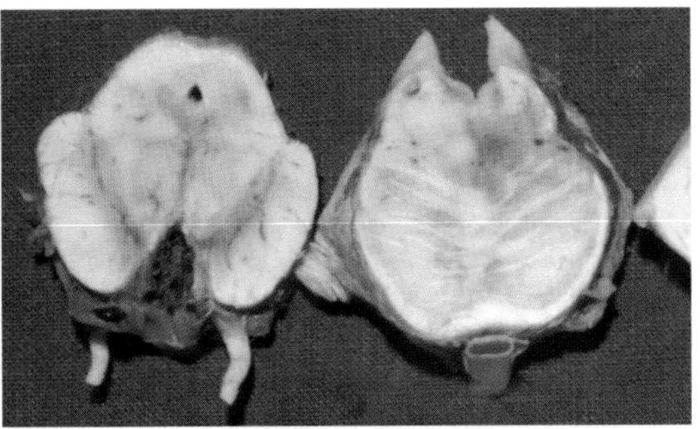

Figure 9.2 Multiple sclerosis. Horizontal sections of brainstem with several plaques of demyelination. They are less easy to see macroscopically than those in the cerebral white matter because of the variegated pattern of the brainstem anatomy.

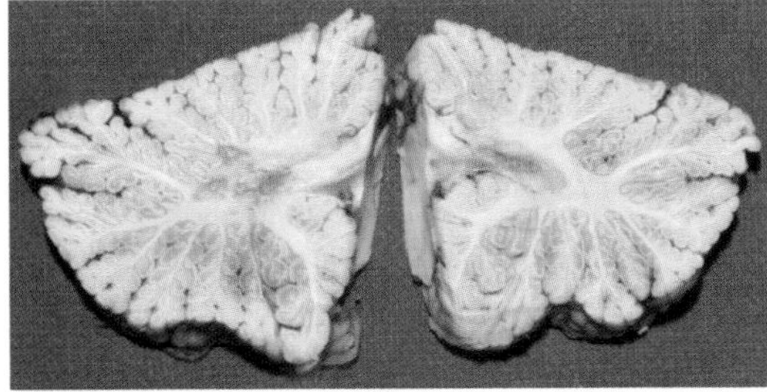

Figure 9.3 Multiple sclerosis. Sagittal sections of cerebellum with several plaques of demyelination in the white matter.

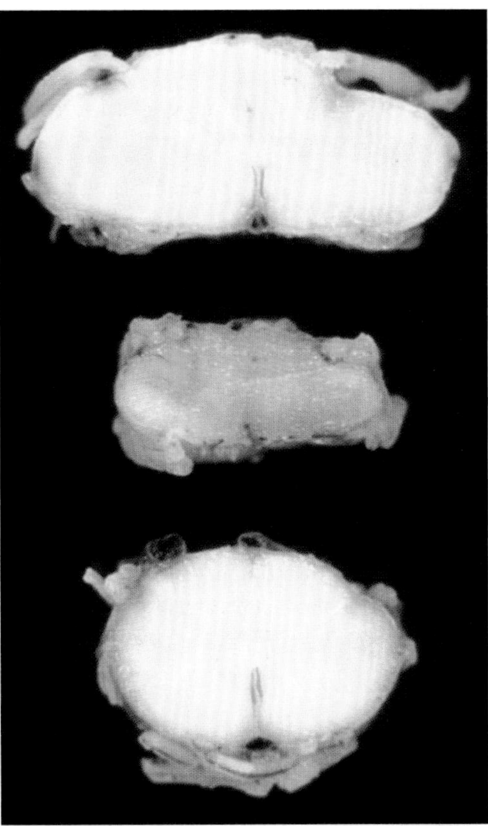

Figure 9.4 Multiple sclerosis. Horizontal sections of spinal cord. There is almost complete demyelination of the cross section of the thoracic cord (center) reflected by brown discoloration and atrophy. The cervical (upper) and lumbar (lower) spinal cord is preserved.

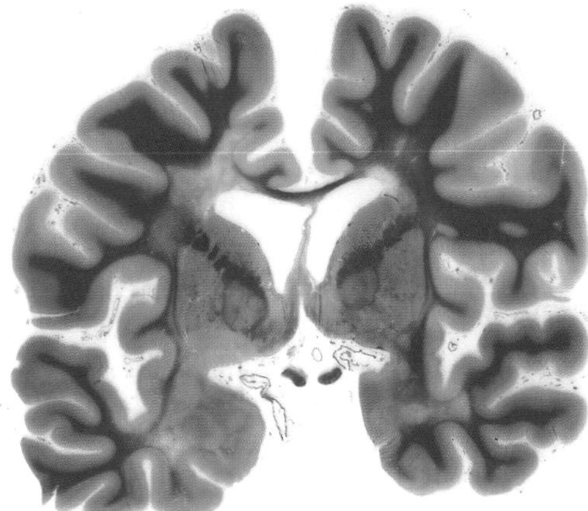

Figure 9.5 Multiple sclerosis. Plaques in the cerebral white matter. Normally myelinated white matter is deep blue in color. The plaques of demyelination appear pale due to the myelin loss. Plaques are particularly prominent around the lateral ventricles. Luxol fast blue/cresyl violet.

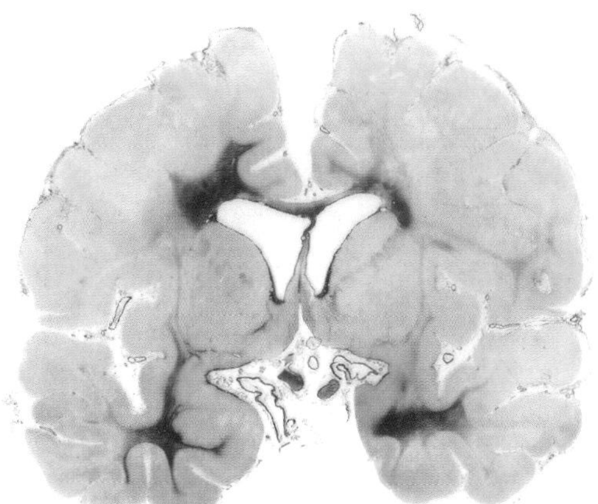

Figure 9.6 Multiple sclerosis. Section corresponding to Fig. 9.5 and stained to demonstrate gliosis (dark blue). The distribution of gliosis corresponds to the locations of the plaques in Fig. 9.5. Holzer stain.

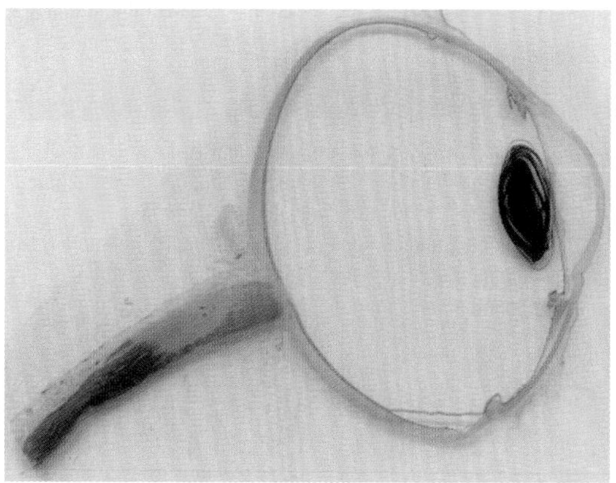

Figure 9.7 Multiple sclerosis. Eye with longitudinal sectional of optic nerve showing a plaque. Demyelination in the optic nerves is common in MS.

in the gray matter but are difficult to detect macroscopically. Plaques in the brainstem and spinal cord (Figs 9.2, 9.4, 9.8–9.10) are also difficult to see with the naked eye because of the variegated color of the cut surface. Some plaques have a clear perivascular location.

Histologically, three distinct plaque types are recognized: acute plaques, chronic or 'burnt out' plaques, and shadow plaques. The features of these different forms of plaque are described below.

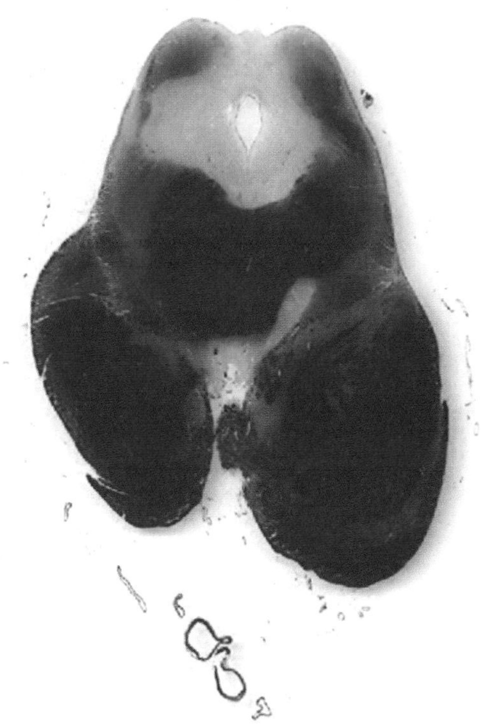

Figure 9.8 Multiple sclerosis. Periaqueductal demyelination in the midbrain. Luxol fast blue/cresyl violet.

Chronic or 'burnt out' plaque

In autopsy practice the lesion most commonly encountered is the chronic plaque in which the active process of inflammation and phagocytosis of myelin occurred many years before. It is a well-circumscribed lesion of complete myelin loss (Figs 9.11 and 9.12). Oligodendrocytes are markedly reduced in density or are absent in the demyelinated zone. Axons in the lesion have no myelin sheaths (i.e. they are demyelinated axons). The density of axons in the plaque may be similar to the adjacent unaffected white matter or, particularly in longstanding lesions, may be somewhat reduced. There is little residual inflammation, although there may be a thin rim of continuing active demyelination at the plaque margin (Fig. 9.13). Abundant chronic reactive astrocytes are present. This fibrillary gliotic reaction gives the lesion its characteristically firm texture in the unfixed brain which led to the term MS.

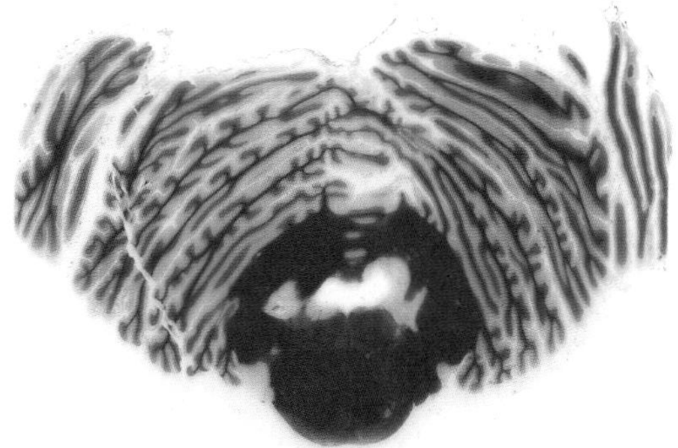

Figure 9.9 Multiple sclerosis. Horizontal section of pons and cerebellum. Plaques of demyelination are present bilaterally at the trigeminal root entry zones and in the cerebellar peduncles. Luxol fast blue/cresyl violet.

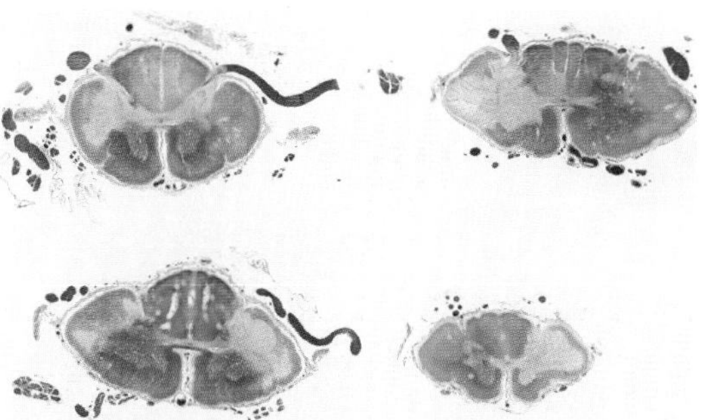

Figure 9.10 Multiple sclerosis. Horizontal sections of spinal cord. There are plaques of demyelination which affect different tracts of the cord at different levels. Luxol fast blue/cresyl violet.

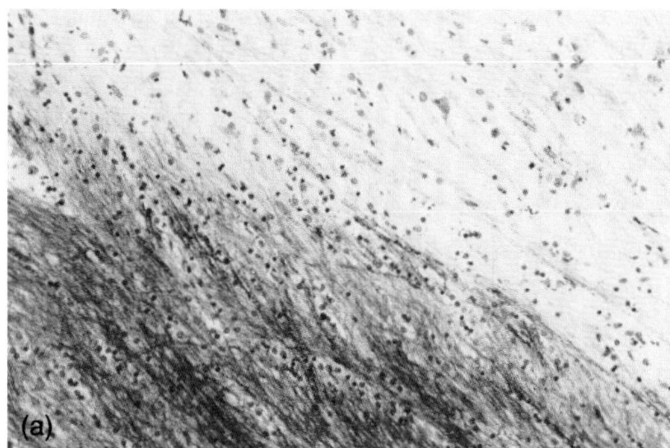

Figure 9.11 Multiple sclerosis. Edge of a chronic inactive plaque stained to show myelin, axons and cell nuclei, respectively. The normal white matter is bottom left and the plaque is top right. (a) Luxol fast blue stain showing complete loss of myelin in the plaque.

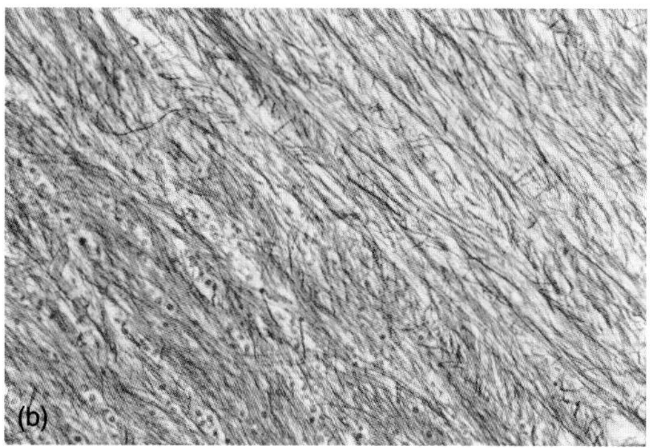

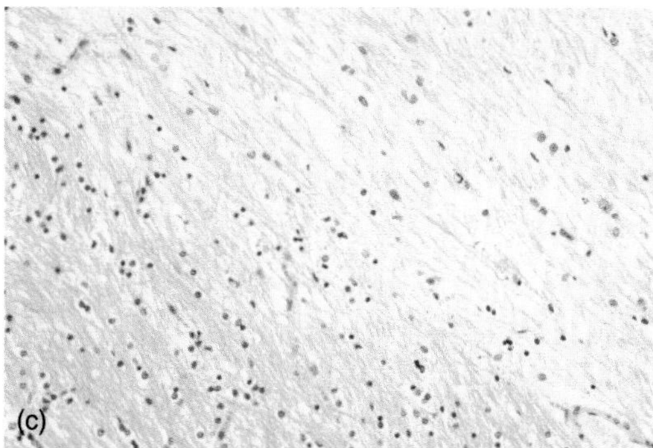

Figure 9.11 (b) Palmgren silver stain demonstrating relative preservation of axons in the plaque, therefore demonstrating selective loss of the myelin sheaths. (c) H&E. The density of nuclei in the plaque is reduced due to loss of oligodendrocytes. Most of the nuclei within the plaque belong to reactive astrocytes.

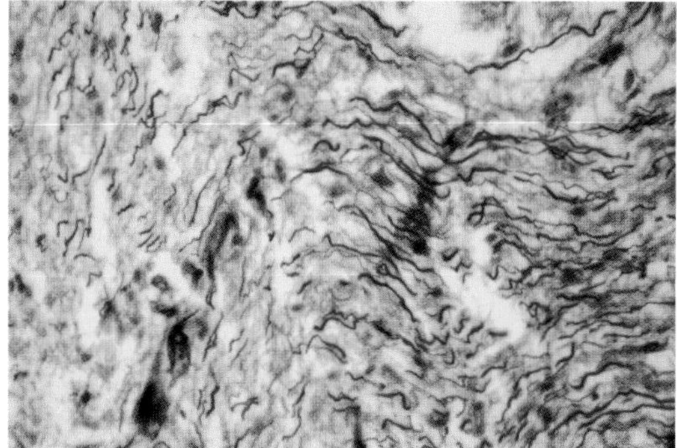

Figure 9.12 Multiple sclerosis. The margin of a plaque. Combined stain to demonstrate axons (Palmgren silver stain) and myelin (Luxol fast blue. Myelin sheaths (blue) can be seen around individual axons (black) in the normal white matter (right) contrasting with the plaque (left) in which axons are visible without myelin sheaths (i.e. they are demyelinated axons).

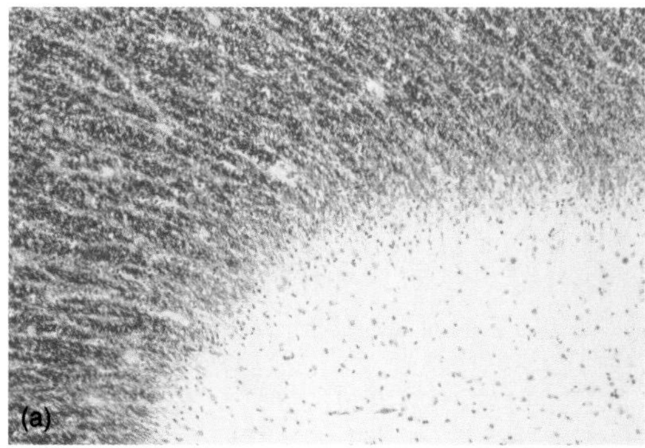

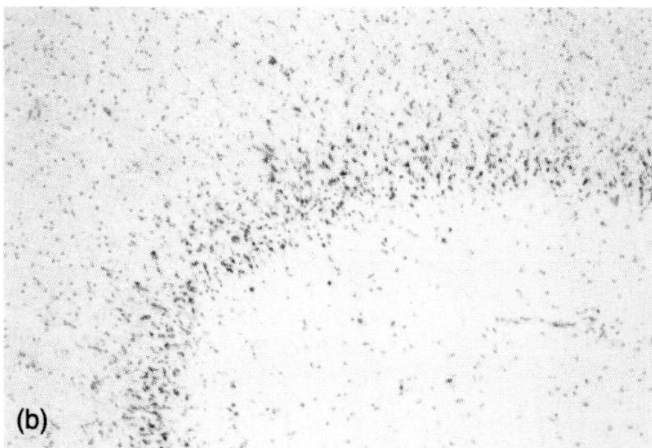

Figure 9.13 Multiple sclerosis. Chronic plaque with an active rim stained to show myelin, macrophages and astrocytes, respectively. (a) Luxol fast blue. The plaque is at bottom right. (b) CD68 immunohistochemistry demonstrates macrophages at the rim of the plaque indicating a rim of active demyelination. (c) GFAP immunohistochemistry demonstrating reactive astrocytes within the plaque.

Acute plaque

In acute plaques there is extensive active demyelination. The margins of acute plaques are typically less sharply demarcated than in chronic plaques. Active demyelination is indicated histologically by the presence within the plaque of macrophages (Figs 9.14–9.17) containing phagocytosed myelin sheath debris. The phagocytosed myelin can be identified on light microscopy by the presence of blue specks within macrophage cytoplasm on Luxol fast blue stained sections, with lipid stains such as oil red O, or by electron microscopy (Fig. 9.17). Macrophages appear to play an active role in stripping myelin from the axons. Although axons are not directly damaged, indirect damage to axons at the plaque margin can be seen in the form of

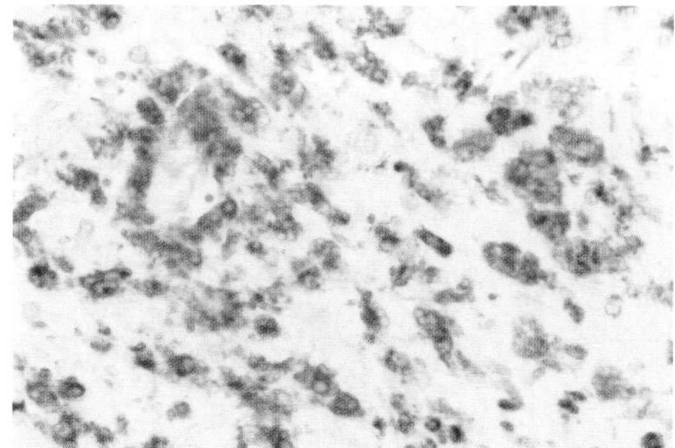

Figure 9.14 Multiple sclerosis. CD68 immunohistochemistry demonstrating numerous actively phagocytosing macrophages within an acute plaque.

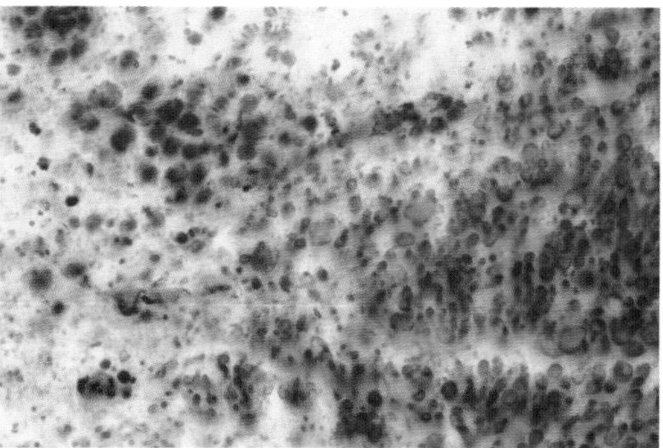

Figure 9.15 Multiple sclerosis. Phagocytosis of myelin lipid in the active rim of a plaque. The phagocytosed lipid within macrophages appears bright red (top left) in contrast to the lipid within intact myelin sheaths which is pale red (bottom right).

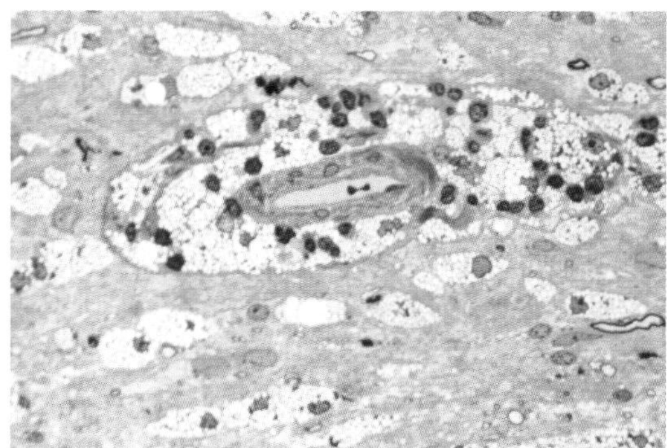

Figure 9.16 Multiple sclerosis. Semi-thin resin-embedded sections of an active plaque showing foamy macrophages aggregated around a blood vessel.

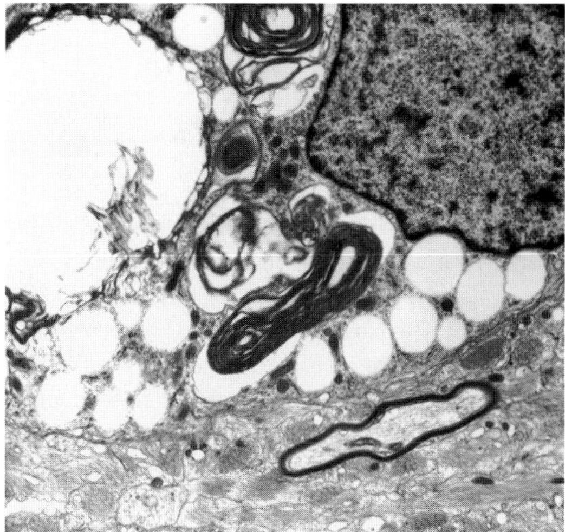

Figure 9.17 Multiple sclerosis. Electron microscopy of an active plaque. There is myelin debris within the lysosomes of a macrophage. ×39 000.

axonal swellings shown by APP immunohistochemistry. Lymphocytes and plasma cells are present in the plaque (Fig. 9.18). There are also abundant reactive astrocytes. Opportunities for histological sampling of the acute phase of the demyelinating process occur relatively rarely, and this has hindered understanding of the pathological process. Active demyelination may be encountered in post-mortem studies of rapidly progressive MS, in neurosurgical biopsies of plaques presenting as space-occupying lesions or in patients who die from an incidental cause during a relapse.

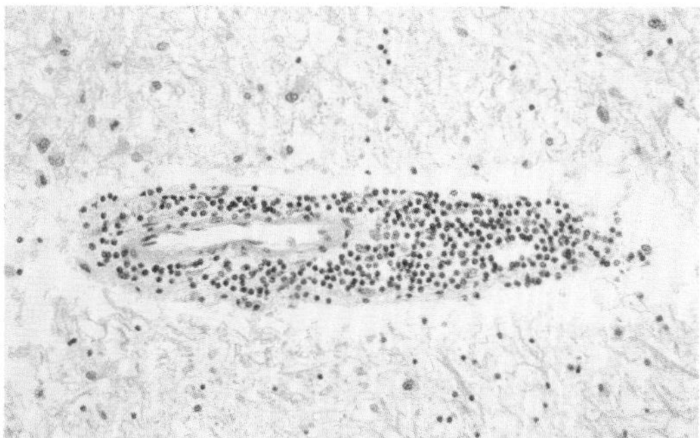

Figure 9.18 Multiple sclerosis. Perivascular cuffing by T lymphocytes in a plaque of demyelination. H&E.

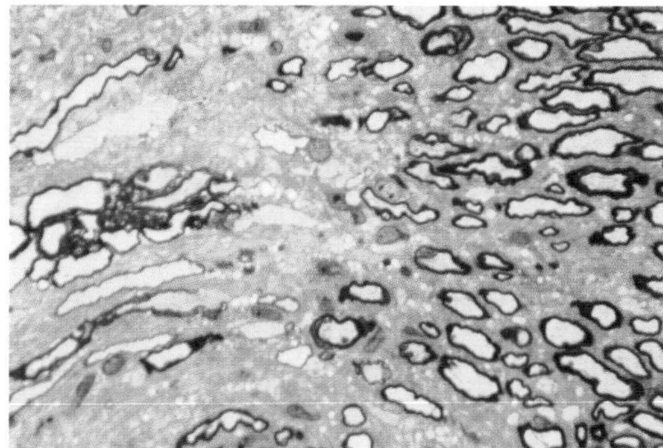

Figure 9.19 Multiple sclerosis. Semithin-resin embedded section of the margin of a plaque of demyelination. The myelin sheaths in the normal white matter (right) are of normal thickness in relation to axon diameter. In the plaque (left) some axons are demyelinated (i.e. they lack myelin sheaths) and some have thin myelin sheaths reflecting remyelination.

MR studies showing contrast enhancement have highlighted blood–brain barrier breakdown as an important feature which may precede demyelination.

Shadow plaque

A shadow plaque is a chronic plaque in which remyelination has occurred. The plaque may show partial or, rarely, complete remyelination. When axons are myelinated during development the number of layers of myelin formed, and therefore the thickness of the myelin sheath, is proportional to the diameter of the axon. A remyelinated axon can be recognized by an abnormally low ratio of myelin thickness to axon diameter (Fig. 9.19). These thinly myelinated axons can be recognized on

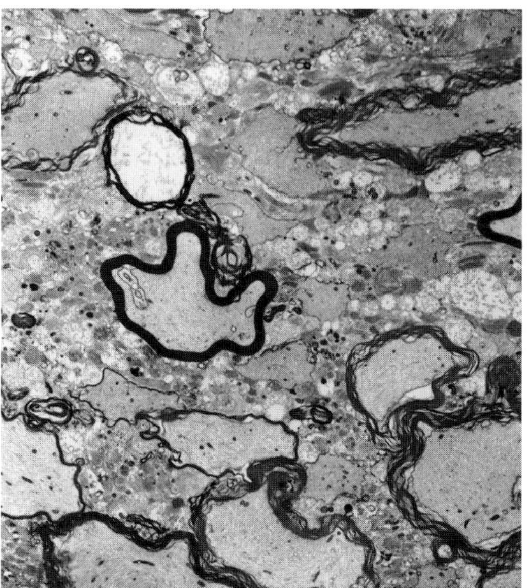

Figure 9.20 Multiple sclerosis. Electron microscopy of the margin of a plaque. Some axons have myelin sheaths of normal thickness, some axons lack myelin sheaths (i.e. they are demyelinated) and some axons have abnormally thin myelin sheaths, reflecting remyelination. ×5000.

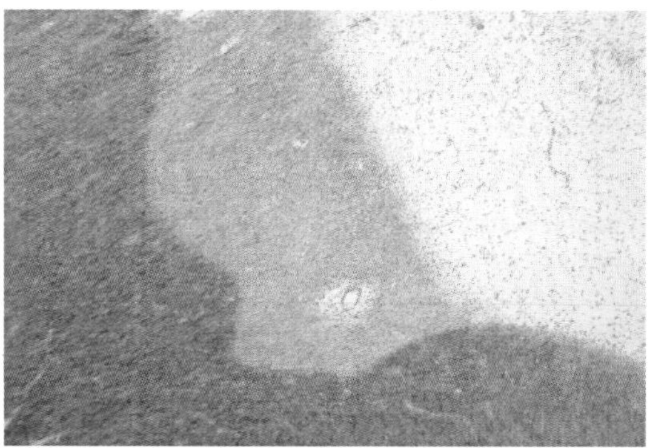

Figure 9.21 Multiple sclerosis. Shadow plaque. The zone of intermediate staining intensity (center) reflects an area of remyelination in the plaque. Luxol fast blue/cresyl violet.

electron microscopy (Fig. 9.20) and also give a characteristic appearance under the light microscope on myelin stains (Fig. 9.21). Normal white matter is stained deep blue, completely demyelinated areas appear white, and remyelinated areas appear intermediate in the degree of staining ('shadow plaque'). In a study of 100 cases of MS in the Glasgow neuropathology archive we identified some evidence of remyelination in 30 cases (30%). Usually this took the form of a relatively thin rim of remyelination at the margin of a few of the plaques in a case, but some cases had very extensive remyelination involving many plaques.

Axonal degeneration

Recent studies have highlighted that, in addition to the selective demyelination, some axonal pathology does also occur in MS plaques. In relatively acute plaques there is evidence of disturbed axonal transport in the form of APP immunoreactive axonal swellings. In chronic plaques quantitative studies have shown a significant reduction in axon density due to axonal degeneration.

Pathological correlates of clinical course

Remission

A striking feature of MS is the relapsing/remitting course with relatively rapid restoration of function, over a period of days, particularly in the early phases of the disease. The biological basis underlying this restoration of function is unknown. Possible mechanisms include remyelination, redistribution of ion channels along the recently demyelinated axon and removal of putative factors which block conduction of the action potential.

Progression

It has recently been recognized that axonal loss may occur in chronic MS. Axonal loss may be responsible for failure of remission and conversion to a chronic progressive clinical course resulting in permanent disability.

Prospects for treatment

Understanding the pathogenesis of MS is important so as to be able to devise prevention or therapy for the disease and in order to better assess prognosis. Potentially fruitful avenues include:

- Identify and prevent environmental trigger (e.g. a virus)

- Prevent immunological attack on myelin (β-interferon, integrin antagonists)
- Promote remyelination (e.g. stem cell transplantation)
- Prevent axonal degeneration
- Identify genetic factors which influence disease susceptibility and the severity of the course of the disease

ACUTE DISSEMINATED ENCEPHALOMYELITIS

Acute disseminated encephalomyelitis (ADEM) is a rare monophasic, self-limiting disorder. In most cases onset is approximately 7–10 days following a non-specific upper respiratory tract infection or other viral infections such as measles, mumps, chicken pox, rubella or pertussis. In some cases a precipitating infection is not recognized. Rarely, ADEM follows immunization, although this was probably more common in the past when vaccines contained CNS antigens as a consequence of their method of preparation. Immune-mediated demyelination occurs as a result of production of antibodies which cross-react with CNS myelin proteins. In its pathogenesis, ADEM closely resembles the animal model experimental allergic encephalomyelitis. The pathology of ADEM is multifocal perivenous demyelination and inflammation scattered throughout the white matter (Fig. 9.22). Macroscopically, there is typically edema and vascular congestion in the acute phase. Microscopically, there is widespread cuffing of small blood vessels (venules) by lymphocytes and macrophages with a small perivascular region of edema and demyelination (Figs 9.23 and 9.24). ADEM is not usually fatal and survival is followed by clinical recovery.

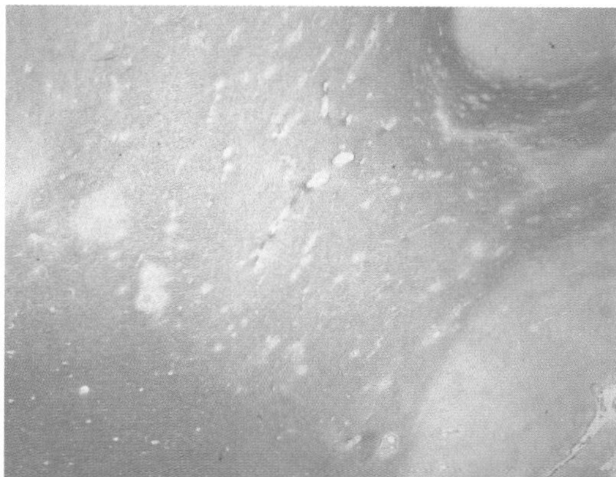

Figure 9.22 Acute disseminated encephalomyelitis. There is multifocal demyelination widely distributed in the cerebral white matter. Luxol fast blue/cresyl violet.

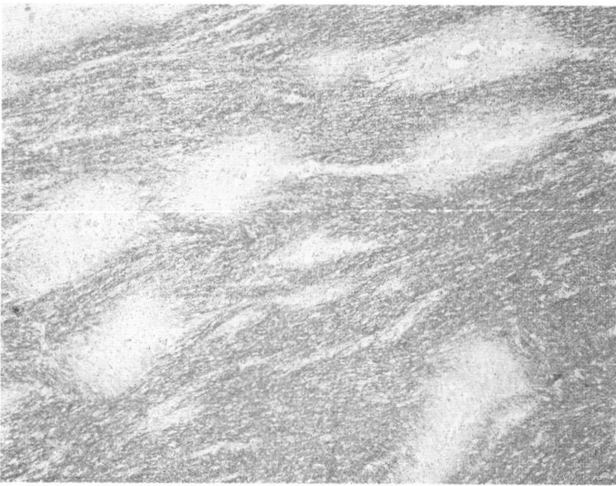

Figure 9.23 Acute disseminated encephalomyelitis. A higher power view of the cerebral white matter show that the foci of demyelination are centered on small veins (venules) Luxol fast blue/cresyl violet.

ACUTE HEMORRHAGIC LEUKOENCEPHALOPATHY

Acute hemorrhagic leukoencephalopathy (AHL) is a very rare disorder in which there are petechial hemorrhages throughout the white matter. There may be fibrinoid necrosis of small blood vessels with perivascular hemorrhages. Perivascular demyelination may be associated with some axonal damage. AHL is rapidly progressive and usually fatal. It probably represents a hyperacute variant of ADEM.

CENTRAL PONTINE MYELINOLYSIS

In central pontine myelinolysis (CPM) there is a symmetrical demyelinating lesion in the center of

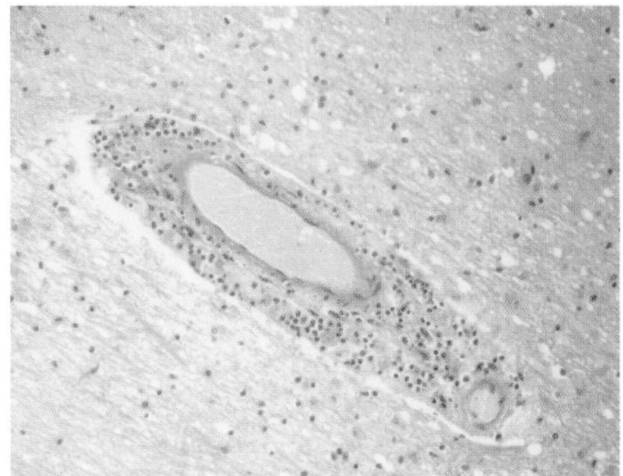

Figure 9.24 Acute disseminated encephalomyelitis. The regions of perivenous demyelination contain a chronic inflammatory infiltrate of lymphocytes and macrophages. H&E.

the basis pontis, usually with a surrounding rim of preserved myelin (see Fig. 13.3, page 244). Occasionally, the demyelination may extend through the brainstem in a rostral or caudal direction. Preservation of axons in the lesion distinguishes CPM from a pontine infarct. The disorder is thought to be due to a metabolic derangement and has specifically been associated with rapid iatrogenic correction of hyponatremia. CPM is a monophasic disorder which is usually fatal.

MARCHIAFAVA-BIGNAMI DISEASE

This rare disorder was originally described in chronic alcoholic Italian men drinking crude red wine, but has subsequently been described in others. It is characterized by demyelination, sometimes accompanied by necrosis, in the central part of the corpus callosum. The etiology is unclear but it seems likely to be due to nutritional deficiency or toxins (Fig. 13.4, page 244).

CHAPTER 10

NUTRITIONAL AND METABOLIC DISORDERS

David I Graham

NUTRITIONAL AND METABOLIC DISORDERS

Within the nutritional component of this chapter aspects of malnutrition, vitamin deficiencies and the various syndromes associated with alcohol abuse, will be described. The next part of the chapter will deal with inborn errors of metabolism such as those associated with amino acids and the porphyrins, together with a description of some of the systemic conditions that have an adverse influence upon the CNS such as those associated with hepatic or renal failure. Finally, an account will be provided of some of the salient features of the paraneoplastic syndromes.

NUTRITIONAL DISORDERS

Malnutrition

The effects of under-nutrition on the CNS depend upon the stage of development or maturity of the brain, and the severity and specificity of the deficiency, and may cause irreparable brain damage at certain critical periods of both prenatal and postnatal development.

It would seem that the brain is particularly vulnerable during the fastest growth periods although in infants it may be difficult to determine the impact of the malnutrition because of associated medical conditions, specially infections, and social and physical deprivation.

In infants there are two principal clinical conditions, one of which is *kwashiorkor* which describes children with a weight for age from 60 to 80% of the standard as a result of inadequate calorie intake, and *marasmus* (marasmic kwashiorkor) in which the weight for age is below 60% of the standard, and is a result of insufficient intake of protein and calories. The situation is complex including protein deficiency, vitamin deficiency, hormonal dysadaptation and aflatoxin intoxication all being proposed to account for the condition.

There appears to be an association between maternal malnutrition and congenital malformations of the CNS such as hydrocephalus, anencephaly, encephalocele and spina bifida. However, more subtle changes have been described including an increased amount of lipofuscin providing further support of the importance of oxidative stress in kwashiorkor. In contrast to the rather uncertain findings in human material, there is experimental data which would suggest, at least in various laboratory models, some of the abnormalities of the brain are permanent, whereas others are reversible, the changes depending on the period of gestation.

Quantitative studies have suggested a disproportionate effect upon the cerebellum, compared with the rest of the CNS.

There is no evidence in adults that once fully developed, the brain is adversely affected in patients with anorexia nervosa.

DEFICIENCY DISORDERS

Among these are disorders associated with vitamin A, the vitamin B complex, and vitamin E.

Vitamin A

Carotene is the precursor of the light-sensitive pigment rhodopsin which is present in the rods of the retina. Vitamin A is also necessary in the synthesis of active sulphate and the formation of myelin. Experimental deficiency in laboratory animals has caused raised intracranial pressure.

Vitamin B Complex

Principal among this group of deficiencies are those due to vitamins B_1, B_2, B_6 and B_{12}.

Vitamin B_1 (thiamine) is water-soluble and plays an important part in the metabolism of carbohydrates, thiamine being a co-enzyme in the glycolytic pathway in the citric acid cycle. The daily requirements in humans are between 1 and 1.5 mg/day and it has been estimated that the body stores can be depleted within about 3 weeks. Deficiency of thiamine impairs the oxidation of pyruvic acid, thereby raising pyruvate and lactate levels and reducing the amount of transketolase in the red blood cells. The vitamin, which is not synthesized in the liver and is only stored in small amounts in the body, is found in many foods and is absorbed through the small intestine. Thiamine deficiency in the western hemisphere is usually due to chronic alcoholism and is responsible for the *Wernicke-Korsakoff syndrome,* and in rice-eating people, for *beriberi.* Deficiency of thiamine, may also be a contributory factor in nutritional *amblyopia.*

Beriberi

Predominantly a disease of the Far East, it is rarely seen in western countries. It is classified as either 'wet' or 'dry' depending on the presence of edema, which is largely a consequence of heart failure. Dry beriberi is characterized by neuropathic changes (see Chapter 18) in which there is axonal degeneration with relative sparing of small myelinated and unmyelinated axons.

A disorder similar to dry beriberi can be produced in pigeons by feeding them polished rice; the affected birds recover rapidly when given thiamine. The disease in horses known as the 'staggers' is due to thiamine deficiency caused by the animals eating fodder being contaminated with bracken; it too is quickly cured by treatment with thiamine.

Wernicke–Korsakoff syndrome

A condition found most commonly in malnourished, chronic alcoholics, it also occurs as a result of excessive vomiting and malabsorption due to gastrointestinal tract disease, and in association with certain tumors such as leukemia and lymphoma (Table 10.1). It is divided clinically into acute and chronic phases. In the acute phase, the Wernicke syndrome is characterized clinically by confusion, ataxia and abnormal eye movements and in the chronic phase (Korsakoff psychosis) by selective impairment of short-term (immediate) memory.

The Wernicke syndrome has been diagnosed in 0.1–0.4% of all hospital admissions, and studies variously carried out in Australia and in North America

Table 10.1 Causes of thiamine deficiency

- Chronic alcohol abuse
- AIDS
- Continuous nausea and vomiting
- Thyrotoxicosis
- Disseminated malignancy
- Long term renal dialysis
- Congestive heart failure treated with diuretics
- Prolonged intravenous therapy without vitamin supplements
- Malabsorption: post gastrointestinal tract surgery

suggest an incidence of about 2.0–2.7% of adult autopsies.

The disease may be acute, subacute or chronic and the principal structures affected are the mamillary bodies, the walls of the third ventricle, the anterior nucleus of the thalamus, the periaqueductal tissues in the midbrain and the floor of the fourth ventricle. In less fulminant cases, abnormalities are restricted to the mamillary bodies.

In acute or subacute Wernicke's encephalopathy, the brain is usually of normal appearance externally. On section there is vascular engorgement and in particular hemorrhages may be seen in the affected areas (Fig. 10.1a and b). On the other hand, in patients who have survived an acute episode the mamillary bodies are characteristically small and on section are often tan/gray in color and granular in appearance (Fig. 10.2).

Histological changes depend on the duration and severity of the condition and is similar in all of the regions affected. In acute cases there is rarefaction of the neuropil and hemorrhage, but with preservation of neurons and axons (Fig. 10.3). Within a short time the changes become subacute, as shown by hyperplasia of capillary endothelial cells (Fig. 10.4a and b). In chronic cases, there is loss of myelin in the central portions of the mamillary bodies, gliosis and more normal looking blood vessels. Evidence of previous hemorrhage is frequently seen in the form of hemosiderin pigment in macrophages. In some 25% of cases structural abnormalities can only be seen histologically. If the Wernicke's encephalopathy is due to chronic alcoholism, there is commonly, atrophy of the superior vermis of the cerebellum (Fig. 10.5) and peripheral neuropathy. Co-existing disease of the liver may give rise to the histological features of hepatic encephalopathy (see below).

The term *Korsakoff psychosis* refers to an amnestic syndrome and is usually secondary to Wernicke's encephalopathy, when it is referred to as the Wernicke–Korsakoff syndrome. The condition can occur with other disease processes that involve the diencephalon or the medial structures of the temporal lobe. The cause of Korsakoff psychosis is uncertain, although there appears to be a correlation of structural abnormalities in the dorsomedial nucleus of the thalamus.

Once the normal temporal sequence of established memory is disrupted the patient begins to confabulate. The overall morbidity remains high, only 25% making a complete recovery and 50% a partial recovery: the remainder make no improvement at all. In the past it was thought the lesions in the

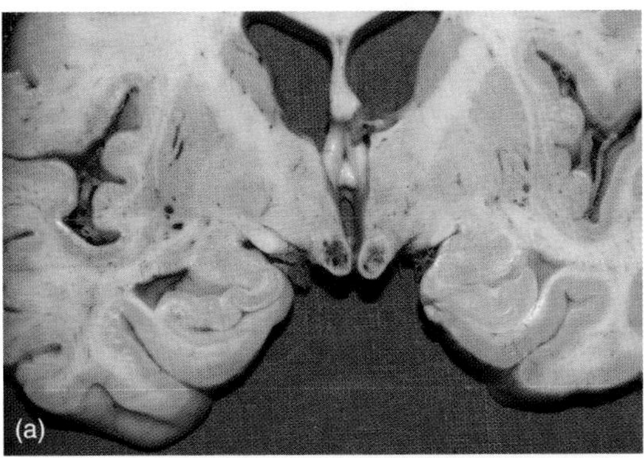

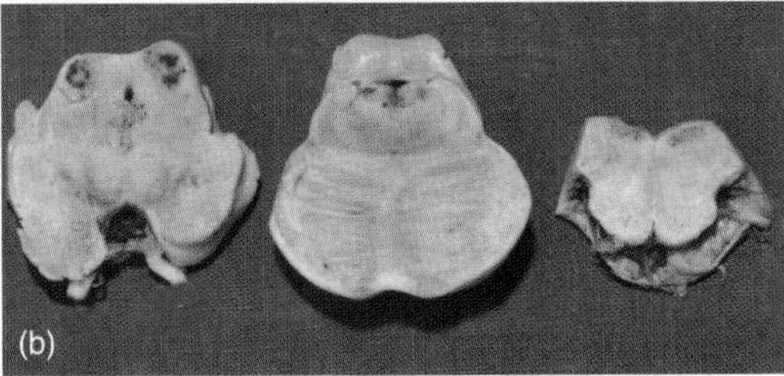

Figure 10.1 Wernicke's encephalopathy. There are multiple petechial hemorrhages (a) in the mamillary bodies and in the walls of the third ventricle, and (b) around the aqueduct and in the floor of the fourth ventricle.

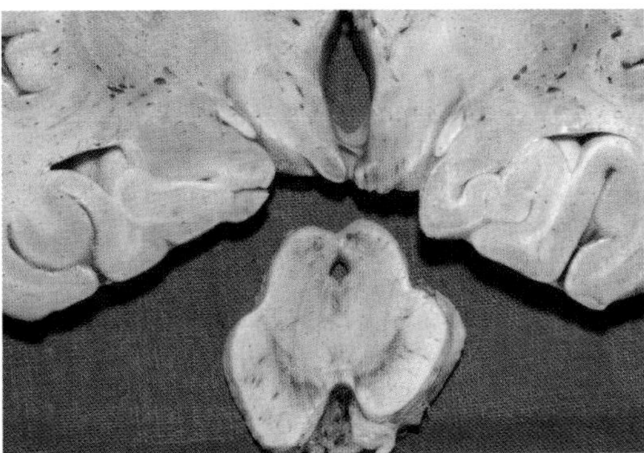

Figure 10.2 Chronic Wernicke's encephalopathy. The mamillary bodies are small, granular in texture and tan/gray in color.

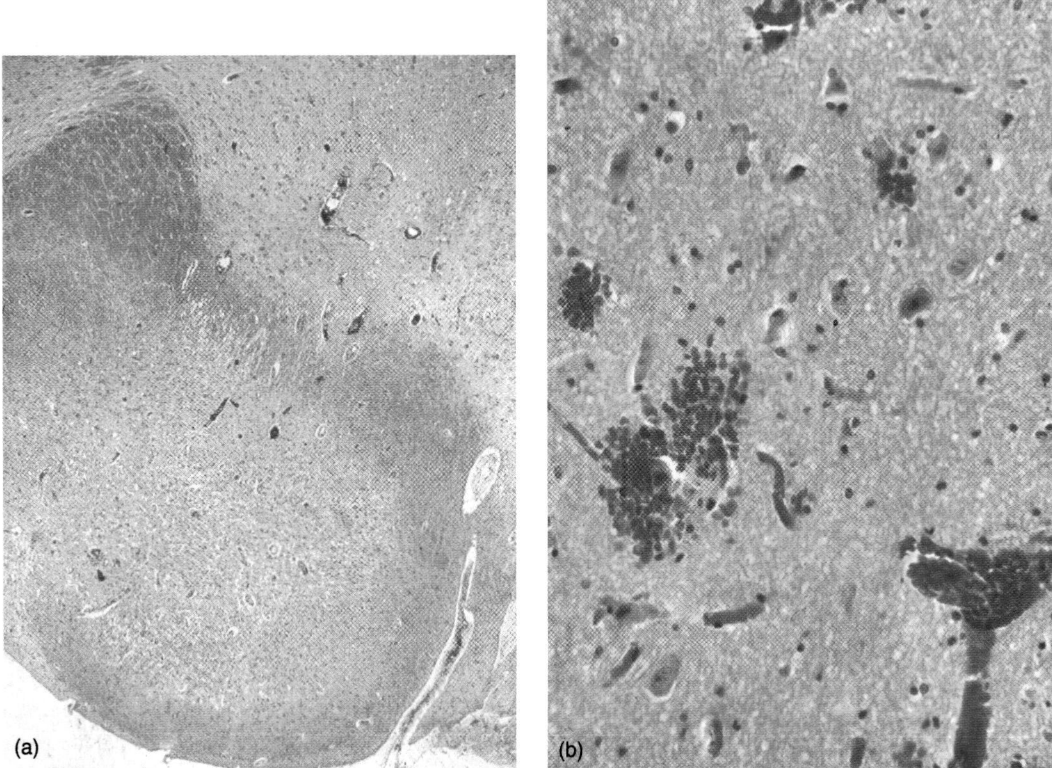

Figure 10.3 Acute Wernicke's encephalopathy. (a) The central part of a mamillary body is rarefied and contains several petechial hemorrhages. (b) Petechial hemorrhages are readily seen. Note preservation of the neuronal population. (a) and (b) H&E.

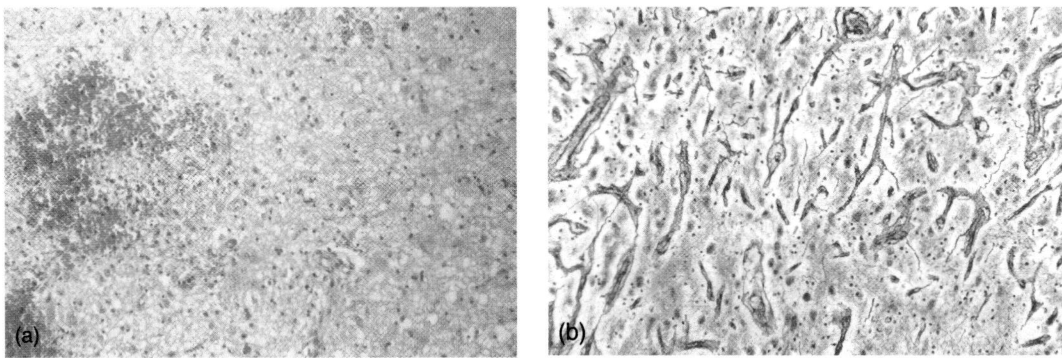

Figure 10.4 Chronic Wernicke's encephalopathy. (a) There is loss of myelinated fibers and prominence of capillaries in the central part of a mamillary body. There are also lipid-containing macrophages, some of which contain hemosiderin, and a prominent reactive astrocytosis. (b) The vascular changes are well seen in a reticulin preparation. (a) H&E, (b) Gordon and Sweet silver preparation.

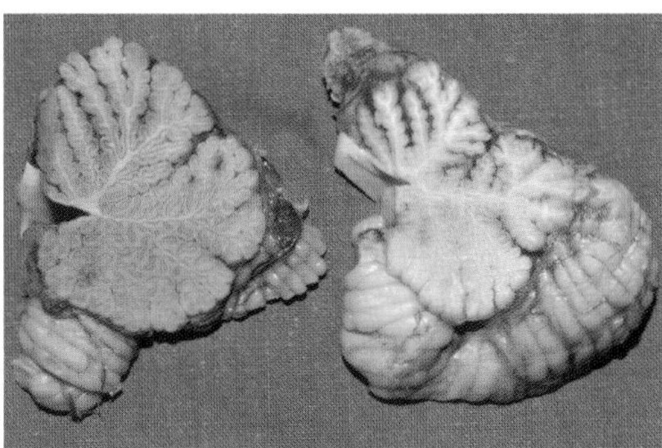

Figure 10.5 Chronic alcoholism. There is partial atrophy of the superior vermis of the cerebellum.

mamillary bodies were responsible for the amnesia, but recent clinicopathological studies provide strong evidence that the structural basis of the amnestic syndrome with which these patients present, is probably due to damage in the anterior nucleus of the thalamus.

Vitamin B2 deficiency

The association of *pellagra* (dermatitis, diarrhea, dementia) in various parts of the world where poverty and subsistence from a diet predominantly of maize, has been known for many years. It is caused by a dietary deficiency of *nicotinic acid* (*niacin*) itself, or of tryptophan, the amino acid precursor of nicotinic acid. Although nicotinic acid itself is important in the diet, it may also be biosynthesized in the intestines. People whose diet is based almost wholly on maize, therefore, are liable to suffer from nicotinic acid deficiency: however, this has now become rare, largely as a result of enriching common foods. Circumstances under which the condition is now found include the modification of the normal bacterial flora of the intestine, certain antibiotics or other drugs, chronic diarrhea and in alcoholism.

The principal histological abnormality in the CNS is the occurrence of central chromatolysis (see Fig. 3.20, page 56) in Betz cells, in various nuclei in the brainstem, in the anterior horn cells in the spinal cord, in Purkinje cells and in the pyramidal cells of the hippocampus. In some cases there is degeneration of the gracile, the spinocerebellar, and the crossed and uncrossed corticospinal tracts of the spinal cord. There may also be a peripheral neuropathy. As many pellegrins also have other nutritional deficiencies, it is possible that at least some of the features of pellagra are due to deficiencies other than tryptophan–nicotinic acid, e.g. pyridoxine.

Vitamin B6

Deficiency of vitamin B_6 (pyridoxine, pyridoxal and pyridoxamine) may be the cause of the peripheral neuropathy that sometimes occurs in patients taking drugs that interfere with the normal metabolism and utilization of vitamin B_6. These drugs include isoniazid, hydralazine and penicillamine.

There are many pyridoxine phosphate-independent enzyme reactions in the nervous system, of particular importance being their role in the decarboxylation of amino acids, and also the formation of amines such as epinephrine, norepinephrine, dopamine and serotonin. It has been suggested that the neuropathy associated with acute intermittent porphyria may be due to deficiency of pyridoxal phosphate as a result of its overuse by D-aminolevulinic acid. In under-developed countries where there is widespread malnutrition, convulsions in children have been attributed to vitamin B_6 deficiency.

Vitamin B12

Humans cannot synthesize this essential vitamin, which must be obtained from dietary sources, principally meat and dairy products. Vitamin B_{12} (*cyanocobalamin*) is absorbed in the distal ileum after combining with the intrinsic factor which is secreted by the parietal cells of the gastric mucosa. Deficiency is almost always due to inadequate absorption, which most often results from inadequate production of intrinsic factor in patients with *pernicious anemia*. Other, rarer causes include inadequate diet as may occur in vegans and impaired absorption from the small bowel as a result of various malabsorption syndromes, or competitive uptake of the vitamin due to tapeworm infestations or bacterial overgrowth in blind loops and diverticulae of the small bowel (Table 10.2).

Deficiency of B_{12} affects particularly the hemopoietic tissue, epithelial surfaces and the nervous

Table 10.2 Causes of vitamin B_{12} deficiency

Inadequate diet
Increased consumption
• Pregnancy
Defective absorption
• Pernicious anemia
• Malabsorption (celiac disease, pancreatic disease, gastric surgery, tapeworm infestation)
Abnormal metabolism

system. It is known to be involved in the conversion of L-methylmalonyl-CoA to succinyl-CoA mutase and folate-dependent methionine synthetase which uses methylcobalamine to synthesize methionine from homocysteine. However, the exact biochemical basis for the various deleterious effects of this particular deficiency upon the nervous system is not known, although the biochemical abnormalities may contribute to the production of non-physiological fatty acids containing an odd number of carbon atoms which are synthesized and incorporated into the membrane of neurons and myelin. Lesions in the spinal cord, similar to those found in human B_{12} deficiency, that have been produced in various laboratory settings, interfere with the biosynthesis of choline (which is an important constituent of myelin), or inhibit methylation of myelin basic protein, as in non-human primates exposed to nitrous oxide, which is thought to inactivate one of the vitamin B_{12} dependent enzymes, thereby causing a depletion of the methionine and a deficiency of the methyl group. There may also be a link between vitamin B_{12} deficiency and cyanide poisoning, and treatment with this vitamin leads to an improvement in tobacco amblyopia.

The principal structural abnormalities in vitamin B_{12} deficiency are in the spinal cord, the optic nerves and the peripheral nerves. The best known is *subacute combined degeneration* in the spinal cord, where there are degenerative changes in the lateral and posterior columns, particularly in the mid-thoracic region. In the cervical region there is more severe involvement of the posterior columns, whereas the lateral columns are more affected in the lumbar region. In early cases there is focal swelling and ballooning of the myelin sheath; these lesions progressively enlarge, thereby imparting a patchy, spongy appearance affecting the white matter (Fig. 10.6). Eventually there is some loss of myelin, degeneration of axons and phagocytosis of the debris by macrophages. Wallerian degeneration ensues and there is an astrocytosis, the degree of which is said to correlate with the duration of the disease. In longstanding severe cases there may be atrophy and discoloration of the posterior and lateral columns. Similar histological appearances are occasionally seen in the deep white matter of the cerebral hemispheres and, more rarely, in the optic nerves. There is also often associated peripheral neuropathy.

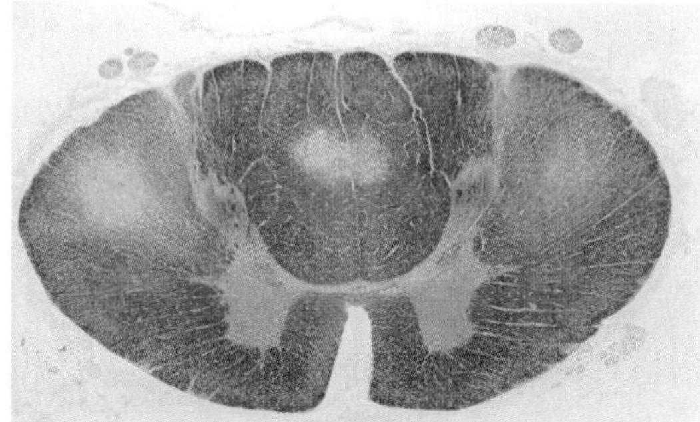

Figure 10.6 Subacute combined degeneration of the spinal cord. There is focal pallor of myelin staining in the posterior and lateral columns. Luxol fast blue/cresyl violet.

The vacuolar myelopathy found in some patients with AIDS is not due to low B_{12} levels which are normal: in African or poverty-associated AIDS the etiology of the spinal cord changes is likely to be multifactorial.

Folic acid

Folate is crucial for the synthesis and methylation of DNA during fetal and early post-natal development. Such is its importance during pregnancy that folate deficiency has been confirmed, in various studies, to be associated with an increased incidence of fetal malformation and mental retardation. Indeed, supplements of folic acid given during pregnancy have now been shown to reduce both the occurrence and recurrence of neural tube defects in babies. Somewhat similar effects can be induced by certain anti-epileptic drug therapy such as phenytoin and primidone and by anti-folate drugs such as methotrexate, trimethoprim, and triamterene. More recently, inborn errors of folate absorption and metabolism have been described. There is continuing controversy about whether the alleged neurological sequelae of folate deficiency are due to a low serum folate *per se* or from associated conditions from which these patients also suffer.

Vitamin E

This vitamin is important in the maintenance and function of the nervous system, in its role as an antioxidant, possibly preventing the peroxidation of phospholipids.

Conditions causing chronic malabsorption or reduced concentration of bile salts in the small intestine may lead to vitamin E deficiency. An inborn error of vitamin E metabolism has also been described, associated with which is a degenerative neurological disorder. Vitamin E deficiency occurs in *abetalipoproteinemia*, in which there is a failure of synthesis of apoprotein BD, an essential component of chylomicrons. Electrophysiological findings and the neuropathology of those with a distal axonopathy demonstrate changes affecting both the central and peripheral axons of sensory ganglion cells. Experimental studies in rats and non-human primates confirm that vitamin E deficiency produces a 'dying back' neuropathy in both central and peripheral central neurons.

Tobacco amblyopia

The cause of this condition remains unknown but it is possibly due to more than one nutritional deficiency, or a combination of nutritional deficiencies. Like alcohol, tobacco is primarily responsible for this condition but well documented cases of this type of amblyopia have occurred in patients who neither smoked tobacco nor drank alcohol. This is probably the result of a deficiency of several vitamins.

Neurological complications of steatorrhea and related gastrointestinal disorders

Neuropathological findings in *celiac disease* (gluten-induced enteropathy) are different from those associated with Wernicke's encephalopathy, subacute combined degeneration, vitamin E deficiency or pellagra. About 10% of patients with celiac disease develop neurological complications attributed to focal neuronal loss and associated reactive changes in the cerebellum, basal ganglia, the nuclei of the brainstem and the spinal cord. Peripheral neuropathy is not uncommon. Etiology of the neurological involvement in this disease is not known, but nutritional, toxic, infective, autoimmune and genetic factors have been implicated. Peripheral neuropathy may also be a feature of *post-gastrectomy states* after surgery for peptic ulcer.

Neurological complications also occur in *Whipple's disease*, a disorder in which PAS-staining granular material is present in macrophages in the wall of the small bowel; focal collections of similar cells are also found in the brain. The PAS-positive material has been shown by ultrastructural studies to be bacterial in nature, caused by the Gram-positive actinomycete *Tropheryma whippleii*. Diagnosis can be achieved by ultrastructure when the better-preserved bacilli may be seen in macrophages, astrocytes and pericytes.

METABOLIC DEFECTS

This category comprises disorders in which there is a known inherited metabolic defect, others are a consequence of systemic disease, and there is a miscellaneous group of disorders in which there is uncertainty about their pathogenesis.

Inherited metabolic defects

Although not common, these conditions are important because some can be detected by screening tests in infants, and brain damage can be prevented or reduced either by replacement therapy or by excluding precursor substances from the diet.

Disorders of amino acid metabolism

There are many different types of disorder due to specific enzyme deficiencies which result in an increase in the amount of a specific amino acid. This may be accompanied by systemic acidosis, hypoglycemia and hyperammonemia. Although, some are potentially treatable, many are associated with mental retardation. In general, they are characterized by status spongiosus of white matter, partial loss of myelin and an astrocytosis. The peripheral nervous system is generally spared. Most are autosomal recessive disorders and different mechanisms are involved in the pathogenesis of the neurological disorders as amino acids have a role in neurotransmission, protein and lipid metabolism, and mitochondrial function. A direct toxic effect may ensue by the abnormal accumulation of byproducts. Diagnosis is usually made by identification of elevated amino acids or their byproducts in serum or urine.

The hyperphenylalanine syndromes comprise phenylketonuria (phenylalanine 4-mono-oxygenase deficiency), or a deficiency of its essential co-factor tetrahydriobiopterin.

Phenylketonuria (PKU) is the most common type of amino aciduria that if not detected and treated, may result in microcephaly, severe mental retardation and epilepsy and in the second or third decade the development of a motor disorder. Clinically, there is decreased hair pigmentation and biochemically the excretion of large amounts of phenyl pyruvate acids. It is not a single disease entity and encompasses a number of subtypes, the most common of which is impaired hydroxylation of phenyalanine to tyrosine due to defects in the activity of phenylalanine hydroxylase and, in some rare cases, a deficiency of the co-factor, tetrahydrobiopterin. The relationship between mental retardation and the biochemical findings, and the occasional occurrence of spongiform change in white matter is not clear, but there is general agreement that increased amounts of phenylalanine retard the development of the nervous system. Once development of the CNS is complete, elevated levels of phenylalanine do not affect intellectual capacity. Screening programs for the detection of phenylketonuria depend on the recognition of the raised concentration of phenylalanine in the blood in the first few days of life. The aim of treatment is to lower the circulating level of phenylalanine to a level just slightly higher than that found in normal individuals by dietary restriction of protein and by use of synthetic substitutes.

Other types of amino-aciduria

These include *leukinosis* (*maple syrup urine disease*) caused by mis-sense mutation of the E_3 subunit of the branched chain oxo-acid dehydrogenase complex. The gene is located on chromosome 19q13.1–13.2. Leukinosis is identified by the presence of sotolone in the urine, which has a characteristic caramel odor. *Homocystinuria* is caused by deficiency of cystathionine β-synthase activity which normally couples homocysteine to serine to form cystathionine. The gene is located on chromosome 21q22.3 and the disease may cause changes in the walls of blood vessels with fibrosis of the intima, degeneration of elastic fibres and thrombosis. *Hartnup disease* is caused by a disorder of tryphophan absorption and produces a picture similar to pellagra with clinical features of dermatitis, dementia and diarrhea and neuropathological features of cortical atrophy and neuronal loss especially in the occipital cortex and the cerebellum. The relevant gene is located on chromosome 5p15. Other examples include *hyperglycinemia* and the *urea-cycle disorders* which are related to hyperammonemia and result from a defect of conversion of ammonia to urea, most commonly due to deficiency of ornithine carbamyltransferase which is an X-linked disorder.

Disorders of trace metal metabolism

Principal among this group of disorders are Wilson's disease (*hepato-lenticular degeneration*) and *kinky hair* (*Menkes*') disease.

Wilson's disease

This is an autosomal recessive disorder of copper excretion with variable expression related to mutation of the Wilson gene on chromosome 13, which usually presents in young adults as an extrapyramidal syndrome or hepatic insufficiency. Copper is deposited in the liver which may become cirrhotic, in the cornea to form Kayser–Fleisher rings, in the kidneys causing impaired tubular absorption and transport, and in the CNS. The copper-binding protein ceruloplasmin is low and increased amounts of copper are excreted in the urine.

In rapidly progressive fatal cases there is cavitation in the lentiform nucleus. In the more common chronic form there is atrophy and often light-brown discoloration of this nucleus. Histologically, there is neuronal loss, astrocytosis and hemosiderin-containing macrophages in the basal ganglia and distinctive changes in the protoplasmic astrocytes. These changes also occur in the cerebral cortex and take two forms, namely Alzheimer type 1 and type 2 astrocytes. Alzheimer type 1 cells, which are much less frequent than type 2, consist of hypochromatic irregular nuclei often having a rim of pink cytoplasm studded with small yellow-brown (with H&E stains) or green (with cresyl violet) granules. Alzheimer type 2 astrocytes have enlarged vesicular nuclei due to the accumulation of glycogen, prominent nucleoli and cytoplasm is conspicuously absent (Fig. 10.7). Another feature of Wilson's disease is the presence of Opalski cells in the same locations as Alzheimer type 2 cells, but particularly in the globus pallidus. The cells are globoid, measure up to 35 μm in diameter and have a slightly foamy cytoplasm and an eccentric nucleus. An origin from degenerating neurons and macrophages has been suggested, but recent evidence suggests that they are derived from Alzheimer type 2 astrocytes. They are not unique to Wilson's disease as they occur in non-wilsonian hepatic encephalopathy (see below).

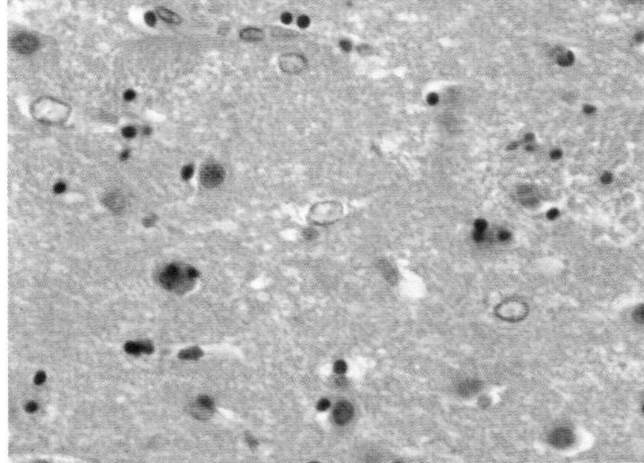

Figure 10.7 Alzheimer's type 2 astrocytes. The nuclei are swollen and vesicular, and usually contain prominent nucleoli. H&E.

Liver damage is a presenting, and often fatal, feature in many cases, of patients dying before any neurological changes are seen. Chelation of copper produces a marked clinical improvement, particularly in the early stages of the disease.

Kinky hair (Menkes' disease)

This is an X-linked disorder of copper uptake. The gene (at Xq13.3) codes for the copper-transporting ATPase 7a. There are low levels of copper and ceruloplasmin in the blood. The disease is characterized by severe systemic neurological abnormalities associated with erect undulating and fragile colorless hair. The disorder is secondary to impaired absorption of copper in the gastrointestinal tract and there is a decreased activity of copper-dependant enzymes, including cytochrome oxidase. In some cases there is atrophy of the brain, particularly of the cerebellum. Abnormalities are also seen in the elastica of blood vessels.

Disorders of purine and pyrimidine metabolism

Lesch–Nyhan syndrome, an X-linked recessive disorder of male infants, is characterized, clinically, by mental retardation, spasticity, movement disorders and compulsive self-mutilation. The deficient enzyme is hypoxanthine guanine phosphoribosyl transferase which results in the systemic accumulation of uric acid and the development of clinical features of gout. There are no specific abnormalities of the brain, suggesting that the disorder is due to changes in functional imbalance between GABA, dopamine and serotonergic neurons.

Disorders of pigment metabolism

The *porphyrias* are a group of disorders of heme biosynthesis: these pigments are normally present in hemoglobin, myoglobin and cytochromes. Classification is based on clinical and biochemical features. The most common is the acquired type (precipitated by drugs or intoxicants) in which there is moderate photosensitivity and increased uroporphyrin and coproporphyrin in the feces at all times. On the other hand, patients with acute intermittent porphyria which has a dominant mode of inheritance, present with episodic attacks (often after the use of barbiturates or sulfonamides) of emotional instability, sleepiness, severe abdominal pain and vomiting, but no cutaneous photosensitivity. The disorder is due to a breakdown in the mechanism of (aminolaevulinic acid synthatase) controlling the rate of heme synthatase in the liver, which results in the accumulation of porphobilinogen and aminolaevulinic acids. Similar neurological manifestations occur in the main forms of porphyria. The most constant finding is that of chromatolytic neurons in the anterior horns of the spinal cord, in motor nuclei and in dorsal root ganglia secondary to axonopathy in the PNS.

Disorders of endocrine metabolism

These include *Addison's disease*, hypothyroidism and abnormalities of calcium metabolism. Patients with Addison's disease may present with clinical signs and symptoms of raised intracranial pressure due to diffuse swelling of the brain. There is a variable increase in skin pigmentation and atrophy of the adrenal gland. *Congenital hypothyroidism* can be detected from a single heel stab between 6 and 14 days of life. If untreated, the infant fails to develop normally and becomes cretinous. Features of hypothyroidism in adults include peripheral mononeuropathy due to entrapment of nerves, psychotic signs and symptoms (myxedematous madness), impairment of higher neurological functions (myxedema dementia), and cerebellar ataxia.

Perivascular mineralization (primarily calcium, phosphorus and iron) is commonly seen histologically in the basal ganglia, hippocampus and dentate nucleus in normal subjects over the age of 40 years. Larger amounts of calcification, again in the basal ganglia in normal subjects, may be seen on CT scanning. Occasionally, the amount is so great that it may be seen on plain X-rays of the skull, and in over 50% of these cases there is an associated deficiency of parathyroid hormone. On slicing the brain, small amounts of calcification impart a gritty resistance to the knife, whereas larger concretions (brain stones) are dislodged and appear as solid lumps with an irregular rough surface. Calcification is seen to be more widely distributed histologically than the microscopy would suggest: it consists of rows of small calcispherites lying along the walls of capillaries and as tubular deposits in the medial coats of medium sized arteries and veins. Brain stones appear to develop by the accretion of these perivascular deposits.

Disorders associated with defective DNA repair

Xeroderma pigmentosum an autosomal recessive disorder is mainly characterized by an abnormal degree of sensitivity of the skin and eyes to ultraviolet radiation and a greatly increased susceptibility to sunlight-induced malignant epithelial tumors. Neurological abnormalities occur in some 20% of patients, most commonly intellectual impairment. There is also involvement of the PNS with demyelination and axonal degeneration with endoneurial and perineurial fibrosis. The underlying defect is the lack of an adequate mechanism to protect or repair environmentally induced damage to DNA caused by a defective nucleotide excision repair mechanism required to repair the cross-linking of pyrimidine residues.

Ataxia-telangiectasia is an uncommon autosomal recessive disorder that combines progressive neurological symptoms including cerebellar ataxia and extrapyramidal and ocular motor disturbances with telangiectatic vascular proliferation in the skin and conjunctiva together with defects in B cell and T cell functioning. These patients are prone to neoplastic disease particularly non-Hodgkin's lymphoma and carcinoma of the stomach. It too is caused by a defect in DNA repair with increased sensitivity to ionizing radiation. Neuropathologically there is diffuse atrophy of the cerebellar cortex, neuronal loss in the anterior horns and degeneration of the posterior columns. In the spinal root ganglia neurons are small and the number of satellite cells is reduced. The relevant gene is located on chromosome 11q22.3 and encodes a phosphatidylinositol-3 kinase protein.

Cockayne syndrome is a very rare autosomal recessive disorder with mental retardation and photosensitivity. There are multiple genes including *CKN1* and *ERCC6* each of which is involved in the repair of DNA following UV radiation. The gene locus is on chromosome 5 (*CKH1*) and is associated with dwarfism, microcephaly, retinitus pigmentosa, deafness and peripheral nerve involvement.

Manifestations of systemic disease in the nervous system

Hypoxic encephalopathy, including brain damage due to carbon monoxide poisoning and hypoglycemia, has already been discussed (see Chapter 5), as has the role of altered serum sodium in the genesis of central pontine myelinolysis (see Chapter 9). In this section the encephalopathies associated with hepatic and renal disease, and with diabetes mellitus will be described in greater detail. Kernicterus is considered (see below) and in Chapter 14.

Hepatic encephalopathy

A metabolic encephalopathy invariably accompanies severe liver failure (Table 10.3). Cases of massive hepatic necrosis, whether viral or drug-induced, are accompanied by *acute hepatic encephalopathy* characterized by rapidly developing coma. On the other hand, in cases of liver disease with cirrhosis, particularly when there is portal–systemic shunting of blood, *chronic hepatic encephalopathy* develops. Both types are potentially reversible so the patient often presents an episodic and relapsing course; they may, however, become chronic and progressive.

There may be no histological abnormalities in the CNS in cases with acute hepatic encephalopathy. In some, however, Alzheimer type 2 astrocytes (see Fig. 10.7) may be present, and a not uncommon finding is diffuse swelling, which may be sufficient to cause internal herniation. The cause of the cerebral swelling is unclear but it has been shown experimentally that there may be alterations in the blood–brain barrier in acute hepatic encephalopathy. Alternately, the cerebral swelling may be secondary to complications of acute liver failure, such as hypoglycemia and hypotension.

Table 10.3 Hepatic encephalopathies

- In fulminant hepatic failure
- Portal–systemic shunts
- Acquired (non-wilsonian) hepatocerebral degeneration
- Familial hepatolenticular degeneration (Wilson's disease)

The principal histological finding in chronic hepatic encephalopathy is the presence of Alzheimer type 2 astrocytes in the deeper layers of the cerebral cortex and in the basal ganglia. In cases of portal–systemic shunting or portal–caval anastomosis, the nuclei of the Alzheimer astrocytes become lobulated, particularly in the globus pallidus, substantia nigra and dentate nuclei. In general, glial fibrils cannot be demonstrated in their cytoplasm. Although a prominent feature, morphometric studies have failed to reveal any increase in the total number of glial nuclei in hepatic encephalopathy. Alzheimer type 2 cell change is not unique to hepatic encephalopathy, similar cells being found in patients dying as a result of hypoxemia and uremia. They are also seen in the brains of children with hyperammonemic syndromes due to genetically determined enzyme defects in various metabolic cycles.

Acquired (*non-wilsonian*) *hepatocerebral degeneration* sometimes occurs as a result of repeated bouts of hepatic encephalopathy, and rather softened gray/tan areas of discoloration maybe seen in the deeper layers of the cortex and in the lentiform nucleus (Fig. 10.8). On histological examination

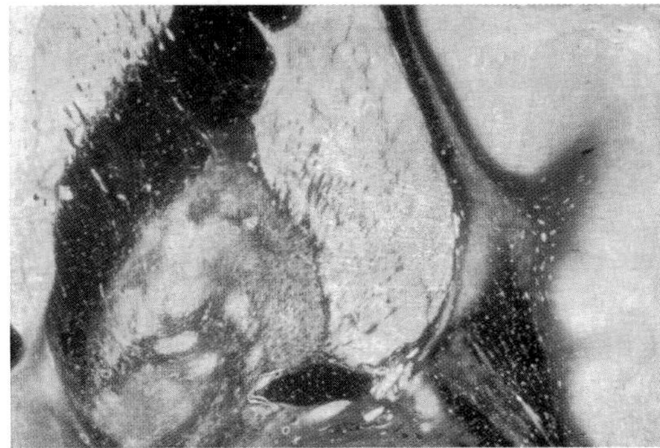

Figure 10.8 Acquired hepatocerebral degeneration. There are rarefied areas in the globus pallidus. Celloidin; Heidenhain for myelin.

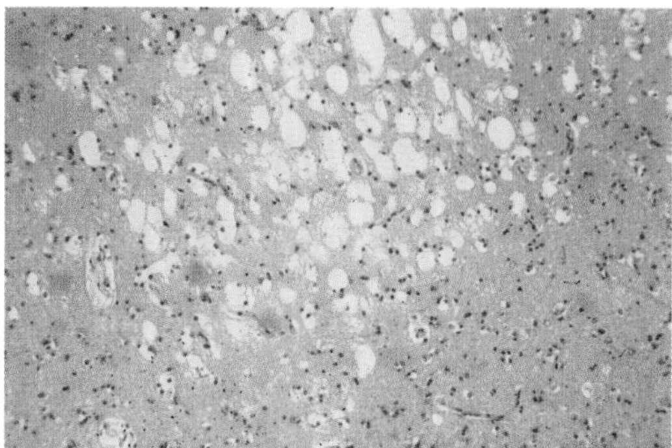

Figure 10.9 Acquired hepatocerebral degeneration. There is spongy degeneration in the globus pallidus. H&E.

there is spongy degeneration (Fig. 10.9), many Alzheimer type 2 astrocytes, loss of neurons and degeneration of myelin and axons: reactive changes are minimal. The structural abnormalities are very similar to those seen in Wilson's disease (see page 204). For example Alzheimer type 1 astrocytes and Opalski cells, which traditionally have been regarded to be specific features of Wilson's disease, are now known to be found in acquired hepatolenticular degeneration.

Patients with a portal–systemic shunt of blood may occasionally develop *hepatic myelopathy*, in which there is symmetrical demyelination of the lateral corticospinal tracts.

It is generally thought that hepatic encephalopathy is due to accumulation of neurotoxic substances in the blood which have an origin in the gastrointestinal tract. Normally, these substances are metabolized by the liver, but in cases of hepatic necrosis, or portal–systemic shunting of blood, they are not detoxified. In general, there is a correlation between the clinical symptoms and the level of blood ammonia, but other substances such as amino acids, biogenic amines (false neurotransmitters), and fatty acids have also been incriminated in the pathogenesis of the encephalopathy.

Uremic encephalopathy

This is a well-recognized complication of renal failure. The pathophysiology is complex and is probably a multifactorial process although there is evidence to suggest that a parathyroid-like hormone may play a role. Because patients with renal failure frequently have co-existing diseases such as hypertension, diabetes mellitus, collagen disease etc. and are subject to intercurrent infections, it is not surprising that most of the neuropathological findings are thought to be non-specific and not to be the cause of encephalopathy *per se*. In between 1 and 3% of cases dying with chronic renal failure, a subdural hematoma is found at autopsy. Histological findings are variable comprising a mixture of hypoxic damage and Alzheimer 2 astrocytes.

Complications associated with dialysis and *renal transplantation* comprise the disequilibrium syndrome, dialysis encephalopathy (dialysis dementia), and features associated with renal transplantation *per se*. The *disequilibrium syndrome* is normally a self-limiting condition, which occurs typically at the end of dialysis. It is more common in children than in adults and is thought to be due to osmotic gradients between brain and blood resulting in brain swelling and an elevation in the intracranial pressure.

Certain patients with renal failure who have been dialyzed for at least 10 years develop a distinct syndrome characterized by dysarthria, dyspraxia of speech, myoclonus and dementia which has been called the *dialysis encephalopathy (dialysis dementia) syndrome*. At first the condition is reversible but later it becomes progressive, although it may be reversed by renal transplantation. Death usually occurs within 18 months. There is an association between this condition and the accumulation of aluminum in blood and brain. The aluminum is derived from the frequent use of phosphate-binding aluminum gels which are in the water used in the dialysis. The pathogenic role of the aluminum, however, has not been universally accepted. Dialysis may also be complicated by subdural hematoma, which is presumably due to anticoagulation and clotting abnormalities associated with renal failure rather than to the hemodialysis *per se*.

As a result of immunosuppressive treatment, patients who have undergone *renal transplantation* are susceptible to a variety of opportunistic infections – viral (cytomegalovirus or herpes simplex) bacterial, fungal (*Candida*, *Aspergillus*) and protozoal in origin. Microglial nodules (see Chapter 3) are the most common microscopic abnormalities in the brain, and they have been ascribed to infection by either cytomegalovirus or herpes simplex virus. Prior to the use of cyclosporin and other modern immunosuppressives, some 70–90% of transplant patients surviving for more than 2 months showed virological and immunological evidence of infection, by cytomegalovirus, and this presumably accounts for the occurrence of inclusion bodies in the brain. The lack of a florid inflammatory cell response is attributed to the impaired immune response.

Neoplasia is another important complication of transplantation, the risk of developing a *de novo tumor* being approximately 100 times greater than an equivalent-age-and-sex-matched control. Lymphoid tumors are particularly prone to develop and have a propensity for the CNS. There is also an association with carcinoma of the skin, lips and cervix. The interval between transplantation and the development of tumor varies between 5 and 46 months. Possible mechanisms for this increased incidence are impairment of the immunological surveillance system, the effects of repeated antigenic stimulation from the transplanted kidneys and activation of an oncogenic virus. In some patients the possibility that the tumor was present at the time of transplantation cannot be completely ruled out. A further complication of renal transplantation is the development of central pontine myelinolysis (see Chapter 9).

Encephalopathy and diabetes mellitus

Complications of diabetes mellitus in the CNS are usually attributable to *cerebrovascular disease* (see Chapter 5). Clinical epidemiological studies have shown that hypertension and atheroma occur at an early age and are of greater severity in diabetic than in non-diabetic patients. It is also thought that the poorer outcome in diabetics with cerebral infarction is due to the high glucose level and the associated increase in lactate production.

The initial favorable response to treatment of *diabetic ketoacidosis* in young patients is occasionally followed by sudden deterioration and evidence of raised intracranial pressure. The sudden drop in glucose after insulin therapy is believed to be the cause of brain swelling which may be contributed to by the vascular changes of disseminated intravascular coagulation.

A common histological finding is demyelination of the posterior columns of the spinal cord. The changes can be so marked that the cord acquires a distinctive shape, referred to as '*pseudotabes*'. Demyelination of the lateral columns have been reported in *diabetic amyotrophic lateral sclerosis*. Pathogenesis of the demyelination is not known; possibilities include primary demyelination, a toxic metabolic factor or microangiopathy due to thickening of the basement membrane and changes of the blood–brain barrier. Neuropathy of peripheral, autonomic and cranial nerves is also common in patients with diabetes mellitus (see Chapter 18).

About 10% of cases of mucor (*Rhizopus*) infections in the nose, orbits and in the base of the brain occur in diabetics (see Chapter 7).

Pancreatic encephalopathy

Patients with acute pancreatitis may develop neurological dysfunction as a result of various complications that include electrolyte imbalance, hypocalcemia, liver disease, hypotension, hypoglycemia and hemorrhagic shock. However, a syndrome apparently independent of these metabolic changes has been described, characterized by acute delirium, seizures and multiple focal neurological signs occurring between the second and fifth day after the onset of acute pancreatitis.

Neuropathological findings include petechial hemorrhage, perivascular edema and astrocytosis, particularly in the basal ganglia and periventricular structures. These findings have been attributed to toxic vasoactive peptides, hormones and enzymes produced during the acute pancreatitis. A similar mechanism may cause CNS complications of the pancreatitis caused by mumps.

MISCELLANEOUS METABOLIC DISORDERS

There are several metabolic and neurodegenerative diseases of childhood of undefined pathogenesis which need to be considered here and which presumably, as the biochemical and molecular understanding of them becomes better understood, will fall into more carefully defined nosological entities. Included are *Rett syndrome* and *Reye syndrome*.

Rett syndrome

This is an X-linked dominant disorder in which the *MECP2* gene encodes methyl-CpG-binding protein-2 that recruits histone deacetcylase to repress gene transcription. Early development may be relatively normal, the child then undergoes a period of rapid regression that includes loss of language and social skills and the development of various hand stereotypes and epilepsy: by the age of 10 years both upper and lower motor neuron signs with a decreased mobility become evident. Pathologically, the most obvious changes are in somatic and brain growth both of which are decreased. Various neuropathological features have been described including pallor of the substantia nigra, reduced neuronal size and packing density in the neocortical ribbon and reductions in the number of dendritic spines. Findings include variable loss of Purkinje cells and associated gliosis.

Reye syndrome

This is an acute non-inflammatory encephalopathy characterized by diffuse cerebral swelling and very severe microvesicular fatty change in the liver. Children between the ages of 2 and 16 years are most susceptible and the disease carries a high mortality. Many survivors are disabled with mental impairment, epilepsy and neurological deficit. Hyperammonemia is a rule and hypoglycemia may also be present. What causes Reye syndrome is not known but there is a strong clinical association with viral illness, and the taking of salicylates, which may contribute to the disorder. A number of cases, which clinically present as Reye syndrome have been found to have underlying inherited metabolic defects including hereditary organic acidemias, urea cycle disorders, mitochondrial disorders, fulminant hepatitis and other rare conditions. The most common denominator in these patients is a deficiency of medium-chain acyl-coenzyme dehydrogenase deficiency. Biochemical findings have shown that mitochondrial permeability translation may be the underlying disorder which results in swelling, depolarization and uncoupling of oxidative phosphorylation. Structural changes are seen in the mitochondria, some of which show morphological changes similar to those seen in liver mitochondria. At the time of brain cutting the most consistent finding is that of diffuse brain swelling and there may be evidence of herniation and secondary damage to the brainstem. Histologically, depending on the degree and duration of hepatic failure, there are variable numbers of Alzheimer type 2 astrocytes.

Bilirubin encephalopathy (kernicterus)

This is a clinico-pathological condition characterized by acute dysfunction of the CNS due to selective damage of the brain in a jaundiced, oftentimes male neonate. The principal risk factor is that of hyperbilirubinemia due to excessive formation or insufficient conjugation and excretion of bilirubin occurring in association with prematurity, hypoxia, sepsis and acidosis. The classical form due to ABO or rhesus incompatibility when the bilirubin levels reached 30 mg/dL has now largely been eradicated. Hereditary disease such as glucose-6-phosphate-dehydrogenase deficiency and Crigler–Najjar syndrome also contribute to the pool of at risk babies. Additional contributing factors include a dysfunctional blood–brain barrier due to hypoxia and reduced binding of bilirubin to albumin due to liver damage or due to treatment with certain drugs. Under these circumstances unconjugated bilirubin produces kernicterus only after the child has been made hypoxic. Increased hemolysis *per se* may also result in bilirubin encephalopathy if there has also been damage to the blood–brain barrier by hypoxia, sepsis, etc.

The typical findings at brain cut is yellow discoloration of the globus pallidus, mamillary bodies, subthalamic nuclei and the hippocampi. In the hindbrain there may be staining of the dentate nuclei, the substantia nigra and nuclei related to the floor of the fourth ventricle (Fig. 10.10). Histologically, the

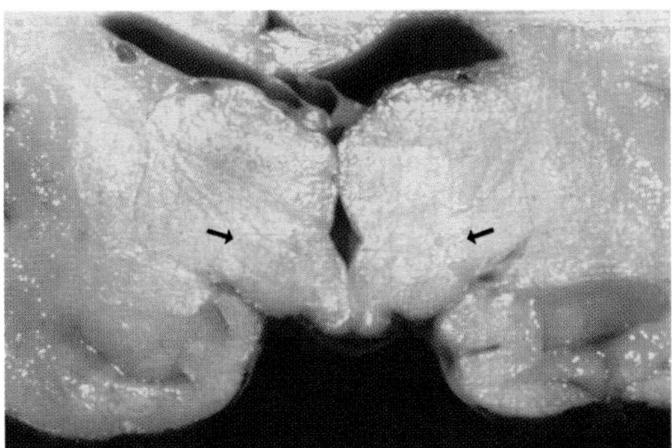

Figure 10.10 Bilirubin encephalopathy (kernicterus). Note selective staining of the subthalamic nuclei (arrows) and the hippocampi.

features are those of acute necrosis – similar to the pink neurons of hypoxia–ischemia: bilirubin is not seen. With survival there is neuronal loss and gliosis.

In contrast to perinatal tissue, the BBB in the adult brain does not allow the passage of bilirubin and, with the exception of the choroid plexus, the pineal gland, and the area postrema in the fourth ventricle, is not stained although the patient may be deeply jaundiced. However, in cases where the BBB is deficient due to infarction, tumor, or abscess, bilirubin becomes extravasated and stains the tissue.

NON-METASTATIC (REMOTE) EFFECTS OF CARCINOMA

The nervous system is frequently involved by malignant tumors arising elsewhere in the body. Metastases may occur in the brain, the spinal cord and peripheral nerve, or the spinal cord may be compressed by extradural deposits of tumor. Many tumors, however, particularly carcinoma of the bronchus and lymphoma may have indirect (remote) effects upon neurons, myelin, the myoneural junction and muscle. The central and peripheral nervous systems may be affected at various levels, singly or in combination. The various neurological syndromes have an approximate incidence of 6% of all patients with carcinoma. There is not a consistent relationship between the course of the neurological disorder and that of the carcinoma. They may develop concurrently, but the neurological disorder may antedate objective evidence of tumor. Furthermore, the severity of the neurological disease is not related to the size of the tumor.

Table 10.4 Paraneoplastic syndrome

Encephalomyelitis • Limbic encephalitis (medial temporal) • Brainstem encephalitis (rhombencephalon) • Spinal cord (necrotizing myelopathy)
Cerebellar degeneration
Sensory neuropathy
Myasthenia (Eaton–Lambert)
Opsoclonus–myoclonus

The *paraneoplastic syndrome* (non-metastatic or remote effects of carcinoma) by definition are a group of neurological disorders associated with systemic malignancy that do not directly involve the nervous system by compression, invasion, or by metastasis. Also excluded are the complications of radiotherapy or chemotherapy, opportunistic infections related to immuno-depression secondary either to the neoplastic process itself or to treatment or to both, and also excluded are the metabolic or deficiency disorders and vascular disorders linked to the development of malignancies.

Current evidence suggests that the paraneoplastic syndromes occur when a systemic tumor aberrantly expresses antigens that are normally found only in neurons. This is particularly true for an autoimmune mechanism found in cases of the Lambert–Eaton myasthenic syndrome (page 380) in which patients develop antibodies against voltage-gated calcium channels in neuromuscular junctions. Another consideration is that the antibodies are not directly pathogenic and the neuronal degeneration may be mediated by cytotoxic T cells. However, individual paraneoplastic antibodies are often but not exclusively associated with specific tumors and neurological syndromes (see page 330).

The principal paraneoplastic syndromes are *encephalomyelitis*, *cerebellar degeneration*, *neuropathy*, *myasthenia* and *opsoclonus–myoclonus* (Table 10.4).

Some 75% of patients with these syndromes harbor an underlying small-cell carcinoma of the bronchus, only a minority having been described in association with carcinomas arising in other organs including the breast, ovary, gastrointestinal tract and in testicular germ cell tumors. The syndrome is almost invariably associated with the presence of a high titer in both serum and CSF with antibody variously designated as anti-Hu. Other antibodies identified include PCA-2 in patients with bronchial carcinoma who presented with limbic encephalitis and anti-TA, anti-Ma1 and anti-Ma2 have been identified in patients with testicular tumors who presented with features of either limbic encephalitis or brainstem encephalitis.

Within this group of patients the histological changes predominate in those brain areas that account for the particular presenting features e.g. the medial temporal cortex, rhombencephalon, or in the brainstem or in the spinal cord. The changes consist of lymphocytes and some plasma cells around small blood vessels and small aggregates of microglia. Gray matter is affected more than white matter and the inflammatory changes are associated with loss of neurons and Wallerian degeneration (Fig. 10.11a, b and c).

A second well-recognized paraneoplastic syndrome is that of cerebellar degeneration most commonly associated with carcinoma of the breast or ovary (Fig. 10.12a and b). Patients present with a rapidly developing ataxia with some associated involvement of the brainstem. In 50% of suspected cases anti-Yo antibodies are present. In other cases anti-Ri, PCA-2 and CRMP-5 antibodies have been found. The histological features are those of extensive degeneration, and loss of Purkinje cells and to a lesser extent of the granule cells.

A frequent presentation is that of sensory neuropathy which is often combined with features of an encephalomyelitis. Clinically, it is manifested by numbness, paresthesia, dysesthesia and reduced tendon reflexes, and histologically there is destruction of posterior nerve root ganglia combined with axonal demyelination of peripheral nerve. Perivascular infiltrates may be present and in the ganglia, inflammatory cells are prominent: the number of ganglion cells is reduced and nodules of Nageotte are found where the ganglion cells had been lost. Autonomic ganglia may also be involved. There is a strong association with small cell carcinoma of the bronchus and anti-Hu antibodies. Patients may also present with a mixed sensory–motor neuropathy which may predate the underlying tumor.

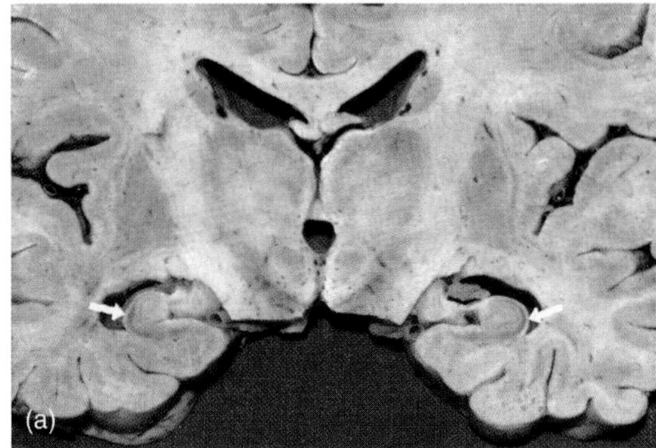

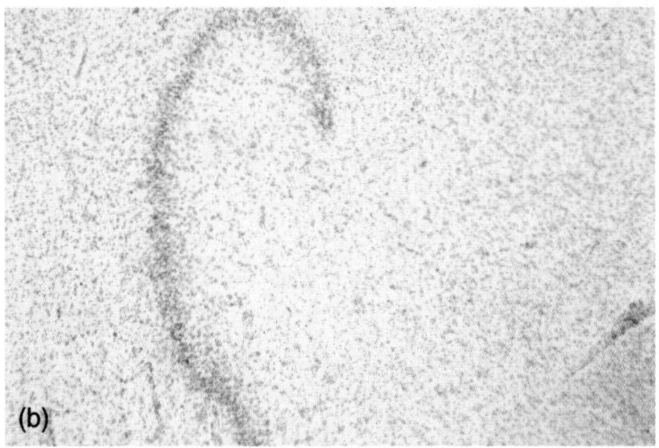

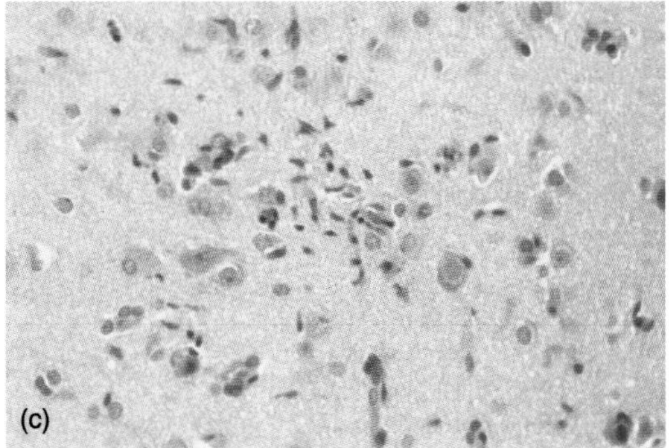

Figure 10.11 Paraneoplastic syndrome: limbic encephalitis. (a) There is partial atrophy and discoloration of the medial portions of each temporal lobe (arrows). (b) There is increased cellularity of the hippocampus with blurring of anatomical boundaries. (c) Focus of inflammation that includes microglia and lymphocytes. (b) Luxol fast blue/cresyl violet. (c) H&E.

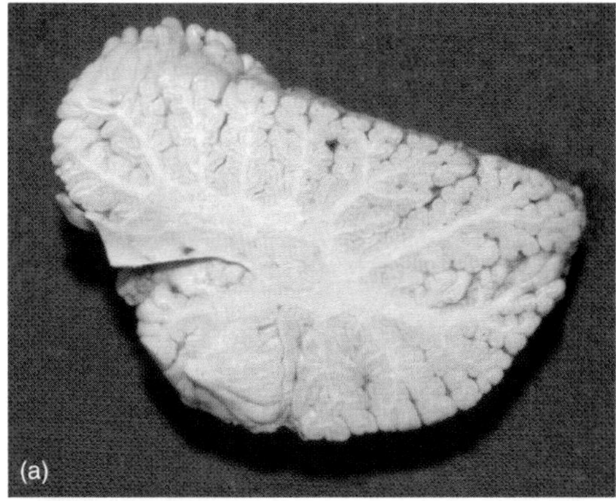

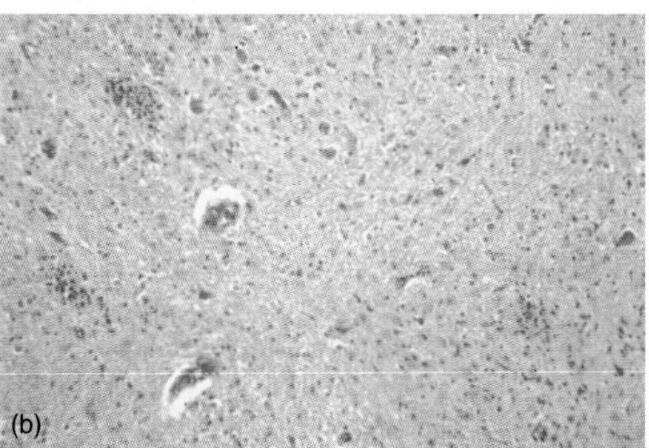

Figure 10.12 Paraneoplastic syndrome: subacute cerebellar atrophy. (a) There is a degree of atrophy with slight exaggeration of the folial pattern. (b) Subacute inflammation with neuronal loss and astrocytosis. (b) H&E.

The myasthenic syndrome of *Eaton–Lambert* is an autoimmune disorder of the neuromuscular junction in which IgG antibodies are raised against the voltage-gated calcium channel. These block the cholinergic synapse resulting in reduced acetylcholine release.

Some patients present with a *myopathy* comprising either proximal limb muscle weakness, inflammatory myopathy (polymyositis/dermatomyositis) or myopathy due to ectopic hormone production of ACTH by a small-cell carcinoma of bronchus. In terminally ill patients cachectic myopathy is also present.

An unusual presentation is that of *opsoclonus–myoclonus* which is best known in association with neuroblastoma in children although it may occur with small cell carcinoma of the bronchus or carcinoma of the breast. As with the other paraneoplastic syndromes, abnormalities may be limited to mild perivascular cuffing of blood vessels and relatively little loss of associated neurons.

CHAPTER 11

PEROXISOMAL AND MITOCHONDRIAL DISORDERS

David I Graham

INTRODUCTION

Peroxisomal and mitochondrial disorders are characterized by an involvement in the β-oxidation of fatty acids and the oxidation of phytanic acid. It has been estimated that these disorders are responsible for approximately a third of human metabolic diseases and that mitochondrial disorders are about twice as common as peroxisomal disorders.

There are similarities between disorders of peroxisomes and mitochondria. For example, in both there is multiple organ involvement, the brunt of the disease in disorders of peroxisomes being borne by the CNS, eyes, skeleton, liver and adrenal glands whereas in mitochondrial disorders, it is the CNS, skeletal muscle, eyes, heart, liver and kidney that are primarily affected. Involvement of the CNS is somewhat similar in both in so far as there is optic atrophy, pigmentary retinopathy and sensory neural deafness, phenotypic heterogeny is common, fatty/organic acids are important in the pathogenesis of both disorders and in some peroxisomal disorders there are also mitochondrial abnormalities, e.g. Zellweger syndrome. Although there are similarities between these disorders there are also differences reflecting involvement of either gray or white matter and changes in the liver, and perhaps the most important difference is that mitochondria possess their own DNA, while peroxisomes do not.

PEROXISOMES AND PEROXISOMAL DISORDERS

Found in all human nucleated cells, peroxisomes are characterized electron microscopically by a granular, electron-dense matrix surrounded by a unit membrane, of variable shape and size ranging from 0.1 to 1 μm and characterized by the presence of catalase within the matrix (Fig. 11.1). In the mature mammalian CNS peroxisomes appear to be largely restricted to oligodendrocytes, while in the developing CNS they are present in neuroblasts, immature neurons and oligodendrocytes. In the human fetus catalase-positive neurons are seen in the basal ganglia, thalamus and cerebellum at 27–28 weeks and in the frontal cortex at 35 weeks of gestation, this reactivity decreasing with increasing post-natal age.

Biochemically, the peroxisome is characterized by a variety of oxidases that generate hydrogen peroxide and is decomposed by catalase (Fig. 11.2). The principal peroxisomal disorders are given in Table 11.1. Group 1 comprises disorders of peroxisome biogenesis and multiple peroxisomal functions, and in group two the peroxisomes are morphologically intact with a single enzymopathy.

With the exception of adrenoleukodystrophy/adrenomyeloneuropathy (ALD/AMN) which is an X-linked disorder, all the peroxisomal disorders are

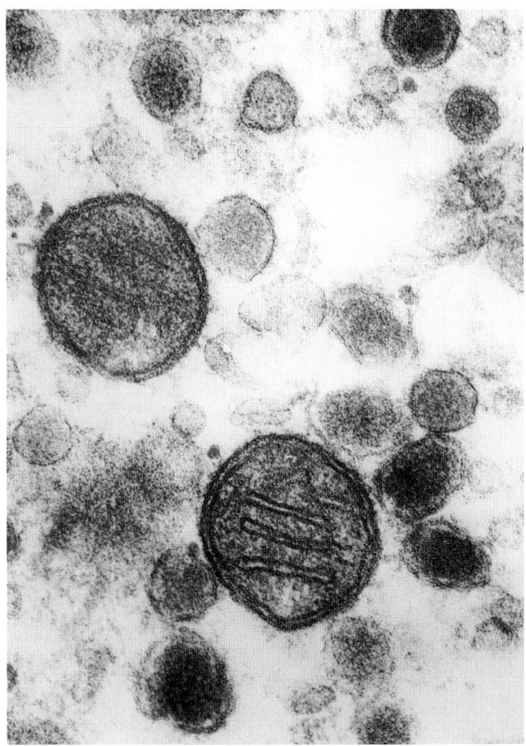

Figure 11.1 Normal CNS peroxisome and mitochondria. The peroxisome has a single limiting membrane that envelopes a homogeneous granular matrix. The mitochrondion is limited by a double membrane the inner of which shows cristae formation in a matrix that has electron-dense granules. Electron microscopy × 60 000.

transmitted by an autosomal recessive pattern of inheritance, neonatal patients presenting with dysmorphic facies, shortening of forelimbs particularly when accompanied by hypotonia, and seizures: later in life there is involvement of central white matter with myelopathy and neuropathy in male children and adults. Plasma very long chain fatty acid (VLCFA) levels, particularly C_{26}, are raised in virtually all peroxisomal disorders. While characteristic, other fatty acids may need to be measured and in typical cases it may be necessary to undertake liver biopsy to demonstrate portal fibrosis or even micronodular cirrhosis and steatosis, PAS-positive macrophages within angulate lysosomes containing trilaminar spicules, and striated adrenocortical cells containing lamellae and lamellar-lipid profiles by electron microscopy. The membrane-bound angulate lysosomes contained in rigid-appearing trilaminar spicules consists of two electron-dense leaflets of 3–5 nm separated by an irregular electron-lucent space of 6–12 nm and is characteristic of such structures occurring in brain, adrenal and retina although it is now apparent that they are not specific having been reported in a number of other degenerative metabolic diseases. They contrast morphologically with the most characteristic inclusions of ALD–AMN which are linear to gently curved lamellar lipid profiles lying free in the cytoplasm of adrenocortical, Leydig and Schwann cells and brain macrophages: the lamellae are not membrane-bound and fundamentally consist of two 2.5-nm electron-dense leaflets separated by a variable electron-lucent space of 1–7 nm. These structures are birefringent and are thought to consist of the accumulation of saturated VLCFA.

Neuropathologically, peroxisomal disorders consist of three major types. First, abnormalities in neuronal migration, a feature that is particularly common in Zellweger syndrome; secondly, defects in the formation or maintenance of central white matter, the latter being a particular feature of ALD–AMN and neonatal adrenoleukodystrophy (NALD); and thirdly, post-developmental neuronal degeneration which is most frequent in AMN and Refsum's disease. The main features of the principal disorders are given in Table 11.2.

Group 1: Disorders of peroxisome biogenesis and multiple peroxisomal functions

'Classical Zellweger syndrome'

The clinical features of dysmorphic facies, seizures, severe hypotonia and profound psychomotor retardation usually allow a diagnosis in the neonatal period. Additional features include cataract, pigmentary retinopathy, optic atrophy, sensorineural hearing deficits and various gray matter abnormalities, and a life expectancy of about 6 months. Abnormalities are also present in many other organs including the liver, heart and kidneys: within the cortex of the adrenal glands there are scattered and infrequent cortical striated cells with lamellar-lipid profiles, and PAS-positive macrophages. Malformed

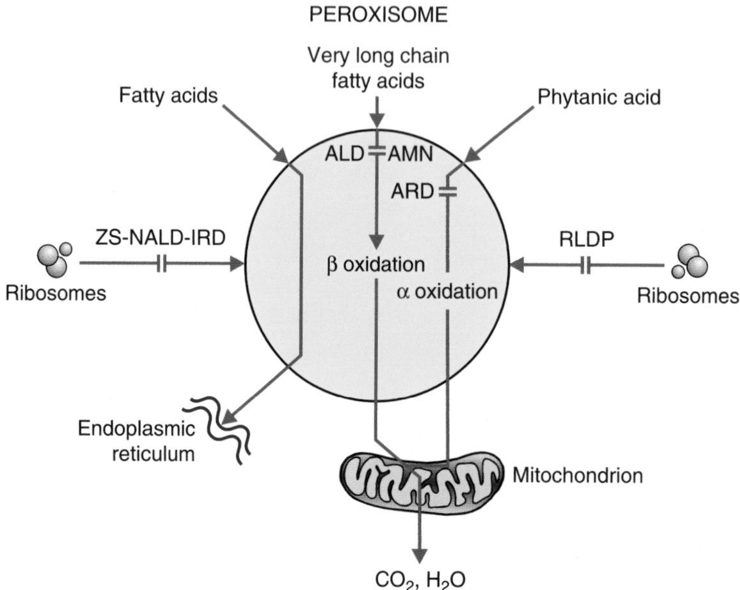

Figure 11.2 Metabolic pathways of peroxisomes and mitochondria in a greatly abbreviated form. The figure shows the anatomical and biochemical relationships between peroxisomes, mitochondria, ribosomes and endoplasmic reticulum with regard to the α and β oxidation of very long-chain fatty acids (VLCFAs), phytanic acid and fatty acids. Absence or malfunction of key enzymes in the metabolic pathways are causally related to adrenoleukodystrophy and adrenomyeloneuropathy (ALD/AMN), adult Refsum's disease (ARD), rhizomelic chondrodysplasia punctata (RCDP), and cerebrohepatorenal (Zellweger) syndrome (ZS) – neonatal adrenoleukodystrophy (NALD) – infantile Refsum's or phytanic acid storage disease (IRD).

Table 11.1 Classification of the principal peroxisomal disorders

Group 1
- Cerebrohepatorenal (Zellweger) syndrome (ZS)
- Neonatal adrenoleukodystrophy (NALD)
- Infantile Refsum's disease (IRD)

Group 2
- Pseudo-peroxisome biogenesis
- Adrenoleukodystrophy and adrenomyeloneuropathy (ALD/AMN)
- Miscellaneous including glutaric aciduria and hyperoxaluria

peroxizomes in the liver cause multiple biochemical defects with elevations in VLCFA.

As a consequence of abnormal neuronal migration there is a unique combination of centrosylvian or parasylvian pachygyria and polymicrogyria (Fig. 11.3a and b). These features differ from those of classical four-layered polymicrogyria or lissencephaly–pachygyria in that all neuronal classes seem to be affected with those destined for the outer layers tending to be the most impeded. Dysplasias may be present in the cerebellum and the hindbrain. In addition, there may be abnormalities in CNS white matter but not of the classical inflammatory type seen in ALD. The changes are thought to be dysmyelinative with hypomyelination so little sudanophilic lipid is present in macrophages, and there is an associated astrocytosis.

Neonatal adrenoleukodystrophy

Clinically, these infants resemble Zellweger syndrome but usually survive until the age of 36 months, although survival into adolescence has been recorded. It is an autosomal recessive trait in which hepatic abnormalities are common, the peroxisomes being reported as either missing, decreased in size or enlarged. There are multiple biochemical abnormalities in all peroxisomal functions and there is atrophy of the adrenal cortex

Table 11.2 Main features of peroxisomal disorders

Disorder	Age of onset	Inheritance pattern	Clinical features	Other organ involvement	Storage product	Biochemical defect	Molecular defect
Group 1							
Zellweger syndrome	Neonatal	Autosomal recessive	Hypotonia Psychomotor retardation; dysmorphic facies; seizures	Liver Heart Kidney Adrenal	Phytanic acids; very long chain fatty acids (VLCFAs)	Multiple	*PEX 1* import
Neonatal adrenoleukodystrophy	Neonatal	Autosomal recessive	Hypotonia; failure to thrive	Liver, adrenal PNS	Not known	Multiple	*PEX 1* import
Infantile Refsum's disease	Neonatal	Not known	Mental retardation; dysmorphic facies; retinitis pigmentosa; deafness; failure to thrive	Liver, adrenal	Phytanic acid	Multiple	Not known
Group 2							
Adrenoleukodystrophy	Juvenile	X-linked	Change in behavior; loss of vision; gait disorder; Addison's disease	Adrenal, gonad	VLCFA	Acyl-CoA synthetase	Xq28
Adrenomyeloneuropathy	Adult	Not known	Spastic paraparesis	None	VLCFA	Not known	Not known
Refsum's disease	Adult	Not known	Pigmentary retinopathy; ataxia; PNS	Heart ichthyosis	Phytanic acid	Phytanic acid α-hydroxylase	Not known

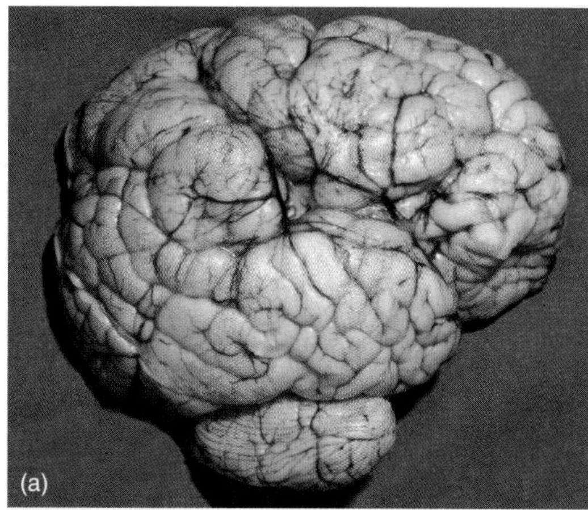

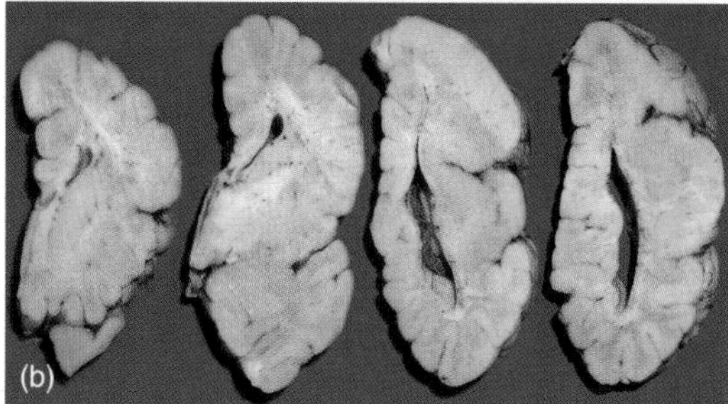

Figure 11.3 Zellweger syndrome. (a) Lateral view of cerebral hemisphere. Note abnormality in region of the Sylvian fissure. (b) Same case as (a) the coronal slices providing more detail of the structural abnormality.

with striated adrenocortical cells that mimic the adrenal lesion of ALD. Also, there are widely distributed PAS-positive macrophages with angulate lysosomes containing spicules throughout many organs and somewhat similar changes have been seen also in the peripheral nervous system. Compared with Zellweger syndrome, the CNS in NALD is more widely affected with abnormalities in neuronal migration. In association with the white matter change in the cerebral and cerebellar hemispheres there is often a prominent perivascular inflammatory reaction, a feature in common with ALD.

Infantile Refsum's disease

These patients manifest mental retardation, dysmorphic facies of a minor degree, retinitis pigmentosa, sensorineural hearing deficits, failure to thrive and hypocholesterolemia: biochemical peroxisomal parameters are abnormal, the peroxisomes being either deficient or greatly reduced in number. Patients present usually in the neonatal period and may survive to be teenagers. PAS-positive macrophages containing angulate lysosomes are a prominent feature in the liver, and in the CNS there are descriptions of hypoplasia, heterotopia and reduced numbers of myelinated axons.

Group 2: Intact peroxisomes with single enzymopathy

Adrenoleukodystrophy (ALD) and adrenomyeloneuropathy (AMN)

ALD is an X-linked juvenile disorder and AMN is its adult variant. There are a number of additional subtypes and genotype–phenotype correlations are poor, the same genetic defect apparently being associated with juvenile ALD, AMN and other variants. This heterogeny probably reflects the influence of a modifying gene and/or environmental factors that account for the phenotypic variation. Further it is unclear how the genetic defect is related to the major biochemical abnormality identified in ALD, i.e. decreased activity of VLCFA acyl-CoA synthetase with resultant elevation of VLCFAs.

The *ALD* gene is localized to the Xq28 region and a large number of mutations have been identified, a particular mutational hot spot being known to be present on exon 5. The X-linked juvenile form usually presents between 6 and 9 years of age, with changes in behavior, hearing, sight and gait disorders of addisonian features. Due to the progressive nature of the disease, death usually occurs within 3 years, longitudinal neuroimaging studies showing the progression of the lesion from the parieto-occipital to the frontal lobes. The adrenal cortex and testes are the only two non-neural organs that show changes. In the former the cells of the fasciculate–reticularis become ballooned and striate due to accumulation of lamellae, lamella–lipid profiles and fine lipid clefts: atrophy ensues in the absence of any significant inflammatory cell response. Similar qualitative changes are seen in the adrenocortex of AMN. The testes in AMN and adult cerebral ALD show the same abnormalities in the Leydig cells as those described in childhood ALD, comprising degenerative changes and loss of the seminiferous tubules and various forms of maturation arrest of spermatocytes.

The principal neuropathological feature of ALD is loss of myelin seen most prominently in the parieto-occipital region which over time extends anteriorly with a leading edge that blends imperceptibly into normal white matter (Fig. 11.4a). There is relative sparing of the arcuate U-fibers with some involvement but to a lesser extent of the white matter of the cerebellum and brainstem: the spinal cord is spared except for descending fiber tract degeneration. Gray matter, in general, is intact and in the most severe cases there is cavitation and calcification. Histologically, there is marked loss of myelinated axons and oligodendrocytes. At the advancing edges of the myelin loss there is intense perivascular inflammation particularly by lymphocytes, macrophages and associated astrocytosis (Fig. 11.4b). The macrophages have either granular or vacuolated cytoplasm that is sudanophilic and PAS positive or have striated cytoplasm due to the presence of clear clefts. The inflammation shows a mixed cell population that is usually T-cell dominant. Plasma cells are much less frequent.

Microscopy shows degeneration of the long spinal tracts with which there are also foci of perivascular lymphocytes and striated macrophages.

The histopathological changes have been interpreted as perhaps indicting a two-stage process: first, biochemical defect in the myelin membrane leads to its breakdown, and second an inflammatory immune response directed towards the CNS exposed during this demyelination. The role of various cytokines including tumor necrosis factor-alpha (TNF-α) and interleukin-1 (IL-1) is unclear although TNF-α may initiate a secondary phase of inflammatory demyelination in which macrophages and T lymphocytes are the main effector cells. The extent and intensity of CNS white matter pathology in ALD do not correlate with clinical or pathological involvement of the adrenal cortex, this lack of correlation perhaps suggesting that testosterone may trigger the onset of AMN or the AMN/ALD transition.

Patients with AMN usually present in the third or fourth decade with a slowly progressive onset of severe spastic paraparesis. There is loss of both ascending and descending fibers in the spinal cord, a pattern that is consistent with a distal axonopathy, being particularly marked in the lumbar corticospinal and the cervical gracile and dorsal spinocerebellar tracts; there is a degree of astrocytosis and inflammation is minimal or absent and perivascular accumulation of striated and granular PAS-positive macrophages.

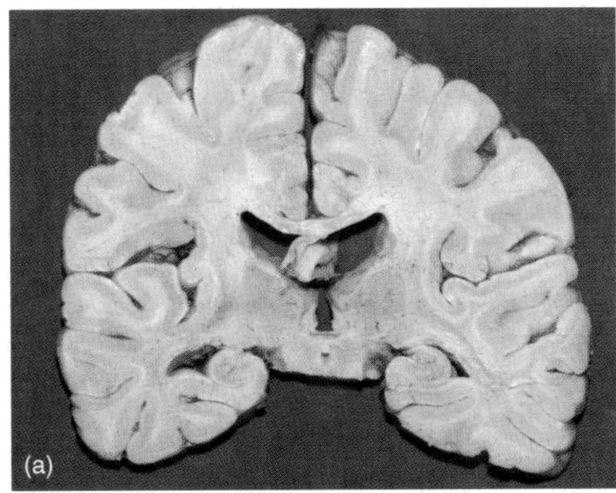

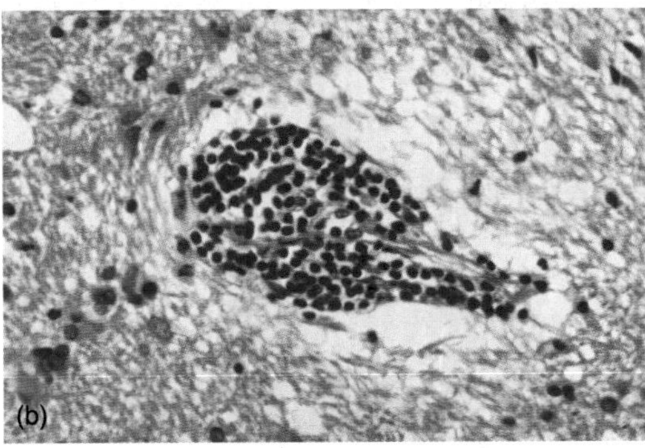

Figure 11.4 Adrenoleukodystrophy. (a) There is some loss of myelin in the parietal lobes and the posterior limbs of the internal capsule. (b) Subacute perivascular inflammation and early loss of myelin. (b) H&E.

Refsum's disease

Typically, patients with classical or adult Refsum's disease present before the age of 20 years with decreased visual acuity due to pigmentary retinopathy and on examination have the additional features of peripheral neuropathy, cerebellar ataxia, sensoryneural hearing deficits, cardiac problems and ichthyosis.

The biochemical defect is the absence of phytanic acid, a hydroxylase, the effects of which can be partially nullified by dietary restriction of phytanic acid. Neuropathological studies have shown onion bulb formation and within Schwann cells osmiophilic granular, granulomembranous and crystaloid bodies. Various system degenerations with loss of myelin have been described in the brainstem and cerebellum, a pattern of involvement in adult Refsum's disease that resembles that seen in AMN and MERRF (see below) in which there is considerable white matter involvement in the PNS but sparse or absent in the CNS.

Pathogenesis of peroxisomal disorders

At present VLCFAs are believed to play a central role in the pathogenesis of ALD/AMN in so much as they are thought to increase the viscosity of various membranes including myelin, this in turn leading to instability and dysmyelination in neuronal and axonal membranes that may result in atrophy and axonal loss affecting migration of radial glia and growth cones. A similar mechanism has been proposed for phytanic acid in the PNS myelin of adult Refsum's disease.

MITOCHONDRIAL DISORDERS

The majority of mitochondria are larger than peroxisomes, the round form in man usually varying between 0.5 and 1 μm in diameter. They have a characteristic ultrastructural morphology comprising a double-unit membrane separated by the intermembranous space and the inner-most matrix, the latter being subdivided by the infoldings of the inner mitochondrial membrane, the cristae. The principal functions of mitochondria are the oxidation of pyruvate, ketone bodies, fatty acids and amino acids, and the synthesis of adenosine triphosphate. Additional functions include the sequestration of calcium and the detoxification of ammonia in the urea cycle. Acetyl-CoA is central to the domains of intermediary metabolism and a particular feature of mitochondria is the need to translocate metabolites and proteins from the intermembranous space into the matrix, a process that is energy dependant and requires the help of chaperone proteins such as 'heat shock proteins and 'stress proteins'.

Mitochondria contain their own DNA all of which is derived from the fertilized ovum (mtDNA). Therefore, mtDNA characteristics are an inheritance exclusively from the mother and it has been estimated that more than 10 000 copies of mtDNA may exist in each cell. The mitochondrial genome requires its own transcription and translation factors for synthesis of mitochondrial proteins and contains 37 genes of which 13 code for structural proteins in the respiratory chain. The mitochondrial genome also contains 24 genes for protein synthesis including two ribosomal RNAs and 22 transfer RNAs. Directly or indirectly, mitochondrial function is effected to a much greater extent by nuclear-encoded genes. It has been suggested that the proximity of mtDNA in the matrix to the respiratory chain embedded in the inner mitochondrial membrane, which is the major source of free radicals in a cell, is one factor that predisposes mtDNA to spontaneous mutation. A further suggestion is the limited ability of mitochondria to repair mtDNA mutations.

Mitochondrial genotype may be either homoplasmic in which case the thousands of mtDNA genomes per cell are identical, or heteroplasmic in which case the genome is made up of a mixture of wild-type (normal) and mutated (abnormal) types. The cellular phenotype is determined by the proportion of wild-type and mutated genomes so that the severity of any given mitochondrial disease is often directly proportional to the percentage of mutant mtDNA genome. It is believed that once the proportion of wild-type mutated genome exceeds a 'threshold' then abnormalities become apparent. It has been estimated that the threshold in MELAS (see below) and MERRF (see below) may be as high as between 90 and 95% compared with other mitochondrial disorders in which the threshold may vary from 60 to 70%. This threshold is influenced by a number of factors that include the age of the patient, and the energy demands of the tissue or organ, brain and muscle cells having a high energy demand as do the tissues of a developing child.

The principal features of the mitochondrial disorders are given in Table 11.3 and the biomolecular

Table 11.3 Main features of mitochondrial disorders

Disease	Age of onset	Inheritance pattern	Clinical features	Other organs involved	Storage product	Biochemical defect	Molecular defect
Leigh syndrome (LS)	Infantile	Sporadic X-linked; autosomal recessive	Psychomotor retardation; seizures; ataxia; loss of vision	Liver Heart	None	Pyruvate dehydrogenase; complex I and IV	Multiple nDNA; also mtDNA
Kearn–Sayre syndrome (KSS)	Juvenile	Not known	Retinitis pigmentosa; ophthalmoplegia; heart block; cerebellar syndrome	Heart	None	Respiratory chain	4977bp deletion mtDNA
Mitochondrial, encephalomyopathy, lactic acidosis, and stroke-like episodes (MELAS)	Young adults	Autosomal dominant or recessive	Exercise intolerance; stroke-like episodes; seizures; dementia	Heart	None	Respiratory chain	Point mutation tRNAleu mtDNA
Myoclonus epilepsy with ragged red fibers (MERRF)	Juvenile adult	Autosomal dominant or recessive	Myoclonus; ataxia; deafness; visual loss; dementia	Heart Liver	None	Respiratory chain	A8344G tRNA mtDNA

classification of mitochondrial disorders is given in Table 11.4. Clinically, there are three main categories of patients, the symptoms and signs of which are due to defects of fatty acid oxidation, pyruvate metabolism, and the respiratory chain. Patients with defects of fatty acid oxidation typically experience metabolic decompensation during fasting, these patients' presenting with cardiac and skeletal muscle symptoms. The brain is only secondarily affected by hypoketotic hypoglycemia or brain swelling. This category includes defects of carnitine, defects of the inner mitochondrial membrane system including very long-chain acyl-CoA and long-chain 3-hydroxy acyl-CoA dehydrogenase deficiencies, and defects in the mitochondrial matrix or β-oxidation system. Their clinical picture is often indistinguishable from Reye syndrome and elevated serum free fatty acids, hypoketonemia, primary or secondary carnitine deficiency, hypoglycemia and dicarboxylic aciduria occur in association with defects of fatty acid oxidation.

Lacticacidosis is the laboratory hallmark of defects involving pyruvate metabolism and of the respiratory chain. The clinical spectrum ranges from life-threatening congenital lactacidosis to a benign clinical syndrome with intermittent weakness or ataxia. Such defects are associated with elevated serum and tissue concentrations of pyruvate, lactate and alanine. Defects of the respiratory chain show wide-ranging phenotypes which include the well-characterized neuropathological entities of Leigh syndrome (LS), MELAS, MERRF and Leber's hereditary optic neuropathy.

Leigh syndrome may be the result of nuclear DNA abnormalities involved in substrate utilization of the respiratory chain, or may result from mtDNA abnormalities such as point mutations.

The unique interplay of nuclear and mtDNA genomes on the respiratory chain results in numerous patterns of inheritance, although classical Mendelian inheritance patterns exist in most mitochondrial diseases. However, there is often maternal intervention because mitochondria were from the cytoplasm of the ovum. Expression is determined by replicative segregation and by the threshold effect, and diagnosis is therefore based initially on the clinical presentation which is usually based on the organ(s) which shows the greatest amount of dysfunction, which in turn depends upon oxidative metabolism. Imaging is of great value in recognizing the various disorders.

The demonstration of ragged red fibers in fresh frozen sections of skeletal muscle using the Gomori one-step trichrome stain is characteristic, but increasingly immunohistochemistry directed against mtDNA or nuclear DNA encoded proteins has been introduced. Abnormal mitochondria can also be studied by the polymerase chain reaction and cultured skin fibroblasts or lymphocytes can be analyzed biochemically for the activities of respiratory chain enzymes.

The major organ systems involved in mitochondrial disorders are the CNS, eyes, skeletal muscle, heart, liver and kidneys. The PNS can also be affected. Systemic involvement includes the presence of ragged red fibers in skeletal muscle, lipid accumulation in skeletal muscle, hypertrophic cardiomyopathy, hepatic steatosis and portal fibrosis. Mitochondria show abnormal variations in size and shape and often contain intramitochondrial protein paracrystalline inclusions (Fig. 11.5).

Mitochondrial disorders can affect both neurons and oligodendrocytes and hence both gray and white matter are typically involved in most mitochondrial encephalomyopathies. Characteristically, there is white matter involvement which varies from rarefaction and spongy change through neuronal loss and astrocytosis to areas of ischemia-like necrosis. White matter involvement usually varies from myelin pallor through a spongiform myelinopathy due to the accumulation of intramyelin edema, to cystic necrosis. In general there are three main patterns: first, widespread damage to brain tissue resulting in microencephaly and ventriculomegaly; this is usually associated with congenital lacticacidosis, urea cycle defects and some diseases of fatty acid oxidation. The localization maybe principally that of poliodystrophy or polio-encephalopathy (white matter), or a leukoencephalopathy (white matter) or combined gray and white matter lesions. The second pattern is limited to gray matter and is best typified by LS in which there is symmetrical subcortical damage particularly affecting the brainstem, cerebellar roof nuclei, basal ganglia and thalamus, and histologically there is rarefaction of the neuropil, neuronal

Table 11.4 Biomolecular classification of the principal mitochondrial disorders

Inherited disorders

Nuclear DNA defects

- Pyruvate dehydrogenase or carboxylase deficiency (Leigh syndrome)
- Respiratory chain (Leigh syndrome)

Mitochondrial DNA defects

- Sporadic large-scale rearrangement (e.g. KSS)
- Point mutation affecting structural genes (e.g. Leber's hereditary optic neuropathy)
- Point mutations affecting structural genes (e.g. MELAS, MERRF, Leigh syndrome)

Acquired conditions

- Infection (Reye syndrome)
- Toxic (e.g. MPTP)
- Drugs (e.g. zidovudine)
- Aging (e.g. hypoxia-induced oxidative stress)

loss with a corresponding decrease of myelin, reactive astrocytosis and proliferation or swelling of small blood vessels. In some disorders, particularly in MELAS, multifocal ischemic-like necrosis develops, whereas in MERRF a more selective neuronal loss and tract degeneration predominate. The third pattern is one of a spongy myelinopathy (leukoencephalopathy), a feature most commonly seen in Kearns–Sayre syndrome (KSS).

Inherited conditions associated with nuclear DNA defects

Increasing knowledge of these disorders has allowed their characterization into defects of substrate transport, defects of substrate utilization, defects of the Kreb's cycle, defects of oxidative phosphorylation, defects of the respiratory chain (oxidative phosphorylation), defects of protein importation, and defects of intergenomic signaling. The number of cases reported within each category ranges from a few to several hundred with considerable heterogeny. As a result it is not always clear which of the neuropathological findings represent the primary disease process and which are the secondary complications of hypoxia and ischemia.

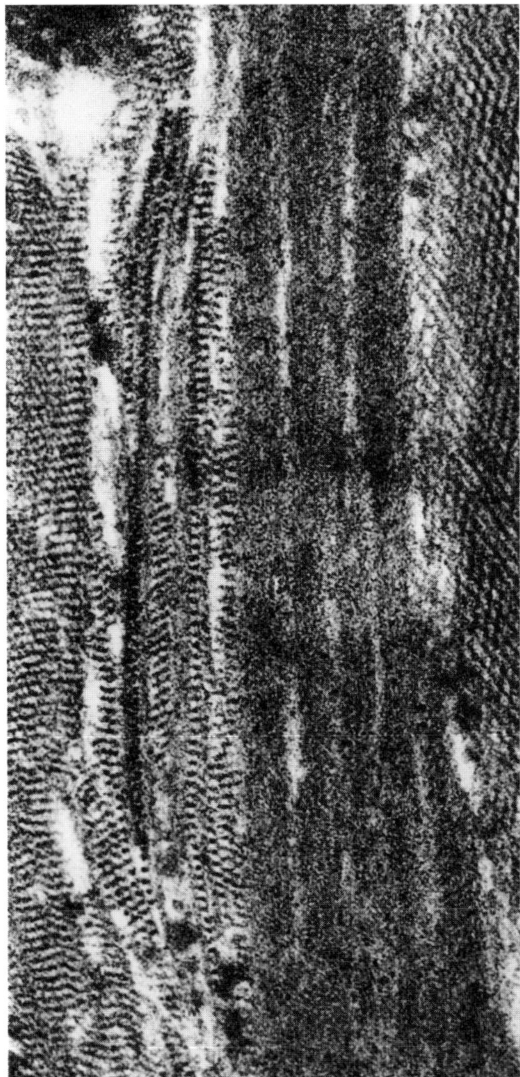

Figure 11.5 Mitochondrial disorder. Paracrystalline inclusion. Electron microscopy ×200 000.

Leigh syndrome

Leigh syndrome (subacute necrotizing encephalopathy) is seen most often in males and has an autosomal recessive pattern of transmission in some 50% of cases, although sporadic linked, and maternal modes of transmission also occur. Recent molecular genetic studies have confirmed the heterogeny of the disease, defects occurring in linked pyruvate dehydrogenase complex deficiency, defects in nuclear genes of complexes I and IV and abnormalities of

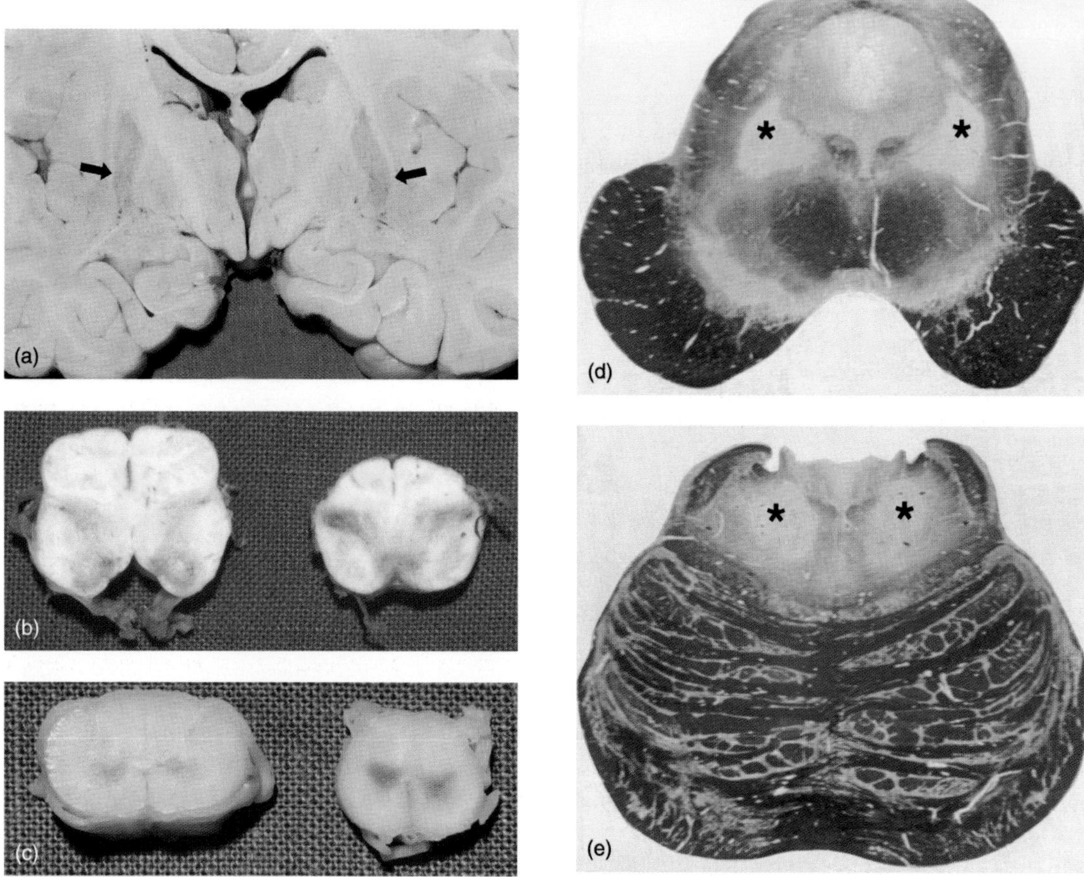

Figure 11.6 Leigh syndrome. (a) There is symmetrical necrosis of each putamen (arrows). (b) Similar symmetrical changes are seen in the medulla of the brainstem. (c) Again note the symmetrical involvement of the spinal cord. (d) The symmetry of the lesions is especially well seen in the periaqueductal gray matter and each substantia nigra (asterisks). (e) As in (d) there is symmetry of lesions in the tegmentum of the pons (asterisks). (d) and (e) celloidin: Heidenhain's for myelin.

mtDNA genes coding for ATPase 6. Hepatic lesions and hypertrophic cardiomyopathy are seen in some cases. Although some of the patients have features reminiscent of KSS, in the great majority abnormalities are restricted to the CNS and include the presence of abnormal mitochondria.

Within the CNS, Leigh syndrome is characterized by symmetrical spongy necrotizing lesions which affect both gray and white matter predominantly near midline structures such as the basal ganglia, thalami, substantia nigra, subthalamic nuclei, tegmentum of the midbrain, the inferior olives of the medulla, and the posterior columns of the spinal cord (Fig. 11.6a–e). There is relative sparing of neurons, endothelial hyperplasia and an astrocytosis, the appearance closely resembling Wernicke's encephalopathy. Eventually cystic cavitation occurs.

Inherited conditions associated with mtDNA defects

Principal among these are sporadic large-scale rearrangements and deletions such as found in the Kearns–Sayre syndrome (KSS), transmitted large-scale rearrangements, point mutations affecting structural genes such as Leber's heredity optic neuropathy, and point mutations affecting genes of the type found in MELAS, and MERRF.

Kearns–Sayre syndrome

Defined as progressive external opthalmoplegia and pigmentary retinopathy with an onset before the age of 20 years, this triad of CNS symptomatology must be accompanied by either cardiac conduction block, a cerebellar syndrome or a CSF protein greater than 100 mg/dL. Overlap occurs with other clinically distinct syndromes such as MELAS.

The principal neuropathological findings are varying degrees of spongy change, neuronal loss, infarct-like necrosis, mineralization, astrocytosis and tract degeneration. The spongy vacuolation and leuko-encephalopathy may be restricted to the brainstem but generally it is more widespread, the appearances ranging from mild pallor with spongy change to coarse vacuolation. Axons and oligodendrocytes are relatively well preserved. Gray matter is also relatively normal although neuronal loss has been reported in both the cerebellum and in the brainstem. In contrast to KSS vascular changes are common, but in both mineralization of the subcortical gray matter including the basal ganglia and thalami, are common. Leber's hereditary optic neuropathy typically presents with an acute to subacute painless bilateral blurring or clouding of vision with central scotoma in young adults or unilateral blindness followed by visual loss in the other eye within weeks or months. An early onset at 5 years of age is also seen. Patients with the most common mutation, *G11778A*, usually have uncomplicated optic atrophy, but a typical presentation also occurs in some patients: features of Leigh syndrome and MELAS may also be present.

MELAS (mitochondrial encephalopathy, lacticacidosis and stroke-like episodes)

This is relatively common with most patients becoming symptomatic before the age of 40 years with the onset of exercise intolerance, 'stroke-like' episodes, seizures and dementia often in the first decade of life. Neuroimaging reveals mineralization in the basal ganglia. In about 80% of patients there is a heteroplasmic point mutation in the small tRNA leucine gene. Overlap with LS, KSS and MERRF occurs and at autopsy findings may include hypertrophic cardiomyopathy, hepatic steatosis, and a generalized mitochondrial microangiopathy.

The neuropathological hallmarks are multi-focal symmetrical infarct-like lesions of the cortex and in the subcortical white matter (especially of the posterior halves of the cerebral hemispheres) but without preferential involvement of arterial territories or boundary zones. In the acute to subacute stage microscopy shows 'pink' neurons, astrocytosis and swelling that affects gray or white matter or both. In most cases, the crest of gyri are preferentially involved although increased vascularity is a frequent finding in the deep cortex. The blood vessels are patent. Ultrastructure has shown abnormalities in the size and shape of mitochondria within the endothelium of the choroid plexus and small blood vessels that have been hypothesized to be responsible for the infarct-like lesions of MELAS. However, other data suggests that microvascular changes are the consequence of, rather than the cause of, brain necrosis. In cases with chronic lesions there is loss of tissue, atrophy, cyst formation and an associated astrocytosis. Mineralization in the basal ganglia is common but subcortical gray matter rarely contains infarcts. Changes in the optic nerves are mild and within the spinal cord there may be neuronal loss and long-tract changes together with mild spongy myelinopathy in the lateral and posterior columns.

MERRF (myoclonus epilepsy with ragged red fibers)

Less common than MELAS, this maternally inherited condition presents with cerebellar ataxia, generalized seizures, myoclonus, dementia, hearing loss, impaired deep sensation, optic atrophy, short stature and lipomas. The age of onset usually varies from childhood to the fifth decade. It has been associated with point mutations in the tRNA lysine gene and there is a degree of overlap with LS. General autopsy findings include muscular wasting (Chapter 18), hepatic steatosis, myocardial fibrosis and abnormal mitochondria in cardiac myocytes.

The principal finding is that of a neuronal system degeneration particularly involving the dentatorubral fibers which may be seen at the time of brain cutting by brown discoloration of the dentate nuclei when neuronal loss is usually severe. There are marked changes in the inferior medullary olives and in the spinal cord the gracile, cuneate and Clarke's nuclei show a reduction in neurons. Abnormalities in the cortices of the cerebral and the cerebellar hemispheres are mild. Findings to date include abnormally large mitochondria with vesicular cristae and mitochondria with equivocable paracrystalline inclusions in the cerebellar cortex and dentate nucleus.

Acquired conditions

These include Reye syndrome (page 210), MPTP toxicity (page 338), zidovudine toxicity, aging and oxidative stress (see Table 11.4).

CHAPTER 12

LYSOSOMAL DISEASES AND THE LEUKODYSTROPHIES

David I Graham

INTRODUCTION

Many of these disorders are due to deficiencies of a particular *lysosomal enzyme*, which plays an essential role in the degradation of various normal metabolites or the breakdown products of cells. As a result, the undegraded material accumulates in, and causes enlargement of, the lysosomes of certain cells. The distribution of structural abnormalities depends on the particular enzyme deficiency, some of the disorders affecting the CNS, others the peripheral nervous system or muscle, and others both the nervous system and visceral organs such as liver, spleen and lymph nodes. Affected cells become enlarged and have a ballooned appearance (Fig. 12.1), hence the previous term of *neuronal storage disorders*. Stored material can be detected histochemically: frozen sections are essential because lipids dissolve in alcohol and mucopolysaccharides in water. Stains required include oil red O and Sudan black B for lipids; Luxol fast blue, which is traditionally regarded as a stain for complex lipids; PAS with and without diastase for glycogen and other carbohydrate-containing constituents; toluidine blue, or acidified cresyl violet for metachromatic leukodystrophy; and toluidine blue for mucopolysaccharides. A range of histochemical techniques, both non-specific and highly specific, is now available for the identification of the stored material. It is often necessary, however, to correlate the histochemical findings with the clinical and morphological features so as to identify a clinicopathological pattern of a particular disease. In many instances, the precise diagnosis can be made on a block of unfixed tissue frozen for biochemical analysis, including thin-layer and gas–liquid chromatography and enzyme assays. Electron microscopy is also essential since this will demonstrate grossly enlarged lysosomes containing non-metabolizable residue. At one stage it was considered that the distinctive ultrastructural features of some disorders were such that morphology could be used to

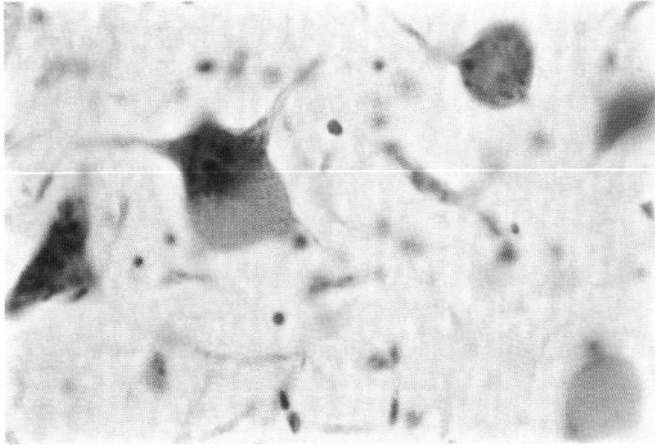

Figure 12.1 Mucopolysaccharidosis. The neurons are greatly distended by stored material. PAS.

diagnose a specific disorder: this is now known not to be so.

It is generally agreed that there are racial differences in the incidence of certain forms of mental retardation and, in particular, Tay–Sachs and Niemann–Pick disease and the adult form of Gaucher's disease which are more common in Jews than in non-Jews. Although reservations have been expressed about the validity of this in view of the genetic heterogeneity of Jews and the probability that the incidence of these disorders has been underestimated in non-Jews, there is now considerable evidence that these disorders are more common among patients with Ashkenazi Jewish ancestry. For example, as determined by enzyme assay, the carrier rate of Tay–Sachs' disease is about 1 in 30 in Ashkenazi Jews, compared with a frequency of about 1 in 300 in other races.

The metabolic disease leads first to dysfunction and then the defective cells ultimately die, resulting in atrophy of the brain, and gliosis in gray and white matter. On the other hand, there may be megalencephaly as in the early stages of Tay–Sachs' disease. In Tay–Sachs' and Niemann–Pick disease the immediate post-natal development is often normal, but in the first 12 months the infant fails to thrive, and there is retardation or progressive deterioration of mental and motor functions, spastic or flaccid paralysis, epilepsy and ultimately coma and death. Affected children often develop a cherry-red spot in the retina because the photoreceptors (cone cells) of the macula die, leaving a defect in the retina through which the choroid is visible. Many of the diseases can be diagnosed by assay of lysosomal enzymes in blood, urine, leukocytes, amniotic fluid and cultured skin fibroblasts. Histological examination of bone marrow, liver, rectum, muscle, peripheral nerve or brain may be required, however, to establish the diagnosis. Antenatal diagnosis may be achieved on a sample of chorionic villi from fibroblasts cultured from amniotic fluid. At autopsy in addition to the retention of frozen samples from the affected organs there should also be comprehensive examination of fetal and placental tissue for confirmation and diagnosis after termination of pregnancy.

There is an appreciation that enzymes are not usually specific for a single substance, and so the lysosomal theory of storage disorders has been modified, in that defective enzyme activity may result from a variety of causes, each having its own individual genetic control.

Principal pathological features

The CNS may appear normal to the naked eye; it may be enlarged or as in many disorders may be atrophic. Macroscopically, whereas gray matter may appear relatively normal, there are usually gross abnormalities of white matter due to either widespread or a more localized loss of myelin, though invariably there is preferential sparing of the arcuate or perivascular fibers. The principal histopathological features are two-fold: namely, the accumulation of abnormal products in the nervous system and other cells, and the vacuolation of white matter with loss of myelin.

The great majority are inherited as autosomal recessive diseases, although in a few there is X-linked recessive inheritance. Therefore, genetic counselling should be made available to families in which these diagnoses are made.

Diagnosis

It will be apparent from the foregoing that in many of these disorders it is now possible to achieve an accurate diagnosis by identifying the enzyme deficiency and the accumulating product. While gene therapy may offer hope for those diagnosed the multi-disciplinary team approach allows consideration of antenatal diagnosis of at-risk fetuses and the management of patients whose presentation ranges from the classic in childhood to the atypical in later life.

LYSOSOMAL DISORDERS

Principal amongst these are the CNS lipidoses, neuronal ceroid lipofuscinoses, the mucopolysaccharidoses, mucolipidoses, glycogen storage disorders, and a miscellaneous group that include I-cell disease, and Wolman's disease (Table 12.1).

Table 12.1 Sphingomyelinosis and disorders of glycosamioglycan metabolism

Disorder	Enzyme defect	Substances stored	Staining methods and other tests
Sphingolipidoses			
GM1-gangliosidosis (two types)	β-galactosidase	GM1-ganglioside, oligosaccharides, ceramide tetrahexoside	PAS, β-galactosidase, TLC, EM LFB
GM2-gangliosidosis (several types including Tay–Sachs' and Sandhoff)	Hexosaminidases	GM2-ganglioside, ceramide trihexoside	PAS, LFB, TLC, EM
Cerebrosidosis (Gaucher's disease (3 types))	β-glucocerebrosidase	Glucocerebroside	PAS, TLC, EM
Sphingomyelinosis (Neimann–Pick) groups 1 and 2	Sphingomyelinase (in group 1 only)	Sphingomyelin, cholesterol	PAS, Sudan black B, acid hematein, TLC, EM
Farber's disease	Ceramidase	Ceramide	PAS, Sudan, EM
Fabry's disease	α-galactosidase A	Trihexosyl ceramide, glycolipids	PAS; Sudan, EM
Batten's disease (neuronal ceroidlipofuscinosis)	Not known	Lipofuscin-like substances	PAS, Sudan black B, autofluorescence, EM
Mucopolysaccharidoses			
Hurler (MPS I-IH)	α-L-iduronidase	Acid mucopolysaccharides	Toluidine blue, PAS, LFB, Sudan black B, EM
Hunter (MPS II)	Sulfoiduronate, sulfatase	Heparan sulfate, chondroitin sulfate, keratan sulfate and several gangliosides	
Sanflippo (MPS III) (4 types)	Various		
Morquio (MPS IV) (2 types)	Various		

PAS = Periodic acid–Schiff; LFB = Luxol fast blue; EM = electron microscopy; TLC = thin-layer chromatography.
(Reproduced in modified form with permission of the author and publisher from Lake BD, Metabolic disorders of the central and peripheral nervous system. In: *Histochemistry in pathology*. Filipe MI, Lake BD (Eds). Edinburgh: Churchill Livingstone, 1983: 53–69.)

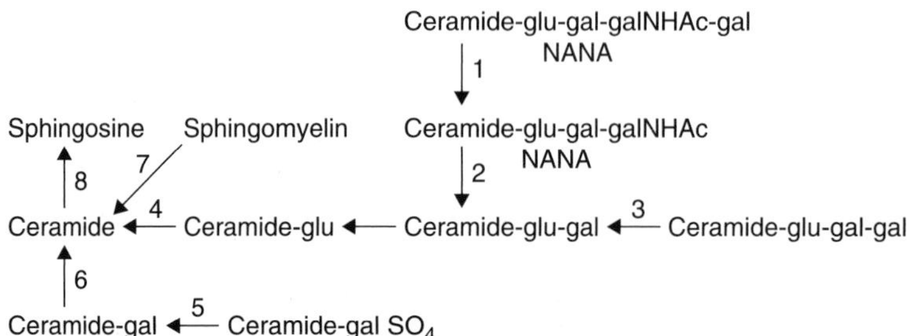

Figure 12.2 Interrelations between lipid components and enzyme difficiences in the lipid storage diseases. (1) β-galactosidase; GM-gangliosidosis; (2) β-hexosaminidase A; GM-gangliosidosis (Tay–Sachs); (3) α-galactosidase A, Fabry; (4) glucosylceramidase; Gaucher; (5) arylsulfatase A; metachromatic leukodystrophy; (6) galactosylceramidase; Krabbe leukodystrophy; (7) spingomyelinase; Niemann–Pick; (8) acid ceramidase; Farber. gal = galactose; glu = glucose; NHAc = *N*-acetylgalactosamine; NANA = *N*-acetyl neuraminic acid (sialic acid). Modified and reproduced with permission of authors and publisher from Lake BD. Metabolic disorders of the central and peripheral nervous system. In: *Histochemistry in Pathology.* Filipe MI, Lake BD (Eds). Edinburgh: Churchill Livingstone, 1983: 53–69.

CNS lipidoses (lipid storage disorders)

Sphingolipidoses

This is probably the most important group of metabolic disorders that affects the nervous system. The sphingolipids include gangliosides, cerebrosides, sulfatides and sphingomyelins, all of which are important constituents of the normal cell. The interrelationship between lipid components and enzyme deficiencies in the lipid storage disorders is shown in Fig. 12.2.

Gangliosidosis

These are composed of ceramide, hexose molecules, sialic acid and hexosamine. There are two main types, GM1 and GM2, both of which contain one sialic acid residue per molecule.

GM1 gangliosidosis may present in infants (type 1), in children (type 2) and, rarely, in adults (type 3). GM1 accumulates in the brain and viscera because of a deficiency of β-galactosidase. In type 1 the clinical course is rapid, with failure to thrive, hepatosplenomegaly and psychomotor retardation at birth or soon after. Characteristically, these patients show many of the clinical and radiological features of mucopolysaccharidosis (see page 219), with coarse facial features, abnormally thick and misshapen bones and hepatosplenomegaly. The type 2 form of the disease has a slower clinical course and usually does not become manifest until the end of the first year of life, progressing thereafter to spastic quadriplegia by about 10 years. The diagnosis can be achieved by staining for β-galactosidase.

There are several types of *GM2 gangliosidosis* resulting from deficiencies of the isoenzymes, hexosaminidase A and B. The most common type is *Tay–Sachs' disease* (type B) in which hexosaminidase A is deficient. Hexosaminidase has now been shown to be made up of α and β subunits and that hexosaminidase B has only B subunits. In type B Tay–Sachs' disease there is no synthesis of the α subunit, resulting in deficient hexosaminidase A activity. The β subunit is not present in type O (Sandhoff's disease), in which neither hexosaminidase A nor B activity is present. The diagnosis may be established prenatally by amniocentesis and the carriers may be detected by examining leukocytes.

At autopsy, depending on the duration of survival, the brain may be enlarged or normal (short survival), or small and firm with atrophic gyri (long survival). The white matter may appear swollen or have a grayish discoloration as a result of loss of the myelin (Fig. 12.3). The cerebellum and optic nerves are often atrophic. The brainstem and spinal cord are usually normal.

Evidence of neuronal storage is seen throughout the central and peripheral nervous system. Stored neuronal material in frozen sections stains positively with PAS and Luxol fast blue, but poorly with the Sudan dye. Similar material is also seen in

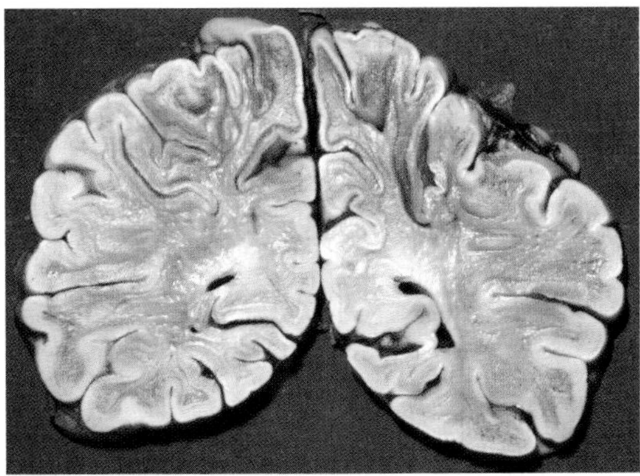

Figure 12.3 GM2-gangliosidosis. (Tay–Sachs disease). There is grayish discoloration of the white matter due to loss of myelin.

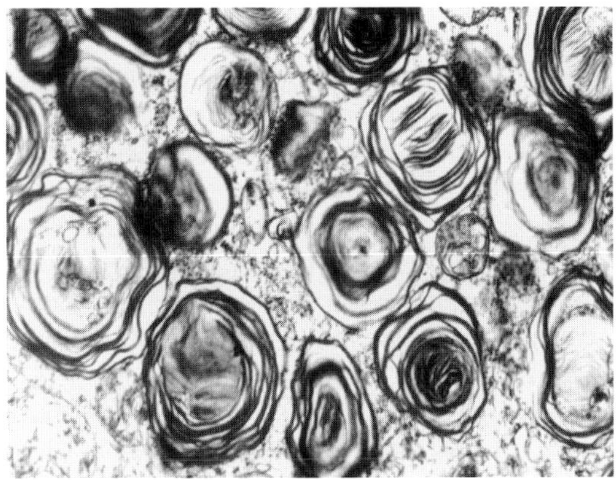

Figure 12.4 GM2-gangliosidosis. (Tay–Sachs disease). Membranous cytoplasmic bodies in a neuron.

astrocytes and macrophages. Electron microscopy shows membranous cytoplasmic bodies (Fig. 12.4) which, although identical ultrastructurally in the GM1 and GM2 gangliosidoses, are biochemically distinct. In longer surviving cases there is loss of neurons, an astrocytosis, and a progressive loss of myelin.

Cerebrosidosis

The two main disorders of cerebroside metabolism are *Gaucher's disease* and *Krabbe's disease* (see page 235 for description under the leukodystrophies). Gaucher's disease is a systemic lipidosis that may present in adults (type 1), infants (type 2) or juveniles (type 3). Most commonly in the adult type 1 form of the disease, the patients present with hepatosplenomegaly, bone pain and hypersplenism: there is no neurological involvement. Hepatosplenomegaly with hypersplenism and neurological symptoms predominate in the infantile and juvenile forms of the disease. The basic defect is a deficiency of β-glucocerebrosidase (one of the β-glucosidases). An association between Gaucher's disease and leukemia, lymphoma and glioma has been reported.

Whereas the brain in the adult form of the disease is usually normal, in the infantile and childhood forms it is often smaller than normal. There is atrophy of the cortex and basal ganglia and an unusually sharp demarcation between gray and white matter. Neuronal storage is particularly evident in the deep gray matter, the cerebellum and in the brainstem: the affected neurons are moderately distended with a PAS-positive material. Perivascular PAS-positive cells are also seen throughout the neuraxis. These may be typical Gaucher cells (20–100 μm in diameter, with a small nucleus and cytoplasm with the appearance of crinkled tissue paper), non-specific lipid-laden cells or multinucleate macrophages (the latter cells resembling those seen in Krabbe's disease). There is neuronal loss and an astrocytosis affecting both the cortical mantle and the subcortical gray matter, especially the dentate nucleus and the tegmentum of the brainstem. Myelin is preserved.

Sphingomyelinosis

Principal among the disorders of sphingomyelin metabolism is *Niemann–Pick disease* in which there is storage of a large amount of sphingomyelin, a normal component of myelin and of cell membranes. Two main types are recognized: group I in which there is sphingomyelinase deficiency, and group II in which sphingomyelinase activity is essentially normal. Both groups are further subdivided into neurovisceral and visceral forms. In group I, the neurovisceral form, which at least in its very early stages is remarkably similar to Gaucher's disease, presents only with hepatosplenomegaly, failure to thrive and mental retardation, whereas the visceral form is characterized by hepatosplenomegaly and hematological problems in the absence of neurological involvement. Group II cases present with various symptoms and signs which tend to be similar in any one family: these include failure to thrive, hepatosplenomegaly and severe prolonged neonatal obstructive jaundice.

The most striking abnormality at post mortem in group I is gross hepatosplenomegaly. There may be some atrophy of the brain. The histological features are very similar to those of a gangliosidosis, stored material in neurons staining positively with PAS, oil red O, Sudan black B, Luxol fast blue, acid hematein and by the ferric–hematoxylin method. Foamy cells are seen in the meninges, the choroid plexus, around blood vessels and in their endothelium, sites which help to distinguish this condition from the gangliosidoses. With time, there is neuronal loss, an astrocytosis and pallor of myelin staining. Systemically, the characteristic feature is the foam cell, or Niemann–Pick cell, which measures between 20 and 90 μm in diameter and may be uni- or multi-nucleated; this is present in most tissues of the body and has a 'mulberry like' appearance due to multiple small cytoplasmic vacuoles.

In cases of group II disease, there is often some degree of cerebral atrophy: myelin is preserved, and there is an astrocytosis. Ballooning of neurons is seen in all regions and is accompanied by axonal swellings. On electron microscopy there are membrane-bound cytoplasmic bodies that measure 3 μm across and contain loosely packed lamellae.

Other types of sphingolipidoses include *Farber's lipogranulomatosis* which is a disorder resulting from deficient activity of acid ceramidase. The disease is characterized by the development of periarticular and perivascular nodules composed of lipid-filled macrophages typically accompanied by a granulomatous inflammatory reaction. The nodules are often first detected in the skin, where they form readily visible subcutaneous nodules, similar nodules involving the joints, bones and kidneys. In the CNS, the larger neurons of the anterior horns of the spinal cord and their homologue in the brainstem are distended with lipid inclusions and are the main structures affected. Sensory and autonomic peripheral ganglion cells are similarly affected and characteristic inclusions (curvilinear tubular structures) are also seen in capillary and endothelial cells in the CNS. *Fabry disease* (*angiokeratoma corporus diffusum* or *α-galactosidase deficiency*) is a rare X-linked recessive disorder due to a deficiency of the hydralase enzyme α-galactosidase, which results in the accumulation of glycosphingolipids, especially in vascular endothelium and smooth muscle cells of the kidneys, heart and cerebral blood vessels leading to renal or cardiac failure or multiple strokes. Common symptoms suggesting involvement of the PNS are recurrent attacks and severe pain in the hands or feet especially in the presence of heat, and the absence of sweating. The stored material is sudanophilic, PAS positive and bi-refringent under polarized light. By electron microscopy inclusions are often seen in a myelin-like lamellated structure, sometimes in parallel arrays, and sometimes in concentric layers with a periodicity of 5 nm: some of them are membrane-bound, others are not. CNS involvement is usually limited to the amygdala, hypothalamus, hippocampus, entorrhinal cortex and brainstem nuclei.

Neuronal ceroid lipofuscinosis

Also known as Batten's disease and Kufs's disease and previously as amaurotic familial idiocy, it is characterized by a progressive hereditary neurological illness associated with blindness. These disorders are autosomal recessive in nature, occur as high as 7 per 100 000 live births in some populations, are characterized by intra-lysosomal accumulation of lipid pigments, that react positively for acid phosphatase and are autofluorescent under light microscopy. Classified according to clinical subtypes (infantile, late infantile, juvenile and adult forms) this group of disorders is now recognized by genetic defects numbering CLN1 to CLN8. The principal neuropathological findings are in the cortex of the cerebral and cerebellar hemispheres resulting in almost complete depletion of neurons in the infantile form at autopsy, lesser depletion in the late infantile form, some neuronal depletion in the juvenile form and a little neuronal loss in the adult form. Therefore, depending on the age of the patient there is variable brain atrophy that correlates with the onset and duration of the disease. There are associated secondary changes in axons and myelin with hydrocephalus. The principal microscopical appearances are those of neuronal loss, proliferation of astrocytes and macrophages and intracellular accumulation of lipopigments that are PAS-positive and stained by Luxol fast blue. As the lipopigments show different ultrastructural patterns, diagnosis may be achieved by electron microscopic examination of circulating lymphocytes that have distinctive ultrastructural profiles.

Mucopolysaccharidosis (disorders of glycosaminoglycan metabolism)

This group of autosomal recessive disorders is due to genetic deficiencies of enzymes involved in the catabolism of mucopolysaccharides which share the accumulation of glycosaminoglycans that are excreted in large amounts in urine. The glycosaminoglycans are large polysaccharide molecules that are found predominantly in skin, cartilage, bone, blood vessels, heart valves and tendons. They are made up of repeating disaccharide units, either glucosamine or galactosamine, usually linked to hexuronic acid. Classification is based on specific enzyme defects and analysis of urinary glycosaminoglycans. Clinically, these diseases of children are characterized by coarse facial features (*gargoylism*), multiple organ involvement and multiple skeletal abnormalities. Death from respiratory tract infections and heart disease within the first decade of life is usual.

The nervous system is only involved in certain forms of mucopolysaccharidosis and in such cases the features are akin to a neuronal storage disorder. The swollen neurons are a particular feature of the cerebral cortex and cerebellum. Appearances are akin to those seen in the gangliosidosis as are the zebra bodies and other structures that are intermediary to the membranous cytoplasmic bodies of Tay–Sachs' disease. Vacuoles are present, not only in the nervous system but also in various visceral organs including the liver, the heart and bone marrow and in circulating lymphocytes. These vacuoles appear to be lysosomal in origin as suggested by the demonstration of acid phosphatase.

There are three main types of mucopolysaccharidosis that involve the central nervous system. First, *Hurler's disease* due to a deficiency of α-L-iduronidase, which is required for the degradation of both heparan sulfate and dermatan sulfate. The same deficiencies are found in the Scheie and Hurler/Scheie subtypes of mucopolysaccharidosis. At autopsy, the brain tends to be rather small due to the loss of both gray and white matter. The ventricular system is enlarged and there is often prominent perivascular spaces in the white matter (Fig. 12.5). Neuronal storage of gangliosides is seen to a variable extent in all areas, the material staining with PAS, the Sudan dyes, and Luxol fast blue. Associated features include loss of neurons, an astrocytosis and partial loss of myelin. A well recognized but nonspecific feature in neurons on electron microscopy is an inclusion called the zebra body, which consists of irregular arrays of transverse lamellae of alternating dense and clear lines, with a periodicity of 5–7 nm, enclosed by a single membrane (Fig. 12.6). Hepatocytes and Kupffer cells store variable amounts of acid mucopolysaccharide in all forms of mucopolysaccharidosis. Second, *Hunter's disease* resembles Hurler's disease but is generally less severe. It is the only known X-linked recessive mucopolysaccharidosis and is due to a deficiency of iduronate sulfatase which results in storage of dermatan sulfate and heparan sulfate. Third, *Sanfilippo disease* due to heparan sulfate *n*-sulfatase deficiency which results in storage of heparan sulfate: histologically, it is similar to both Hurler and

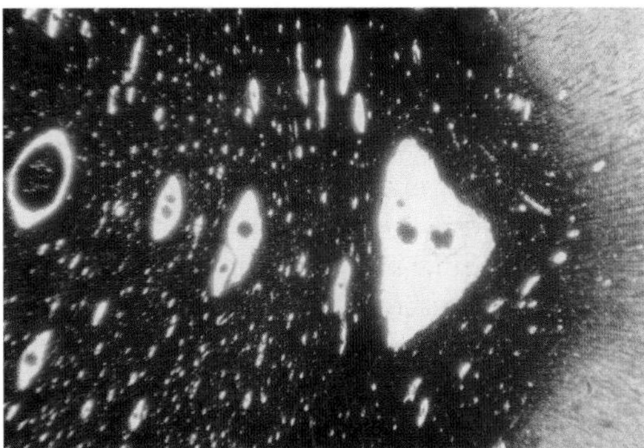

Figure 12.5 Mucopolysaccharidosis (Hurler's disease). Perivascular spaces are distended with cells containing water-soluble mucopolysaccharides.

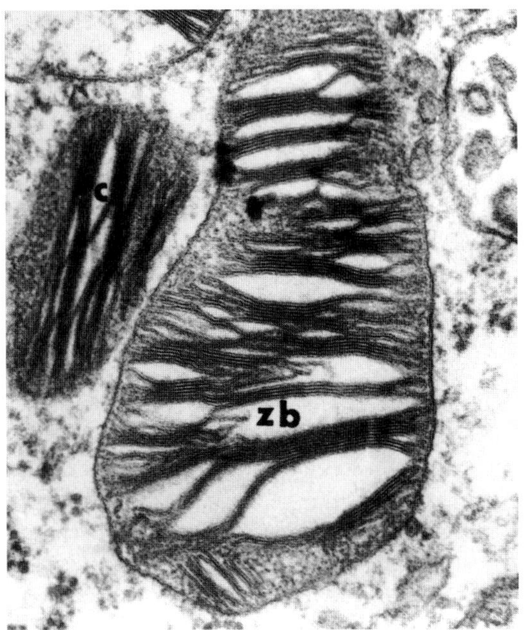

Figure 12.6 Mucopolysacchardosis. Membrane-bound collections of lipid lamellae (zebra bodies, zb) are present in the cytoplasm of an astrocyte. Electron microscopy ×30 000.

Hunter's disease but only heparan sulfate accumulates in large amounts. Other types of mucopolysaccharidosis include *Morquio's disease* in which there is deficiency of sulfatase galactosidase, which results in the accumulation of keratan sulfate and *Maroteaux–Lamy disease* in which dermatan sulfate accumulates as a result of sulfatase deficiency.

Mucolipidoses (glycosaminoglycans and lipid storage disorders)

There are four principal disorders that affect the nervous system, all of which are autosomal recessive and present clinically with dysmorphism similar to mucopolysaccharidosis sometimes associated with skeletal deformity and mental retardation and resembling GM1 gangliosidosis. There is variable involvement of systemic organs such as the liver, spleen and the skeleton. In *sialidosis* (*mucolipidosis 1*) the enzyme deficiency results in sialic-rich oligosaccharides whereas in *I-cell disease* (*mucolipidosis 2*) there are several acid hydrolases that are deficient that result in the storage of mucopolysaccharides and glycolipid. In *mannosidosis* there is a deficiency of α-mannosidosase A, which results in mannose-rich oligosaccharides to be stored, and in *fucosidosis* there is deficiency of α1-fucosidase, which results in the storage of fucose-rich polysaccharides, glycosphingolipids and oligosaccharides.

Glycogen storage disorders

These are glycogen storage diseases that result in the intracellular accumulation of glycogen. They can present in many ways, mainly brain damage or as disorders primarily of the liver, heart or musculoskeletal systems. All are rare and mostly of autosomal recessive inheritance: type 8 is X-linked. There are eight major types of which types 2 and, rarely, type 4 primarily affect the brain, and types 2–4, 5 and 7 affect muscle (see Chapter 18). Brain damage is most likely caused by severe recurrent bouts of lactacidosis and hypoglycemia. New feeding regimens have resulted in considerable improvement in the clinical outcome.

Type 2 (*Pompe's disease*) is due to a deficiency of α-1,4-glucosidase (acid maltase). The infantile form is rapidly progressive and fatal, death usually occurring by the age of 2 years. It is a generalized condition and there is profound hypotonia, cardiomegaly and sometimes hepatomegaly. Juveniles present with the symptoms and signs of muscular dystrophy, and adults with weakness and respiratory difficulties due to involvement of skeletal muscles. Excessive amounts of glycogen can be demonstrated in neurons of ganglia, in neurons in the ventral horns of the spinal cord and in motor nuclei in the brainstem. There may be limited involvement of other nuclei in the brainstem. There is positive staining with PAS and methenamine silver, and it is sensitive to salivary amylase. Skeletal muscle is affected in all forms of the disease. In the infantile form the heart is enlarged, all fibers are vacuolated and contain excess glycogen. Similar changes are seen in hepatocytes and in Kupffer cells and in cells of the lymphoreticular system. Ultrastructurally, glycogen accumulates in greatly distended lysosomes.

Other disorders

Wolman's disease (lysosomal acid lipase deficiency)

This is an autosomal recessive disease of infants who present with hepatosplenomegaly, gastrointestinal tract signs, and progressive neurological deterioration caused by mutations in the gene for lysosomal acid lipase (chromosome 10q24–q25) which results in an accumulation of cholesterol and triglyceride.

Tangier disease (hypo-α-lipoproteinemia)

This is an autosomal recessive multi-organ disease affecting cells of the lymphoreticular system, the cornea, and the peripheral nervous system. The disease is characterized by near or total absence of circulating α lipoproteins. Patients present with hypertrophy of the tonsils, hepatomegaly and splenomegaly due to the accumulation of cholesterol ester in tissue histiocytes, particularly of the lymphoid tissues and bone marrow. There is usually a degree of neuromuscular dysfunction, patients presenting with peripheral neuropathy, distal symmetrical polyneuropathy or a syringomyelia-like illness.

Abetalipoproteinemia

This is a rare disease, characterized by a combination of malabsorption of lipids, chronic progressive peripheral neuropathy, pigmentary degeneration of the retina and acanthocytosis. Signs of cerebellar dysfunction are frequently seen in association with peripheral neuropathy, the disease resulting from mutations of a gene on chromosome 4q22–q24 that encodes the microsomal triglyceride transfer protein.

LEUKODYSTROPHIES

This group of disorders is characterized by dysmyelination due to an inability to form completely normal myelin. This is in contrast to the demyelinating disorders (see Chapter 9) in which, after the formation of normal myelin injury, there is a loss of myelin sheaths with relative sparing of the axons. It is therefore necessary for the pathologist to have knowledge of the pattern and timing of normal myelination of white matter tracts within the developing brain (see page 244). Principal milestones in this regard include myelination of white matter within the spinal cord between 14 and 24 weeks' gestation, myelination of the internal capsules, optic nerves and pons between the 35th and 40th weeks of gestation, myelination of the corticospinal tracts within the brainstem between birth and 3 months of age, and myelination of the central white matter of the cerebral hemispheres between the ages of 1 and 2 years.

The leukodystrophies are a complex group of uncommon disorders which have in common diffuse symmetrical loss of myelin and gliosis of the white matter of the cerebral hemispheres, and sometimes also of the cerebellum, the brainstem and the spinal cord. There are several different types of leukodystrophy, some of which are genetically determined with a known enzyme defect leading to the accumulation of myelin-associated proteins. They occur most commonly in childhood. Whereas *metachromatic leukodystrophy* and *Krabbe's disease* are primary leukodystrophies due to disorders of lipid metabolism, enzyme defects in the other (idiopathic) types of leukodystrophy are not known (Table 12.2).

Lysosomal and peroxisomal related disorders

Metachromatic leukodystrophy

This, the most common of the leukodystrophies, can be divided by age of onset and clinical presentation into three main types, late infantile (onset before 2 years), intermediate (onset 4–6 years) and, juvenile (onset 6–10 years): adult cases also occur. In general, however, the disease pursues a relentless clinical course over a period of 1–2 years. This autosomal recessive disorder is a systemic lipidosis due to a deficiency of arylsulfatase, an enzyme that is responsible for cleaving the sulfate radical from the sulfatide. Myelin in this condition is not broken down into neutral fat or cholesterol esters but into metachromatic material containing sulfatides. The gene for arylsulfatase is located on chromosome 22q13.31–qter and the variable

Table 12.2 Principal types of leukodystrophy

Disorder	Enzyme defect	Substances stored	Staining methods
Lysosomal or peroxisomal related disorders			
Metachromatic	Arylsulfatase A mapped to chromosome 22	Sulfatides	Acidified CV, TLC
Krabbe's	Galactocerebroside β-galactosidase 14q31	Galactocerebroside	PAS, TLC, EM
Adrenoleukodystrophy and adrenomyeloneuropathy	ATP-binding transporter Xq28	Very long chain fatty acids	Sudan, PAS, EM
Other related disorders			
Alexander's disease	Not known	Glial fibrillary acidic protein	IHC, EM
Canavan's disease	Aspartoactylase	—	EM
Pelzaeus–Merzbacher disease	Xq21.33-22	Myelin proteolipid protein	Sudan
Cockayne's disease	Defective DNA repair mapped to chromosome 5	—	Sudan
'Burnt-out' cases	—	—	—

IHC: immunohistochemistry, CV: cresyl violet. Other abbreviations as in the footnote to Table 12.1.

clinical expression of this disorder is thought to be related to the residual enzyme activity associated with the two mutations affecting each allele, with the least enzyme activity associated with the late infantile form of the disease.

At autopsy the brain may appear normal externally: on section it may be firm to touch and the white matter may be somewhat grayer and more translucent than normal (Fig. 12.7). Histologically, there is widespread loss of myelin in the white matter, including the subcortical arcuate fibers, and the fiber tracts which mature last are the most severely affected. Within the demyelinated areas there are large amounts of both intracellular (prominent in oligodendrocytes and astrocytes) and extracellular metachromatic granules, and small amounts in neurons and in perivascular macrophages. Sulfatide deposits accumulate in many tissues including the PNS, liver, pancreas and kidney and can easily be recognized as 20–30 μm deposits of PAS-positive and metachromatic material which stains brown with acidic cresyl violet and pink with acidified cresyl violet (Fig. 12.8). Electron microscopically, some of the cytoplasmic inclusions have a characteristic pattern – a herringbone

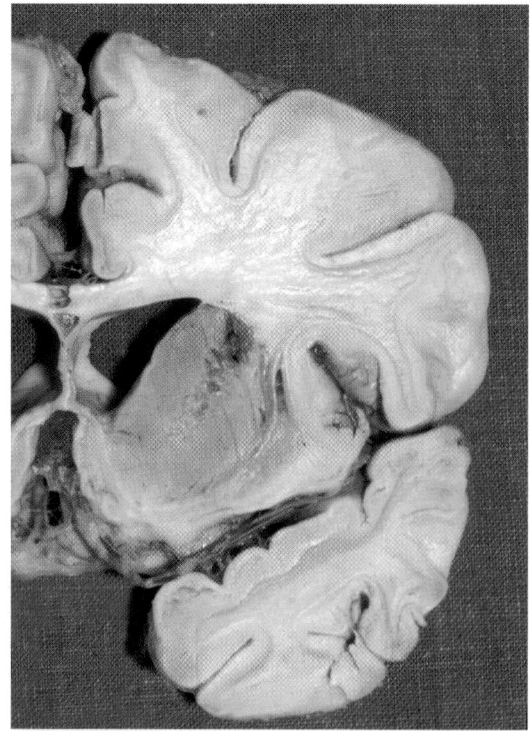

Figure 12.7 Metachromatic leukodystrophy. The white matter is gray due to demyelination.

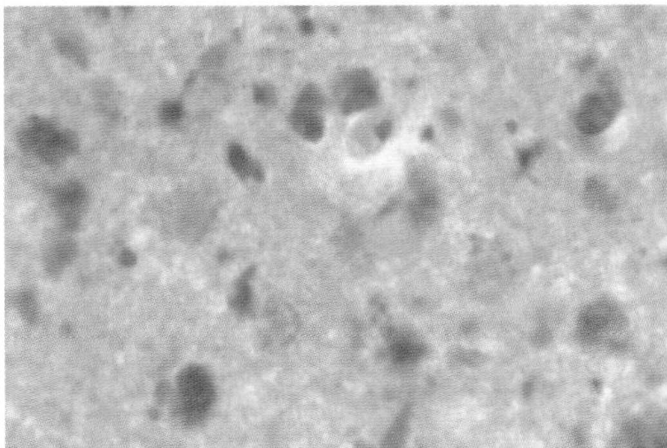

Figure 12.8 Metachromatic leukodystrophy. Cryostat section showing metachromatic macrophages in the white matter. Acidified cresyl violet.

appearance in longitudinal section and a honeycomb structure in cross section.

Initial screening can be easily carried out by the examination of urinary sediment for metachromatic deposit. Confirmation can be achieved by enzyme assay in white blood cells, cultured fibroblasts, or by sural nerve biopsy.

Krabbe's disease

This is an autosomal recessive leukodystrophy caused by deficiency of the enzyme, galactosylceramidase which is necessary for the catabolism of galactosyl ceramide, an integral component of myelin. Usually, the onset is before the age of 6 months and the clinical course is rapidly progressive with death occurring within the first few years of life.

The brain is generally small and has a normal external appearance. On section the white matter, with exception of the subcortical arcuate fibers, is grayish in color and firm to touch (Fig. 12.9a, b and c). Histologically, the cortex is normal but there is widespread loss of myelin, with more or less preservation of axons and an astrocytosis. The characteristic feature is perivascular clusters of multinucleated globoid cells within the areas of loss of myelin. The globoid cells measure some 20–50 μm in diameter and are thought to develop from smaller mononuclear (epithelioid) macrophages that become filled with galactocerebroside (Fig. 12.10). The cytoplasm is moderately positive with PAS, and stains only weakly with oil red O and Sudan

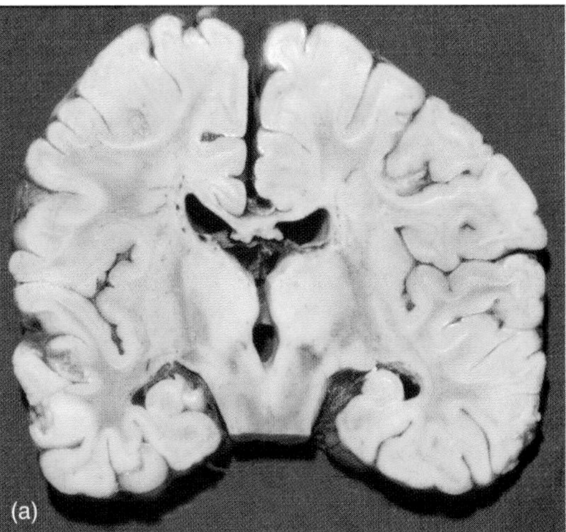

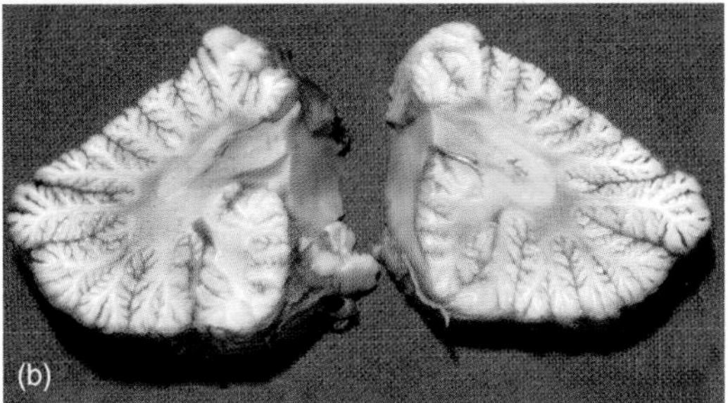

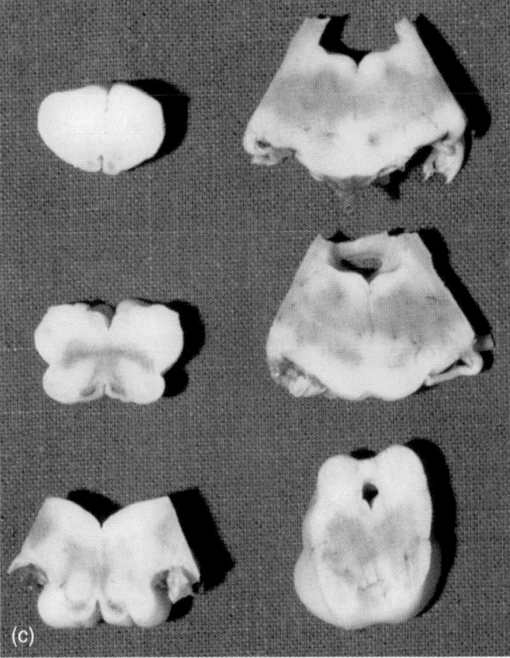

Figure 12.9 Krabbe's leukodystrophy. There is symmetrical gray discoloration of white matter in (a) cerebral hemispheres, (b) cerebellum, (c) brainstem.

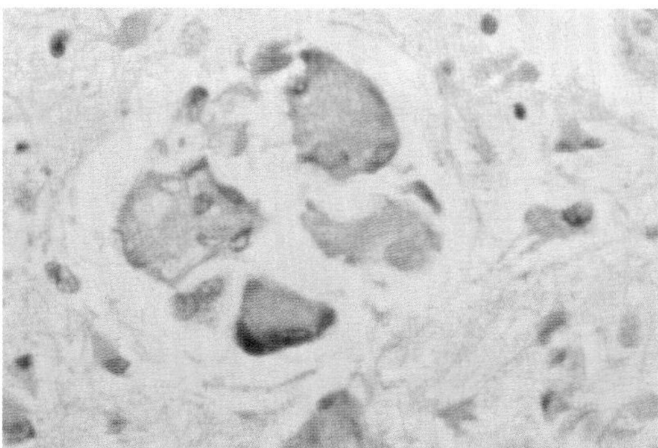

Figure 12.10 Krabbe's leukodystrophy. There are globoid cells in the white matter. H&E.

black B. As the loss of myelin becomes more severe, a point is reached where there is marked loss of axons, intense astrocytosis and only a few scattered clusters of globoid cells. A diagnosis can be established by enzyme assay using leukocytes or cultured fibroblasts.

Adrenoleukodystrophy and adrenomyeloneuropathy

These disorders have been already described (see Chapter 11). It is now considered that the overwhelming majority of males thought to have sudanophilic leukodystrophy are, in fact, examples of adrenoleukodystrophy, and patients with this type of dysmyelination in whom the adrenal glands are normal have a variant of multiple sclerosis. The term *Schilder's disease* has been used in the past for leukodystrophy of sudanophilic types. If the term has to be retained, it should be restricted to cases of adrenoleukodystrophy.

Other related disorders

Alexander's disease

This is a rare autosomal recessive disorder caused by mutations of the glial fibrillary acidic protein gene. The patient usually presents with mental retardation, seizures, spasticity and megalencephaly with death occurring within 10 years of onset. At autopsy the brain is heavy and appears enlarged; on section there may be hydrocephalus, the cortex is ill-defined and the white matter is soft and gray in color. Histologically, the most striking feature is the presence of large numbers of homogenous elongated hyaline bodies measuring up to 200 μm long (Rosenthal fibers) arranged radially around blood vessels and at right angles to both the surface of the brain beneath the pia and the ependyma. The Rosenthal fibers stain red with H&E, dark purple with PTAH and blue with Luxol fast blue. Immunohistochemistry has shown that their peripheral portions are made up of glial fibrillary acidic protein. Their central portions do not stain and, on electron microscopy, consists of non-fibrillary and densely osmiophilic masses without limiting membrane. There is continuity of the filaments with the granular masses. The relationship between Rosenthal fibers and glial fibers is therefore uncertain. In general the number of Rosenthal fibers correlates with the severity of myelin lost but the cause of the demyelination in a disease that principally affects astrocytes is not known.

Canavan's disease

Congenital, infantile and juvenile types have been described and are characterized clinically by mental deterioration and megalencephaly. This condition is due to deficiency of aspartoacylase, an enzyme necessary for the catabolism of *N*-acetyl-aspartate and *N*-acetyl-spartate glutamate. At autopsy, the white matter is soft to touch and 'edematous'. Histologically, the most striking feature is the spongy change in white matter, loss of myelin, relative preservation of axons and a reactive astrocytosis. Sudanophilic macrophages are seen and there are many Alzheimer type 2 astrocytes in the cerebral cortex and in subcortical gray matter. Neurons are normal in the early stages of the disease. Ultrastructural studies have shown that the spongy change is due to vacuolation of myelin sheaths, and swelling of astrocytic cytoplasm the latter frequently containing greatly enlarged mitochondria with a peculiarly arranged matrix and cristae. In some cases the diagnosis can be established by finding abnormal mitochondria in a muscle biopsy.

Pelizaeus–Merzbacher disease

This X-linked recessive leukodystrophy is caused by mutations involving the protolipid protein-1 gene which regulates the chief structural protein of central compact myelin. There is a male predominance, boys presenting with nystagmus, cerebellar ataxia, progressive spastic paraparesis and a movement disorder without evidence of a peripheral demyelination. Death usually occurs in late adolescence and, as in other leukodystrophies, the disease is characterized by loss of myelin in the white matter. Due to the sparing of a few small islands of normal myelin, often in a perivascular distribution, the appearance of perivascular myelin sparing has been known as the 'tigroid leukodystrophy'. There is relative sparing of axons and a marked gliosis. Microscopy shows relative preservation of gray matter and an almost complete absence of myelin in which there is a marked reduction in oligodendrocytes.

Cockayne syndrome

This rare autosomal recessive disorder presents in infants with mental retardation and photosensitivity. There are multiple genes that can give rise to the syndrome each of which is involved in the repair of DNA following UV light radiation. The classic Cockayne syndrome with the gene locus on chromosome 5 is associated with dwarfism, macrocephaly, retinitis pigmentosa, deafness and peripheral nerve involvement. The brain is small, especially in the cerebellum and the brainstem. There is hydrocephalus and microscopy confirms the relative preservation of gray matter and an almost complete absence of myelin. Oligodendrocytes are markedly reduced in number or may be absent and there is diffuse astrocytosis.

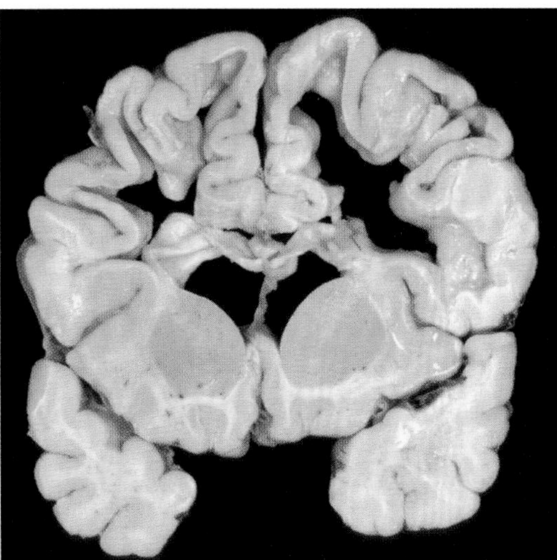

Figure 12.11 Burnt-out case of leukodystrophy with marked cavitation of central white matter.

'Burnt-out' cases

Rare and usually reported as autosomal recessive. Recognizable with widespread cavitation of oftentimes green-colored central white matter. Histologically, macrophages contain large amounts of lipofuscin. In some cases there are excessive numbers of oligodendrocytes and yet, in others, features include calcification and meningeal angiomatosis (Fig. 12.11).

CHAPTER 13

INTOXICATIONS

David I Graham

INTRODUCTION

There is increasing awareness that from a mechanistic point of view there are considerable similarities in the cellular and molecular events that take place after head injury, 'stroke' and in various neurodegenerative disease that is shared within the disciplines of neurotoxicology and neurodegeneration. This implies that although triggered by different events there are certain final common pathways that are ultimately expressed as abnormal metabolism that may culminate in structural damage to the nervous system. Broadly speaking neurotoxicology separates *neurotoxicants* which are exogenous agents from *neurotoxins* which are endogenous agents and through which the exogenous agents cause damage to the nervous system. Although the mechanisms of action of some of the neurointoxicants are known, there are many other circumstances in which the precise mechanism is not known so that it is hypothesized that one or more of the known mechanisms of cellular damage, *viz.* the production of free radicals, excessive amounts of excitatory amino acids, trace elements, lipid peroxidation and glycation end-products, have been operating.

The neuropathology of neurotoxicants is somewhat similar regardless of the nature of the injurious agent in that in the acute phase, swelling of either gray or white matter predominates. Such may be its degree that the features of raised intracranial pressure are seen. Histologically, there may be pallor of staining and the vascular consequences of internal herniation may be identified. In some instances, there is selective neuronal loss whereas in other cases, the damage is more diffuse. In either event it is possible to recognize that irreversible neuronal damage has occurred associated with which there will be a microglial response and an astrocytosis. Specific changes in myelin may be evident and if there has been associated liver damage Alzheimer type 2 astrocytes may be present. A not uncommon finding, but particularly in the PNS, is axonal damage with a pattern that is referred to as 'dying-back' axonopathy. If there have been repeated episodes of intoxication, although initially the changes may have been reversible, then there may come a time when these are irreversible and are reflected in cavitation, scarring and various neurodegenerative changes.

TOXIC GASES

Carbon monoxide

The clinical features of acute carbon monoxide intoxication can be correlated with the concentration of caboxyhemoglobin in the blood, which, in turn, is a product of the duration of the exposure to, and the concentrations of carbon monoxide in the environment. A previously healthy individual will experience severe headache and dizziness at 20–30% saturation; impaired vision, hearing and mental function at 40–50% saturation; coma and seizures at 50–60% saturation; and cardiorespiratory failure and death at over 70% saturation. The outcome is often influenced by pre-existing cardiovascular disease, many of the acute deaths resulting from myocardial dysfunction.

Carbon monoxide may give rise to structural brain damage because its affinity for hemoglobin is about 250 times that for oxygen. The remaining normal hemoglobin has a normal oxygen saturation and blood oxygen tension is normal when the oxygen content is reduced. Furthermore, the dissociation curve of oxyhemoglobin is shifted to the left so that less oxygen is available to the tissues at a particular oxygen tension.

When death occurs within a few hours, the blood, brain, muscles, skin and viscera have the pink/red color characteristic of carboxyhemoglobin. The brain and leptomeninges are usually congested and petechial hemorrhages are frequently seen in white matter, particularly in the corpus callosum. If the patient survives in coma for a few days, microscopic evidence of necrosis may be seen in the cerebral cortex, the hippocampi and in the basal ganglia, particularly the globus pallidus (Fig. 13.1). The pattern and damage is very similar to that seen in other types of hypoxia–ischemia (see Chapter 5). In contrast, alterations within the white matter may result from carbon monoxide intoxication, although the extent is not necessarily proportional to the damage in gray matter, so the latter may appear normal even when there is extensive myelin breakdown. White matter damage takes the form of *peri-axial demyelination* (see Chapter 9) and is a well-recognized feature of the brains of patients presenting with delayed-onset neurological symptoms after an episode of intoxication (Fig. 13.2). The pathogenesis of carbon monoxide encephalopathy is multifactorial, and includes the high affinity of carbon monoxide for oxyhemoglobin, its binding to brain cytochromes, and the various vascular mechanisms due to systemic circulatory factors. The concentration of damage in white matter is thought to be due to a local cytotoxic effect of carbon monoxide, with an additional reduction in blood flow.

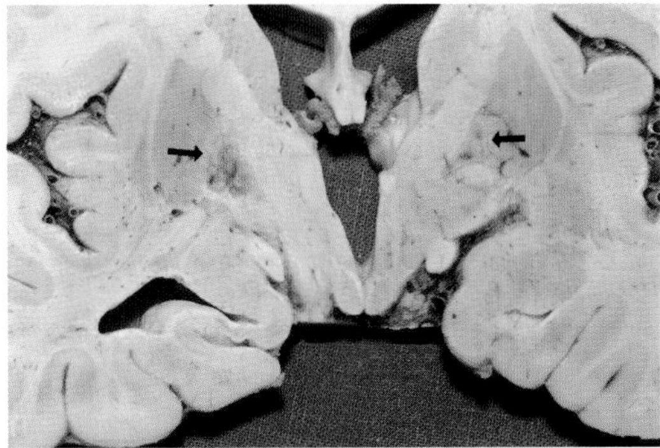

Figure 13.1 Carbon monoxide poisoning. There are foci of necrosis in each globus pallidus (arrows).

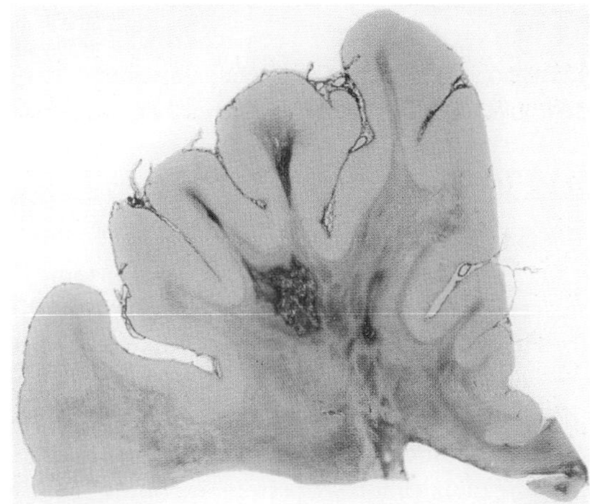

Figure 13.2 Carbon monoxide poisoning. Patient lived in coma for 9 months after acute poisoning. Note extensive astrocytosis throughout the white matter. There was associated loss of white matter. Celloidin. Holtzer for astrocytosis.

Nitrous oxide

Nitrous oxide, as with other inhalation anesthetics, may occasionally lead to accidents during which the patient becomes hypoxic. If resuscitation is successful, then the patient may manifest various degrees of disability as a result of ischemic brain damage (see Chapter 5).

The gas has been used as an intoxicant with individuals inhaling it from whipped-cream dispensers. Because of the similarity with subacute combined degeneration of the spinal cord it has been suggested that nitrous oxide interferes with vitamin

B_{12} metabolism. However, the relationship between exposure to nitrous oxide and the development of *myeloneuropathy* is not clear particularly as whipped-cream dispensers contain many potentially neurotoxic contaminants whereas the anesthetic gas is pure.

An uncommon and sometimes fatal complication of general anesthesia is that of *malignant hyperthermia* characterized by a dramatic rise in core temperature and generalized muscle rigidity (see Chapter 15). It has been associated with exposure to a variety of anesthetic gases, including nitrous oxide, and is more common when succinylcholine is used as a premedication. A positive family history is present in about 30% of patients. Malignant hyperthermia, however, has also been reported in certain muscle diseases, such as Duchenne muscular dystrophy, myotonia congenita and central core disease.

Cyanides

The effects of the cyanide ion are due to the inhibition of cytochrome oxidase, the terminal enzyme in the respiratory electron transport chain which utilizes the oxygen derived from dissociation of oxyhemoglobin. There is no essential difference between the neuropathological effects of sodium potassium cyanide, hydrocyanic acid and cyanogen chloride. In acute intoxication death from respiratory failure rapidly ensues and is often preceded by seizures. The brain may be congested and swollen and occasional petechial hemorrhages are seen, but there are no significant microscopic changes. If death is delayed, there may be structural changes in both gray and white matter. Experimental studies have shown that cyanide can damage myelin sheaths after administration by any route. Damage to gray matter usually follows cardiorespiratory complications and/or seizures.

ALCOHOL-RELATED DISORDERS

Ethanol

After absorption via the small intestine into the blood, ethyl alcohol is rapidly distributed to all parts of the body and equilibrates with body water compartments. Eventually, most of the alcohol is oxidized in the liver through acetaldehyde to acetic acid; a small proportion – less than 10% – is secreted unchanged from lungs, kidneys and skin. An average adult can metabolize about 10 mL of pure ethyl alcohol, hourly. Blood alcohol levels above 100 mg/100 mL usually are associated with the signs of intoxication in a non-habituated person: levels above 400 mg/100 mL are associated with a stupor or coma, regardless of the degree of tolerance: levels above 500 mg/100 mL are often fatal.

The pathological effects of chronic alcohol abuse on the liver are well established, yet in many instances abnormalities in the nervous system are not due to a direct toxic effect of alcohol but rather to an associated nutritional deficiency. A wide range of histological changes had been attributed to alcoholism, but most are now regarded as non-specific. There are, however, a number of conditions that fall within the domain of the neuropathologist (Table 13.1).

Fetal alcohol syndrome

It is now recognized that alcohol consumption during pregnancy can cause a variety of CNS abnormalities that range from gross morphological changes with mental retardation (fetal alcohol syndrome – FAS) to more subtle cognitive and behavioral disorders (fetal alcohol effect – FAE). Because of the difficulties in making a diagnosis of FAS the precise estimates of the incidence and prevalence are difficult to determine, but large numbers of epidemiological studies have suggested an incidence of about 0.33 cases per 1000. Therefore, it is thought

Table 13.1 Ethanol-related disorders

- Fetal alcohol syndrome
- Acute intoxication and withdrawal syndrome
- Alcoholic dementia
- Alcoholic cerebellar degeneration
- Central pontine myelinolysis
- Wernicke–Korsakoff syndrome
- Peripheral neuropathy
- Alcoholic myopathy
- Hepatic encephalopathy

that fetal alcohol syndrome is now a more common cause of mental retardation than either Down syndrome or the fragile X syndrome.

The degree of maternal alcoholism, at a critical stage in gestation for the development of this disorder, is not known precisely, and it is still not clear whether it is the alcohol *per se*, or its metabolites or an associated nutritional deficiency that is the actual cause of the teratogenic effects. The most common abnormality is microcephaly. Hydrocephalus, agenesis of the corpus callosum, generalized disorganization of neuronal migration, hypoplasia of the mid-face and limb malformations have also been reported. Abnormalities also include cardiac defects and various joint and limb abnormalities have been noted. Studies have broadened the syndrome to include ocular abnormalities, hearing disorders and cerebellar symptoms and behavioral disorders. However, the phenotype of FAS is not specific and is also thought to occur after exposure to other agents.

Acute alcohol intoxication and the withdrawal syndrome

There are no specific neuropathological features, but head injury and subarachnoid hemorrhage due to rupture of a saccular aneurysm are more common in intoxicated than sober individuals, and there is an increased risk of cerebral infarction after an 'alcoholic binge'. There are no characteristic features in fatal cases of *delirium tremens* or *withdrawal seizures* other than those associated with terminal hypoxia and electrolyte imbalance.

Alcoholic dementia

In chronic alcoholics neuropsychological impairment can usually be linked to CT scan evidence of atrophy. Whether the features on imaging reflect the state of hydration and/or neuronal loss is not clear as the CT changes are said to be reversible with abstinence. Therefore, it may be that these changes are not a direct result of alcohol *per se* but reflect a variety of associated nutritional deficiencies.

The frequency, severity and relation of the atrophy to the alcoholism is controversial. There is increasing evidence from CT scans and autopsy studies that both cerebral atrophy and ventricular enlargement are common in alcoholic patients, in the absence of significant hepatic disease. Studies have suggested that cerebral atrophy is not due to loss of gray matter but rather to a reduction in the volume of the deep white matter. The abnormalities may be reversed by abstinence from alcohol. Perhaps an appropriate term for the reversible abnormalities would be '*thiamine-deficiency dementia*'.

Alcoholic cerebellar degeneration

Probably the most common cause of acquired ataxia is in alcoholic patients who are either developing the syndrome as a sequel of Wernicke syndrome, or as a distinct clinical entity. Males are more affected than females in whom there is a gradual onset of existing signs of peripheral neuropathy.

There is often selective atrophy of the anterior portion of the superior vermis of the cerebellum in chronic alcoholics (see Fig. 10.5). Microscopically, within the atrophic cerebellar cortex there is loss of Purkinje cells, a variable loss of granular cells, and associated reactive proliferation of Bergmann astrocytes and an isomorphic gliosis of the molecular layer. Clinicopathological studies have shown that these changes correlate with truncal instability, leg ataxia and with a widespread stance and gait. The cerebellar degeneration has been attributed to the direct toxic effects of ethanol, a more likely explanation is that it is secondary to nutritional deficiency, particularly as a similar atrophy may be seen in malnourished patients in whom there is no history of alcohol abuse.

Central pontine myelinolysis

This demyelinating disease is seen most commonly in association with alcohol abuse but also in various debilitating diseases or after the rapid correction of hyponatremia. Diagnosis can be achieved by MRI, the recognition of the condition being important in view of its potential reversibility.

At the time of brain cutting, a typical lesion appears as a midline, essentially symmetrical, discolored area in the basis pontis that may have undergone a degree of cavitation. The lesions are often triangular, T-shaped or diamond-shaped. They vary from a few millimeters across to lesions that may involve the entire basis pontis. There is usually a rim of entrapped myelin that separates the lesion from the lateral and ventral aspects of the pons, damage being maximal in the middle and rostral portions of the pons (Fig. 13.3a). Histologically, central pontine myelinolysis is characterized by demyelination and relative preservation of axons and neuronal perikarya (Fig. 13.3b). In acute lesions there may be many lipid-laden macrophages with remarkably few inflammatory cells. In severe cases extrapontine lesions may involve the subcortical white matter, the striatum, anterior commissure, internal and external capsules and the lateral geniculate bodies.

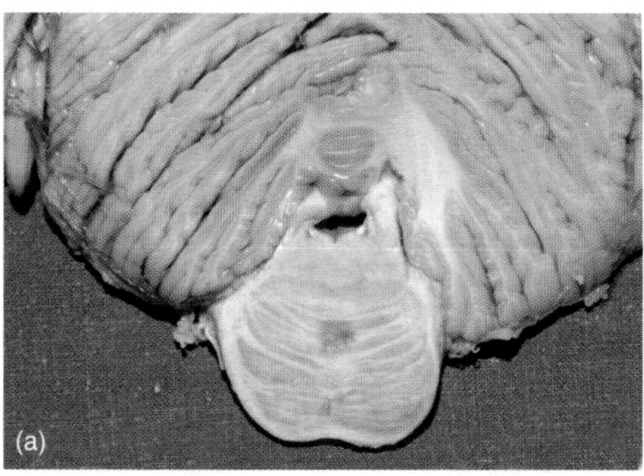

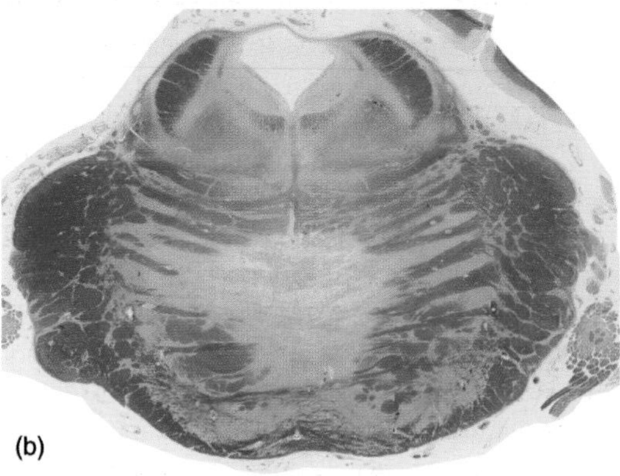

Figure 13.3 Central pontine myelinolysis. (a) Note well demarcated area of loss of myelin in midline of basis pontis. (b) There is a centrally placed symmetrical area of demyelination in the pons within which there is sparing of neurons. Luxol fast blue–cresyl violet.

Corpus callosum demyelination

Also known as *Marchiafava–Bignami disease* this rare disorder may also occur in patients with chronic alcoholism. Occasionally, it occurs in association with Wernicke's encephalopathy or central pontine myelinolysis characterized by a focal loss of myelin within the corpus callosum (Fig. 13.4) and occasionally by similar involvement of the optic chiasm, anterior commissure, middle cerebellar peduncles and in the centrum semiovale: the involvement is maximal in the genu and body of the corpus callosum.

An associated feature is that of Morels' *laminar sclerosis* in which there is a band-like proliferation of astrocytes localized to the third cortical layer especially in the lateral frontal cortex.

Other associated disorders

The features of the Wernicke–Krosakoff syndrome (see page 199) and peripheral neuropathy (see page 388) and alcohol-induced liver disease with the formation of Alzheimer's type 2 astrocytes in the brain are described elsewhere (page 207).

Alcohol myopathy is said to be not uncommon. Acute necrotizing myopathy after binge drinking or a chronic myopathy which takes the form of painless promixal weakness is sometimes associated with cardiomyopathy. The cause of alcoholic myopathy is uncertain, hypotheses including

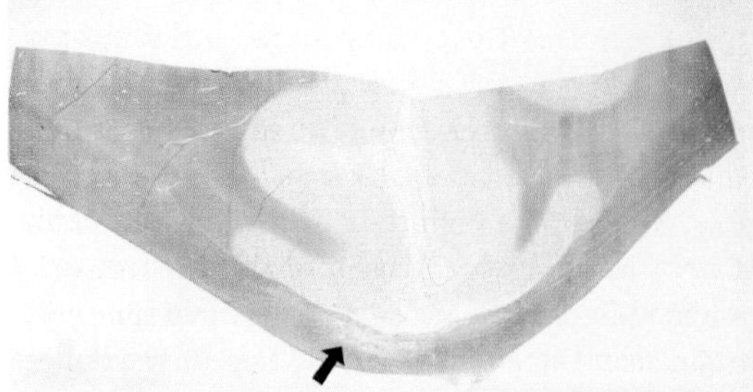

Figure 13.4 Marchiafava–Bignami disease. Patient was a chronic alcoholic. Note symmetrical loss of myelin in the central position of the corpus callosum (arrow). Luxol fast blue–cresyl violet.

mitochondrial disturbances, potassium depletion, and rhabdomyolysis.

Methanol

There is considerable variation in individual susceptibility to ingested methanol, either in the form of cheap intoxicants or as solvents. More serious sequelae, however, are produced by its catabolites formaldehyde and formic acid. Blindness occurs frequently in methanol intoxication and has been attributed to either degeneration of the retinal ganglion cells and photoreceptors, or to swelling of the optic disc, thought to be due to swelling of axons in which there is stagnation of axoplasmic flow, possibly related to the diffusion of formic acid from choroidal blood vessels. Abuse may also induce parkinsonism. The neuropathological features in acute deaths are not specific, but in patients who survive, necrosis of the basal ganglia and in particular in the putamen, and of the deep white matter of the cerebral and cerebellar hemispheres, have been described. It has been suggested that the changes in the white matter and in the optic nerves represent a toxic form of loss of myelin caused by formates.

Ethylene glycol

This dihydroxy alcohol is widely used as a solvent and is a component of certain antifreezes and coolants. Intoxication is encountered most often when it is consumed as an ill-advised substitute for ethanol, or is used as a means of suicide. The minimum lethal dose is thought to be in excess of 100 mL. Ethylene glycol is progressively oxidized into a series of toxic compounds, including glycoaldehyde, glycolic acid and glyoxylic acid; a small proportion is oxidized eventually to oxalic acid. In fatal cases there is swelling, congestion and occasional petechial hemorrhages in the brain. Histologically, there is infiltration by neutrophil polymorphs in the meninges and in relation to the intracerebral blood vessels. Deposits of crystalline calcium oxalate may be seen in and around the blood vessels of the meninges, the brain and choroidal plexus: they are best seen with polarized light.

INDUSTRIAL TOXINS

Carbon disulfide

Exposure is an occupational hazard in the production of viscose, rayon and film. Fortunately, acute toxicity no longer occurs, and attention is now directed to complications of long-term exposure to low concentrations of carbon disulfide – it is, for example, a constituent in the fumigants used for treating grain – which include peripheral neuropathy and an increase in cardiovascular disease. In long-term survivors various neuropsychiatric symptoms and parkinsonism may develop, neuropathological correlates of which are widespread neuronal loss in the cerebellar hemispheres but particularly in the basal ganglia. In addition, there is a central-motor peripheral distal axonopathy which closely resembles the hexacarbon neuropathies. It has been suggested that carbon disulfide acts by binding to neurofilament proteins, thereby affecting axoplasmic transport. Carbon disulfide is a metabolite of disulfiram, a drug used in the treatment of chronic alcoholism and occasionally associated with a toxic neuropathy. Neurotoxicity of disulfiram is probably due to its conversion to carbon disulfide in the body.

Solvents

Toluene is both an important solvent in many different industries and an important base compound in the synthesis of other substances. It is a prominent substance in solvent abuse. It is readily absorbed from the lungs, and rapidly distributed through, and metabolized in the body. Acute toxicity depends upon the concentration and duration of exposure. Chronic exposure produces cerebellar ataxia due largely to damage of the white matter. Chronic exposure results in a peripheral neuropathy.

Carbon tetrachloride is a common solvent that has been used in certain types of fire extinguishers. Acute intoxication results in damage to the CNS, liver and kidneys. In cases where there is hepatic or renal failure, the neural dysfunction may be secondary to metabolic encephalopathy. In addition, there are changes in the white matter referred to as carbon tetrachloride-induced vasculopathy.

Another important solvent is *trichloroethylene* used in dry-cleaning procedures. Acute intoxication produces multiple cranial nerve palsies, particularly of the Vth and VIIth cranial nerves.

The hexacarbon compounds *n-hexane* and *methyl n-butyl ketone* have been employed extensively as organic solvents in the production of adhesives and cement. These two substances and their common metabolite, 2,5-hexanedione, produce a distinctive form of peripheral neuropathy which may occur in 'glue sniffers' as well as a result of industrial exposure. Histologically, the hexacarbon neuropathies are characterized by a distal neuropathy in which there is the formation of focal swellings on axons prior to degeneration of the more distal regions of the affected nerves. These swellings tend to develop proximal to nodes of Ranvier and are filled with masses of neurofilaments. Their formation may be related to impairment of axoplasmic transport due to inhibition of the glycolytic enzyme or, alternatively, as a reaction of hexacarbons with amino groups of neurofilaments, causing them to form aggregation. Similar axonal enlargements have been seen in other forms of intoxication, namely *acrylamide* and *carbon disulfide.* In hexacarbon neuropathy there is distal axonal degeneration in both the central and peripheral nervous systems, and changes are therefore found in the gracile, corticospinal, and spinocerebellar tracts.

Organophosphorous compounds

Exposure to organophosphates occurs in the manufacture and formulation of the compound, and in the large-scale spraying operations of insecticides. Acute poisoning results from the accumulation of endogenous acetylcholine in neural tissue and effect organs because of the inhibition of choline esterase, with subsequent signs and symptoms that mimic the muscarinic, nicotinic and CNS actions of acetylcholine. These can usually be controlled and there are no long-term effects. Some organophosphates, however, cause a delayed peripheral neuropathy which develops between one and three weeks after a single dose. One such agent, tri-orthocresyl phosphate (TOCP), is used as a plasticizer and lubricant and has been responsible for accidental neurotoxicity, well-documented cases occurring in 'ginger jake paralysis' which followed the consumption of alcoholic extracts of ginger contaminated with TOCP during prohibition in the USA, and after contamination in Morocco of cooking oil by aircraft lubricating oil. TOCP causes distal degeneration of peripheral nerves, particularly affecting the longest and largest fibers; long fiber tracts in the cord are also involved. Degeneration gradually progresses towards the parent cell body. It has been suggested that this 'dying back' type of neuropathy is caused by impairment of perikaryon metabolism whose affects are most marked upon the largest and longest fibers. Experimental studies with another organophosphorous compound, di-isopropyl fluorophosphonate (DFP) however, have shown focal and non-terminal fiber changes which suggest a direct affect upon the axon rather than on the perikaryon.

Microbiological and plant-derived neurotoxins

Botulism is caused by intoxication of the protein neurotoxin produced by the organism *Clostridium botulinum.* Food-borne botulism is caused by ingestion of a neurotoxin preformed in foods contaminated with the organism. The illness is now relatively rare in most developed countries. However, there are cases that continue to be reported, largely caused by home-processed food or improperly cooked or uncooked meat. Botulinum toxins block transmission at cholinergic synapses by preventing the release of acetyl choline. There is neither an effect on the production of impulses along the axon into the presynaptic terminal node nor the excitability of muscle fibers in cells. Morphological studies demonstrate binding of labeled toxin to presynaptic membranes. Wound botulinum is now very rare and occurs when wounds become contaminated by the micro-organism.

Despite a widespread immunization program, *tetanus* continues to occur and has a high mortality. The toxin is a protein produced by *Clostridium tetani,* the primary clinical manifestations of which are caused by a blockade of inhibitory input to spinal motor neurons. The toxin probably gains access via retrograde axonal transport along the nerve fibers and perhaps along the endoneurium as well, originating at the portal of entry. The effects of the toxin may remain localized to the motor neuron pool supplying the affected muscles (local tetanus), e.g. 'lock jaw' or 'risus sardonicus'; however, the effects become generalized if enough toxin is present to enter the bloodstream and affect the nervous system diffusely, resulting in generalized muscle spasm.

Diphtheria is now an uncommon illness in most parts of the world as a result of widespread active immunization. It is due to a protein neurotoxin released by *Corynebacterium diphtheria,* which is believed to act by preventing the elongation of polypeptide chains. The condition may be life threatening because of either the local pharyngeal infection or systemic intoxication, which primarily affects the heart and nervous system. The predilection of diphtheria toxin for the peripheral nervous system is unexplained, but it has been shown to inhibit synthesis of myelin proteolipids and basic proteins, causing a segmental demyelinating neuropathy.

In 1987 in the maritime provinces of Canada there was an outbreak of *domoic acid* intoxication, a potent structural analogue of glutamate which had been concentrated in mussels. Neuropathological findings included neuronal loss in the hippocampus, thalamus and cerebral cortex.

Lathyrism occurs when large amounts of the seeds of *Lathyrus* are eaten, usually at times of drought and famine. The characteristic clinical features are spastic paraplegia, which neuropathologically is due to symmetrical degeneration of the corticospinal tract. The substance at present considered most likely to be responsible is β-*N*-oxalylamino-L-alanine (BOAA), the neurotoxicity of which is similar to another plant-derived amino acid, L-β-methylaminoalanine (BMAA).

Animal poisons

Bites and stings by venomous animals include those from snakes, spiders, scorpions, jelly fish, bees and wasps. It has been estimated that about 100 000 persons per year die from envenomation, the peripheral signs and symptoms of which result from the action of three major groups of toxins: *viz.* post-synaptically active neurotoxins that bind to acetycholine receptors at the neuromuscular junction thus blocking neuromuscular transmission; presynaptically active neurotoxins that bind to motor nerve, and cause the delayed degeneration of the motor nerve terminal; and myotoxic agents such as the phospholipases A_2 that may result in acute renal failure. Other syndromes include *tick paralysis* and *seafood poisoning.*

NEUROTOXIC METALS

More than 25 metals can be detected in human tissues, but of these only 13 are considered to be 'essential'. The deficiency of certain of these essential elements may lead to neurological dysfunction, the basis of which is often the absence of the metal in critical metallo-enzymes, loss of stabilization in membranes or impaired release of neurotransmitters. On the other hand, certain of the essential and non-essential metals, if given in sufficient concentration and appropriate form, are known to be toxic, affecting multiple systems in the body, including the nervous system.

Aluminum

Aluminum was for a long time considered to be a non-absorbable, non-toxic element, the health hazard of which was restricted to the occupational inhalation of aluminum-contaminated dust. In recent years, however, it has been implicated as an etiological factor in *dialysis encephalopathy* (see Chapter 10, page 208). The source of the increased levels of aluminum in the brains of these patients was originally identified as the aluminum-containing phosphate binders. Later studies have suggested there is a relationship between the encephalopathy and the aluminum content in the water used to prepare the dialysis fluid.

At one time aluminum was implicated as a factor in the pathogenesis of dementia of Alzheimer type (see Chapter 17). The neurofibrillary tangles that can be produced in experimental animals by aluminum, however, are quite different electron microscopically from the paired helical filaments seen in the naturally occurring Alzheimer's neurofibrillary tangles in humans; furthermore, senile plaques, granulovacuolor degeneration and amyloid angiopathy are not seen. The significance of the increased amounts of aluminum in the brain is also uncertain, as accumulations of this element take place with increasing age. The predominant current opinion is that aluminum is not causal in Alzheimer's disease.

Arsenic

Toxicity can be caused by exposure to a variety of arsenic-based compounds such as pesticides, mordents, paints, wood preservatives and medical agents. Inorganic and organic arsenical compounds may be toxic.

Inorganic arsenic

Acute inorganic arsenic poisoning manifests first as a gastrointestinal disturbance, and thereafter by circulatory collapse, and hepatic and renal failure. There may then be a transient encephalopathy. Peripheral neuropathy is a well-known and often disabling sequel of both acute and chronic arsenic intoxication. Occupational exposure to inorganic arsenic occurs mainly in the smelting industry and in the manufacture and application of arsenic-based pesticides. Patients with mild sensory-motor disturbances recover completely and quickly, but recovery from an acute attack or after cessation of exposure during chronic poisoning may take as long as three years, and residual disability is to be expected in those severely affected initially. Nerve biopsy shows axonal degeneration with regeneration after acute exposure and demyelination with chronic exposure.

Organic arsenic

Organoarsenic toxicity in the form of an *acute hemorrhagic encephalopathy* was a serious complication of the treatment of syphilis with organic arsenicals (arsenobenzene derivatives). The problem was recognized soon after the introduction of arsphenamine and its wide use in the 1930s and 1940s, about 10% of patients developing an acute neurological illness. It is currently a major problem in the treatment of human African trypanosomiasis ('sleeping sickness'). The clinical onset of organoarsenic encephalopathy is rapid, and the mortality rate is over 50%. At post mortem there are multiple hemorrhages of varying size, particularly in the white matter of the brain. Autopsy shows varying degrees of endothelial damage and occasional thrombi in venules and capillaries: perivascular infiltrates are rare (Fig. 13.5a and b). There may be focal demyelination. The pathogenesis of this condition is unclear, though a direct toxic effect of arsphenamine on the endothelial cells is possible. There are, however, similarities between arsphenamine encephalopathy and acute hemorrhagic leukoencephalopathy (see Chapter 9). There is, however, no evidence that organoarsenic encephalopathy is an immune response, and it seems more likely that, particularly with trivalent forms of arsenic, the encephalopathy is related to the binding of arsenic to thiol groups.

Lead

There is no known biological requirement for lead and it must therefore be viewed purely as a toxicant. Lead poisoning has afflicted humans since antiquity, and although many of the occupational and domestic environmental sources have been eliminated or reduced, raised blood levels still occur in large numbers of children, especially among lower socioeconomic groups. Lead can enter the body through the gastrointestinal and respiratory tracts and occasionally through the skin: many systems of the body are affected adversely by an excessive amount of lead. Most modern-day exposure is from industrial sources in the manufacture of organo-leads, such as fuel additives, or the manufacture of lead-based pigments, solder or batteries. There is also a potential source from deteriorating housing with lead furnishings and lead-based paints. It is also a consequence of the consumption of lead-contaminated alcohol.

Inorganic lead poisoning

The systemic pathological features of *plumbism* include basophil stippling of red cells, lead lines in the metaphases of long bones in children, and

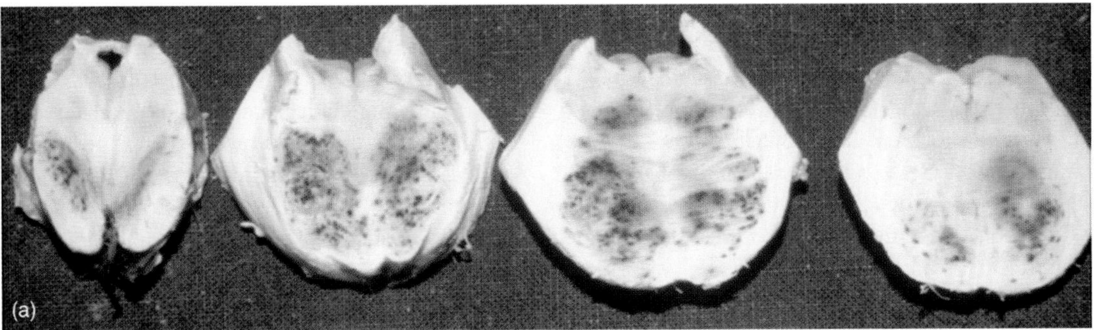

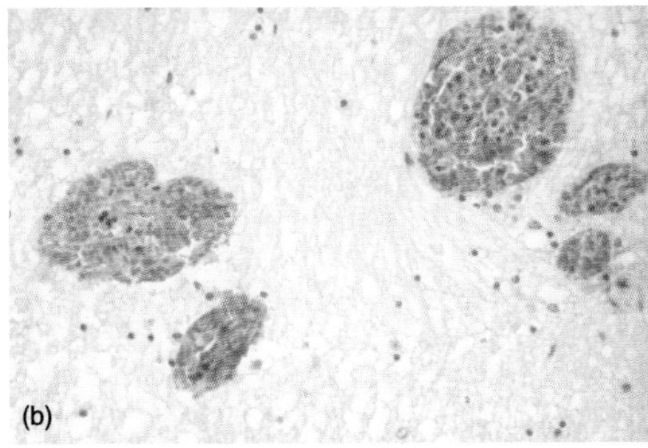

Figure 13.5 Organoarsenic intoxication. Patient was treated for sleeping sickness (trypanosomiasis). (a) Multiple hemorrhages in the brainstem. (b) Confirmation of petechial hemorrhage formation in the pons. (b) H&E.

lead-containing intranuclear inclusion bodies in the proximal tubules of the kidneys. By contrast, the changes in the CNS in acute lead encephalopathy are less specific. There may be generalized swelling of the brain, diffuse vascular congestion, and petechial hemorrhages in both gray and white matter. Histologically, capillaries may be dilated, necrotic or occluded by thrombus, and around many there is a protein-rich exudate that stains positively with PAS which often appears as discreet perivascular PAS positive droplets, which appear to be within astrocytic processes. A similar proteinaceous exudate may also be seen in the meninges. Endothelial proliferation and/or enlargement also occurs, and from within the affected areas there are enlarged astrocytes, and changes in neurons that are difficult to distinguish from hypoxia and macrophages. These changes are particularly marked in the cerebellum: they are more frequently seen and severe in children than in adults. Experimental studies suggest that lead causes selective damage to capillary endothelial cells. Developing blood vessels appear to be particularly susceptible. Recent evidence suggests that there is an association between chronic lead poisoning and mineralization of the dentate nuclei of the cerebellum (see Chapter 10).

Of contemporary concern is the possibility of subclinical neurological manifestations of lead toxicity and, in particular, potential consequences of low-level lead exposure on mental development of infants and children. Certainly, there are clinical studies that suggest a correlation between undue lead burdens during the post-natal period, and learning and behavior disorders. The potential for low levels of lead to cause latent brain dysfunction or minimal brain damage is a contentious issue, possible sources for the lead being the breathing of vehicular exhaust fumes and ingestion of domestic water conveyed in lead pipes. The biochemical basis for lead toxicity and neurotoxicity is not known, although there is some evidence that lead affects enzymes involved in oxidative phosphorylation and in heme formation, and that lead possibly replacing such biologically important divalent cations as calcium. It is also known that lead, by its inhibition of aminolevulinic acid dehydrogenase, creates a pool of *δ-aminolevulinic acid* which, because of its structural similarity to *γ-aminobutyric acid* (*GABA*), may act as a putative neurotransmitter. Other proposed mechanisms of lead encephalopathy are related to the effects of the vasculopathy.

Peripheral neuropathy is now an uncommon manifestation of lead neurotoxicity in the adult. Before improvements in industrial conditions, however, lead caused a remarkably pure motor neuropathy, often selectively severe in the radial nerve. Experimental studies show species variation in the type of neuropathy: guinea pigs and rats generally develop demyelination, whereas in rabbits an axonal type of neuropathy occurs. In humans the neuropathy appears to be of demyelinating type. Endoneurial edema is a conspicuous feature of lead neuropathy.

Organic lead

Organolead poisoning is usually due to either tetraethyl or tetramethyl lead compounds, which are either inhaled or absorbed through the skin. Most cases of organolead toxicity are industrial, exposure occurring in workers wearing inadequate protective clothing when cleaning out petrol storage tanks when tetraethyl lead had been added to the petrol as an anti-knock agent. This is no longer the case. Acute toxicity is characterized by brain swelling, congestion and petechial hemorrhages. Repeated episodes of acute organolead toxicity are the basis of chronic petrol-sniffing encephalopathy, in which the neuropathological findings are similar to those seen in acute encephalopathy with the additional feature of atrophy of the cerebellar folia. In experimental studies, neuronal loss has been identified in neurons and in the limbic system. Unlike inorganic lead, organic lead does not damage capillaries or myelin.

Manganese

This is an occupational hazard of mining and processing of manganese-containing ores. Manganese is absorbed through the lungs and may induce psychiatric disturbances ('*manganese madness*') and a parkinsonian-like extrapyramidal dysfunction. Once the chronic stage develops, the neurological dysfunction is irreversible, the cessation of exposure at this stage does stop the progression of the disease. In patients with an extrpyramidal syndrome, there is neuronal loss in the lentiform and subthalamic nuclei and, to a lesser extent, in the substantia nigra. Both the clinical and pathological features identified in man can be reproduced in experimental animals. Biochemical studies suggest that, at high concentrations, manganese ions act as powerful synaptic transmitter inhibitors producing the release of norepinephrine from synaptic nerve endings and the release of acetylcholine at the neuromuscular junction. PET shows preservation of presynaptic and postsynaptic nigrostriatal dopaminergic function.

Mercury

Together with lead and cadmium, mercury is among the most toxic of the heavy metals. It is used in a large number of industrial processes and, depending upon its form, has many commercial uses. The organic compounds, such as methyl mercury and ethyl mercury, have biocidal properties, methyl mercury being a cheap and effective fungicide. Inorganic mercury is a waste product of some industrial processes, most notably in the manufacture of paper and in the chloralkaline industry. Factory effluent is sometimes discharged into nearby rivers or into the sea. Some micro-organisms in water have the capacity to convert inorganic mercury salts into methyl mercury salts, these compounds then enter the food chain and accumulate in fish to an extent that, if eaten, they become toxic to humans or animals. Mercury is still used as a preservative in childhood vaccines, but is not considered to be in amounts that are harmful.

Inorganic mercury poisoning

Acute mercury poisoning is characterized clinically by gastrointestinal disturbances and acute renal failure. On the other hand, neurotoxicity is a prominent manifestation of chronic inorganic mercury poisoning, initial symptoms often consisting of bizarre behavioral changes called 'erethism'. Occasionally, patients develop a peripheral neuropathy, which is also one of the major manifestations of 'pink disease'; this disorder is thought to result from chronic mercury poisoning from teething powders and antihelminthic agents. It is also now thought to be a potential danger to dentists preparing amalgam for filling teeth. There is atrophy of the cerebellum, with a loss of granule cells and some Purkinje cells.

Organomercury poisoning

Cases are generally due to methyl mercury or ethyl mercury intoxication. Methyl mercury is a fungicide that is particularly useful in treating wheat seeds to produce a healthy crop. The first recognized outbreak of disease due to methyl mercury resulted from industrial effluent and occurred in Minamata in Japan in the early 1950s; 56 people were affected, of whom one third died. There was also an episode of poisoning in Iraq in 1971, where over 6000 people were affected and at least 500 died when treated wheat seed was mistakenly eaten. There is a triad of clinical signs which is unique to adults with methyl mercury poisoning, namely, parasthesia around the mouth and in the extremities, ataxia and concentric constriction of the visual field. Congenital methyl mercury neurotoxicity may occur from exposure *in utero,* affected children then presenting with psychomotor retardation. Whatever the route of administration, the neuropathological changes are consistent, comprising severe focal atrophy in the calcarine cortex, precentral cortex, and less severe atrophy in the postcentral and temporal cortex. In these areas there is neuronal loss especially from the outer cortical layers, and astrocytosis. The cerebellar cortex is always affected, there being selective loss of granule cells, particularly in the depths of sulci. Purkinje cells are usually spared but axonal swelling (torpedoes) may develop. There is an astrocytosis.

In experimental studies on organic and inorganic mercury neurotoxicity, similar ultrastructural changes affecting ribosomes are found, suggesting a common mechanism of toxic action affecting protein synthesis. The possible mechanism is impaired phosphorylation of uridine, leading to inhibition of RNA synthesis.

Thallium

The use of thallium sulfate as a rodenticide and ant killer presents the most serious hazard of accidental, suicidal and homicidal poisoning. Clinical effects are dose-dependent. A single large dose in rodents may cause death due to gastroenteritis, shock and dehydration; smaller doses result in a peripheral neuropathy associated with severe pain and extreme restlessness. An early and characteristic sign is dark pigmentation of hair roots, followed some weeks later by alopecia. The mode of action of thallium is uncertain but, like other metals, it may combine with sulfhydryl compounds. Neuropathologically, in acute cases there is cerebral swelling and, with survival, there is a peripheral neuropathy and chromatolysis of motor neurons.

Tin

Inorganic tin is not known to be neurotoxic. Of the many organotin compounds known, only two have *neurotoxic* properties. The neurotoxicity of tri-ethyl tin became only too evident in the early 1950s as a result of an outbreak of metal intoxication in France. A total of 290 people were poisoned and 110 died after using an oil preparation containing diethyltin iodide. At autopsy there was diffuse swelling on the white matter of the cerebral hemisphere. Histologically, there is a characteristic form of intramyelinic edema due to separation of the myelin lamellate at the intraperiod line. In long-term exposure, demyelination may occur in association with reactive astrocytosis. Experimental studies have established that peripheral nerve myelin is less susceptible to vacuolation than is central myelin.

Intoxication with *trimethyl tin* produces an entirely different type of brain damage. Unlike triethyl tin, trimethyl is not myelotoxic, but mainly causes neuronal loss in the pyriform cortex, specific regions of the hippocampal formation and the amygdaloid nuclei.

DRUGS AND DIAGNOSTIC AGENTS

The principal drug-induced neurological syndromes are detailed in Table 13.2 and include confusion–delirium, seizures, movement disorders

Table 13.2 Principal drug-induced neurological syndromes

Confusion–delirium
- Anticholinergics
- Anticonvulsants
- Antimicrobials: isoniazid, rifampicin
- Antineoplastics: vincristine
- Dopamine agonists
- Tranquillizers

Seizures
- Antidepressants
- Antimicrobials: cycloserine, isoniazid, penicillin, metronidazole
- Antineoplastics: vincristine, methotrexate
- Analgesics: fentanyl, opiates
- Anesthetics: ketamine, halothane
- Sympathomimetics

Movement disorders
- Antiemetics: metoclopramide
- Butyrophenones: haloperidol
- Dopamine agonists
- Phenothiazines: chlorpromazine
- Tricyclic antidepressants

Ataxia
- Anticonvulsants: phenytoin, primidone, carbamazepine
- Antineoplastics: cytosine arabinoside, fluoracil
- Phenothiazines; sedatives: barbiturates, chloral hydrate

Eye and cranial nerve damage
- Retinopathy
- Antimalarials: choroquine, mepacrine
- Optic neuritis
- Antimicrobials: dapsone, isoniazid, streptomycin
- VIII cranial nerve damage
- Aminoglycoside antibiotics: gentamicin, kanamycin, neomycin, streptomycin

Peripheral neuropathy
- Antimicrobials: ethambutol, isoniazid, nitrofurantoin, dapsone
- Antineoplastics: cytosine arabinoside, cisplatin, procarbazine, vincristine
- Antirheumatics: colchicine, D-penicillamine, gold, indometacin

Muscle pain and weakness
- Antineoplastics: cytosine arabinoside, methotrexate, thiotepa

and ataxia, eye and cranial nerve damage, peripheral neuropathy, muscle pain and weakness. A few examples will be discussed in more detail.

Phenytoin (diphenylhydantoin)

Manifestations of toxicity include drowsiness, nystagmus, cerebellar ataxia, encephalopathy and peripheral neuropathy. Some appear in relation to high serum drug levels and resolve when the levels are decreased. Occasionally, however, the symptoms and signs do not resolve even after withdrawal of the drug, and this has led to the longstanding controversy about the pathogenesis of the *cerebellar syndromes* attributed to atrophy in the cerebellum brought about by diffuse loss of Purkinje cells (Fig. 13.6a, left and right). Opinions differ about the role of phenytoin in their pathogenesis because the cerebellum is particularly sensitive to hypoxia, and epilepsy alone may be a cause of Purkinje cell loss. Even experimental studies of phenytoin neurotoxicity have yielded conflicting results, and although there is considerable evidence to suggest that phenytoin *per se* can cause cerebellar degeneration, no definite conclusion can be reached.

The administration of anticonvulsants, including phenytoin, to pregnant women has been implicated in the production of various congenital anomalies, namely the so-called *fetal hydantoin syndrome*: the spectrum of malformations in the CNS include hydrocephalus, microcephaly and defects in the neural tube. It is necessary, however, to consider a whole range of possibilities, such as the effects of maternal infections and possible prenatal exposure to other teratogens before directly attributing any fetal abnormalities to anticonvulsants.

Neuroleptics

Drugs such as the phenothiazines and butyropherones are important in the long-term treatment of psychosis. An untoward complication is that of *tardive dyskinesia*: this is more common in females and increases with age, the duration of treatment and with the total dose of the agent given. Neuropathological studies in these patients have shown that there is an increase in the amount of neuronal loss, satellitosis and increased neuronal lipofuscin

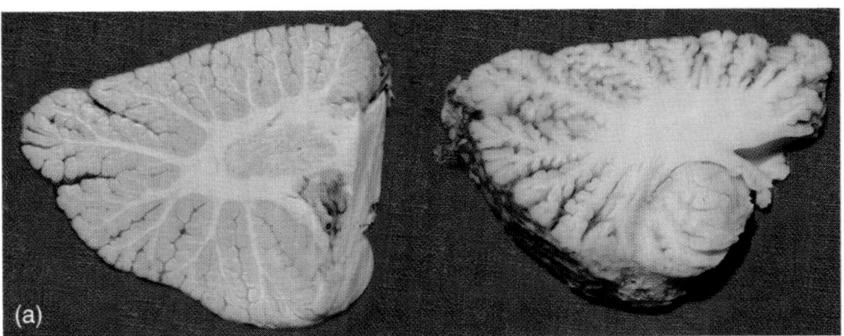

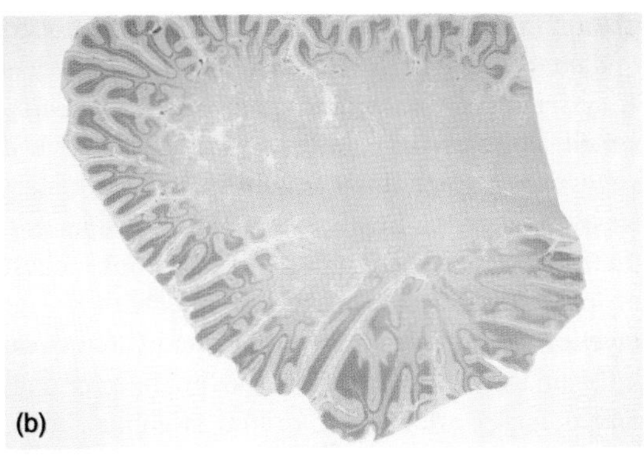

Figure 13.6 Phenytoin intoxication. (a) In comparison with the normal cerebellum on the left, there is atrophy of folia (b) Microscopy confirms the naked-eye appearances. Luxol fast blue–cresyl violet.

in the basal ganglia, substantia nigra and midbrain compared with age-matched controls.

Clioquinol

This drug has been used for many years in the treatment of intestinal amebiasis. It has also been used less discriminately for a variety of 'chronic non-specific diarrheas and traveller's diarrhea'. There is considerable circumstantial evidence that it may cause *toxic encephalopathy*, *isolated optic atrophy*, and *subacute myelo-optic neuropathy* (*SMON*). The toxic syndrome has, for reasons unknown, been restricted almost exclusively to the Japanese. Post-mortem studies in human cases of the SMON syndrome has revealed lesions in the spinal cord, spinal nerve roots, dorsal root and autonomic ganglia, optic and – less severely – peripheral nerves. There is axonal degeneration of the gracile tract and, to a lesser extent, of the spinocerebellar and distal parts of the distal corticospinal tracts of the spinal cord. Neuronal loss and proliferation of satellite cells in the dorsal ganglia, with evidence of axonal degeneration and demyelination in the posterior spinal root and the peripheral nerves, are also seen. Similar changes are seen in the optic nerve. Experimental studies have produced similar changes in the CNS and in the optic nerve. There is distal degeneration of centrally directed fibers and dorsal root ganglia cells, with sparing of peripheral fibers.

Antibiotics, antiviral and antifungal agents

The antibacterial agents *dapsone*, *nitrofurantoin* and *chloramphenicol* are recognized, but are rarely causes of peripheral neuropathy in humans. On the other hand, isoniazid may cause peripheral neuropathy in some 30–40% of cases, depending on dose and genetic factors: it causes a disturbance of vitamin B_6 metabolism, which can produce distal axonal degeneration. Pyridoxine supplementation reduces the incidence of neuropathy. Neurotoxicity, manifested by ototoxicity, encephalopathy and psychosis, has also been associated with the use of *gentamicin*.

Neuropathological studies have demonstrated widespread central chromatolysis and necrosis of neurons in the brainstem of patients treated with *adenine arabinoside,* after treatment of herpes simplex encephalitis and disseminated varicella infection.

Dementia and akinetic mutism have followed the intravenous use of *amphotericin* for the treatment of fungal infections. The principal findings are diffuse cerebral encephalopathy with relative preservation of axons. Experimental studies confirm that the methyl ester of the drug is particularly neurotoxic.

Recreational drug abuse

There is an increased risk of cerebral and spinal infarction and intracerebral hemorrhage from the use of all recreational drugs. Mechanisms include drug-induced hypertension, coagulopathies, foreign body (talc) embolization, and septic emboli from infective endocarditis. Furthermore, all intravenous drug abusers are at risk of HIV infection and its complications (see Chapter 7). The principal neurological syndromes associated with more commonly used recreational drugs are given in Table 13.3.

Table 13.3 Neurological complications of recreational drug abuse

Cocaine
- Headache, tremor, myoclonus, seizures

Metamphetamine and ecstasy
- Chorea, intracranial hemorrhage

Heroin
- Myelitis, neuropathies and plexopathies

Phencyclidine
- Dystonia, athetosis, seizures, rhabdomyolysis

Anti-neoplastic agents

Various neurological complications may occur as a result of systemic or intrathecal chemotherapy with various antineoplastic agents. Of particular interest have been those associated with *methotrexate*, a widely used folic acid antagonist. Methotrexate neurotoxicity may take several forms, principal amongst which are a *chemical arachnoiditis* and a disseminated *necrotizing leukoencephalopathy* (see Chapter 8). Occasionally, the intracarotid infusion of a high dose of methotrexate has been associated with multiple hemorrhagic infarcts in the brain. Of particular concern has been the delayed encephalopathies which most often follow a combination of high-dose, long-term systemic and/or intrathecal methotrexate therapy, and cranial irradiation in children with leukemia. Several patterns of damage have been identified. The best known is a *disseminated necrotizing leukoencephalopathy* which consists of multiple well-circumscribed yellowish-gray granular lesions in the white matter of the cerebral hemispheres, the brainstem and the spinal cord. Histologically, the lesions consist of focal areas of coagulative necrosis with loss of myelin, axons and oligodendrocytes. There is no inflammatory cell infiltrate and lipid-containing macrophages are sparse. Axonal swellings, some of which may be mineralized, are frequently seen at the periphery of the lesions in association with vacuolation of the white matter and a reactive astrocytosis (Chapter 8). In many cases there are no vascular changes but in some there is fibrinoid necrosis of small blood vessels. The etiology of this condition is unknown, as most patients with necrotizing leukoencephalopathy have received both methotrexate and irradiation to the CNS. The neuropathological features, however, are not those typically associated with radiation necrosis; it may be that the radiation, by damaging the blood–brain barrier, permits methotrexate to diffuse into the brain to produce damage to white matter. Milder cases of encephalopathy have also been described in which there is imaging evidence of cerebral atrophy, with ventricular dilation and intracerebral calcification.

Acute encephalopathies, degeneration of the cerebellum and necrotizing encephalomyelopathy have all been described after treatment with various antineoplastic agents that include *cytosine arabinoside, 5-fluorouracil, hydrogen mustard, cyclophosphamide* and various *nitrosourea compounds.* On the other hand, the *vinca alkaloids, vincristine and vinblastine*, which are mitotic spindle inhibitors, are particularly associated with peripheral neuropathy. A rare complication of vincristine neurotoxicity is myeloencephalopathy, when it has been accidentally administered intrathecally. Histologically, there are marked changes in the neurons of the brainstem and spinal cord, consisting of large amounts of interwoven neurofilaments with loss of microtubules and the formation of crystalline masses. The changes have been attributed to the action of the alkaloids on microtubule protein (tubulin) and consequent changes in axoplasmic transport.

CHAPTER 14

DEVELOPMENTAL AND PERINATAL DISORDERS

Jeanne E Bell and Jean W Keeling

PRACTICAL ASPECTS OF REMOVING AND EXAMINING THE IMMATURE CENTRAL NERVOUS SYSTEM

Introduction

Removal of the brain in the fetus, neonate and infant needs to be carried out with particular care. At this stage, the brain is frequently very soft for three reasons: firstly, myelination is poorly advanced; secondly, hypoxic stress may have been present for hours or even days prior to death; and, thirdly, in many fetal deaths, softening attributable to maceration will supervene during the period between death and refrigeration after delivery. In early life the dural membrane is closely applied to the skull and fused with fibrous sutures. The dural folds may be damaged during delivery. All of these factors necessitate a different approach to removal of the developing brain.

Scalp

The head circumference and biparietal diameter are recorded. The presence of any scalp injury is noted. The scalp is reflected following incision from behind the ear, curving upwards and medially over the posterior fontanelle and down behind the opposite ear. This incision makes reconstruction easier and, in most cases, the incision line will not be noticed by the family at any subsequent viewing.

The scalp is reflected forwards as far as the nasion so that the reflected skin is well clear of the inferior part of the frontal bone. Posteriorly the skin is reflected to the level of the cervical spine. The atlanto-occipital membrane is incised, following which gentle pressure on the parietal bones will allow inspection of the cerebrospinal fluid (CSF). If the fluid is blood stained, or if meningitis is suspected, a sample of CSF should be aspirated through the atlanto-occipital membrane at this stage of the post mortem examination. This sample can be submitted for microbiology or examined for xanthochromia in cases of injury. Caudal displacement of the cerebellar tonsils is noted if present and the cervico-medullary junction is divided.

Skull

The skull bones are inspected for fracture or abnormal development. The size of the fontanelles and the width of sutures is observed. Both will be enlarged when the intracranial pressure is raised. The anterior fontanelles may be small when brain volume is unduly low. The skull is best opened by a modified Beneke technique (Fig. 14.1). The anterior fontanelle is incised parasagittally on both sides.

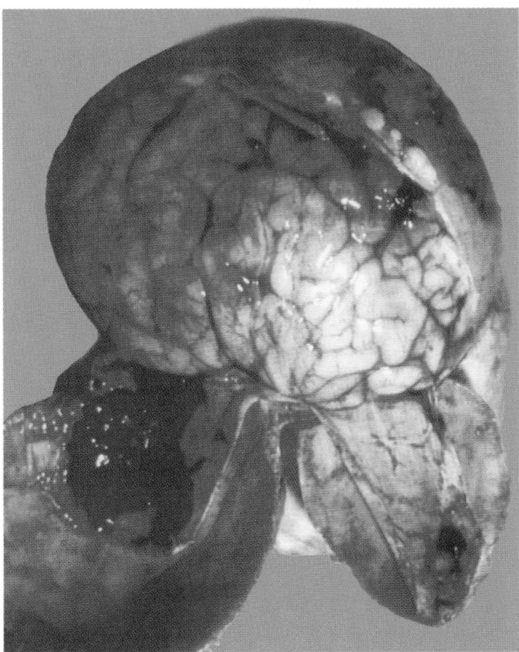

Figure 14.1 Cranial cavity of a 1-month-old child, opened by the Beneke technique. The frontal and parietal bone flaps are seen in the lower part of the field. There is evidence of subdural bleeding on the dura mater lining the parietal bone.

With tapered, rounded scissors, this incision is extended forwards towards the nasion, taking care not to damage the sagittal sinus. The frontoparietal suture line is divided, then the original incision is extended posteriorly to the posterior fontanelle and the parieto-occipital suture line is opened. The parietal flap is reflected and the surface of the brain examined for hemorrhage. The complexity of the gyral pattern is observed. The head is tipped forwards so that one occipital pole can be gently elevated to expose the posterior falx and tentorium which are examined for injury. The occipital pole is gently replaced. This procedure is repeated on the other side. Right-handed prosectors will find it easier to approach the left side first.

The sagittal sinus is divided anteriorly, the sinus and attached falx pulled backwards and cut through at the posterior fontanelle. It is convenient to remove the brain directly into a pre-weighed container of fixative, which is not a problem with a down draught table. An assistant supports the body and steadies the head by holding the scalp. The prosector lowers the occipital bones into the fixative so that the hemispheres are half submerged. The head is tipped backwards to expose the first and second cranial nerves. The former are detached from the skull base, the latter divided. The head is progressively tipped so that nerve and vascular connections are divided sequentially, the hemispheres being supported by the fixative and not by the prosector's fingers. The tentorium is incised on either side and the posterior fossa contents are eased out using a scalpel handle. The base of the skull is inspected and the pituitary removed.

The Circle of Willis is fragile in the very young. Saturating the formalin with sodium chloride will keep the brain afloat but may affect microscopic appearances. The brain is optimally fixed for 2–4 weeks but even overnight fixation is preferable to slicing the unfixed brain of an infant.

When the fetus is macerated, the periosteum over the skull vault bones can be incised and skull bones lifted off. The brain can be removed within the dura. Histological examination of such cases is often rewarding despite the discolored, semi-liquefied state of the brain tissue.

Spinal cord

The spinal cord is readily approached anteriorly in early life. Subsequent reconstruction is quicker. A lower lumbar cartilage is incised and the pedicles are divided on each side with heavy scissors or bone cutting forceps. The spinal canal is large and cord damage is unlikely. Nerve roots are divided sequentially as far laterally as possible. The filum terminale is divided and elevated and the cord eased out, cutting any tethering blood vessels with a small scalpel. The cord is laid out on firm card, allowed to adhere for two or three minutes and fixed with the brain.

Yates' method for examination of the cervical spinal cord

This method permits examination of the cervical spinal cord with its membranous and bony coverings intact, together with the vertebral arteries. It is the method of choice when trauma is suspected. Clinical indications are difficult forceps or breech delivery. The pathologist should consider using it when there is no intracranial pathology in a mature baby who was unresponsive at birth. It can also be adapted following trauma to a different spinal region.

Following brain removal and neck and thoracic evisceration, the cartilage at C8/T1 or T1/T2 is divided together with the spinal cord, cartilage and muscle attachments back to the paraspinal muscle. The spinal block is freed by dissecting off the muscles laterally and posteriorly working in a cephalad direction. The freed block is fixed for at least a week, decalcified and cut horizontally into slices of 2–3 mm. These are arranged sequentially, examined with a magnifying lens looking for hemorrhage and injury to the cord, arteries and joints. Arterial dissection or thrombosis is found in only a small minority. Joint damage, hemorrhage and cord infarction are more likely findings. Any abnormality is photographed and those slices processed whole for microscopy. The body can be reconstituted using any stiffening material appropriate for the size of the infant.

Examination of the brain *in situ* offers the best opportunity of observing the pathology of encephaloceles, Dandy–Walker malformation (Fig. 14.2), Chiari malformations and of hydrocephalus. Careful removal of the coverings of the central nervous system (CNS), particularly at the level of the foramen magnum, reveals abnormal displacement and cystic dilation of brain structures which may be no longer apparent once the brain has been removed and fixed (Fig. 14.2). Photography of structures *in situ* is extremely helpful. If a spina bifida lesion is present, photography, X-ray examination and removal of the affected region of the vertebral column to include the open or covered lesion, all help to delineate the neuropathology accurately.

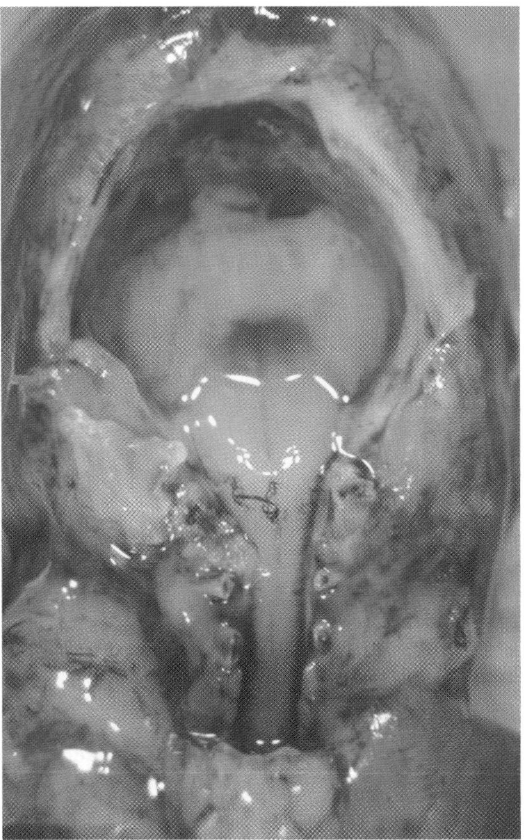

Figure 14.2 The occipital bone has been removed in a fetus of approximately 19 weeks gestation to display the posterior fossa contents. There is a Dandy–Walker malformation with upward displacement of the cerebellum and an open fourth ventricle. The actual cyst has been de-roofed in removing the occipital bone.

Removal in forensic cases

If the cause of death is not established by the end of the systemic, non-CNS examination in an infant who has died suddenly, the brain should be fixed in formalin for a minimum of 1–2 days and preferably for 2 weeks or more prior to sampling. The presence of subdural hemorrhage (Fig. 14.1) should be recorded with photographs. If hemorrhage has been detected in the retina, it may be necessary to retain the globes in fixative. Detailed protocols and guidelines have been published for the investigation of sudden unexpected death in infancy. In this controversial area of forensic pediatric neuropathology, detailed examination, objective reporting and evidence gathering, as well as further research, is mandatory.

NORMAL AND ABNORMAL CENTRAL NERVOUS SYSTEM DEVELOPMENT

Development of the CNS

The CNS is formed from the neural tube, the development of which is induced by the notochord. The

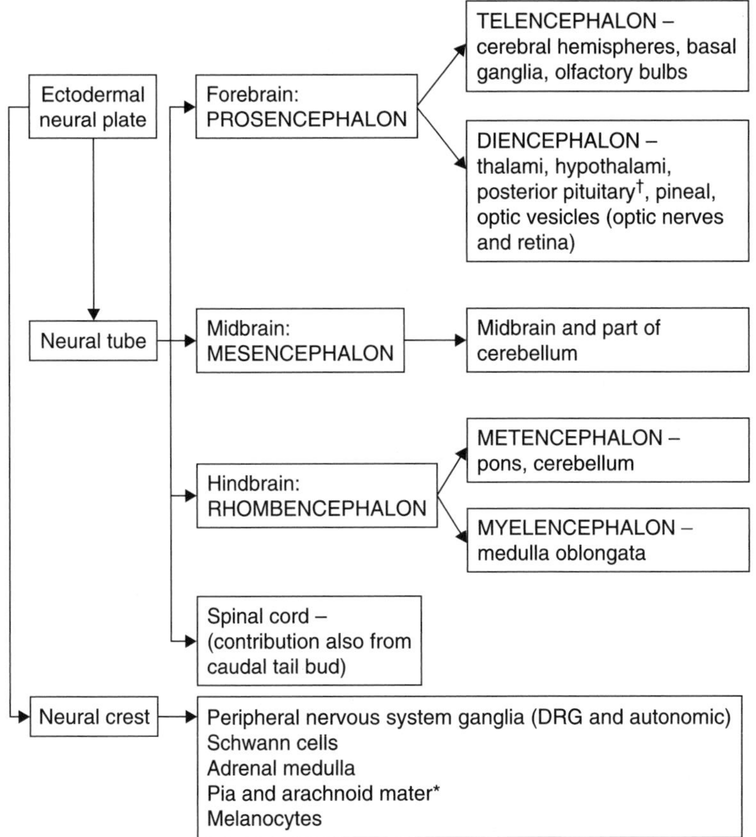

Figure 14.3 Derivatives of the neural tube. † Anterior pituitary develops from the roof of the mouth. * Dura mater is a mesodermal derivative. DRG = dorsal root ganglia.

neural tube closes first in the centre and subsequently at cranial and caudal ends. The stages of nervous system development are shown in Fig. 14.3. During closure of the neural tube the dorsolateral lip of neuroectoderm is sequestered on each side between the closing tube and the overlying ectoderm, giving rise to the neural crest from which develops the peripheral nervous system. The most caudal portion of the spinal cord is derived from the caudal tail bud rather than the neural tube proper.

The neural tube is normally closed by the end of the fourth week of development. The wall of the tube increases in thickness due to mitosis in neuroectodermal cells, particularly in the cells lining the tube, the so-called germinal zone (Fig. 14.4). Newly born cells move outwards from the lumen and this movement is facilitated by the presence of radial glia which are among the earliest cells to appear and which span the thickening wall of the neural tube (Fig. 14.5). The first wave of migrating cells forms a two layer zone outside the ventricular zone, made up of an outer layer of Cajal–Retzius cells adjacent to the pia mater and an inner layer, the subplate, which is adjacent to the ventricular zone. During the first half of gestation the majority of developing cells are destined to become nerve cells. Many of these neuroblasts move outwards from the germinal matrix in successive waves of migration along the radial glia. In the developing brain the later born neuroblasts move past earlier migrants to take up their position at the surface, only to be buried beneath later arrivals until migration is complete. The developing cortex is normally confined between the original Cajal–Retzius cell layer and the inner subplate and is arranged ultimately in six layers. The outward migration of neuroblasts is arrested by a protein, reelin, expressed by the Cajal–Retzius cells. In the brain, gray matter containing the neuronal cell bodies lies at the surface while the white matter, made up of tracts of

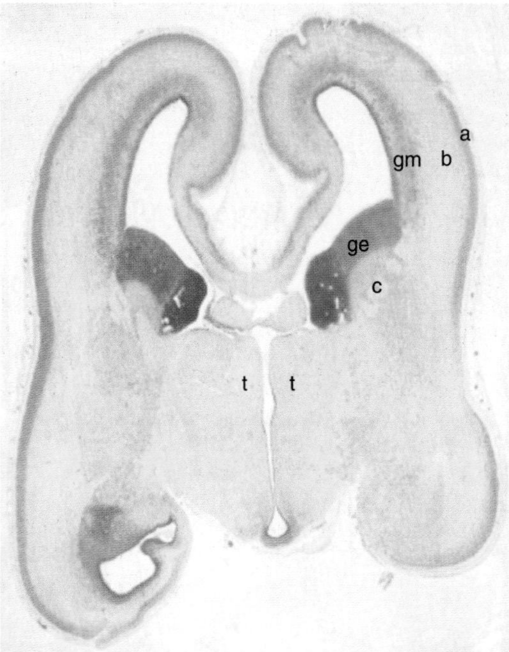

Figure 14.4 Coronal slice of a normal fetal brain at 15 weeks' gestation. The layers of the cerebral hemispheres are displayed including cortex (a), intermediate zone (b) and germinal matrix (gm). The germinal eminence (ge) overlies the developing caudate nucleus (c). The thalami (t) lie either side of the lateral ventricle and are comparatively well developed.

Figure 14.5 Section of fetal cerebral hemisphere at 15 weeks gestation showing radial glia traversing the wall. The radial glia are positive for glial fibrillary acidic protein, ×200.

neuronal processes, is more deeply placed. This arrangement is reversed in the spinal cord where neuroblasts remain close to the germinal zone, their processes forming the peripherally placed white matter. Not all neuronal migration occurs in a radial pattern. Neuroblasts destined to become inhibitory interneurons migrate from the germinal eminence (Fig. 14.4) in a tangential manner, using developing neuronal processes as a scaffold for route finding. These inhibitory neurons ultimately secrete somatostatin, calbindin and calretinin.

The cerebellar cortex shows a different pattern of development with surface tangential migration followed by centripetal migration of neuroblasts to the internal granular layer.

On completing their migration, nerve cells differentiate by developing axonal processes and dendritic trees, establishing specialized contacts and secreting a variety of neurotransmitters. Many prospective nerve cells fail to fully differentiate and die by apoptosis during development. It has been estimated that approximately half of the original neuroblasts are lost in this way. Despite this massive cell loss, the brain ultimately possesses a huge number and variety of neurons.

In the second half of gestation most of the cells arising in the germinal matrix are destined to become glial cells, both astrocytes and oligodendrocytes. These cells have important functions in the mature nervous system and share some properties with neurons, reminiscent of their common origin from neuroectodermal cells. Astrocytes form complex associations, both structural and functional, with neurons and with blood vessels. Oligodendrocytes serve to wrap and insulate axonal processes, forming myelin sheaths in relation to larger axons.

Microglia make up another major component cell type of the CNS. These cells are not derived from the neuroectoderm but from the bone marrow, arriving in the CNS with the blood vessels which penetrate the developing neural tube at an early stage of development. These immigrant cells give rise to the long lived parenchymal microglia of the brain which do not participate in ongoing exchange with blood-derived cells. In contrast, perivascular microglia continue to undergo slow turnover with blood monocytes throughout life.

Until recently it was held that because fully differentiated neurons cannot divide, their replacement following loss for whatever cause was not possible. In the last few years it has become evident that the mature brain does retain a quota of neuronal stem cells which are found predominantly around the lateral ventricle in the temporal lobe. There is evidence that radial glial cells may persist as neural stem cells, whereas at one time they were thought to differentiate only into mature astrocytes. The functional capacities of neuronal stem cells, both in regard to normal CNS upkeep and in potential repair of injury, are only beginning to be understood.

The original neural tube cavity gives rise ultimately to the ventricular system of the brain, lined by ependymal cells which are derived from residual neuroectoderm. In the spinal cord the central cavity is frequently occluded and may disappear in adult life. The choroid plexuses are formed by invaginations of ependyma with vascular stroma derived from the mesoderm surrounding the neural tube. The fetal choroid plexus epithelium is glycogen-rich leading to striking vacuolation of cells in the first and second trimester.

The arrangement of brain gyri and sulci in the fully mature fetus should be recognizably similar to an adult brain although the brain is far from mature in other ways. In infants born prematurely, the brain appears very different in terms of gyral development. At 24 weeks, the brain surface is almost entirely smooth apart from the Sylvian fissure since gyral development is maximal in the third trimester (Fig. 14.6). At this stage the cortical ribbon is also generally smooth in section although artefacts such as cortical tufting may lead to a mistaken diagnosis of polymicrogyria. Judgements of abnormalities such as heterotopias are also much more difficult at these early stages of development. The germinal matrix is more prominent in the second trimester reflecting an earlier phase of cell migration. This highly cellular zone contains very thin walled and poorly supported blood vessels which are prone to hemorrhage if the immature infant has respiratory difficulties (Fig. 14.6).

The brain is poorly myelinated at birth and cell differentiation is incomplete. Myelination is largely complete by three years of age. Perivascular foci of migrating undifferentiated cells are often to be seen in the deep white matter where they are sometimes mistaken for inflammatory cells (Fig. 14.7). The cerebellar cortex is also immature and the folia display a surface layer of undifferentiated, pre-migratory cells called the external granular layer, which does not disappear until sometime during the second year after birth (Fig. 14.8). The developing leptomeninges are more vascular than in adult life and the subarachnoid space contains many more cells, mostly

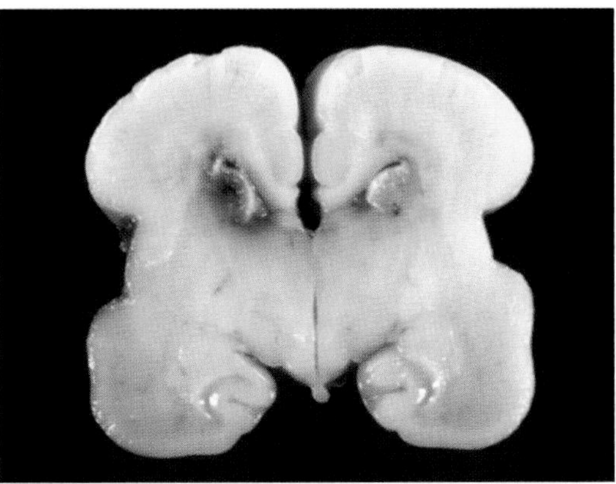

Figure 14.6 Coronal brain slice from an infant born at 23 weeks' gestation who survived for 10 days. At this stage there is very little gyral development and the cerebral hemisphere is smooth. An organizing subependymal hemorrhage is present in the germinal matrix, particularly on the left side.

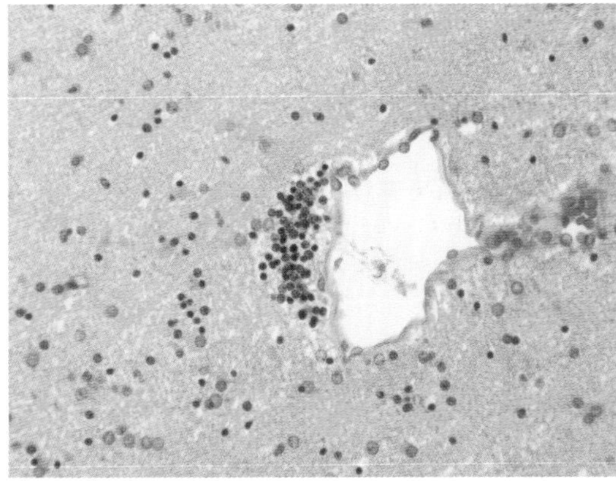

Figure 14.7 Section from the central white matter of a fetus of 38 weeks' gestation showing a clump of undifferentiated migrating cells alongside a small parenchymal blood vessel. H&E, ×200.

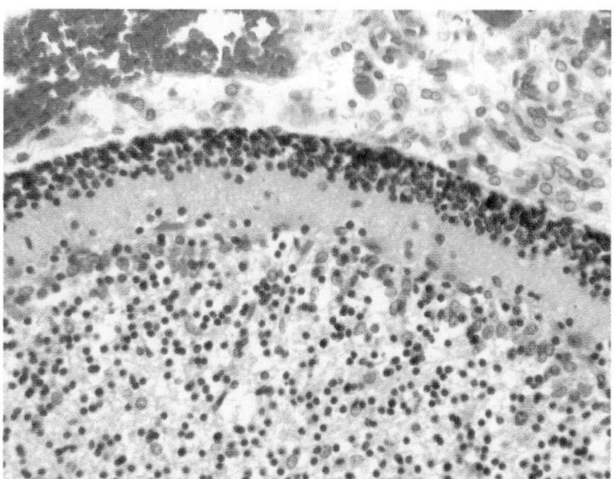

Figure 14.8 Cerebellar cortex in a fetus of 27 weeks' gestation. The surface of the folium is covered with vascular meninges which abut on the external granular layer. Damaged Purkinje cells have been largely replaced by glial cells in this fetus which had suffered hypoxic/ischemic injury. H&E, ×200.

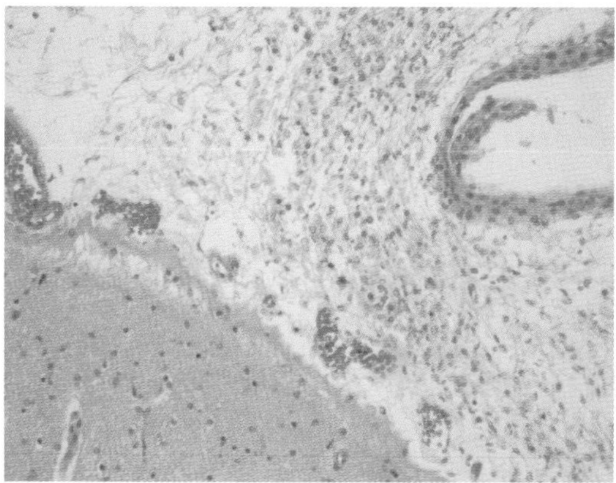

Figure 14.9 Meninges and cortex from a mature fetus. The cellularity of the subarachnoid space is normal and is composed largely of macrophages. H&E, ×100.

macrophages, than are seen in the adult subarachnoid compartment (Fig. 14.9). Although lipofuscin begins to accumulate in neurons from infancy, neuromelanin is not generally visible in the substantia nigra or locus caeruleus until about the fifth year of life.

Differentiation occurs at a faster pace in the spinal cord than in the brain. However, the pyramidal tracts, comprising the descending motor fibers, are not fully myelinated until two years of age.

Genes and proteins influencing normal CNS development

The orderly development of the CNS is under the control of a very large number of genes, the expression of which coordinates the process. These genes, and their associated proteins, may be active for only a short period of time during development and may exert quite different effects at different functional stages. Single or multiple gene mutations give rise to CNS disorders and syndromes. These genes may be dominant or recessive, may vary in penetrance and encode proteins which act as signalling molecules, transcription factors or membrane receptors.

The genetic control of early neural tube development is now becoming known. Sonic hedgehog protein produced by the notochord induces shape changes in the overlying ectoderm, thus bringing the neural tube into being. Development of the forebrain is critically dependent on *Sonic hedgehog* whereas *Wnt-1* influences midbrain and hind brain development. Normal radial migration of neuroblasts is under the control of reelin which also provides the stop signals just beneath the surface meninges of the developing cortex. The *Hox* genes specify segmental differentiation in different regions of the spinal cord. The *trkB* gene acts as a receptor for brain-derived neurotrophic factor (BDNF) which is required for normal neuronal arrangement in the cortex and motor nuclei. Fibroblast growth factor (FGF) is also required for normal development of the brain and skull.

A variety of trophic factors produced by neuronal nuclei serve as attractants for appropriate incoming axons. Nerve cell adhesion molecules (NCAMs) assist axons to bundle together. Migration of neuroblasts along glial or axonal processes is dependent upon a number of different proteins, and their receptors, expressed by migrating and scaffold cells. These include cell adhesion and extracellular matrix molecules such as tenascins and integrins, as well as neuoregulin and ERB4. Cell proliferation in the germinal zone is promoted by cyclins. The balance of cell numbers which is achieved in the mature CNS is also influenced by pro- and anti-apoptotic genes. The genes *Bcl-2* and *Bcl-x* prevent apoptosis whereas *Bad*, *Bax* and caspase 3 promote cell death.

GENETIC AND CHROMOSOMAL ABNORMALITIES

The chromosome abnormalities which are likely to come to the attention of a neuropathologist are listed in Table 14.1. A much wider range of chromosomal abnormalities is observed amongst early pregnancy losses. For this reason the prevalence of these conditions is always quoted as a proportion of live births. Infants with autosomal trisomies other than Trisomy 21 do not generally survive beyond infancy. In addition to the aneuploidies listed in Table 14.1, certain chromosomal deletions and translocations are also compatible with postnatal survival. Small deletions of chromosomes 3, 4, 5, 9, 11, 13, 18 and 21 are variably associated with mental retardation although no characteristic neuropathological abnormalities have been described in any of these conditions. Mental and physical development may appear normal in affected individuals. However, deletions of the short arm of chromosome 4 (Wolf–Hirschhorn syndrome), the short arm of chromosome 5 (cri du chat syndrome) and long arm of chromosome 11 (Jacobsen syndrome) are very regularly associated with severe mental retardation and developmental delay. Balanced translocations, in which exchange of genetic material occurs between two chromosomes, may be clinically silent if no important genes have been lost in the chromosomal switch. Chromosomal deletions and/or translocations are not themselves predictive of the clinical phenotype nor of the presence or otherwise of brain abnormalities. Paediatric pathologists and neuropathologists should be alert to the importance of genetic and chromosomal investigation of any infant who has an abnormal phenotype, particularly if this is associated with mental retardation and microcephaly (Fig. 14.10). Referral to a geneticist may be of paramount importance for other members of the family. The genetic basis of a number of well recognized syndromes is becoming clearer in recent years. For instance, FDF-receptor-2 mutations are associated with Aperts' syndrome which is characterized by abnormalities in the skull. Other genetic syndromes are considered elsewhere in the chapter.

Table 14.1 Chromosomal aneuploidies encountered in live births

Trisomy 21 – Down syndrome
Trisomy 18 – Edwards syndrome
Trisomy 13 – Patau syndrome
Triploidy 69 XXX or XXY
45XO – Turner syndrome
XXY – Kleinfelter syndrome
Multiple copies X or Y
5p– Cri du chat syndrome
4p+, 8+, 9+, 20+ – microcephaly

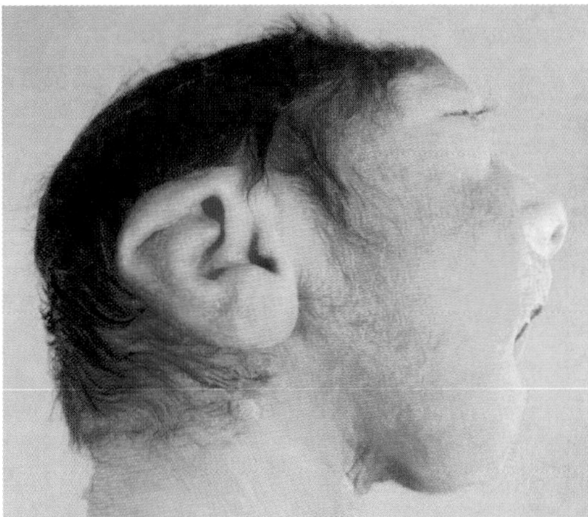

Figure 14.10 Third trimester fetus with significant microcephaly.

Trisomy 21 (Down syndrome)

This condition occurs with a prevalence of 1.3 per thousand live births and becomes more common with advancing maternal age. Antenatal screening is available for older mothers but unexpected cases may be born to young mothers. Individuals with Down syndrome generally possess three copies of chromosome 21 in its entirety or of its long arm. Some Down syndrome subjects are found to be mosaics in that not all their somatic cells possess an extra chromosome 21. Chromosome 21 is one of the shortest chromosomes but it carries important genes on the long arm, including those for β-amyloid precursor protein (β-APP), superoxide dismutase (SOD) and S-100 protein. A diagnosis of trisomy 21 can be established using the fluorescent *in situ* hybridization (FISH) technique in which nucleated cells show

Table 14.2 Features of Down syndrome

General
- Characteristic rounded facies with hypertelorism
- Congenital cardiac malformations common
- Tendency to infection and leukemias

Genetic
- Chromosome 21 trisomy or mosaic
- Triple gene dose of β-APP, SOD-1, S-100

Neuropathology
- Apparently normal fetal brain development
- Failure to attain adult brain weight
- Failure to attain mature dendritic arborizations
- Premature appearance of Alzheimer disease pathology
- May also be associated with serious or lethal CNS malformations e.g. holoprosencephaly and spina bifida

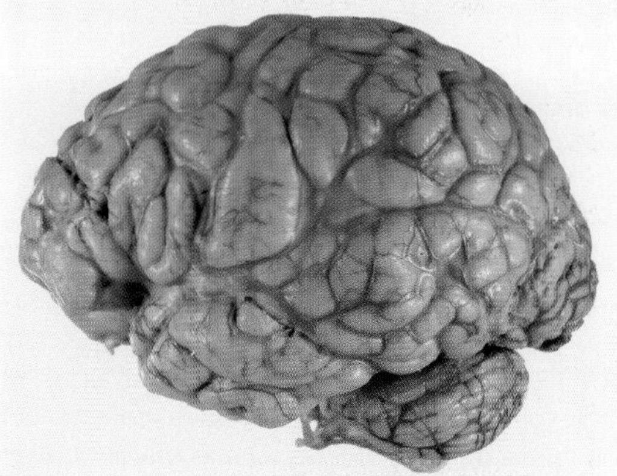

Figure 14.11 Brain from a woman of 46 with Down syndrome. The characteristic small superior temporal gyrus is noted below the Sylvian fissure.

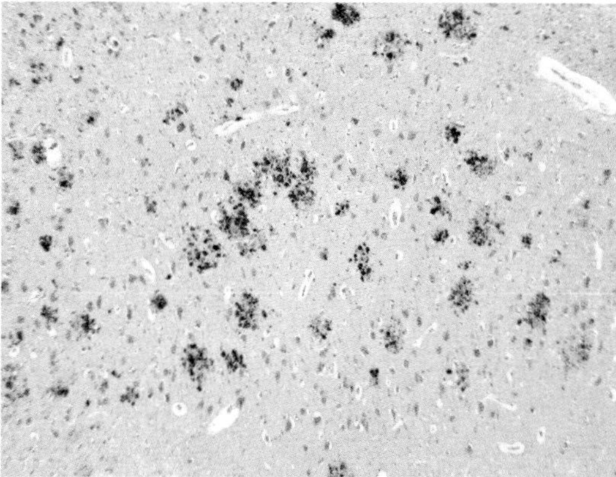

Figure 14.12 Section of the occipital cortex from the brain shown in Fig. 14.11, stained immunohistochemically for β-amyloid precursor protein. The presence of numerous amyloid plaques is confirmed. ×100.

three rather than two fluorescent signals when a chromosome 21 probe is applied. The Down syndrome phenotype (Table 14.2) may not be easy to detect immediately after birth. The characteristic facies and rounded head become more obvious as the infant grows. Investigation has shown that brain development may be surprisingly normal during fetal life despite the over-expression of proteins encoded by genes on chromosome 21. However, abnormalities of brain growth and development become apparent soon after infancy. In the mature Down syndrome brain, the superior temporal gyrus is often abnormally narrow (Fig. 14.11). At the molecular level, overexpression of β-APP stimulates microglial cells which release neurotoxic cytokines and which contributes to the premature appearance of Alzheimer changes in Down syndrome brains (Fig. 14.12). Amyloid plaques and neurofibrillary tangles are generally present in such cases from the third decade, leading to symptomatic neurodegenerative disease by the age of 50 or so. The association between trisomy 21, β-APP genetic load and Alzheimer pathology formed one of the early leads in deciphering the genetic background to neurodegenerative dementias.

Trisomy 18 (Edwards syndrome)

Trisomy 18 occurs with a prevalence of 1 per 3000–5000 live births and affected individuals show systemic abnormalities as well as defects of the face, eyes, skull and brain. Severe retardation is the norm. Likely brain abnormalities are listed in Table 14.3.

Trisomy 13 (Patau syndrome)

Trisomy 13 infants have a prevalence of 1 in 15 000 live births approximately. Holoprosencephaly is the most severe abnormality to be associated with this chromosomal defect (Fig. 14.13). It should be noted that holoprosencephaly has a number of causes, as described later in this chapter. Holoprosencephaly is

Table 14.3 Neuropathology of Trisomy 18 and 13

Trisomy 18
- Microcephaly
- Agenesis of the corpus callosum
- Migrational defects in the cerebral hemispheres
- Cerebellar hypoplasia
- Spina bifida in some cases
- Anencephaly in some cases

Trisomy 13
- Holoprosencephaly
- Absent first cranial nerves
- Agenesis of the corpus callosum
- Hydrocephalus
- Myelomeningocele in some cases

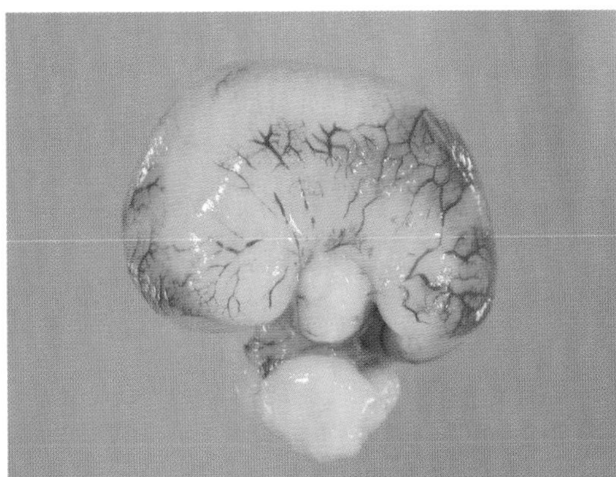

Figure 14.13 Posterior view of a fetal brain displaying holoprosencephaly at approximately 20 weeks gestation. The single cerebral vesicle overlies the brainstem and small cerebellum.

neither characteristic of, nor exclusive to, trisomy 13, being found also in individuals with an apparently normal karyotype. Midline facial abnormalities serve to alert clinicians to the underlying brain defect. The possible neuropathology findings are listed in Table 14.3.

Fragile X syndrome

This syndrome, causing mental retardation, occurs in males only, being inherited by means of an X-linked gene. This syndrome appears in up to 1 in 1000 live births and is one of the commonest causes of mental retardation, along with Down syndrome. Affected individuals may have microcephaly and a characteristic long facies with large ears. Examination of the brain may reveal heterotopias, indicative of impaired neuronal migration and abnormal dendritic spines with immature synaptic connections.

Triploidy (69 XXX or 69 XXY)

These individuals may display holoprosencephaly, hydrocephaly, Chiari type II malformation, microcephaly or myelomeningocele. Postnatal survival is usually limited. Hydatidiform degeneration of the placenta is frequently associated with triploidy.

Turner syndrome (45 XO)

There is no characteristic neuropathology in this condition but subtle abnormalities of the basal ganglia and cerebellum may be present. Affected individuals may display mental retardation or may be intellectually normal. Long term survival is usual but infertility and sexual immaturity is the norm since the developing ovaries regress in this condition. The brain is deprived of the effects of estrogen.

STRUCTURAL ABNORMALITIES

Open neural tube defects

The prevalence of neural tube defects (NTDs) varies in different populations for reasons which remain unclear and may be as high as 2 per 1000 live births. NTDs are detected more frequently amongst early spontaneous abortions and are more common in female fetuses. Abnormalities of the neural tube and its derivatives are listed in Table 14.4. The more severe neural tube defects, including anencephaly (Fig. 14.14), are caused by failure of the neural tube to close either in part or its entirety. By late gestation there is usually little residual neural tissue left on the exposed skull base or in the vertebral gutter. Despite the major brain abnormality in anencephaly,

Table 14.4 Abnormalities affecting the neural tube

Condition	Pathology
Anencephaly	Brain represented by area cerebrovasculosa (vascular cystic mass of tissue with glial, ependymal and choroid plexus remnants). Absence of skull vault
Craniorachischisis	Anencephaly combined with complete spina bifida. Absence of skull and all vertebral arches
Myelocele	Open spina bifida lesion, usually restricted to the lumbosacral region. Absence of related vertebral arches
Myelomeningocele	Localized spina bifida lesion covered in part by a cystic mass of meninges distended with CSF usually in the lumbosacral region. Absence of related vertebral arches.
Meningocele	More nearly normal spinal cord and lesion covered by distended meninges and a thin layer of epithelium. Focal deficit of vertebral arches
Encephalocele	Hernia of cranial meninges and brain tissue, usually occipital or frontal in position and associated with defects in the vault of the skull
Diplomyelia	Duplication of the central canal of the spinal cord
Diastematomyelia	Division of the cord into two separate halves, often associated with a cartilagenous or bony spur
Hydromyelia	Dilation of the central canal of the spinal cord
Syringomyelia	Cavitation of the spinal cord dorsal or ventral to the central canal
Spinal bifida occulta	Focal absence of vertebral arches but covered with intact skin. Spinal cord usually normal or near normal
Hydrocephalus	Distended ventricular system. Causes shown in Table 14.6
Arnold Chiari malformation	Displacement of medulla and/or cerebellar tonsils into the upper cervical vertebral canal, often in association with hydrocephalus

the globes and optic nerves are comparatively well formed as is the anterior pituitary gland. In anencephaly, the foramen magnum is most often incomplete posteriorly and the upper end of the cervical vertebral canal is open (Fig. 14.14). In some cases, remnants of the medulla and cerebellum may be identifiable histologically in the posterior cranial fossa. The fetal adrenal glands are much smaller than normal in anencephaly, owing to incomplete pituitary development. The spinal cord is narrower than normal and the descending corticospinal tracts are absent. The spinal meninges are hypervascular and may contain heterotopic neural tissue (Fig. 14.15).

Spina bifida affecting the cervical and thoracic regions is associated with shortening of the vertebral column. The normal curvatures of the spine are lost and the neck is extended, with consequent upward tilting of the face. In the localized spina bifida lesions, including myelocele and myelomeningocele (Fig. 14.16), the spinal cord is represented as a flat disc of neural tissue which merges laterally with the surrounding skin (Fig. 14.17). Dorsal root ganglia and spinal nerves may be present. Surgical biopsies of lesions removed at birth may reveal very little neural tissue but staining for glial fibrillary acidic protein (GFAP) is helpful in detecting remnants of glio-ependymal tissue. Fetuses with apparently localized open spina bifida lesions often show CNS abnormalities elsewhere, including diplomyelia, diastematomyelia or hydromyelia (Fig. 14.18 and Table 14.4). Cavitation of the spinal cord, which does not involve the central canal and is termed syringomyelia, may be present with NTDs or may be found in isolation. Fetuses with spina bifida have hydrocephalus more often than not, usually accompanied by a Chiari type II malformation in which a kinked medulla is displaced downwards into the upper cervical canal, often with related displacement of parts of the cerebellum (Fig. 14.19). The different types of Chiari malformation are shown in Table 14.5. Despite the presence of ventriculomegaly, the head size may actually be reduced in mid-gestation in affected fetuses, owing probably

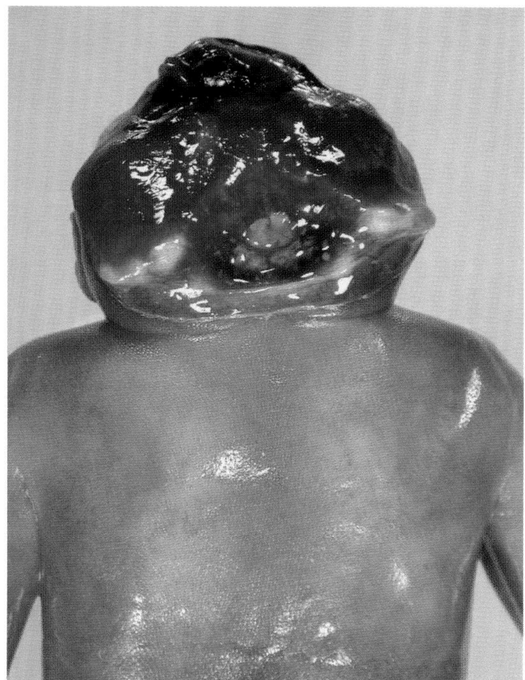

Figure 14.14 Posterior view of a fetus with anencephaly. The foramen magnum and cervical vertebral column are deficient posteriorly and the remnants of brainstem are seen in the base of the posterior fossa.

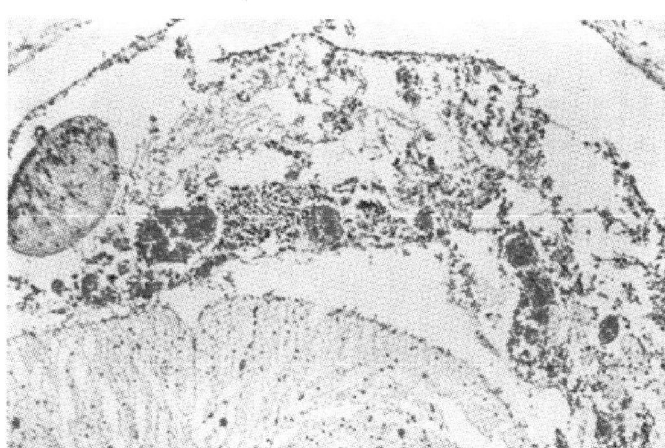

Figure 14.15 Section of the spinal cord from a 20 week fetus with anencephaly. The subarachnoid space contains heterotopic undifferentiated neural tissue and the meninges are more vascular than normal. H&E, ×100.

to reduced brain growth and the relatively large subdural space normally present in the second trimester. Only later in development does the head size enlarge if the ventricles are dilated.

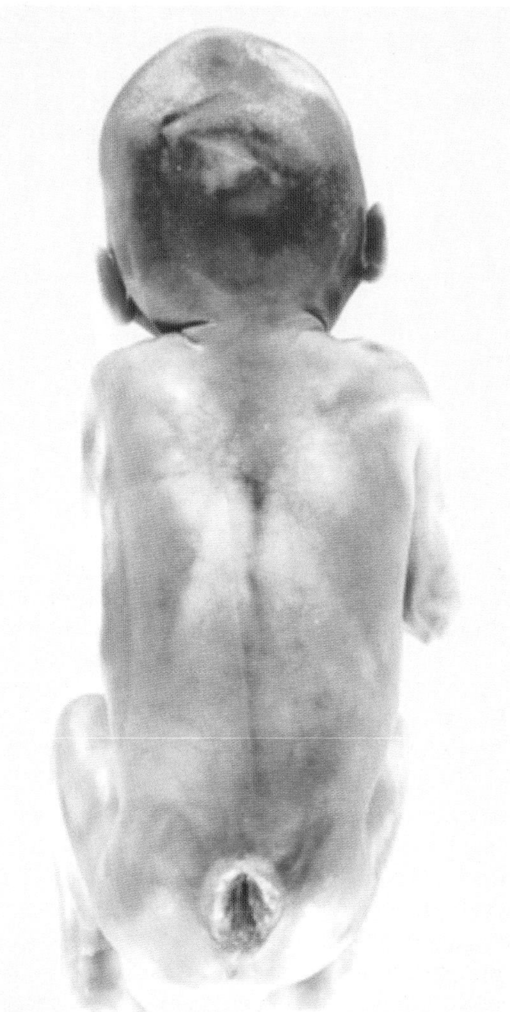

Figure 14.16 Fetus of 20 weeks' gestation with a lumbar meningomyelocele. The spinal cord lesion is visible in the base of the defect.

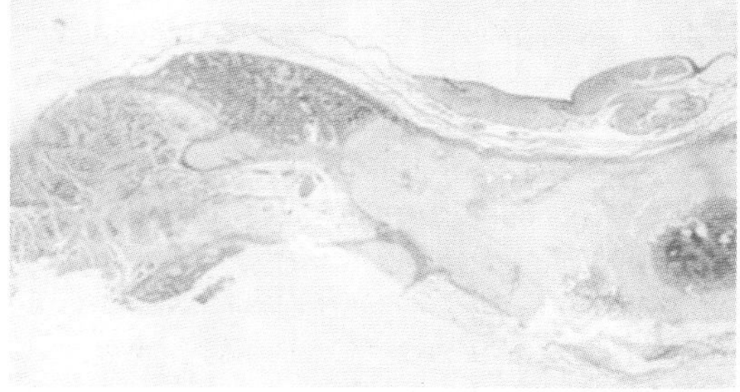

Figure 14.17 Section through an open spina bifida lesion in a fetus of 21 weeks. The spinal plaque is laid open on the dorsum of an abnormal vertebra and is in continuity laterally with thin skin. H&E, ×20.

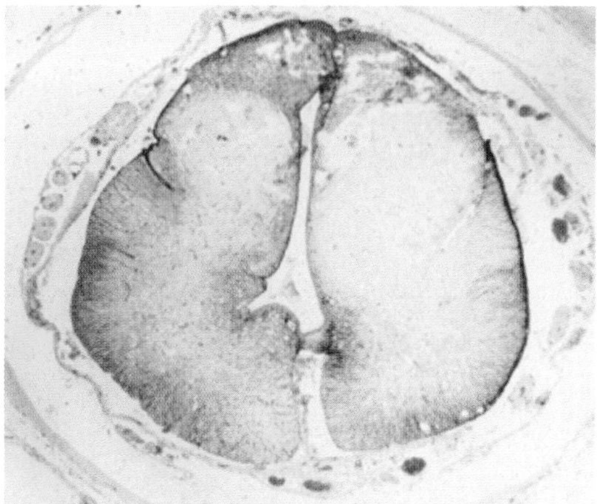

Figure 14.18 Section through the spinal cord in a fetus with lumbar spina bifida. Section taken at the thoracic level in the enclosed part of the spinal canal. The cord displays hydromyelia with gross dilatation of the central canal which is ependymal lined. The cord has been stained for glial fibrillary acidic protein. ×40.

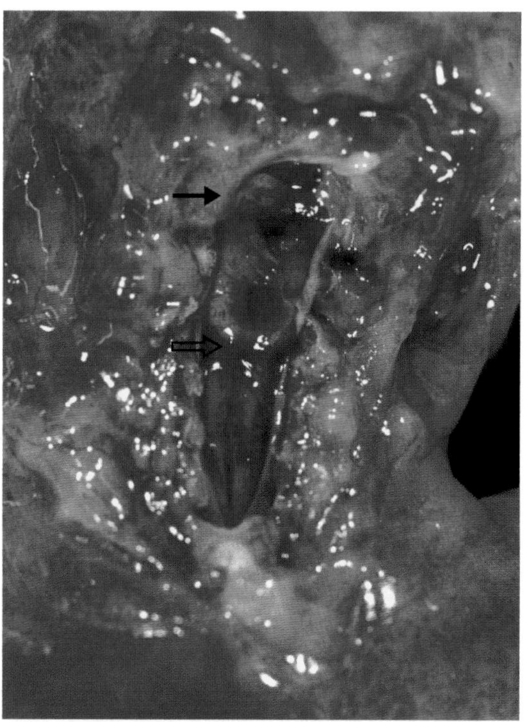

Figure 14.19 Fetus of 22 weeks with an Arnold Chiari malformation accompanying lumbar spina bifida. The cervical vertebral arches have been removed. The medulla is present within the spinal canal to the level of C2–3 (open arrow). The level of the foramen magnum is indicated by the intact arch of C1 (arrowed).

Open NTDs allow the escape of fetal CSF into the amniotic fluid. Unlike adult CSF, fetal CSF has a high protein content, including fetal specific alphafetoprotein (AFP), at least in the first half of gestation. The leak of fetal CSF results in higher than normal levels of protein in the amniotic fluid. These proteins pass into maternal blood and a high maternal serum AFP level is one of the diagnostic tests used to detect the presence of NTD in pregnancy. Most affected fetuses are terminated following detection of the defect. Folic acid supplements administered before and during pregnancy have helped to reduce the prevalence of neural tube defects.

The causation of human neural tube defects remains unknown but is believed to be multifactorial. The genetic factors have not been identified. A variety of genetic loci have been identified in mouse NTD models. The most important of these is Sonic hedgehog which influences neural and axial bending and hence the ability of the neural tube to close. Maternal diabetes and treatment with certain drugs used in epilepsy, such as valproate and carbamazepine, are associated with a higher risk of NTDs. Myelomeningocele is not uncommon in trisomy 18.

Table 14.5 Chiari malformations

Lesion	Pathology
Type I	Displacement of tonsils into the upper cervical spinal canal – may be associated with cervical syringomyelia. NB the tonsils normally lie at the foramen Munro in the very young and are retractable
Type II (Arnold Chiari malformation)	Cerebellar vermis displaced into the upper cervical canal, associated with abnormalities of the brainstem and usually with a lumbosacral spina bifida lesion and hydrocephalus
Type III	Displacement of cerebellum or of occipital lobe in conjunction with an encephalocele

Covered neural tube defects

Defects such as encephalocele (Fig. 14.20) and meningocele are not the result of a failure of neural tube closure. In these cases part of the vault of the skull or of the vertebral arches has failed to develop, resulting in herniation of meninges and neural tissue. Encephaloceles are usually associated with more widespread abnormalities within the CNS than the external lesion would suggest. An occipital encephalocele is frequently a feature of the Meckel–Gruber syndrome, together with polydactyly, polycystic kidneys and hepatic fibrosis. This is an autosomal recessive condition associated with a gene(s) on chromosome 17. Other types of neural tube defect and fourth ventricular cysts are found less commonly in the Meckel–Gruber syndrome.

The Dandy–Walker malformation may be detected on a prenatal scan. This abnormality occurs with a prevalence of 1 in 5000 live births and consists of a dilated fourth ventricle with a small or absent vermis. Since the roof of the fourth ventricle appears to be imperforate, hydrocephalus is also present. It can be difficult to confirm the presence of this lesion once the brain of an affected fetus has been removed and careful examination in the post mortem room is particularly helpful (see introduction and Fig. 14.2, page 244). The cause of this condition is unknown.

Spina bifida occulta lesions occur at the caudal end of the neural tube and are found in the lumbosacral region, covered by normal skin. The lower end of the abnormal cord may be tethered within the abnormal region of the vertebral canal, leading to problems as the child grows and the spine lengthens. Abnormalities of the pelvic viscera may also be present. These abnormalities are thought to arise from maldevelopment of the caudal tail bud which, though not part of the early neural tube, contributes to the development of the low lumbar and sacral segments of the spinal cord.

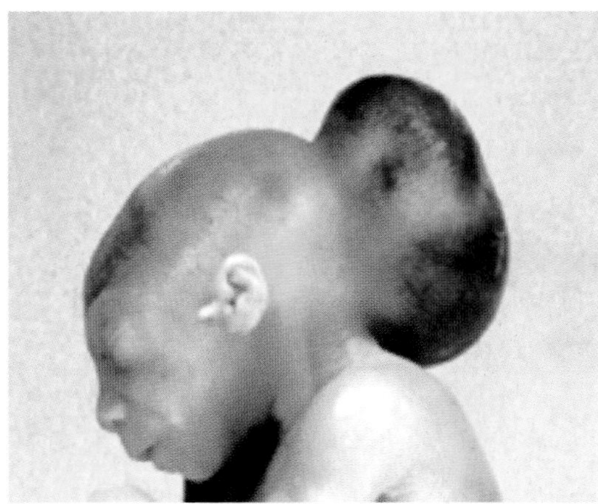

Figure 14.20 Fetus with large occipital encephalocele. There is concomitant microcephaly because much of the brain is within the encephalocele. A skin tag is present in front of the left pinna.

Table 14.6 Causes of ventricular enlargement

A. Hydrocephalus
(caused by obstruction to CSF circulation or possibly by CSF overproduction)
Genetic
- X-linked recessive: aqueduct stenosis
- Autosomal recessive

Spina bifida/Chiari type II malformation
Other congenital malformations
e.g. Dandy–Walker malformation
Infection eg fetal CMV, rubella, toxoplasmosis
Intraventricular hemorrhage
(prematurity associated)
Tumors, e.g. ependymomas, astrocytomas, colloid cyst, choroid plexus

B. Hydranencephaly
(hydrocephalus *ex vacuo* due to failed development, or destruction, of the cerebrum
Hypoxic ischemic encephalopathy
Twin–twin transfusion
Proliferative glomeruloid vasculopathy (genetic)

Hydrocephalus

This condition is characterized by a dilated ventricular system in which there is a disturbance of CSF circulation due to one of a variety of causes, listed in Table 14.6 (Figs 14.21 and 14.22). The overall prevalence of hydrocephalus is 2–3 per 1000 births. CSF is secreted into the ventricular system by the choroid plexuses at a rate of 400–500 mL per day. The fluid escapes from the roof of the fourth ventricle through the foramina of Luschka and Magendie, enters the subarachnoid space and is subsequently absorbed through the arachnoid granulations and

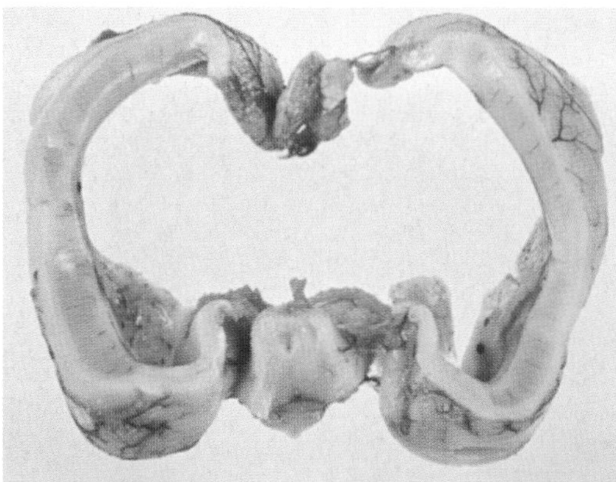

Figure 14.21 Coronal slice from the brain of a neonate with gross hydrocephalus. The brainstem shows a patent aqueduct and the cause of the hydrocephalus was unclear.

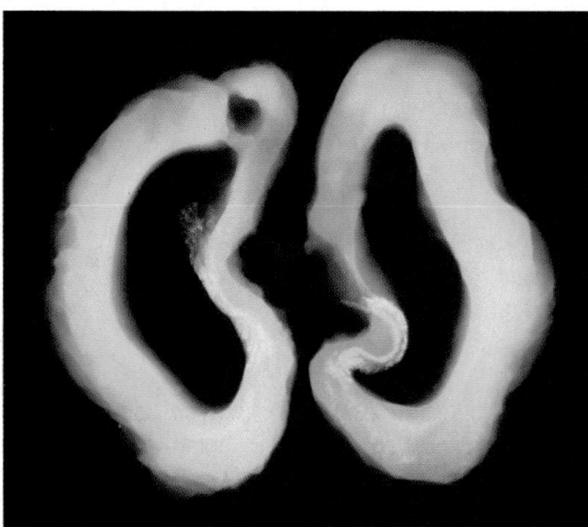

Figure 14.22 Radiograph of a brain slice removed from a fetus at 32 weeks' gestation. There is ventriculomegaly and periventricular calcification due to congenital cytomegalovirus infection.

back into the venous system (superior sagittal sinus). In addition, two-way flow of CSF likely occurs between brain tissue and the ventricular cavities. Over-production or decreased absorption of CSF results in hydrocephalus. Two types of this condition are described. In the non-communicating type, CSF accumulates within the ventricular system and fails to reach the subarachnoid space. In communicating hydrocephalus the obstruction usually lies within the subarachnoid space leading to a failure of CSF resorption. Hydrocephalus may occur in isolation but is seen with X-linked aqueduct stenosis or more commonly in association with NTDs and prematurity-associated intraventricular hemorrhage. This latter condition is probably the most important since it is increasing in prevalence as more very low birth weight infants survive. These infants are likely to have respiratory difficulty and fluctuating cerebral blood flow, which may cause subependymal hemorrhage in the richly vascularized germinal matrix (Fig. 14.6) and subsequent rupture into the ventricular cavity. A proportion of the surviving infants develop both hydrocephalus and white matter damage. Traditionally, post-hemorrhagic hydrocephalus has been ascribed to occlusion of arachnoid granulations. Recent work has highlighted the probable contribution of factors such as transforming growth factor β (TGFβ) which promote the deposition of collagen and extracellular matrix protein, not only in the subarachnoid space but also within brain tissue leading to significantly reduced ependymal resorption of CSF. A better understanding of the complex and multiple mechanisms causing hydrocephalus suggests that a division into communicating and non-communicating types is too simplistic. The increased pressure of hydrocephalus leads to secondary ischemic and mechanical injury in the periventricular white matter with consequent loss of axons, myelin and oligodendrocytes. Hydranencephaly is the term given to ventricular enlargement resulting from maldevelopment or damage which is primarily within cerebral tissue (Table 14.6B).

X-linked aqueduct stenosis (Fig. 14.23a and b) is linked to genetic mutations in the gene for L1 neural cell adhesion molecule in some cases. Because this gene is recessive, carrier females do not manifest the effects of the gene but can pass it to male offspring who develop X-linked hydrocephalus (Fig. 14.21). However, these mutations are not present in all cases of aqueduct stenosis and in these the etiology remains to be fully elucidated. The pathology of aqueduct stenosis includes duplication or forking of the channel (Fig. 14.24) with evidence of gliosis or hemosiderin laden macrophages in some cases. Other causes of hydrocephalus are listed in Table 14.6. Ventricular dilation may result from primary pathology within brain tissue (Fig. 14.22).

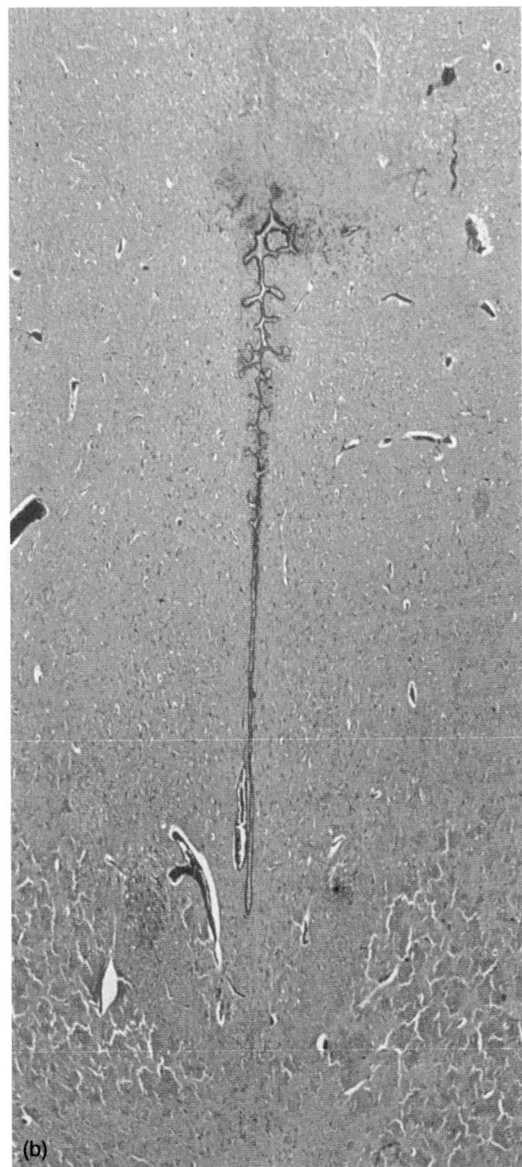

Figure 14.23 (a) Normal profile of the aqueduct of Sylvius in third trimester. (b) Aqueduct in X-linked hydrocephalus. Fetus gestationally matched with the case shown in (a). The aqueduct is narrow and elongated in the anteroposterior plane. H&E, ×40.

Holoprosencephaly

The prevalence of holoprosencephaly is approximately 1 per 5000 live births. This defect affects the forebrain or prosencephalon which to a variable degree fails to separate into two hemispheres, resulting in a single ventricular cavity and absent corpus callosum (Fig. 14.13, page 265 and Fig. 14.25). The malformed prosencephalon may be partially divided into two hemispheres or represented by a single vesicle (semilobar or alobar forms). The basal ganglia and thalami are variably fused. The olfactory bulbs and tracts are absent. There is a spectrum of associated facial abnormalities, ranging

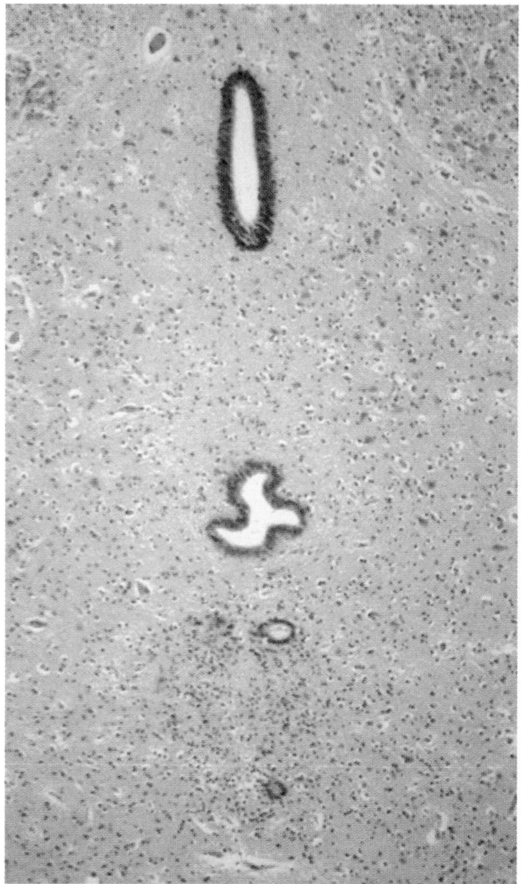

Figure 14.24 Multi-channelled aqueduct in a fetus with marked hydrocephalus detected at about 20 weeks of gestation. H&E, ×100.

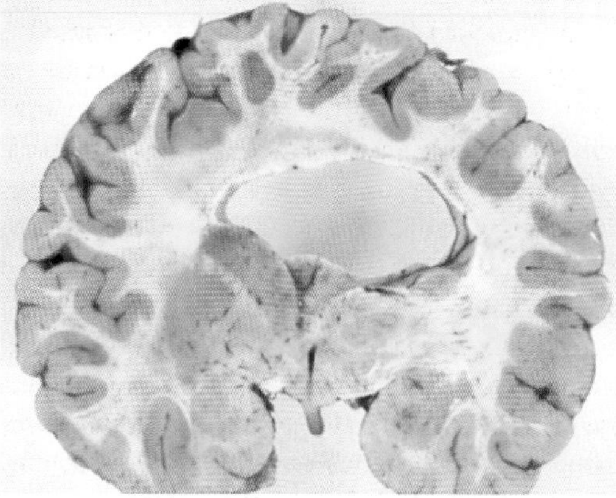

Figure 14.25 Coronal slice from the brain of a 4-year-old girl who proved to have holoprosencephaly. There is a single ventricle and the basal ganglia are partially fused. The corpus callosum is absent.

from cyclopia in which the nose is represented as a proboscis in the midline above a single orbit, to varying degrees of midline facial narrowing. Midline cleft lip and palate are often present.

The causation of holoprosencephaly appears to be multifactorial. Some cases are genetic with an autosomal dominant pattern although with variable penetration in an individual family. Mutations in sonic hedgehog play a central role in some cases. Holoprosencephaly is found in the majority of Trisomy 13 individuals. Holoprosencephaly is a feature of certain syndromes such as the Smith–Lemli–Opitz and Labotte syndromes. In the Smith–Lemli–Optiz syndrome there is a defect of cholesterol synthesis resulting in low serum cholesterol, which may lead to abnormal sonic hedgehog signalling. However, holoprosencephly is usually sporadic and a significant number of cases have no recognizable genetic defects.

Agenesis of the corpus callosum

This condition may be present in association with other malformations of the CNS or may be found as an isolated phenomenon. Partial absence of the posterior fibers is sometimes seen. An anteroposterior longitudinal tract of white matter may occupy the position of the corpus callosum and is called the bundle of Probst (Fig. 14.26). If the absent corpus callosum is an isolated finding, it may be completely asymptomatic and discovered only on neuroimaging or at autopsy.

Migrational defects

Cell migration defects include lissencephaly and cerebral heterotopias, most of which may be diagnosed in life by magnetic resonance imaging (MRI).

Two types of lissencephaly are described. Both are characterized by partial or complete loss of normal gyral pattern and by a thickened cortex. The terms agyria and pachygyria have also been used to describe these conditions, which are genetic in origin.

Type 1 lissencephaly is due to a genetically caused failure of radial migration although a deficiency of cell proliferation may also be involved. This results

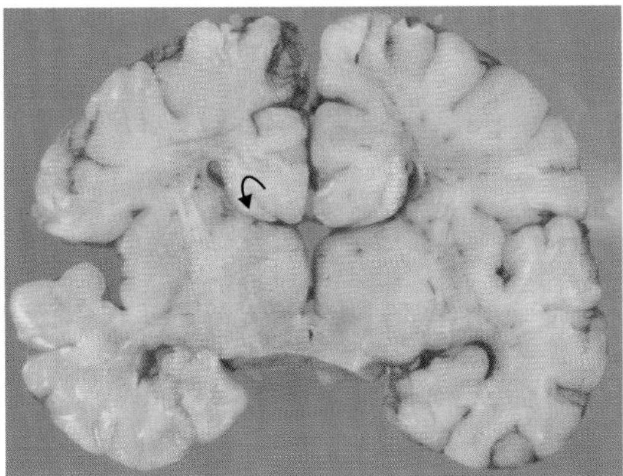

Figure 14.26 Coronal slice of a brain from a term fetus showing absence of the corpus callosum. A prominent bundle of Probst (arrow) is present bilaterally.

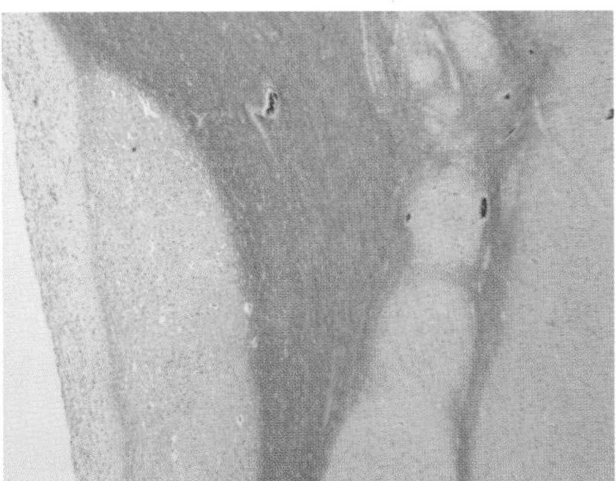

Figure 14.27 Section of the cerebrum from an infant of 2 months with microcephaly and seizures. There are heterotopic nodules of grey matter within the paraventricular and subcortical region, highlighted by staining of the white matter for myelin. Luxol fast blue, ×40.

in microcephaly, developmental delay and motor impairment. The condition may be associated with non-CNS abnormalities. The prevalence of type 1 lissencephaly is of the order of 1 per 500 000 population but partial lissencephaly (pachygyria) may be more common than this. The causes include mutations in the gene for reelin (chromosome 7), in *LIS1* (chromosome 17), doublecortin (*DCX* gene, X chromosome) or *ARX* (X chromosome). Hence type 1 lissencephaly may be autosomal dominant, autosomal recessive, X-linked or sporadic. Microcephaly is usually present and the brain shows a four layer cortex, made up of a myelinated zone lying between layers of poorly orientated neurons. The white matter is considerably reduced.

Type 2 lissencephaly is also characterized by microcephaly and a thickened cortex but has a different origin in that radial migration of neuroblasts occurs as usual but fails to be arrested at the Cajal–Retzius subpial layer. Migrating cells break through the limiting pia mater in an irregular fashion forming a thick layer outside the normal cortex. This results in a cobble-stone appearance on the surface of the brain. Type 2 lissencephaly is associated in all cases with congenital muscular dystrophy and very often with cerebellar and ocular abnormalities. The best known forms are Fukuyama congenital muscular dystrophy (gene on chromosome 9), which is largely confined to Japan and the Walker–Warberg syndrome (gene on chromosome 9). The overall prevalence of type 2 lissencephaly is not known. The basis appears to be an abnormality of glycosylation but the exact genetic background is not established.

Heterotopias consist of collections of gray matter developing in an abnormal position most commonly in one of three locations; in the subarachnoid space, just beneath the normal cortex in the form of a subcortical band, or in the periventricular region (Fig. 14.27). The leptomeningeal form is usually associated with other CNS malformations and may be detected only on microscopic examination of the brain. The other two variants may be diagnosed in life by means of neuroimaging. Heterotopias are the result of migrational abnormalities. Apart from those cases associated with a recognized pathogenic event, such as hypoxic/ischemic injury, most cases of subcortical band heterotopia are isolated defects and have a genetic basis, usually in female carriers of *DCX* doublecortin gene. In contrast, periventricular heterotopias are often associated with other cerebral defects such as polymicrogyria and agenesis of the corpus callosum. The prevalence of all heterotopias is difficult to determine. Clinically, they are usually manifested by mental retardation and seizures. Small, gray matter heterotopias may be present in the cerebellar white matter and these can include both undifferentiated and differentiated

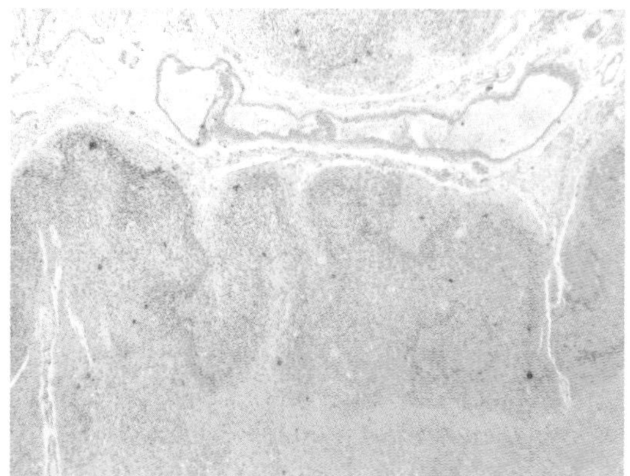

Figure 14.28 Section of the cortex from a fetus of 23 weeks with multiple abnormalities. The cortical ribbon is thrown into numerous irregular folds, amounting to polymicrogyria. H&E, ×40.

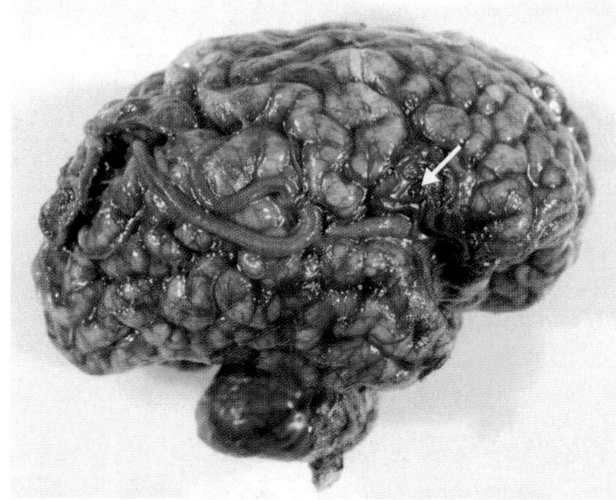

Figure 14.29 Brain from a mature fetus with a large abnormal vessel running horizontally across the hemisphere. Inspection of the region of the Sylvian fissure shows a vascular malformation. Focal irregular gyral atrophy (arrow) of ischemic origin is noted above the Sylvian fissure.

neurons. Whether these give rise to medulloblastomas is not known.

Polymicrogyria and other gyral abnormalities

Polymicrogyria, which is not a migrational disorder, is characterized by excessive folding of abnormally small gyri, usually in a focal distribution (Fig. 14.28). These gyri may be fused so that the external surface appears relatively smooth or only slightly dimpled. Non-layered and four layered variants are described. The antecedents of this condition are varied and include both genetic causes (autosomal dominant, recessive, X-linked and inherited metabolic disorders) and ischemic or inflammatory disorders (Fig. 14.29). Infective causes are often associated with calcification and the infective agents include cytomegalovirus (CMV), *Toxoplasma* and syphilis. Polymicrogyria is characteristically found in Zellweger syndrome, a very long chain fatty acid disorder. The clinical correlates include microcephaly, developmental delay and epilepsy. Neuropathological examination reveals a thickened cortex in which folded and fused gyri can be made out, and which is separated only indistinctly from underlying white matter. Abnormally broad gyri may be present in thanatophoric dysplasia, due to a mutation in fibroblast growth factor receptor 3 (FGFR-3) (Fig. 14.30). Abnormal cerebral

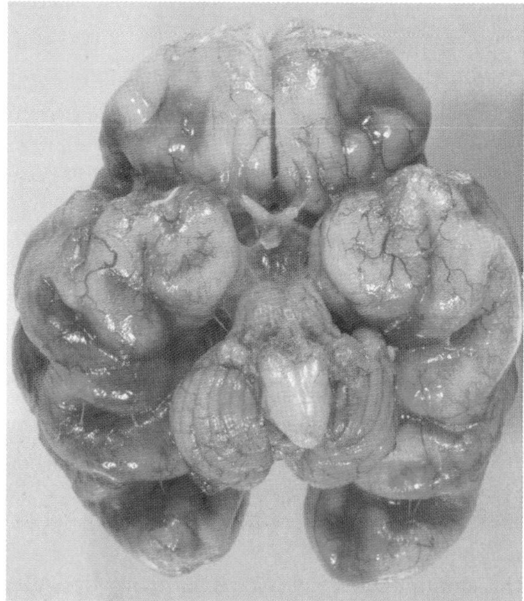

Figure 14.30 Base of the brain in a fetus with thanatophoric dysplasia. The temporal lobe gyri are enlarged and thickened, a characteristic finding in this condition.

patterning is also seen in short ribbed polydactyly syndrome (Fig. 14.31). More subtle abnormalities of cortical architecture are known as cortical dysplasias, in which there is a disturbance of lamination

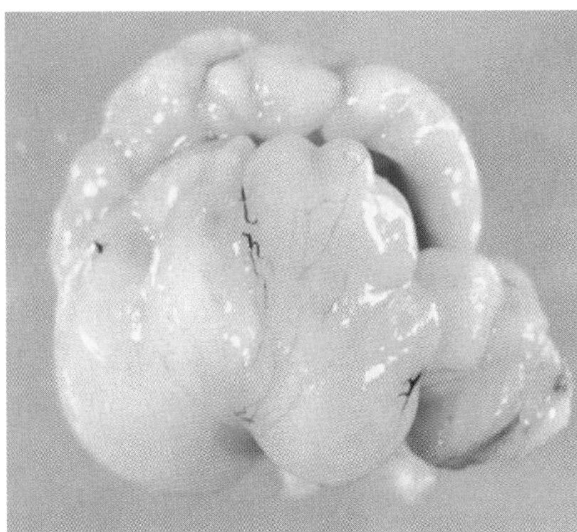

Figure 14.31 An oblique view of the cerebrum from a fetus of 20 weeks' gestation with short rib polydactyl type IV. There is gross irregularity of cortical development and absence of the corpus callosum.

associated in some cases with the presence of abnormal nerve cells. Excessive numbers of neurons may be seen in the white matter although it should be noted that these are always more common in developing white matter than in the adult brain. Cortical dysplasia is a cause of epilepsy especially if it is associated with hippocampal sclerosis (see later). Certain syndromes, e.g. Zellweger syndrome (see Chapter 11) are characterized by cortical dysplasia, migrational abnormalities and polymicrogyria.

MICROCEPHALY AND MEGALENCEPHALY

The multiple causes of microcephaly are listed in Table 14.7. Because skull growth is linked to brain growth, any failure to attain normal brain size results in a reduction in head size compared with mean values for the age and gender of the individual concerned. Megalencephaly is found in conditions such as the leukodystrophies and Alexander's disease. This generalized enlargement of the brain, compared with age-matched standards, is often associated with learning difficulties.

Table 14.7 Causes of microcephaly

Genetic
- Autosomal recessive (e.g. Smith–Lemli–Opitz syndrome)
- Autosomal dominant
- X-linked (fragile X syndrome)
- Chromosomal aneuploidy (e.g. Down [trisomy 21], Edwards [trisomy 18], Patau [trisomy 13] and cri du chat [5p−] syndromes
- Progressive genetic microcephaly (e.g. Rett syndrome, Alpers syndrome)

Ionizing radiation
Fetal alcohol syndrome
Congenital infection (e.g. rubella, CMV, *Toxoplasma*, HIV)
Gross hypoxia/ischemia
Idiopathic
May or may not be associated with other malformations

NEUROFIBROMATOSIS TYPES 1 AND 2

In neurofibromatosis type 1 (von Recklinghausen's disease), children display pigmented lesions of the skin (café-au-lait spots) and subsequently develop neurofibromas on peripheral nerves. There is an increased risk of developing malignant peripheral nerve sheath tumors. This condition is inherited as an autosomal dominant disorder and the gene locus is on chromosome 17. Neurofibromatosis type 2 is similarly an autosomal dominant disorder in which tumors arise. Bilateral acoustic schwannomas are characteristic of this condition.

TUBEROUS SCLEROSIS

Tuberous sclerosis is another autosomal dominantly inherited condition with high penetrance and a prevalence of approximately 1 in 10 000 births. This condition is also characterized by a propensity for non-CNS tumors, in this case rhabdomyomata, particularly in the heart. These may appear in early life. Older patients display cysts and tumors in other

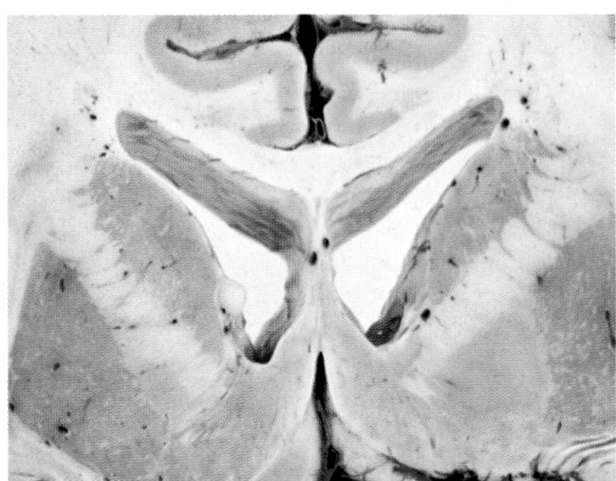

Figure 14.32 Coronal section through the brain of an adult with tuberous sclerosis. A subependymal nodule is noted in the left lateral ventricle. Elsewhere in the brain more subtle abnormalities were found in the cortex.

organs. However, it is involvement of the brain which is most often symptomatic in these patients. The brains of affected individuals display nodules of abnormal neuroglial tissue in the cortex (tubers), in the white matter (heterotopias) and in the periventricular region (subependymal nodules) (Fig. 14.32). These nodules contain enlarged abnormal cells which may show both glial and neuronal characteristics on immunophenotyping. Reactive gliosis is present and mineralization is common. The pathology of subependymal nodules merges with that of subependymal giant cell astrocytomas which possess a low grade growth potential. However the main clinical problems in affected individuals are epilepsy and mental retardation. The disease is determined by mutations in one or other of the two tuberous sclerosis genes, one on chromosome 9 and one on chromosome 16. The lesions of tuberous sclerosis are visible on magnetic resonance imaging.

VASCULAR ABNORMALITIES AND MALFORMATIONS

The blood vessels of the cranial cavity show a range of abnormalities which, although not common in some of their manifestations, are unique to this part of the body (Fig. 14.29). Individuals with the Sturge–Weber syndrome show a port wine stain of the face or scalp with abnormal blood vessels in the meninges of the same side. Abnormalities of the underlying cortex, with calcification, may also be present and these manifest as seizures and stroke-like symptoms. Vascular malformations include abnormal networks of capillary, venous and/or arteriolar channels which usually present with episodes of hemorrhage later in life, if at all. Saccular or berry aneurysms of cerebral arteries present in adult life also, by way of subarachnoid hemorrhage, but the underlying abnormality of the arterial wall is thought to be present from much earlier in development (Fig. 14.33). In contrast aneurysms of the vein of Galen present in infancy, either with focal signs or with cardiac failure due to the size of the lesion. The presence of abnormally proliferated blood vessels throughout the meninges or in the cerebral tissue can be associated with failure of cerebral development in the

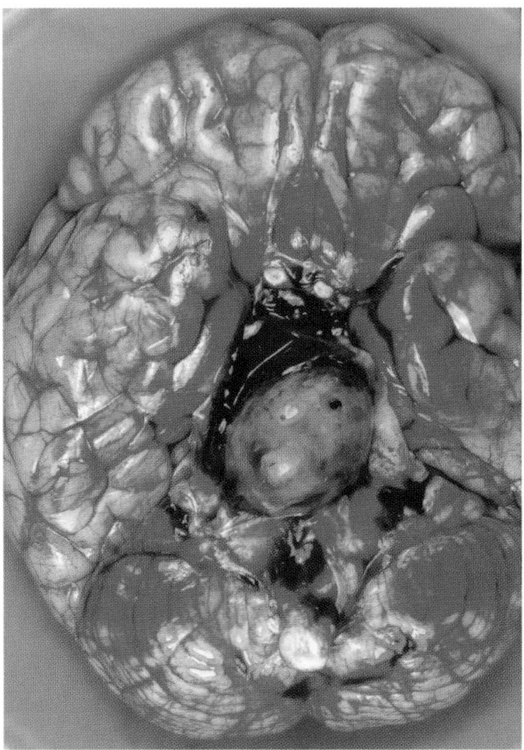

Figure 14.33 A 12-year-old girl who fell, following the rupture of an aneurysm on the Circle of Willis. This aneurysm has arisen on the posterior circulation.

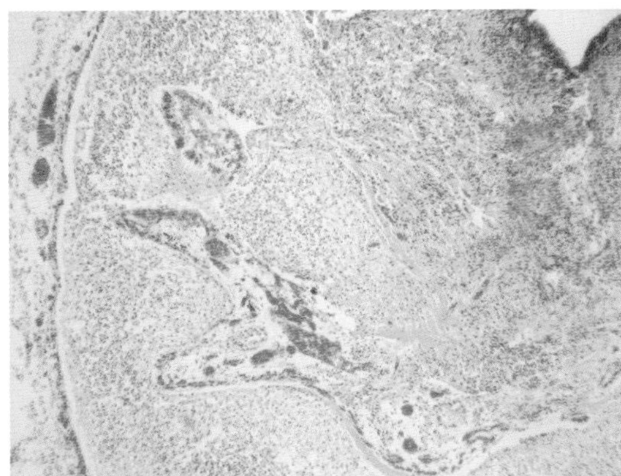

Figure 14.34 Section of the cerebral hemisphere from a 15 week fetus terminated following an antenatal diagnosis of hydrocephalus. Abnormal blood vessels are seen penetrating the full thickness of the cerebrum. The next sibling in this family had a similar but milder manifestion of this glomeruloid vasculopathy (Fowler syndrome). H&E, ×100.

condition of proliferative vasculopathy (Fowler syndrome) (Fig. 14.34). It is worth noting that fetal and pediatric meninges do appear much more vascular than in the adult and if these blood vessels are engorged in the context of hypoxia, there is a risk of over-interpreting these normal or merely reactive appearances as structurally abnormal.

BIRTH-RELATED NEUROPATHOLOGY

Birth-related injury

Potentially, the poorly myelinated brain is at risk of injury in the birth canal. Remarkably, most infants are born without evidence of brain damage. In part this is due to the compressibility of the fetal skull due to movement within as yet unfused cranial sutures. However, precipitate vaginal delivery of premature infants may cause intracranial hemorrhage. Obstructed labor and high forceps delivery resulting in trauma to the head and neck are unusual nowadays. Spinal nerve palsies may result from traction on the neck and pressure from a forceps blade can damage the fetal head. Dural tears, particularly in the tentorium, are one marker of traumatic delivery but are now a very uncommon cause of significant subdural hemorrhage (Fig. 14.35). Hemosiderin staining of the dura mater in a neonate should be interpreted carefully in the light of possible birth-related trauma versus head injury at a later date. Premature babies who become jaundiced in the neonatal period are at risk of kernicterus (Fig. 14.36) due to unconjugated bilirubin entering

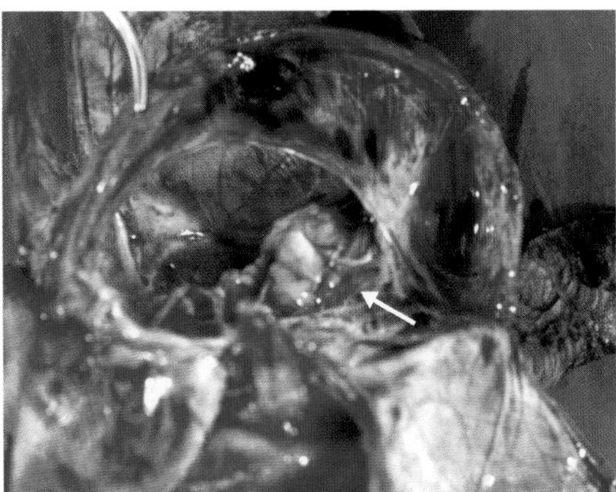

Figure 14.35 Infant who died shortly after birth. Both hemispheres have been removed to demonstrate the relationship between falx and tentorium. There is a tear in the tentorium (arrow) which is the source of considerable falcine and subdural hemorrhage.

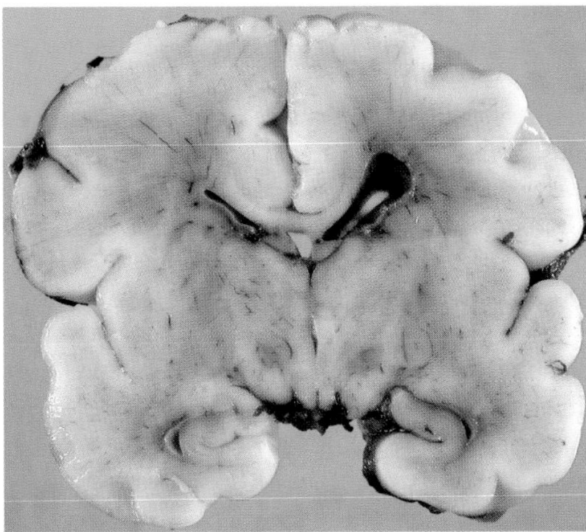

Figure 14.36 Coronal slice from the brain of a premature infant who developed jaundice and marked encephalopathy. Yellow discoloration of the hippocampus and deep brain nuclei with unconjugated bilirubin is well demonstrated, confirming the diagnosis of kernicterus.

brain tissue. This condition is considered in more detail in Chapter 10.

Hypoxic/ischemic encephalopathy

The exact prevalence of birth related hypoxic/ ischemic encephalopathy (HIE) is difficult to establish because it encompasses a wide range of clinical severity but may be around 40 per 1000 live births. The underlying neuropathology is similarly varied. At one extreme, infants may present in the neonatal period with profound hypoxia and seizures. More commonly, affected infants may show few signs in the neonatal period but later display mental retardation and cerebral palsy. The prevalence is in inverse proportion to the gestational age at birth. The cerebral damage is associated with deprivation of blood supply and/or oxygen to the brain. Clearly, infants who have respiratory difficulties will be at greater risk of developing HIE. The observed pathology in the brain, including periventricular leukomalacia, may not be due simply to hypoxic or ischemic injury. Increasingly, cytokines such as interferon gamma are implicated as causative agents and maternal/ fetal infection, which may not be clinically obvious, is thought to be the likely context.

In contrast with the mature nervous system, it appears that developing white matter is more vulnerable to these insults than gray matter. Acute hypoxic ischemic injury may cause brain swelling and characteristic duskiness of the white matter (Fig. 14.37). The range of pathological abnormalities includes periventricular leukomalacia, status marmoratus and diffuse white matter astrocytosis. At the most extreme, the multifocal infarction of white matter may lead to a multicystic encephalopathy in which the cerebral hemispheres are largely reduced to a thin shell of cortical gray matter (Fig. 14.38). Periventricular leukomalacia consists of focal areas of axonal injury and mineralization progressing to infarction and later cyst formation (Fig. 14.39). The surrounding white matter shows a variable degree of damage including vacuolation, microglial activation, infiltration by macrophages and astrocytosis (Fig. 14.40). Oligodendroglia and their precursors are depleted in the damaged area with grave consequences for later myelination in surviving infants. At the mild extreme of HIE, the white matter may show simply a diffuse astrocytosis which is best revealed by GFAP immunocytochemistry (Fig. 14.41a and b). The exact relationship between these pathological lesions, the clinical symptoms of cerebral palsy, and the obstetric history, remains to be elucidated. Although these lesions have been linked in the past to birth-related events, it is now clear that cerebral palsy is more the result of prenatal than of intrapartum injury.

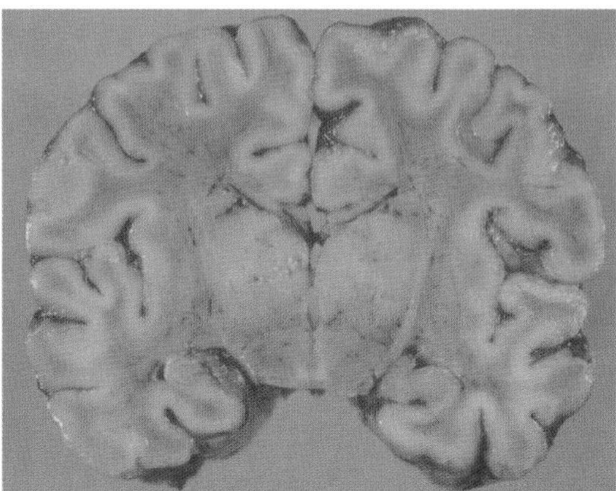

Figure 14.37 A coronal brain slice from a mature stillbirth. There is brain swelling with compression of the ventricles and dusky discoloration of the white matter which contrasts with pallor in the cortical mantle. These findings are consistent with cerebral hypoxia.

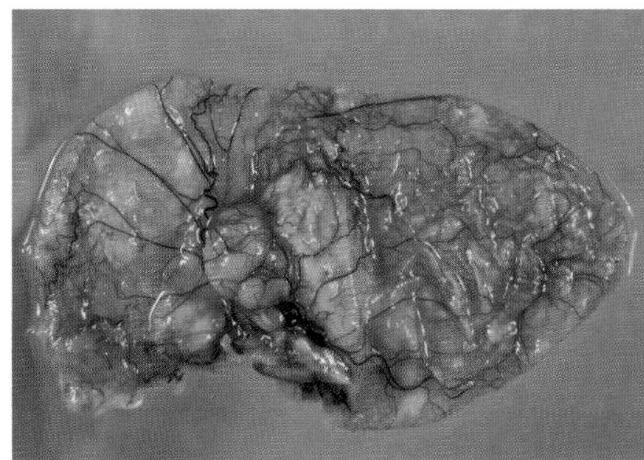

Figure 14.38 Hydranencephaly in an infant born at 35 weeks' gestation who had suffered catastrophic hypoxic/ischemic injury *in utero*. The cortex is reduced to small nodules of tissue adherent to the leptomeninges.

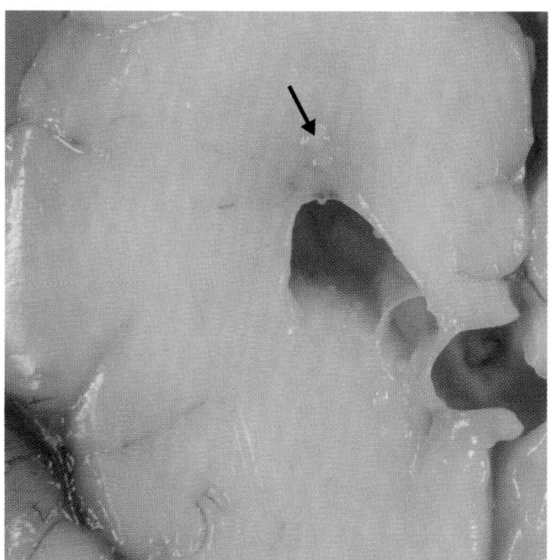

Figure 14.39 Coronal slice of the brain at approximately 30 weeks' gestation. There is a periventricular cyst and a focus of calcification (arrowed), consistent with periventricular leukomalacia.

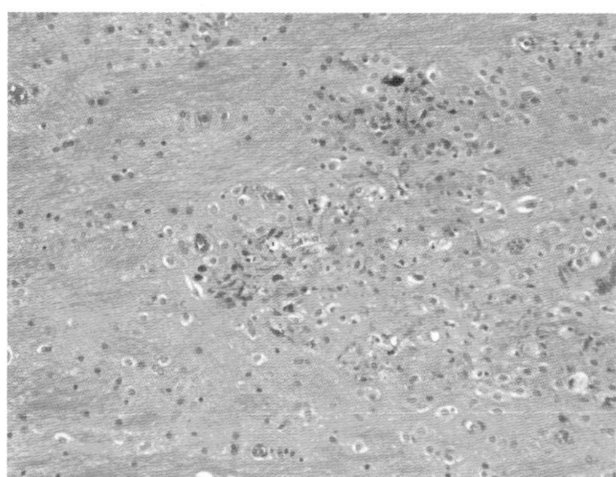

Figure 14.40 Section of a lesion of periventricular leukomalacia showing accumulation of macrophages associated with abnormal mineralized axons in the deep white matter. Severe lesions progress to necrosis and cyst formation. H&E, ×100.

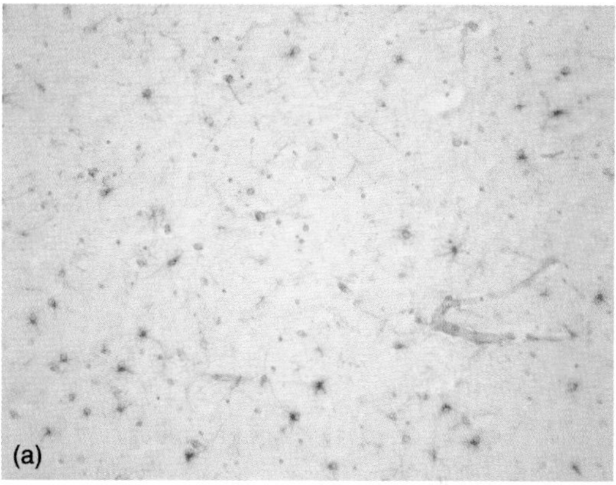

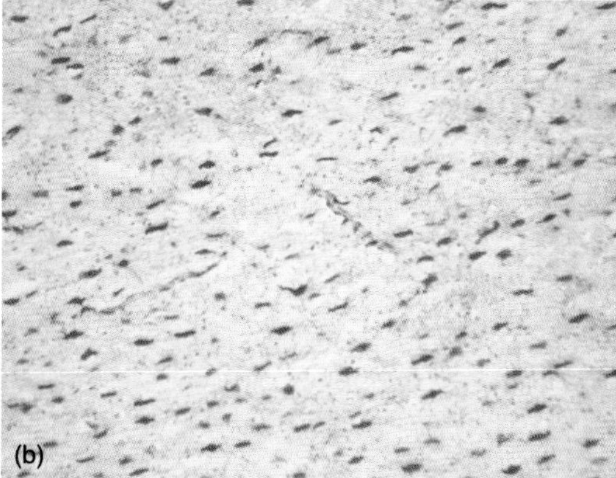

Figure 14.41 (a) Normal white matter from a third trimester fetus stained for glial fibrillary acidic protein. The relationship between astrocytes and small blood vessels is shown. ×100. (b) Reactive astrocytosis in the deep white matter from a fetus age-matched with (a). The cause of the brain injury is unknown in many cases but is assumed to be hypoxic/ischemic. ×100.

Examination of infants who die in the first day or two after birth confirms that prenatal brain injury is present in over 40% of neonatal deaths (Table 14.8). The signs of perinatal asphyxia include a low Apgar score (failing to attain a score of 5 by 5 min after birth), acidosis with an arterial pH of 7.2 or less, and in the worst cases, seizure activity. While the evidence of HIE is often reflected in white matter damage, the gray matter does not escape injury. Focal gyral injury may result from ischemic damage in the developing brain (Fig. 14.42). Certain patterns of neuronal vulnerability are expressed preferentially in the developing brain. Neuronal eosinophilia (Fig. 14.43) or nuclear karyorrhexis (Fig. 14.44) is identified particularly in the subiculum and entorhinal cortex and in the ventral pons, and the lesion is termed pontosubicular necrosis. Macrophage (Fig. 14.45a and b) and astrocyte responses to neuronal injury

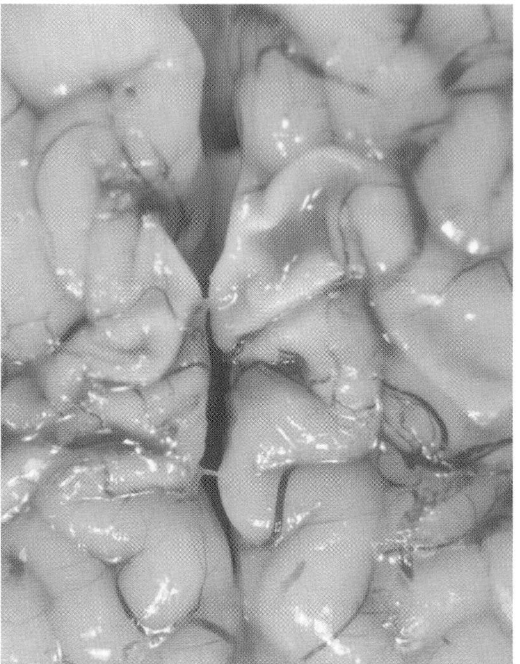

Figure 14.42 Superior view of the brain from a mature fetus. There is collapse of individual gyri close to the sagittal sulcus, resulting from focal ischemic injury.

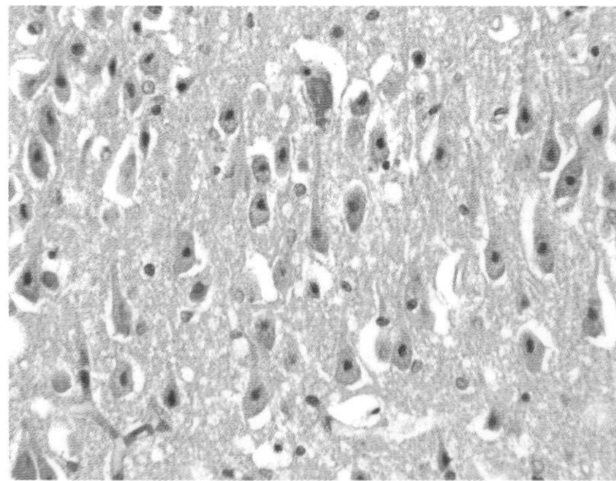

Figure 14.43 Section of the hippocampus from a 2-day-old infant who had suffered perinatal hypoxia. The neurons are brightly eosinophilic, signifying recent hypoxic injury. H&E, ×200.

appear to be more leisurely in the gray matter than in the central white matter. The location of these different features is shown in Table 14.8. The timing of cellular reactions to perinatal brain damage

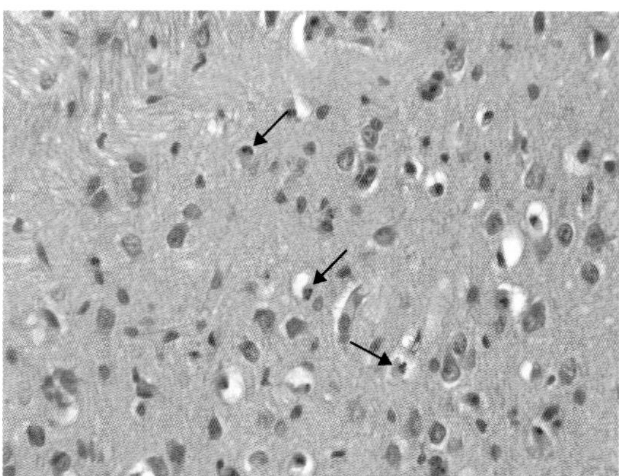

Figure 14.44 Section from the pons of an infant of 1 day who displayed signs of perinatal asphyxia. Many of the neurons are shrunken with karyorrhectic nuclei (arrowed). Similar findings were noted in the subiculum, indicating the presence of pontosubicular necrosis. H&E, ×200.

is listed in Table 14.9, to the extent of present knowledge. Evidence of glial karyorrhexis may be present in damaged white matter (Fig. 14.46). Hypertrophic astrocytes may be difficult to distinguish from so-called myelination gliosis but the application of GFAP immunocytochemistry resolves this matter immediately. Myelination glial cells are oligodendroglia with an unusual quantity of cytoplasm, which are orientated in orderly rows within myelinating white matter (Fig. 14.47a). These cells are not GFAP positive (Fig. 14.47b). Status marmoratus appears in surviving children as streaking of the thalamus signifying abnormal myelination of astrocytic processes (Fig. 14.48).

Hippocampal sclerosis

This lesion is characterized by loss of neurons in the cornu ammonis and replacement by glial cells. The abnormality is maximal in the CA1 sector and is a basis for temporal lobe epilepsy. The granular layer of the hippocampus may also be disorganized. This abnormality resembles the end-stage damage produced by hypoxic/ischemic injury. Since seizures can themselves lead to hypoxic injury in the brain, the exact sequence of events which leads to hippocampal sclerosis remains unclear.

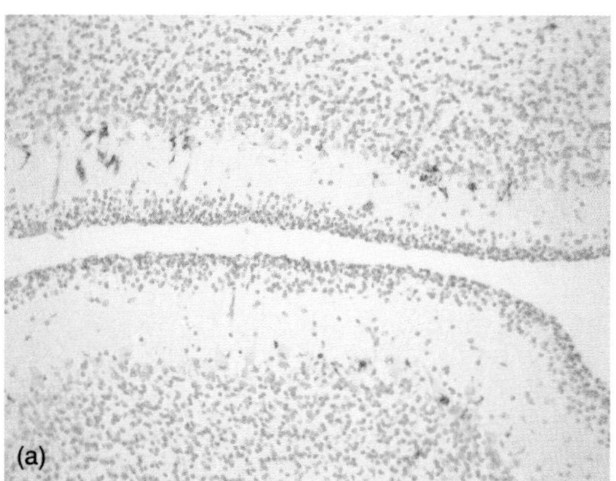

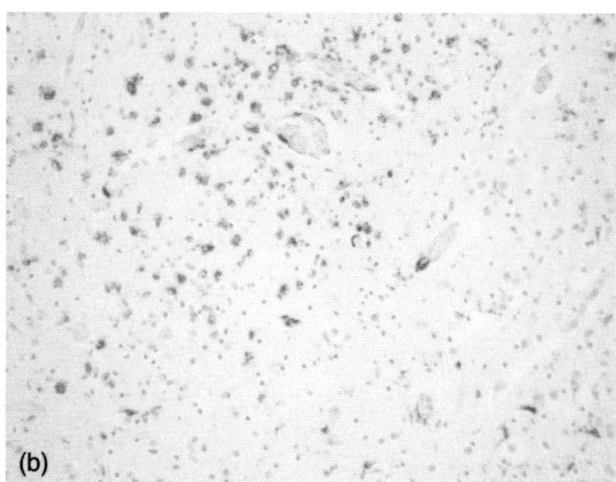

Figure 14.45 (a) Cerebellum from a 32 week gestation infant who survived for 2 days. The Purkinje layer of the cortex is damaged and there is focal infiltration with CD68-positive macrophages, indicating prenatal injury. ×100. (b) Medulla from the same infant showing accumulated macrophages in the nuclei of the floor of the 4th ventricle, consistent with neuronal damage. ×100.

Table 14.8 Microscopic neuropathological abnormalities which may be detected in infants dying in the perinatal period

Abnormality	Likely distribution
Neuronal eosinophilia	Hippocampus, basal ganglia, thalamus, brainstem, dentate nuclei, Purkinje cells or global phenomenon
Neuronal karyorrhexis	Hippocampus and brainstem (pontosubicular necrosis)
White matter necrosis	Central white matter of hemispheres
Macrophage accumulation, gray or white matter	Cerebral and cerebellar cortex, white matter of cerebrum, germinal matrix
Astrocytosis, gray or white matter	Cerebrum, cerebellum
Periventricular leukomalacia	Periventricular white matter
Fresh hemorrhage	Meninges, petechial hemorrhages in gray and white matter of cerebrum and cerebellum, germinal matrix, ventricular cavities
Older hemorrhages and hemosiderin deposition	Germinal matrix, cerebellar cortex
Mineralization	Basal ganglia, cerebral white matter (neurons and perivascular deposits)

Vascular injury in the developing brain

Engorgement of small parenchymal blood vessels is a usual response in hypoxic brain tissue. Endothelial hyperplasia and new blood vessel formation is a feature of ongoing perinatal hypoxic brain injury. Perivascular microhemorrhages are frequent in this context. Vascular damage reaches greater significance in the germinal matrix and germinal eminence where thin-walled blood vessels may break down in response to hypoxic injury, causing germinal matrix hemorrhage (Figs 14.6, page 261 and 14.49). Such hemorrhages may extend and disrupt the ependyma, leading to intraventricular hemorrhage which undergoes organization with post hemorrhage survival (Fig. 14.50). While respiratory difficulties in the premature neonate are a contributory factor, germinal matrix and intraventricular hemorrhages are also found in stillborn

Table 14.9 Timing of birth-related CNS injury after cerebral insult

Pathological feature	Time lapse from insult to appearance
Neuronal	
• Eosinophilia	6–24 h
• Karyorrhexis	12–48 h
Astrocyte	
• Reactive gliosis of white matter	3–11 days
• Reactive gliosis of gray matter	3–5 days
Macrophage	
• Microglial upregulation	3 h to 3 days
• Macrophage infiltration	3–7 days
Vascular	
• Fresh hemorrhage	Minutes
• Hemosiderin deposits	2–3 days
Tissue responses	
• Coagulation necrosis	3–8 h
• Cavitating infarcts	14–42 days
• Mineralization	3–14 days

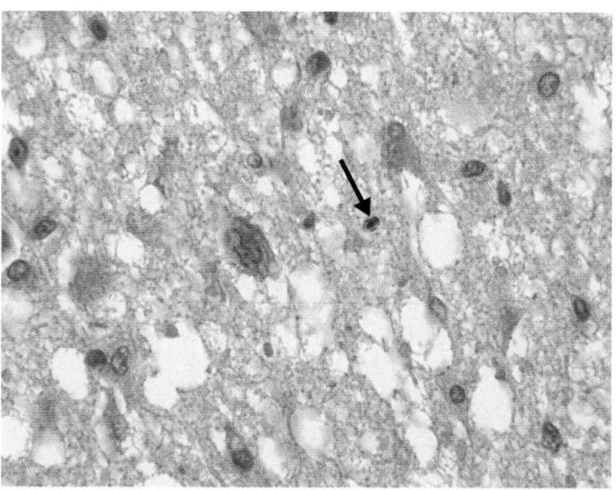

Figure 14.46 Severely damaged white matter in an infant with perinatal asphyxia. The white matter is rarefied and vacuolated and extensive astrocytic hyperplasia is present. Occasional karyorrhectic glial nuclei are noted (arrowed). H&E, ×400.

infants. The grades of germinal matrix and intraventricular hemorrhage are shown in Table 14.10. Intraventricular hemorrhage in the mature infant, older than 35 weeks' gestation, is more commonly traced to a choroid plexus origin.

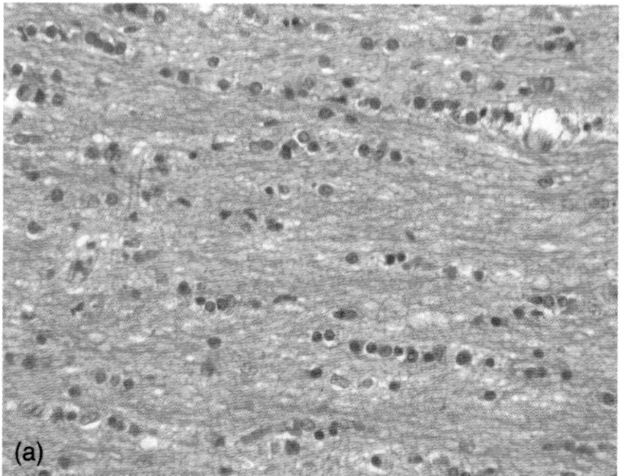

Figure 14.47 (a) Normal white matter from the periventricular region of a term fetus. Glial cells are orientated in rows and display occasional eosinophilic cytoplasm. These are the appearances of 'myelination gliosis' and most of these cells are oligodendroglia. H&E, ×100. (b) Similar brain area stained for glial fibrillary acidic protein. The linear arrays of glial cells are negative for glial fibrillary acidic protein, in keeping with their oligodendroglial lineage. ×200.

Stillbirth, maceration

Significant neuropathological findings can almost always be distinguished from post mortem maceration changes and other artefacts. Hemorrhage, evidence of white matter damage and micromineralization (Fig. 14.51) are readily seen in the brains of stillborns. The changes are not dissimilar from those seen in the neonatal brain and include germinal matrix and intraventricular hemorrhage. Pontosubicular necrosis and other signs of neuronal injury are identifiable in some stillbirths and

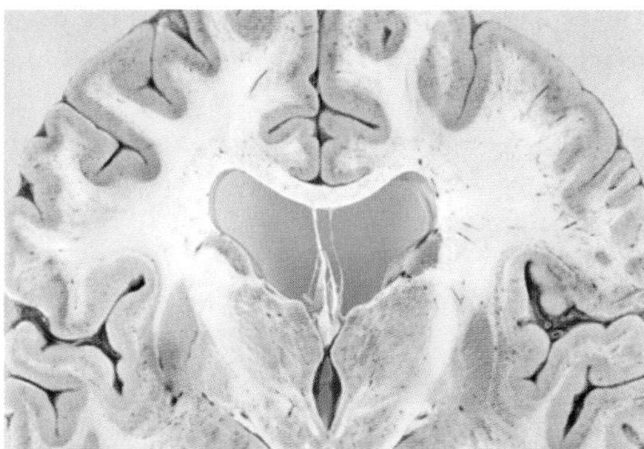

Figure 14.48 Coronal brain slice from a 5-year-old child who suffered from mental retardation and birth injury. The ventricles are dilated and both thalami show pale streaking of grey matter, consistent with status marmoratus.

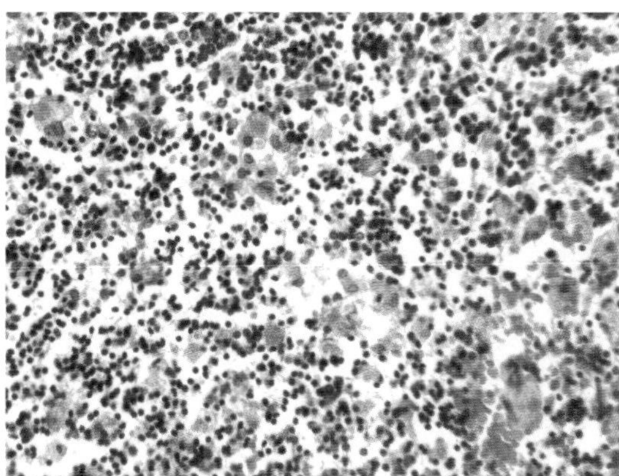

Figure 14.49 Section from the germinal matrix of a 3-day-old premature infant who sustained a subependymal hemorrhage. Fresh hemorrhage is present together with pigment laden macrophages, indicating previous or ongoing hemorrhage. H&E, ×200.

are indicative of fetal brain injury before ultimate fetal death, possibly linked in some cases to failing placental function.

INFECTIONS AND INFLAMMATORY CONDITIONS

Infections which involve the developing nervous system may be acquired during fetal life, around the

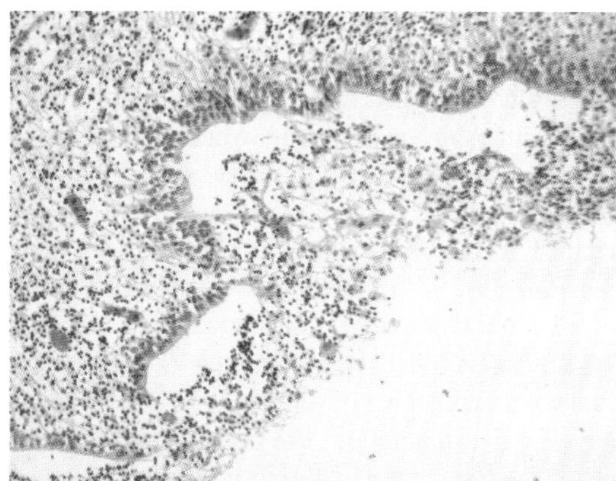

Figure 14.50 Lining of the lateral ventricle in the infant shown in Fig. 14.49 shows the presence of organizing intraventricular hemorrhage attached irregularly to the ependymal surface. H&E, ×100.

Table 14.10 Grades of germinal matrix hemorrhage

Grade	Hemorrhage
I	Subependymal hemorrhage (SEH)
II	SEH plus intraventricular hemorrhage (IVH) without ventricular enlargement
III	SEH, IVH plus ventricular enlargement
IV	SEH, IVH plus intracerebral hemorrhage beyond germinal eminence

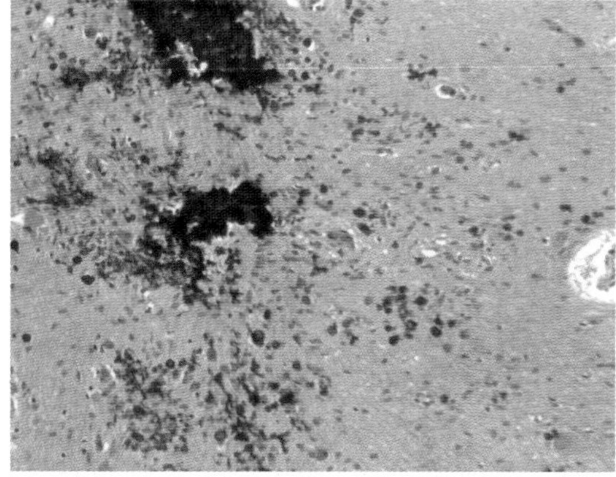

Figure 14.51 Section of the internal capsule from a fetus stillborn at 36 weeks' gestation. Extensive mineralisation of the white matter is present, indicating longstanding prenatal brain injury. H&E, ×100.

time of birth or during early infancy, and in childhood. The developing fetus and the newborn do not have fully developed immune mechanisms and are thus vulnerable to infections which are less of a threat to the mature CNS. Passively acquired maternal antibodies may be insufficient to protect them against acquired infections. Children may also suffer from a defect in their immune system as a result of genetic inheritance, or related to advancing human immunodeficiency virus (HIV) infection or following iatrogenic measures including chemotherapy and transplantation. The CNS is generally protected against contamination from the environment by means of various physical barriers, including the meninges. Just as in adult life, infective organisms may arrive within the CNS by means of the blood stream, by transport along nerve pathways or by breaching barriers. CNS tissue may be exposed to a heightened risk of infection by trauma, by surgical procedures including the placement of shunts and by cannulae to the ventricular system.

The severity of infection, and the effects which are produced, vary according to the microbiological agent involved and the stage of development at which the infection is acquired (Table 14.11). Fetal infections are acquired transplacentally from the mother and may be diagnosed by examination of the amniotic fluid. Infections arising during fetal development often cause fetal death or multi-organ abnormalities including fetal hydrops. Such lethal results are most frequently associated with parvovirus and listeria. Infections which target the brain at these early stages may induce microcephaly from impaired brain growth. There may also be signs of diffuse or multifocal inflammatory changes, often with associated vascular changes and ensuing infarction and mineralization. The causative agent may not be apparent from histological examination of the brain tissue since the damage may be end-stage and represented by necrosis, calcification and gliotic reactions. More commonly there is a microglial/macrophage reaction, often in the form of microglial nodules. Immunocytochemical, tissue culture and polymerase chain reaction (PCR) methods should be used to identify responsible microbiological agents.

The developing infant is also at risk of acquiring infections such as HIV during birth or breast feeding. The neonate is at risk of infection from the environment, particularly following premature birth. Involvement of the CNS usually occurs as a complication of septicaemia. Fungal agents such as *Candida* are a particular risk for premature infants in intensive care. Infections of the CNS during childhood are similar to those seen later in life and reflect the environment in which the child is growing up. Cerebral malaria is often fatal in children in tropical countries. One or two infective agents can lead to a fatal outcome only after a long quiescent period and these are described below.

Cytomegalovirus (CMV)

This virus can cause CNS infection during fetal life (Fig. 14.52), in the neonatal period and in children who are immunosuppressed. Infection of the fetus occurs as a result of maternal primary or reactivated infection or re-infection. The virus targets many fetal organs and can lead to fetal hydrops. Involvement of the brain may give rise to a meningoencephalitis with polymicrogyria, hydrocephalus or porencephaly. Alternatively, fetal infection may be occult at the time of birth with later emergence of CNS signs and symptoms. CMV is entirely promiscuous in cell targets and can infect any of the cells of the CNS (Fig. 14.53). It has a particular propensity for endothelial involvement and this may lead to thrombosis and resulting ischemic damage. Inclusion bodies which are present in both nucleus and cytoplasm of infected cells may be hard to detect in the absence of immunocytochemical staining. Immunosuppressed children who acquire CMV infection only after birth show neuropathological changes reminiscent of those seen in older individuals. These take the form of necrotizing lesions with acute inflammation characterized by polymorphonuclear leukocyte infiltration, or widespread microglial nodular encephalitis in which inclusion bearing cells are often hard to find.

Rubella

Congenital rubella infection has become rare since the introduction of immunization. Congenital malformations may occur in the heart, eye, ear or brain

Table 14.11 Impact of infection at different stages of CNS development

Infective agent	Fetal	Perinatal/neonatal/infancy	Childhood
Viruses			
CMV	Meningoencephalitis/microcephaly and calcification	Meningoencephalitis	Opportunistic
Rubella	Microcephaly/eye and ear abnormalities	o	o
HIV	o	Encephalitis	Encephalitis
Herpes simplex 1	Microcephaly	Encephalitis	Encephalitis
Herpes simplex 2	Microcephaly	Encephalitis	Encephalitis
Measles	o	Meningoencephalitis	Meningoencephalitis
Varicella zoster	Microcephaly	o	Meningoencephalitis
Parvovirus	Hypoxic/ischemic injury	o	o
Enteroviruses	o	Meningitis	Meningoencephalitis
Bacteria			
Trepanema pallidum	Hydrops	Meningoencephalitis	Meningoencephalitis
Listeria monocytogenes	Meningitis	Meningitis	o
Staphylococcus aureus	o	Meningitis	o
Escherichia coli	o	Meningitis	o
Haemophilus influenzae	o	o	Meningitis
Streptococcus pneumoniae	o	Meningitis	Meningitis
Neisseria meningitides	o	o	Meningitis
Mycobacterium tuberculosis	o	o	Tuberculous meningitis
Protozoal			
Toxoplasma	Meningoencephalitis/necrosis/calcification	o	Opportunistic
Plasmodium falciparum	o	o	Cerebral malaria
Fungi			
Candida	o	Meningoencephalitis	Opportunistic
Aspergillus	o	Meningoencephalitis	Opportunistic
Cryptococcus	o	o	Opportunistic
Other			
Hydatid disease	o	o	Cerebral cysts
Ameba	o	o	Meningoencephalitis

o = No reported significant effect.

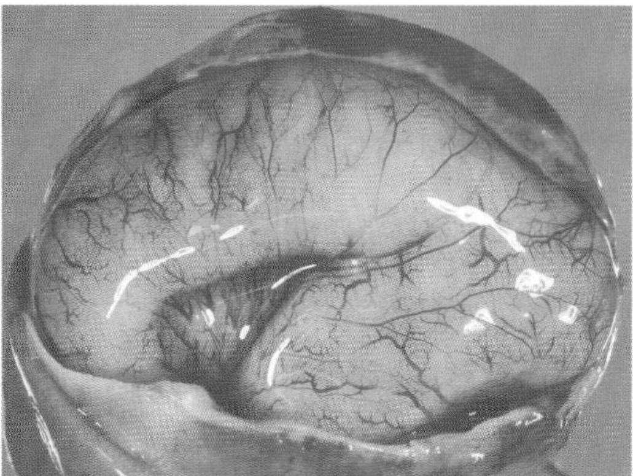

Figure 14.52 Termination of pregnancy at 20 weeks' gestation because of cytomegalovirus infection. The leptomeninges are very congested but thickening is not apparent at this stage. Histological examination confirmed the presence of early meningitis.

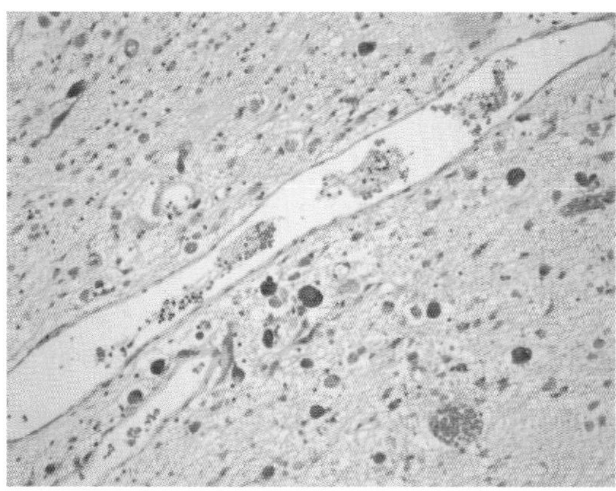

Figure 14.53 Section of the brain from a fetus terminated because of hydrocephalus. Extensive brain damage is associated with widespread cytomegalovirus infection. Infected cells are seen scattered through the parenchyma. H&E, ×200.

as a result of fetal infection in the first trimester. Infection of the brain leads to microcephaly through loss of brain tissue due to rubella-associated vascular problems and mineralization. There is generally little inflammation within brain tissue as a result of the infection. Congenital rubella infection may be far from obvious at birth and the damaging effects may become clinically manifest only later in development.

Human immunodeficiency virus (HIV)

Soon after the start of the HIV/AIDS epidemic, it became clear that transmission could occur in up to 40% of the offspring of HIV infected women. All infants born to HIV positive mothers are themselves HIV positive since they passively acquire the maternal antibody. Detection of the virus by PCR is required to establish the presence of infection in the infant prior to the loss of maternal antibodies. Examination of fetuses from terminated HIV positive pregnancies failed to identify specific HIV-associated fetal abnormalities or evidence of infection. The realisation that the risk of HIV transmission to the fetus is maximal around the time of birth (rather than in fetal life) has led to effective policies for protecting the fetus from vertical HIV transmission, usually by treatment with a single antiretroviral drug such as nevirapine. HIV infection may also be transmitted by breast feeding. HIV-infected infants and children vary considerably in their progress to AIDS even in the absence of all treatment. Before effective therapy was available, the late effects of HIV/AIDS, including HIV encephalitis and CNS opportunistic infections, did occur in children just as in similarly affected adults. HIV encephalitis is characterized by giant cells (Fig. 14.54) and HIV immunopositive microglia/macrophages. If this condition develops in the first year or two of life, brain growth slows and microcephaly results. Most HIV infected children living in parts of the world where treatment is not available die of non-CNS complications of immunosuppression.

Herpes simplex 1 and 2

Infections with the herpes viruses may be intrauterine or perinatal. Intrauterine infections affect multiple fetal organs but may lead to microcephaly through brain involvement and the appearance of meningo-encephalitis. Perinatal herpes infection may be acquired from the birth canal if genital herpes is present. In these infants CNS infection is acquired by retrograde transport along sensory axons. Most neonatal herpes encephalitis is caused by herpes simplex 2. The brain in such cases is

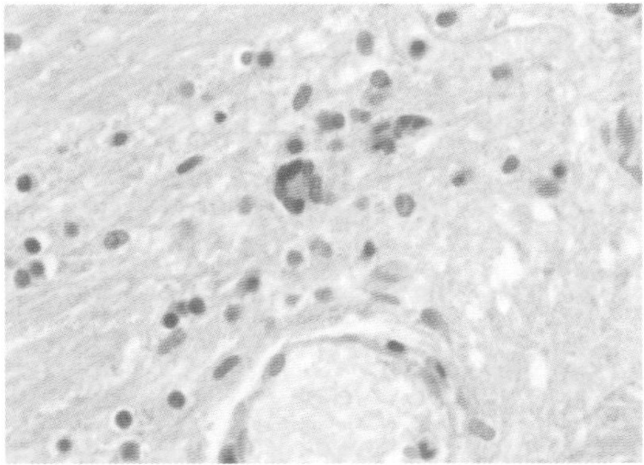

Figure 14.54 Section of the deep white matter from an HIV positive African child of 15 months. Giant cells are seen in relation to a small blood vessel, indicating the presence of HIV encephalitis. H&E, ×400.

swollen and shows necrotic lesions associated with macrophages and lymphocytic infiltrates.

Measles

Infection with this virus is seen in infants and young children following respiratory spread from another infected individual. The acute systemic infection with characteristic skin rash may be associated with an episode of relatively mild viral meningitis or more rarely, acute encephalitis. Very occasionally an attack of measles is followed a number of years later by subacute sclerosing panencephalitis (SSPE). In this condition there is severe neuronal loss and gliosis with variable inflammatory infiltrate. Inclusion-bearing cells, both neurons and glia, are found within the damaged cortex (Fig. 14.55). In SSPE, genetic changes occur in the measles virus which limit its ability to propagate freely but which do not inhibit its tissue damaging properties. The disease proves fatal eventually after progressive cognitive decline.

Varicella zoster

This virus is only rarely transmitted to fetuses and is generally an illness of young children, causing chicken pox. Affected fetuses may show inflammatory and ischemic damage in the CNS associated with a microglial infiltrate. Cortical abnormalities

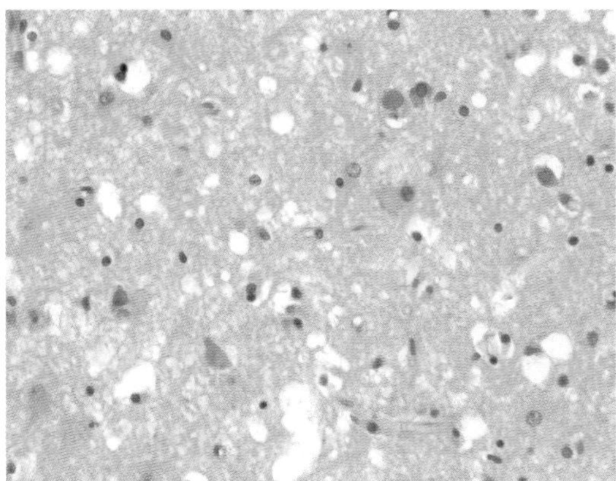

Figure 14.55 Section of the cortex from an HIV negative African child with measles. The changes of measles encephalitis include widespread destruction of the cortex, loss of neurons and status spongiosis. Viral inclusion bodies are noted in neurons and other cells in this case. H&E, ×200.

may be present and there may be motor and sensory nerve cell loss, particularly in the spinal cord.

Parvovirus

Parvovirus can be transmitted during pregnancy and is a cause of fetal hydrops. The ensuing anemia and heart failure can cause cerebral hypoxia/ischemia, leading to destructive lesions in the gray matter and secondary ventricular dilation.

Enteroviruses

These include poliovirus, coxsackie viruses and echoviruses. This group of viruses can cause meningitis in infants and in some cases, meningoencephalitis. Poliovirus has an affinity for gray matter and targets motor neurons, whose destruction is associated with microglial nodules and slight lymphocytic infiltrate. Destruction of motor neuron cells results in paralysis of the innervated muscle fibers.

Syphilis (*Trepanema pallidum*)

Congenital syphilis is rare nowadays since maternal infection is readily detected and treatable in pregnancy. An affected fetus may display multi-organ involvement with hepatosplenomegaly and hydrops.

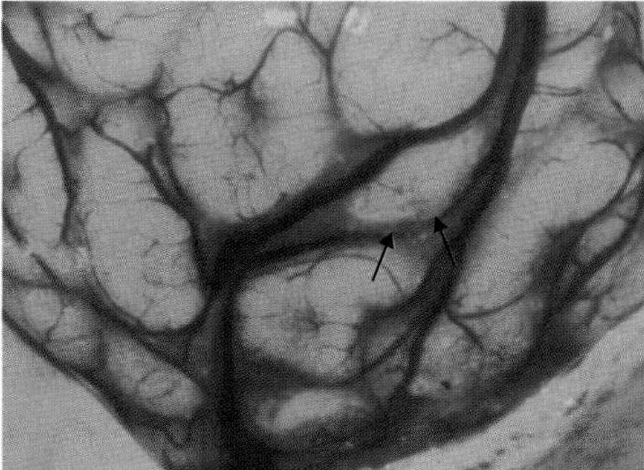

Figure 14.56 Lateral view of cerebrum in a preterm twin. The leptomeninges are congested and multiple microabscesses (arrowed) are present, subsequently confirmed as congenital *Listeria monocytogenes* infection.

There may be no apparent CNS involvement at birth and only later does this become apparent. Late complications include meningitis, meningeal fibrosis leading to hydrocephalus, vasculitis leading to ischemic necrosis and in exceptionally rare circumstances the tertiary stages of tabes dorsalis and general paralysis of the insane (GPI). These conditions display the same pathology as in the adult.

Listeria monocytogenes

Listeria infection is acquired by the mother from eating contaminated food, such as soft cheese and pre-prepared salads. If the infection is passed to the fetus it gives rise to multiple abscesses in many organs. The brain is involved infrequently but may display meningitis (Fig. 14.56) or ventriculitis.

Toxoplasmosis

This protozoan is an important cause of fetal brain damage if it is transmitted during pregnancy. The maternal infection may be primary or reactivated. The brain displays inflammation and tissue destruction associated with free *Toxoplasma* tachyzoites or encysted forms (Fig. 14.57). Microglial nodules may be present together with necrosis, macrophage infiltration and mineralization. Tissue destruction leads to fetal hydrocephalus. Less severe forms may manifest later and are associated with seizures, mental retardation and foci of cerebral mineralization.

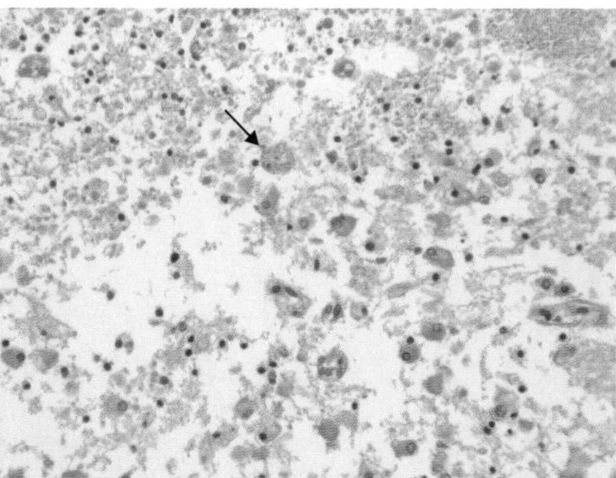

Figure 14.57 Section of the brain from an hydropic fetus with hepatosplenomegaly and extensive cerebral necrosis. Pseudocysts (arrowed) and free organisms indicate the presence of cerebral toxoplasmosis. H&E, ×200.

Malaria (*Plasmodium falciparium*)

This infection is transmitted to young children through mosquito bites. The red blood cells are parasitized and cerebral malaria ensues when the cerebral microvasculature is involved. Seizures and coma may result. The brain is swollen and displays congested meninges with petechial hemorrhages and small infarcts. Microscopic examination reveals malarial pigment within the blood vessels (Fig. 14.58) together with necrotic white matter lesions (Durck granulomata) (Fig. 14.59), which may result from disturbance of blood flow in the microvasculature.

Fungi

Fungi may be acquired as an ascending infection from the birth canal or, in the neonatal period, from the environment, usually via infusion cannulae. Fungal meningo-encephalitis is characterized by foci of macrophages and giant cells containing fungal hyphae and spores, readily identified by PAS or silver staining (Fig. 14.60a and b). *Candida* and *Aspergillus* are the usual fungal agents involved. Cryptococcal infection may be a risk in older infants who are immunosuppressed particularly if this is HIV-associated. *Cryptococcus* involves particularly the meninges and the basal ganglia.

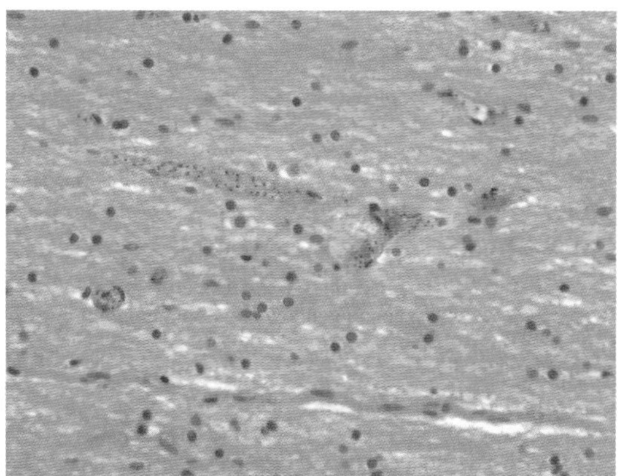

Figure 14.58 Cerebellar white matter from an HIV-positive African child who died of malaria. The small blood vessels contain malarial pigment and parasitized red blood cells. H&E, ×200.

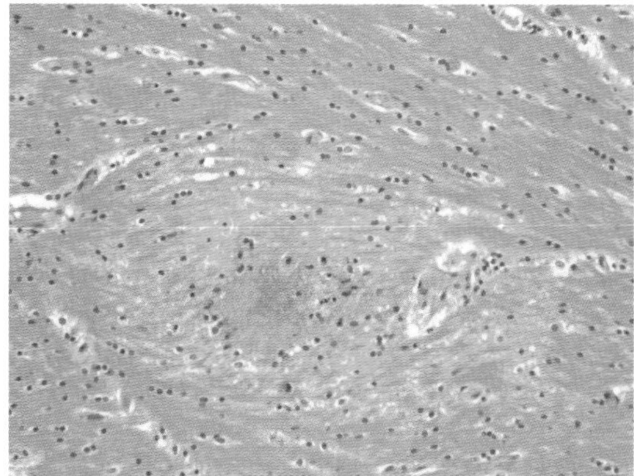

Figure 14.59 African child of 18 months with signs of malaria who lapsed into coma. The cerebral white matter contains ischemic lesions and infarcts centered on small thrombosed blood vessels and associated with microglial infiltration. These lesions are known as Durck granulomata, a hallmark of cerebral malaria. H&E, ×100.

Acute meningitis in children

The organisms causing bacterial meningitis in neonates (Fig. 14.61) are somewhat different from those affecting older children. The causative agents are listed in Table 14.11, page 285. *Mycobacterium tuberculosis* can cause meningitis and tuberculomas in young children if they are environmentally exposed. Meningitis may be particularly hard to diagnose in infants and can be rapidly fatal. The affected brain shows vascular congestion and brain swelling but there may be little or no evidence of purulent exudate on macroscopic examination. It is important to examine multiple blocks histologically for the presence of polymorphs in the subarachnoid space since there may be relatively few present. These are most often seen over the cerebellum and around the brainstem, and over the occipital convexities. More established cases have macroscopically detectable pus in the leptomeninges and are at risk of cortical infarction from involvement of blood vessels crossing the subarachnoid space (Fig. 14.62).

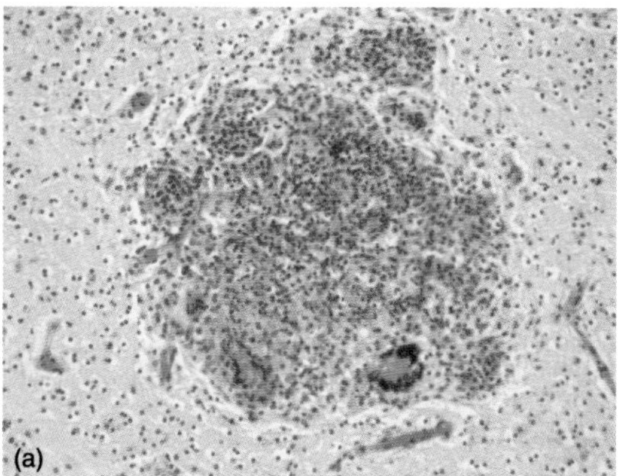

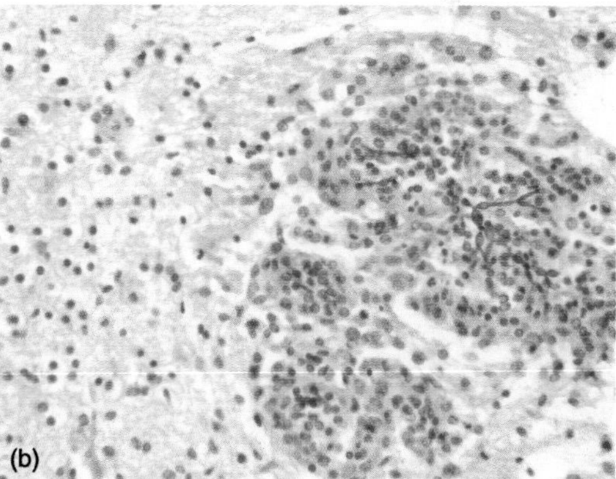

Figure 14.60 (a) Two-week-old neonate maintained in an intensive care unit and who died of septicemia. Granulomata were found in the brain and these contained giant cells. H&E, ×100. (b) Staining of the granulomata shown in (a) reveals fungal hyphae. The appearances are consistent with *Candida albicans* infection. Periodic acid–Schiff reaction, ×200.

Brain abscesses are rare in developed countries but remain a risk following trauma or associated with malformations, dental abscess, mastoiditis or

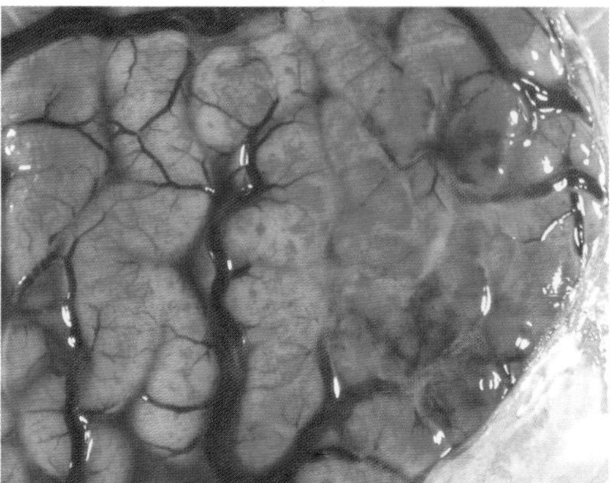

Figure 14.61 Term neonate who died at 3 weeks of age. There is a purulent exudate within extremely congested meninges. A group B streptococcal infection was responsible for the meningitis.

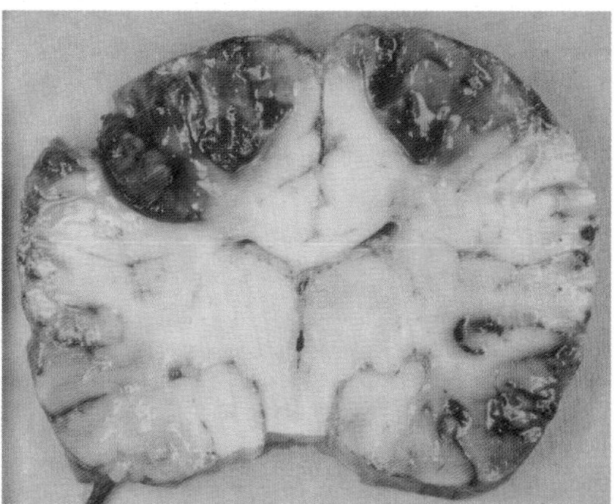

Figure 14.62 Same case as Fig. 14.61. A coronal slice of the brain demonstrates extensive cortical venous infarction.

cranial surgery. Immunodeficiency also predisposes to cerebral abscess. Spinal epidural abscesses carry a risk of spinal cord compression and are likely to be confused with tumors.

Rasmussen syndrome

This syndrome is manifested by a seizure disorder which is unresponsive to therapy. Children under 10 years of age are usually affected. The neuropathological abnormality is confined to one hemisphere and is characteristically inflammatory. Focal lymphocytic infiltrates are present around meningeal and parenchymal blood vessels and the cortex displays microglial nodules and widespread activated microglia. There is ongoing neuronal damage and loss with resulting gliosis and spongy change. The etiology of this curious condition is unknown and both viral and autoimmune causation has been invoked though never proven. Neuroimaging suggests that the inflammatory process commences in the basal ganglia. Hemispherectomy may be necessary to control the seizures.

MATERNAL DRUG AND ALCOHOL USE

Maternal drug abuse may result in the birth of an addicted infant who requires treatment for drug withdrawal. Non-specific effects have been described in the brain, the most severe of which is microcephaly. The effects of alcohol use are also deleterious and are described in more detail in Chapter 13.

INFANCY AND EARLY CHILDHOOD

Sudden infant death syndrome/sudden unexpected death in infancy

Sudden infant death syndrome (SIDS) is the term used to describe the death of an infant or young child which is unexpected by history and where a thorough investigation of the circumstances, and a full post mortem examination, fail to establish the cause of death. If the examination is incomplete for any reason, or if an unexpected potentially significant abnormality is found (Fig. 14.63) thereby rendering a diagnosis of SIDS invalid, the infant may be assigned to the group of sudden unexpected death in infancy (SUDI). The incidence of SIDS varies widely but overall is approximately 1 per 1400 liveborn infants. The age group of infants most at risk for SIDS is 2–4 months and the infant dies during a period of sleep. Although a family history of SIDS,

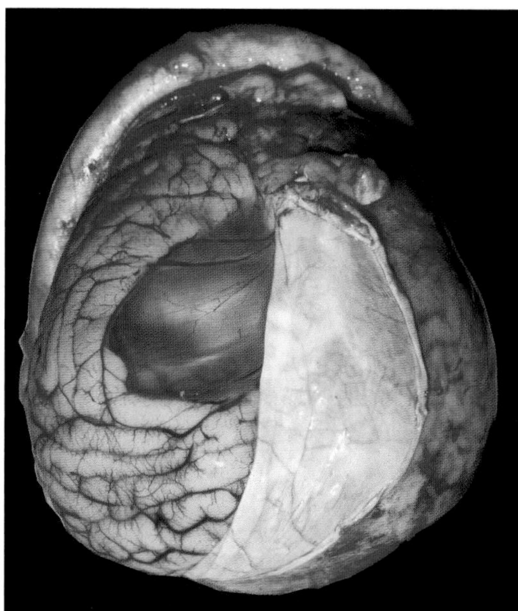

Figure 14.63 Sudden unexpected infant death at home. Left-sided porencephaly was an unexpected finding.

including a similar occurrence in a sibling, is unusual, it is not unknown which focuses attention on possible genetic causes. A recent study has shown that the recurrence rate for unexpected infant deaths may be as high as 6 per 1000 live births, most of these being natural deaths or SIDS. It is also of note that a history of stillbirth is more common in the family of SIDS victims.

A diagnosis of SIDS is arrived at by exclusion of other possible causes. Microscopical examination of autopsy tissue samples and full neuropathological examination are more likely than other laboratory investigations, including microbiology and toxicology, to reveal a cause for the death. The factors contributing to the likelihood of a SIDS death include preterm delivery and low birth weight, sleeping in the prone position particularly at high ambient temperature, co-sleeping with an adult and parental smoking or intake of drugs or alcohol.

The cause of SIDS is unknown but is thought to be multifactorial with a fatal intercept of environmental factors acting on an innately vulnerable infant at a particular developmental age. Cardiac abnormalities, such as a prolonged QT interval and increased susceptibility to apneic attacks are present in a small proportion of cases. There are indications that brain development or function may not be entirely normal in these infants. None of these abnormalities is sufficient to account for the death of the infant and, by definition, examination of the brain in SIDS cases does not show major abnormalities. If these were found to be present, the diagnostic label of SIDS becomes untenable. However, careful investigation of SIDS cases may show subtle abnormal features in the CNS which are listed in Table 14.12. There is a similarity between these subtle neuropathological findings and those seen in the brains of unexplained stillbirths. Detailed research studies suggest that neuronal abnormalities in functionally important areas of the brainstem, including the autonomic and olivary nuclei, are associated with SIDS. The recent report of an association between elevated alphafetoprotein levels in maternal serum during pregnancy and an increased risk of SIDS also suggests that fetal development may not have been optimal in such cases. Rarely, *de novo* mutations in genes controlling the QT interval are present in SIDS. Polymorphisms in the IL-10 gene, controlling anti-inflammatory cytokines, have also been described. The causes of SIDS, including the genetic causes, remain the subject of active investigation.

Table 14.12 Central nervous system findings in sudden infant death syndrome

- Brain weight increased for age
- Gliosis of the cerebral white matter, brainstem and cerebellum in some cases
- Hypomyelination of the cerebral white matter, brainstem and cerebellum in some cases
- Changes in neuronal number and arrangement in the brainstem nuclei

Trauma and non-accidental head injury

Head injury in children is a leading cause of death and of disability in survivors. Mobile children may suffer accidental falls and be involved in road traffic accidents. In both of these circumstances severe head injury may occur, including skull fracture, subdural hemorrhage and cerebral contusions. Infants

Table 14.13 Post mortem findings suggestive of traumatic and non-accidental head injury

Classic triad
- Subdural hemorrhage(s)
- Extensive retinal hemorrhages
- Diffuse cerebral swelling

Features sometimes present
- Skeletal and extra-cranial injuries
- Skull fracture
- Cerebral contusions
- Axonal injury

Table 14.14 Causes of subdural hemorrhage in infants

- Birth-related injury
- Severe accidental injury, e.g. road traffic accident or high-level falls
- Coagulopathies
- Non-accidental injury
- Iatrogenic (complication of neurosurgical procedures)
- Brain shrinkage from any cause, including some genetic metabolic diseases and hypernatremia
- Vascular malformations
- Hypoxic/ischemic injury and short falls have been proposed as possible causes but require further evidence

may also be involved in road traffic accidents but rarely suffer the effects of severe falls since they are relatively immobile. In this age group particularly, the possibility that head injury is of non-accidental origin should be considered. The pathology features of traumatic head injury are shown in Table 14.13. In the context of suspected head injury subdural hemorrhage may be detected on scan. If it is not suspected it is first found at autopsy (Fig. 14.1, page 257). The hemorrhage is usually bilateral and often described as a thin film overlying the cerebral convexities. Extensive bilateral retinal hemorrhages are present in a high proportion of cases and the infant is usually comatose as a result of diffuse cerebral swelling. When the history provided by the infant's carer is inconsistent with the clinical findings, or there is no account of a traumatic event, non-accidental injury (NAHI) should be suspected. Certain physical features contribute to the findings found in injured infants. In this age group the skull has a smooth inner surface to which the dura mater is tightly adherent, thus predisposing to greater stretching and possible rupture of veins which cross the subdural space. Lacerations of the brain surface are less commonly found than in adults. Myelination is far from complete in the infant brain and this confers a different consistency on immature brain tissue.

For the last 50 years, prevailing opinion has held that infants who display subdural hemorrhage(s), retinal hemorrhages and diffuse cerebral swelling have suffered a head injury which is most likely to be non-accidental. It is supposed that the infant has been shaken, perhaps with an additional contact or impact injury to the head. Since the infant head is comparatively large in proportion to the body and neck muscles are poorly developed, uncontrolled movement of the head is thought to result in injury at the cervico-occipital junction. However, the view that these injuries are due to concealed inflicted trauma has been challenged and the hypothesis has been advanced that the pathological findings may stem from hypoxic injury if an infant stops breathing. In this view, hasty attempts at resuscitation may then induce further injury. Others have disagreed with this interpretation or have suggested that short falls can produce these findings. Among other possible causes, birth-related traumatic subdural hemorrhage is now extremely rare. Coagulopathies should always be excluded. It is clear that further evidence is required as to the causes of subdural hemorrhages in infants. These are listed in Table 14.14 according to current evidence.

It is very difficult to determine the prevalence of non-accidental head injury since the origins of most cases are concealed by the perpetrator. A figure of up to 20 severely affected or fatal cases per 100 000 of the population has been quoted. In the past, this condition has been known as the 'shaken baby syndrome' but this term is best avoided since it implies certainty of causation.

Support for a traumatic causation of these pathological findings is provided by the presence in some infants of other skeletal injuries and/or skull fracture. However, the cause of the diffuse cerebral swelling seen in these cases is not well understood.

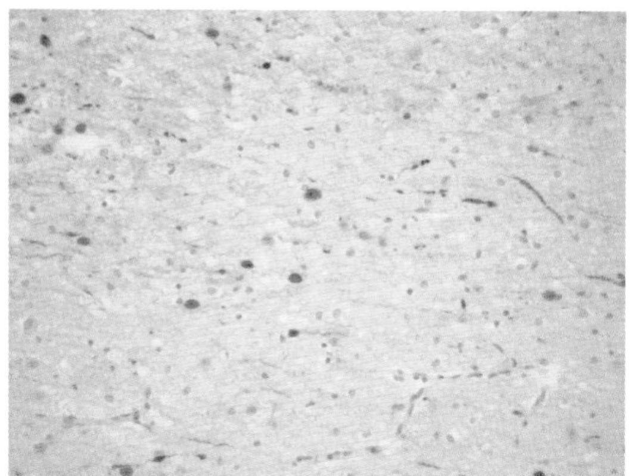

Figure 14.64 White matter from a stillborn infant who suffered hypoxic/ischemic cerebral injury with infarcts in the deep white matter. Axonal damage at the edge of the infarct is revealed by positivity for β-amyloid precursor protein, which highlights the axonal beading. ×200.

Recent studies suggest that axonal injury may be focal rather than diffuse and of hypoxic/ischemic rather than traumatic origin. The brainstem, upper cervical cord and spinal roots are a likely site for axonal injury in these circumstances. How much of this may be due to stretch injury remains problematic. Axonal positivity for β-APP is a useful early marker of axonal injury but does not necessarily distinguish traumatic from hypoxic injury (Fig. 14.64).

CHAPTER 15

TUMORS AND PARANEOPLASTIC SYNDROMES

Colin Smith

INTRODUCTION: CLASSIFICATION, EPIDEMIOLOGY AND CLINICAL FEATURES

There are several large textbooks which provide comprehensive coverage of tumors of the nervous system (see, for example, Bigner *et al.*, 1998; Burger *et al.*, 1994, 2002; Ironside *et al.*, 2002; Kleihues and Cavenee, 2001 in the Further Reading section). Only a brief introduction to the topic will be given here.

The current WHO classification was introduced in 2000 (Table 15.1). As for any classification system it needs to be both reproducible and meaningful. There is little point in endlessly separating entities if they are recognizable only by a small minority of practising pathologists, or if they are of little consequence to the clinicians with regard to treatment. The current classification achieves this, although, as discussed below, the ever-increasing wealth of molecular information may necessitate a revision of the classification in the near future.

Intrinsic tumors of the nervous system are uncommon. It must be remembered that metastatic tumors are by far the commonest group of malignancies encountered within the nervous system. Bronchus, breast and bowel are the most common primary sites but metastases can develop from almost anywhere. In countries where malignant melanoma has an increased frequency, such as Australia, metastatic melanoma is frequently encountered.

The average annual incidence of neuroepithelial tumors, i.e. tumors arising from brain tissue, is estimated at between 3 and 4 per 100 000 population. They account for less than 2% of all malignant neoplasms but approximately 20% of all childhood cancers (Fig. 15.1 and Fig. 15.2). A range of potential environmental risk factors has been suggested but only therapeutic X-irradiation has been unequivocally linked with brain tumors. The time between irradiation and brain tumor presentation may be as little as 7–9 years. The commonest brain tumors seen in this setting are meningiomas, schwannomas and gliomas.

All intracranial tumors have essentially similar effects. They may produce focal dysfunction, e.g. hemiparesis or hemianopia, depending on their site; they may act as an epileptogenic focus resulting in seizures; and they may act as intracranial expanding lesions (Fig. 15.3), leading ultimately to an increase in intracranial pressure (ICP) (see Chapter 4). With regard to the last of these, the effective size of the tumor is frequently contributed to by swelling of the adjacent brain. Furthermore, a high ICP is usually an early feature of any tumor in the posterior cranial fossa because of the frequently rapid occurrence of obstructive hydrocephalus. Spinal tumors, whether extradural or intradural, are

Table 15.1 WHO classification of tumors of the nervous system (2000)

Neuroepithelial tumors

Astrocytic tumors

- diffuse astrocytoma
- anaplastic astrocytoma
- glioblastoma
- pilocytic astrocytoma
- pleomorphic xanthoastrocytoma
- subependymal giant cell astrocytoma

Oligodendroglial tumors

- oligodendroglioma
- anaplastic oligodendroglioma

Mixed gliomas

Ependymal tumors

- ependymoma
- anaplastic ependymoma
- myxopapillary ependymoma
- subependymoma

Choroid plexus tumors

- choroid plexus papilloma
- choroid plexus carcinoma

Glial tumors of uncertain origin

- astroblastoma
- gliomatosis cerebri
- choroid glioma of the third ventricle

Neuronal and mixed neuronal–glial tumors

- gangliocytoma
- dysplastic gangliocytoma of the cerebellum
- desmoplastic infantile astrocytoma/ganglioglioma
- dysembryoplastic neuroepithelial tumor
- ganglioglioma
- anaplastic ganglioglioma
- central neurocytoma
- cerebellar liponeurocytoma
- paraganglioma of the filum terminale

Neuroblastic tumors

- olfactory neuroblastoma
- olfactory neuroepithelioma
- neuroblastoma of the adrenal gland and sympathetic nervous system

Pineal parenchymal tumors

- pineocytoma
- pineoblastoma
- pineal parenchymal tumor of intermediate differentiation

Embryonal tumors

- medulloepithelioma
- ependymoblastoma
- medulloblastoma
- supratentorial primitive neuroectodermal tumor (PNET)
- atypical teratoid/rhabdoid tumor

Tumors of peripheral nerves

Schwannoma

Neurofibroma

Perineuroma

Malignant peripheral nerve sheath tumor

Tumors of the meninges

Meningioma

Mesenchymal, non-meningothelial tumors

Primary melanocytic tumors

Tumors of uncertain histogenesis

Hemangioblastoma

Lymphomas and hemopoietic neoplasms

Malignant lymphomas

Plasma cell tumors

Granulocytic sarcoma

Germ cell tumors

Germinoma

Embryonal carcinoma

Yolk sac tumor

Choriocarcinoma

Teratoma

- mature teratoma
- immature teratoma
- teratoma with malignant transformation

Mixed germ cell tumors

Tumors of the sellar region

Craniopharyngioma

Granular cell tumor

Metastatic tumors

characterized by signs of compression of, or focal damage to, the spinal cord.

The prognosis in patients with a neuroepithelial tumor remains generally poor. There are certain exceptions such as pilocytic astrocytomas, and the rare subependymomas, subependymal giant cell astrocytomas and choroid plexus papillomas, which can be excised without subsequent recurrence. In

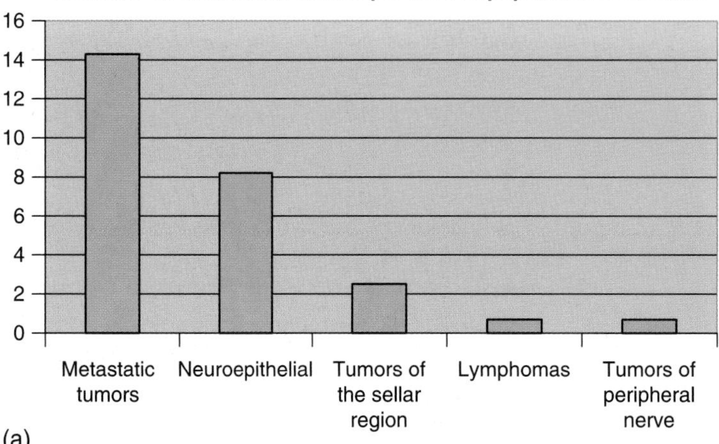

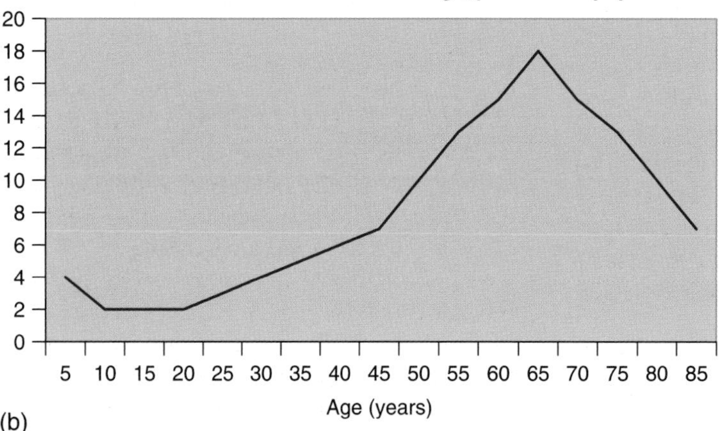

Figure 15.1 (a) The incidence of common intracranial tumors based on Scottish data. Results are given per 100 000 population. Metastatic tumors are almost twice as common as other intracranial tumors. It is likely that the figure for metastatic tumors may be an under-representation of the true figure. (b) Two age-related incidence peaks are seen in intracranial tumors. The first is in childhood and the second occurs in old age. The data are based on Scottish cancer registry publications.

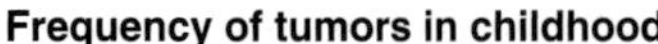

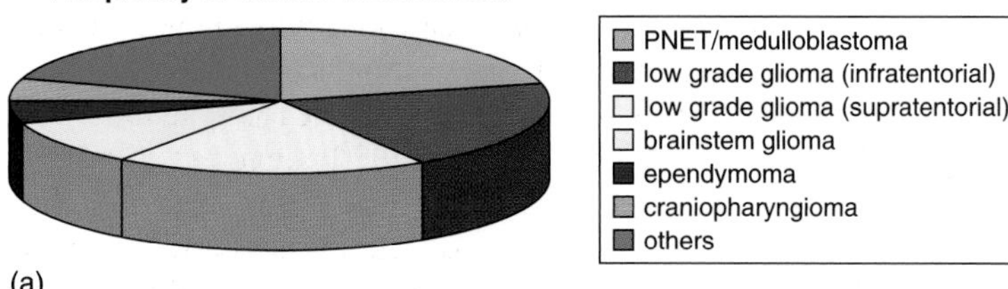

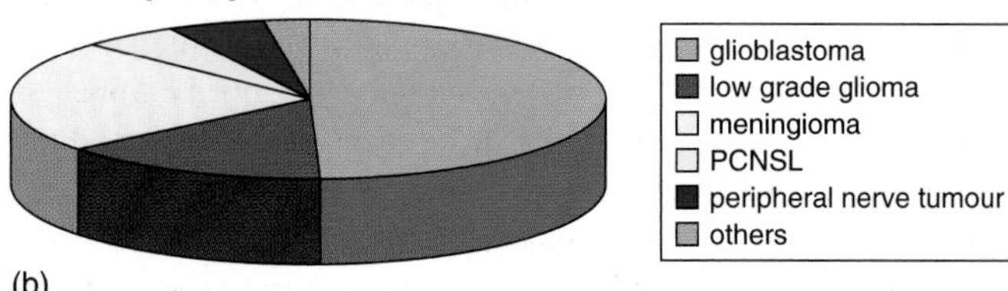

Figure 15.2 (a) Incidence of primary CNS tumors in childhood. A high proportion of tumors are infratentorial. Medulloblastomas are the most frequently encountered tumors within the nervous system and are the commonest solid tumor in pediatric practice. (b) Incidence of the main tumor types, excluding metastatic tumors, in adults.

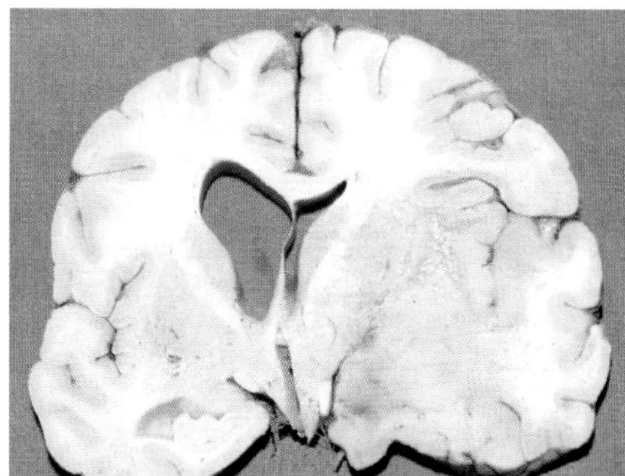

Figure 15.3 Mass effect. A coronal section with a diffuse astrocytoma producing a mass effect with ventricular compression and tentorial herniation.

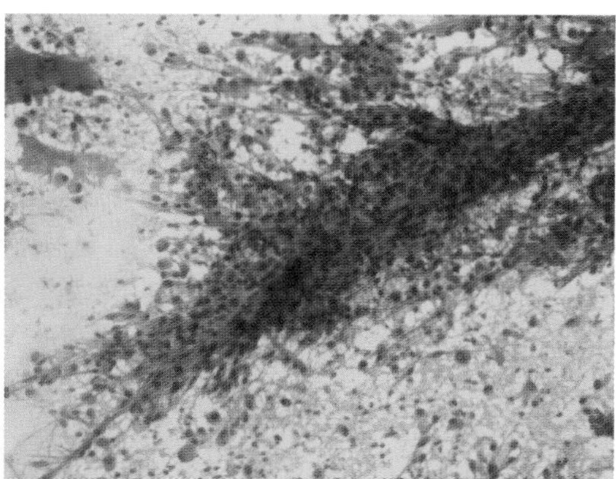

Figure 15.4 The brain smear technique. Stained smear preparation of a glioblastoma. The malignant cells are pleomorphic and show the formation of processes. There is a characteristic perivascular distribution of tumor cells. H&E.

general, however, most neuroepithelial tumors progress inexorably, the duration of survival being in general related to the anaplasia of the tumor. Thus, the median survival for patients with glioblastomas is in the region of 4–6 months, whereas patients with astrocytomas, or other gliomas, that are well differentiated may be for up to several years. There are specific problems of anatomical location and diffuse infiltration, which are discussed later, which make treatment of tumors of the nervous system particularly difficult.

Tumors of the meninges or peripheral nervous system are much more amenable to surgical resection although early diagnosis is important to try and limit the degree of functional deficit produced by the tumor. Complete surgical resection is also more likely with a smaller tumor diagnosed at an early stage.

DIAGNOSIS

The process of diagnosis involves several steps. First, the clinical examination may include malignancy as part of the differential diagnosis. The patient may then be referred for neuroradiological investigation. Neuroimaging is becoming increasingly sophisticated with both CT and MRI investigations providing greater resolution. However, a tissue diagnosis remains the 'gold standard'. The biopsy does have its limitations, however, and pathological examination of a biopsy specimen will not always allow an exact diagnosis in every case. In all biopsy interpretations it is imperative to review the clinical and radiological information before arriving at a final diagnosis, and this is particularly important in those difficult cases in which the diagnosis is uncertain.

With brain tumors the biopsy can be obtained through a burr hole or in the course of an open craniotomy. Modern neurosurgical techniques allow CT-guided biopsies of deeply seated lesions with a high rate of targeting accuracy and a low mortality rate. For spinal tumors, either percutaneous biopsy or laminectomy are required. The surgeon may wish an intra-operative diagnosis, in which case fresh biopsy tissue must be sent rapidly to the pathology laboratory, or may indicate that a rapid diagnosis is not required, in which case the biopsy tissue should be placed in formalin for fixation and transferred to the pathology laboratory for processing. An intra-operative diagnosis can be provided by smear preparations (or touch preparations for tougher, more fibrous specimens) and by frozen sections. The smear technique is particularly valuable in cases with only very small quantities of tissue, such as stereotactic biopsies and pituitary tumors, as preparation of the slides requires only a very small fragment of tissue (Fig. 15.4). An audit of smear preparations undertaken in Glasgow showed that, provided the biopsy had come from the appropriate site, the correct diagnosis (when correlated with the paraffin section diagnosis) had been made in 93% of cases, and in another 5% of cases it was possible to make a positive diagnosis of a malignant tumor although its precise type could not be identified. Despite this degree of accuracy our local policy is that the intra-operative diagnosis is a provisional diagnosis only and that the final diagnosis requires examination of paraffin sections and possibly also some additional investigations, as discussed below. The technique is not restricted to the identification of tumors, since the smear technique can help in the diagnosis of cerebral infarction, cerebral abscess and viral encephalitis. The smear technique is not discussed further in this chapter and the interested reader is referred to the Further Reading section for more information.

Special techniques

As special techniques become increasingly sophisticated then so do we have to modify our system of classification of tumors of the central nervous system. Originally, classification systems were based on assessment of tinctorial stains. Immunohistochemistry allowed for greater insight into phenotypic expression and subsequent reclassification of many tumors. We are now entering a new era of molecular investigation which is providing us with increasing diagnostic and prognostic information in relation to tumors, and which will almost certainly play an ever-increasing role in shaping future classification systems. It is, however, always worth remembering that these special techniques should not be interpreted in isolation. Immunohistochemistry taken out of context may be misleading; neuropathologists will be aware of cases of glioblastoma with cytokeratin expression. The application of molecular investigations to central nervous system tumors is still in its infancy and both neuropathologists and clinicians will require time to fully assess the importance of these additional investigations with regard to patient treatment.

Immunohistochemistry

Immunohistochemistry is now a common first-line investigation of the difficult tumor and, indeed, in these days of 'best practice' many would argue that immunohistochemistry should be undertaken on all tumors. A number of 'markers' have been identified that correlate to the phenotype of the malignant cell. Immunohistochemistry involves the binding of an antibody, either polyclonal or monoclonal, to a specific epitope in the protein of interest, and subsequent identification of the antibody-epitope binding using a secondary marker, most commonly the avidin–biotin complex (ABC). Immunohistochemistry can involve either the application of one or two specific antibodies to confirm a diagnosis, such as GFAP in a glioblastoma, or the application of a panel of antibodies to further characterize a tumor which has a non-specific pattern on haematoxylin and eosin (H&E) staining, such as a spindle cell panel in a sarcoma of the meninges.

A number of the frequently used antibodies in the diagnosis of nervous system tumors are listed below. Table 15.2 provides a quick reference for commonly used antibodies and their profiles in selected tumors.

Glial markers

Glial fibrillary acidic protein (GFAP) is an intermediate filament expressed by a number of glial cells. Strong GFAP immunoreactivity (Fig. 15.5) is seen in astrocytic tumors, although the staining may become increasingly focal as the tumor becomes more anaplastic. Indeed, in glioblastomas composed predominantly of small cells with little cytoplasm the staining may be very focal. GFAP immunoreactivity in other glial tumors is variable and is discussed in the appropriate section below.

Neuronal markers

A range of neuronal markers has been developed. The most widely used are neurofilament protein and synaptophysin. Neurofilaments are intermediate filaments within the neuronal cytoplasm and processes, and synaptophysin is a protein associated with synapse formation. Neuron-specific enolase (NSE) was used as a neuronal marker in the past but is now known to be rather non-specific. A number of newer markers have been developed, such as the neuronal nuclear antigen Neu-N, but the role of these markers in diagnostic neuropathology remains to be defined.

Table 15.2 Immunohistochemical profile of selected brain tumors

Tumor	GFAP	Synaptophysin	NF	EMA	panCK	S-100	Transthyretin	CD45	PLAP
Astrocytoma	+	−	−	−	−	+	−	−	−
Glioblastoma	+	−	−	+/−	−	+	−	−	−
Oligodendroglioma	+/−	+/−	+/−	−	−	+	−	−	−
Ependymoma	+	+/−	−	−	−	+	−	−	−
Choroid plexus tumor	+/−	−	−	−	+/−	+	+	−	−
Medulloblastoma	+/−	+	+/−	−	−	+	−	−	−
Schwannoma	−	−	−	−	−	+	−	−	−
Meningioma	−	−	−	+	−	+/−	−	−	−
Primary CNS lymphoma	−	−	−	−	−	−	−	+	−
Germinoma	−	−	−	−	−	−	−	−	+
Hemangioblastoma	−	−	−	−	−	+/−	−	−	−

GFAP = glial fibrillary acidic protein; NF = neurofilament protein; EMA = epithelial membrane antigen; panCK = pancytokeratin; PLAP = placental alkaline phosphatase.
+ = positive; +/− = variably positive; − = negative.

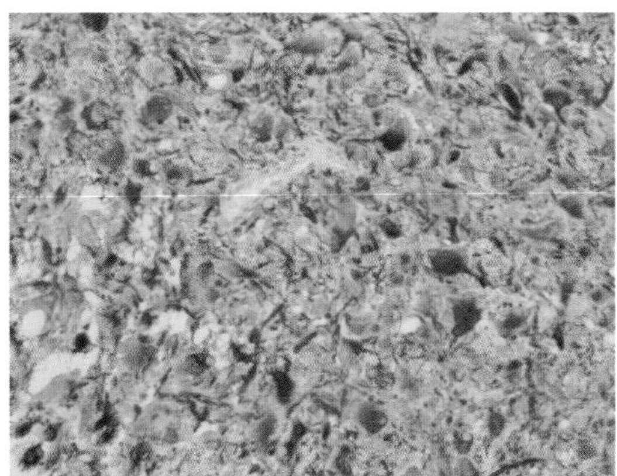

Figure 15.5 Glioblastoma. There is strong cytoplasmic staining and staining of cellular processes. There is no staining of the central blood vessel. Immunohistochemistry glial fibrillary acidic protein (GFAP).

Peripheral nerve sheath markers

S-100 is a calcium-binding protein expressed in a range of cells including schwann cells, astrocytes, melanocytes, chondrocytes and sustentacular cells of paragangliomas. When interpreting the staining pattern only nuclear staining, with or without cytoplasmic staining, should be considered positive.

Proliferation markers

These give an indication of the proliferative index within a tumor. In general high rates of proliferation correspond with a higher grade of tumor. Ki67 and MIB1, markers of the proliferation index, are commonly used in diagnostic practice. Both will stain nuclei in the proliferative cycle. Mini-chromosomal maintenance (MCM) proteins are better characterized in the proliferative cycle and may replace both Ki67 and MIB1 in the future.

Antibody panels

Pituitary panel

This is a panel of anterior hormone proteins and includes prolactin (PRL), growth hormone (GH), adrenocorticotrophic hormone (ACTH), follicle-stimulating hormone (FSH), luteinizing hormone (LH), thyroid-stimulating hormone (TSH), and α-subunit. The current WHO classification of pituitary adenomas requires characterization of the hormones produced by the adenomas.

Lymphoid panel

A lymphocytic infiltrate can be characterized by immunohistochemistry. At the simplest level, B and T lymphocytes can be differentiated by appropriate antibodies such as CD3 (T lymphocyte) and CD20 (B lymphocyte). In neoplastic conditions a larger panel is required including CD5, CD10, CD21, CD23, CD30, CD79a, CD138, Bcl-2 and Bcl-6. Assessment of the pattern of expression of these markers can

Table 15.3 Typical cytokeratin 7 and 20 immunoprofiles in relation to primary epithelial malignancies

CK7+/CK20+	CK7+/CK20−	CK7−/CK20−
Pancreas	Lung	Liver
Bile duct	Breast	Kidney
Urothelium	Thyroid	Adrenal gland
Some upper GI tract carcinomas	Ovary	
	Endometrium	

It should be noted that while this is a useful guide it is not absolute and exceptions are not uncommon.

assist in the diagnosis of non-Hodgkin's lymphomas: CD5, CD20, CD23 and CD79a are expressed in B-cell small lymphocytic lymphomas; CD20, CD79a and cyclin D1 are expressed in mantle cell lymphomas; CD10, CD20, CD79a, Bcl-2 and Bcl-6 are expressed in follicular lymphomas; CD20, CD21 and CD79a are expressed in extranodal marginal zone B-cell lymphomas; CD20 and CD79a are expressed in diffuse large B-cell lymphomas and most intravascular large B-cell lymphomas; CD30 is expressed in anaplastic large cell lymphomas; CD138 is expressed in plasma cell tumors.

Metastatic epithelial malignancy

Pan-cytokeratin will determine the epithelial nature of a metastatic tumor. In the setting of an unknown primary, further information may be available from using low and high molecular weight cytokeratins and more specific markers such as thyroid transcription factor-1 (TTF-1) for bronchial and thyroid, estrogen receptors for breast and carcinoembryonic antigen (CEA) for gastrointestinal tumors. In particular cytokeratins 7 and 20 can be useful in providing information about potential primary sites (see Table 15.3).

Sarcoma panel

Spindle cell sarcomas can arise in the central and peripheral nervous system. A panel to establish the nature of the tumor should include markers for glial tumors (GFAP), vimentin, smooth muscle tumors (smooth muscle actin), nerve sheath tumors (S-100), skeletal muscle tumors (MyoD1 and myogenin), epithelial markers (cytokeratins and epithelial membrane antigen [EMA]), endothelial markers (CD31 and CD34), and a primitive neuroectodermal tumor marker (CD99).

Molecular investigations

A range of molecular investigations are now employed to provide information in relation to protein and gene expression.

Cytogenetics

Cytogenetics is a hybrid science combining cytology and genetics. For many years cytogenetics was limited to analysis of banding patterns of metaphase chromosomes produced by Giemsa staining. In recent years cytogenetics has seen the development of fluorescence *in situ* hybridization (FISH) and comparative genomic hybridization (CGH).

FISH uses colored labels (fluorochromes) which can be visualized under ultra-violet light with microscope filters. FISH can be used to assess DNA deletions and amplification. For each case two probes with different fluorochromes are used together; one corresponds to the area of interest on the chromosome, the other a region on the same chromosome but distant from the area of interest. In a normal somatic nucleus there will be four signals, two of each color. If there has been a deletion on one chromosome there will be three signals.

CGH involves hybridizing differentially fluorochrome labeled somatic and tumor DNA with metaphase chromosomes. Image analysis techniques are then used to quantify the ratio of both fluorochromes along the chromosomes. Amplifications and deletions can be detected by an increase or decrease in the tumor DNA fluorochrome.

Protein expression

Assessment of protein expression ranges from investigation of a single protein, using techniques such as immunohistochemistry and western blotting to the investigation of large numbers of proteins using proteomic analysis. Immunohistochemistry is discussed above. Western blotting separates proteins using a polyacrylamide gel and detects specific proteins on the gel using antibodies. This can be used for serum or CSF analysis in possible cases of paraneoplastic disease.

In situ hybridization (ISH) is used to detect DNA or RNA for a specific protein. ISH uses a labeled probe which has base pairs complementary to the DNA/RNA sequence of interest. ISH can be used to identify specific mRNA expression within cells; for example, kappa or lambda light chain restriction can be demonstrated in plasma cell tumors using ISH techniques.

Flow cytometry

This technique can be used to assess cell surface antigens. Cells bind with a fluorochrome-labeled antibody and are separated by a fluorescence-activated cell sorter (FACS). Labeled cells pass through a laser beam and the emitted light is stored and analysed electronically. The proportion of cells labeled with specific markers within a sample can then be determined. This can be useful in differentiating lymphoma from a reactive cellular infiltrate in CSF specimens.

Proteomics

Proteomics allows the analysis of large numbers of proteins from a tissue sample, provided they are expressed in that tissue at a sufficiently high level. Analysis requires fresh tissue from which proteins are separated on a two-dimensional gel and analyzed using a mass spectrometer. This provides a protein signature for a given tissue.

Gene analysis

DNA can be examined to look for both qualitative and quantitative abnormalities. The former covers gene re-arrangements or mutations, the latter over- or under-expression of genes.

Polymerase chain reaction (PCR) is a common methodology employed in the analysis of DNA. It is a technique which allows the production of large quantities of DNA from a specimen, and is effective in both fresh tissue and formalin-fixed, paraffin embedded material. By choosing appropriate primers, usually 30–50 base pairs in length, a region of DNA can be amplified to produce many copies. PCR can be used in the assessment of genetic markers (CA repeat microsatellites are used in assessment of loss of heterozygosity [LOH]), or can be used to produce large quantities of DNA for mutation analysis.

DNA sequencing can be done in many ways with direct sequencing being the 'gold standard'. Mutational analysis is used in assessing possible genetic syndromes, such as neurofibromatosis.

Large scale gene analysis can be done by DNA microarrays using chips on which thousands of genes can be printed. Complex statistical analysis of the data from many cases allows for clustering of gene expression data and some indication of potentially important genes in certain malignancies.

Epigenetic analysis

It is well known that direct changes to the order of base pairs in human DNA can result in pathological abnormalities; this underlies mutational analysis. Epigenetics refers to how chemical alterations to a single base may also result in, or modify, pathological processes. The main areas of interest are histone binding of DNA, which influences enzyme access to DNA, gene silencing by methylation (and genomic imprinting), and *de novo* cytosine methylation regulating gene expression. Methylation-specific PCR is a technique which can assess methylation status of a specific gene.

Molecular pathology applied to neuro-oncology

The ultimate goal will be to produce a molecular classification for neuro-oncology. This will incorporate histological appearances with specific patterns or protein expression and genetic changes that will be of both diagnostic and prognostic significance. Currently there are a number of diagnostically and prognostically important molecular alterations.

Oligodendrogliomas

LOH at 1p and 19q indicates chemosensitivity, and therefore better prognosis, in both oligodendrogliomas and anaplastic oligodendrogliomas. This

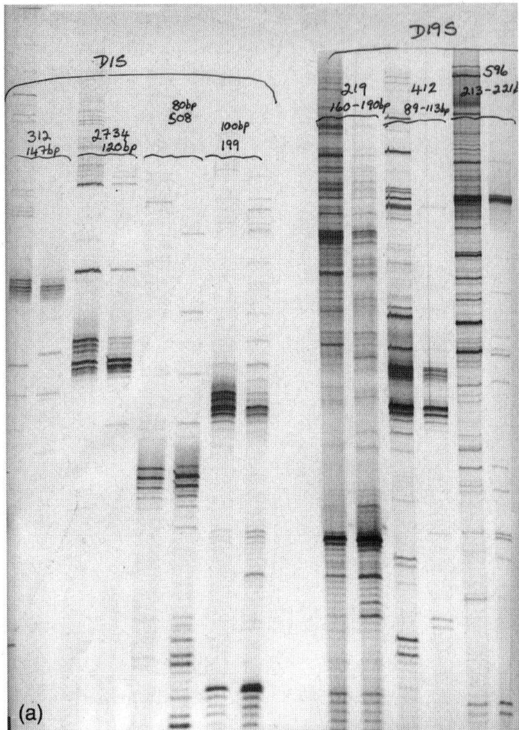

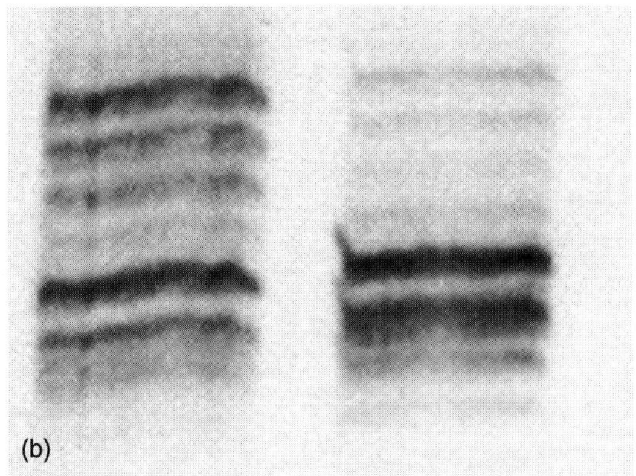

Figure 15.6 (a) Polymerase chain reaction (PCR) gel of an oligodendroglioma. Four different microsatellite markers are used to examine the short arm of chromosome 1 (1p) [D1S312, 2734, 508, 199] and three markers to examine the long arm of chromosome 19 (19q) [D19S219, 412, 596]. The base pair lengths of each fragment is indicated on the gel and this determines the position of the fragments in each ladder on the gel. For each set of primers the left hand column represents somatic DNA, the right tumor. (b) Detailed image of the region of interest from the D1S2734 marker (approximately 120 base pairs in length). On the left is somatic DNA (patient's blood sample). On the right is tumor DNA which has fewer bands indicating LOH at 1p. There is not a complete absence of bands due to somatic DNA from blood vessels and white blood cells being included in the tumor sample.

can be assessed by a variety of techniques including PCR (Fig. 15.6) and FISH (Fig. 15.7).

Glioblastomas

Differing genetic pathways have been found in primary glioblastomas (those that arise *de novo*, usually in the elderly) and secondary glioblastomas (those arising within a low grade astrocytoma). EGFR over-expression is more typical of primary glioblastoma while *p53* mutations are more typical of the secondary tumors. These differing genetic pathways may in the future form the basis of differing treatments. Recent studies looking at epigenetic changes in glioblastomas have found that patients with glioblastoma containing a methylated MGMT (06-methylguanine DNA methyltransferase) DNA repair gene promoter benefited from temozolomide chemotherapy whereas those without a methylated MGMT promoter did not.

Medulloblastomas

C-myc and *N-myc* amplification, and 17p loss are associated with a poor outcome. Over-expression of *TrkC* mRNA has been demonstrated to be a good prognostic indicator.

Future studies

The National Cancer Institute in the USA provides an on-line resource for genome analysis of tumors

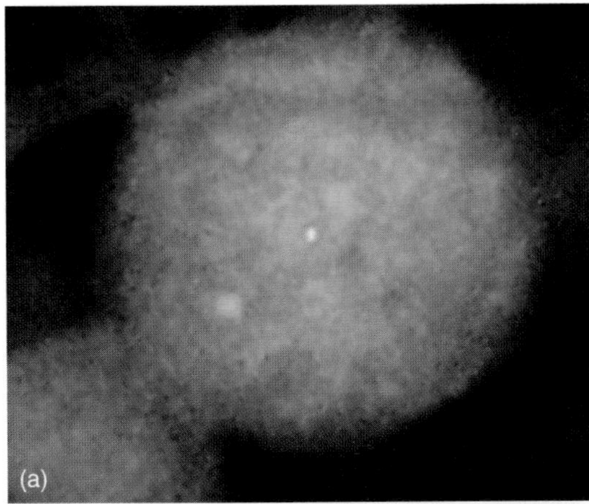

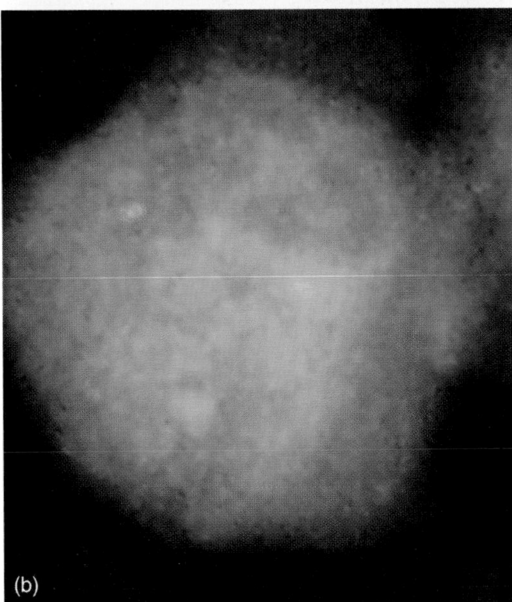

Figure 15.7 (a) Fluorescence *in situ* hybridization (FISH) image of a cell nucleus with two 1p signals. There are two red signals (probe labeling 1p) and two green signals (probe labeling 1q). (b) FISH image from the nucleus of an oligodendroglioma cell showing a deletion at 1p. There is only one red signal but two green signals.

(www.cgap.nci.nih.gov). By pooling data from many laboratories and disseminating molecular information there will be a move towards molecular classification of brain tumors. This can then influence the development of new therapies and clinical trials.

TUMORS OF NEUROEPITHELIAL TISSUE

The frequently used term glioma applies to neoplasms derived from neuroglia: astrocytes, oligodendrocytes and ependymal cells, with the corresponding tumors astrocytomas, oligodendrogliomas and ependymomas. There are differing grades of tumor and specific entities within this group such that the gliomas account for the largest category within the current WHO classification (Table 15.1, page 295). As a group, the gliomas share many common features. Grading is based on pleomorphism, mitotic activity and microvascular proliferation. This grading system is best defined in relation to astrocytic tumors but is also applied to other gliomas. Generally, when discussing gliomas the terms benign and malignant tumors have little meaning. Rather these tumors are described as being of low or high grade. This is due to the fact that, with the exception of one or two specific entities discussed below, a low-grade glioma cannot be completely surgical excised and will continue to acquire genetic mutations and transform to an ultimately fatal high grade tumor. The reasons for the surgical limitations in relation to these tumors are two-fold: anatomical constraints and diffuse infiltration. The neurosurgeon will be severely limited in the approach to a tumor if the tumor is in anatomically sensitive regions (thalamus, motor cortex, brainstem, spinal cord) (Fig. 15.8). In such a situation the neurosurgeon may opt only for stereotactic biopsy in order to establish a diagnosis on which to base subsequent management. It must be remembered that when dealing with a stereotactic biopsy the sample may not be representative of the tumor as a whole. This is usually seen when the diffusely infiltrating edge of a high-grade glioma is biopsied with no high grade features being present in the biopsy. In such situations the term 'at least grade II' is used with management being based on the outcome of the multidisciplinary team (MDT) meeting; clinical and radiological features point to a high grade glioma, pathology confirms the diagnosis of glioma but only the diffusely infiltrating edge with low grade features. In such a situation

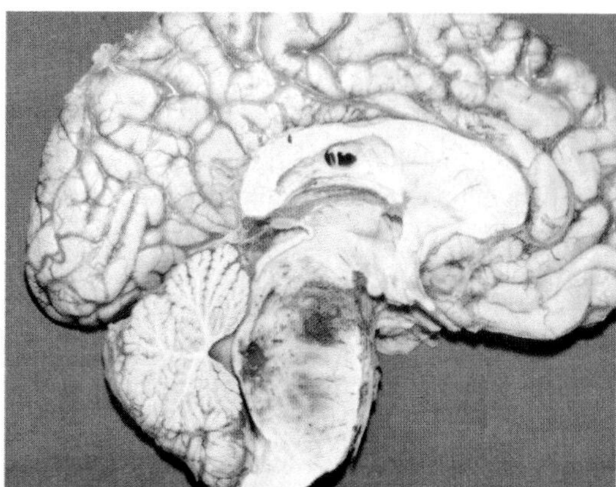

Figure 15.8 Brainstem glioma. The pons is diffusely enlarged by a poorly defined tumor.

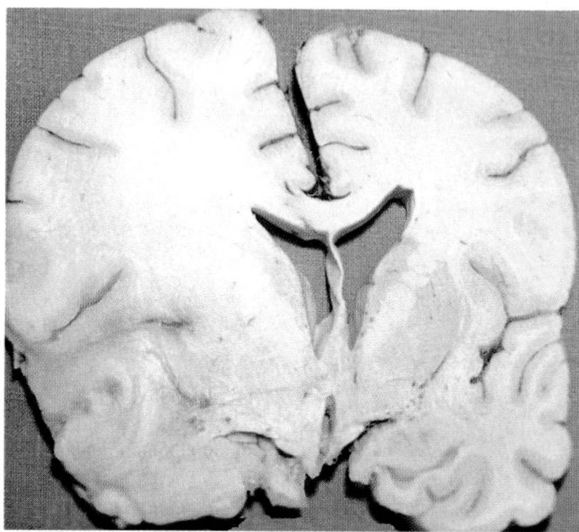

Figure 15.9 Astrocytoma. The tumor is poorly defined, diffusely infiltrating and expanding the white matter.

the value of the biopsy has been in confirming the diagnosis of glioma (as opposed to metastatic tumor or lymphoma for example) and the patient will be treated for a high-grade glioma.

However, even in regions more accessible to surgical intervention, such as the frontal lobe, complete surgical resection is not an option, although the neurosurgeon will aim for debulking and complete macroscopic resection. Glioma cells are capable of binding to the extracellular matrix and migrating from the main tumor mass. Examination of peritumoral tissue will always reveal diffusely infiltrating tumor cells. Therefore, a macroscopically complete surgical resection is likely to leave behind a significant microscopic tumor load.

Gliomas very rarely metastasize outwith the nervous system. This is due in part to the short survival associated with high grade gliomas and in part to the biological inability of the tumor cells to invade the vascular system and spread systemically. Gliomas can, however, infiltrate the subarachnoid space and spread resulting in *meningeal gliomatosis*. Multicentric gliomas probably represent a single tumor which has diffusely infiltrated the brain. On imaging this can give rise to disparate areas of enhancement throughout the brain.

Astrocytic tumors

The majority of gliomas are astrocytomas. They have an incidence of about 3.5 per 100 000 people per year, the bulk being the highly aggressive glioblastoma with lower-grade astrocytic tumors being relatively uncommon.

Macroscopic appearances

Astrocytomas can arise anywhere in the central nervous system but occur principally in the white matter. In general they are poorly demarcated diffusely infiltrating adjacent tissue (Fig. 15.9). Infiltrated tissue is pale and expanded and there may be loss of the gray–white matter interface. In diffuse astrocytoma WHO grade II the infiltrated tissue may be firm. In the brainstem they can show diffuse infiltration or an exophytic growth pattern. There may be considerable swelling in adjacent tissue resulting in further distortion of the surrounding brain. Cyst formation is not uncommon in astrocytic tumors, particularly higher-grade tumors (Fig. 15.10). Glioblastomas often have hemorrhagic areas and areas of necrosis which appear yellow or creamy white in color (Fig. 15.11).

Histological appearances

Astrocytic tumors can have a range of appearances and in one single tumor the architecture and cytological appearances can vary greatly. The old

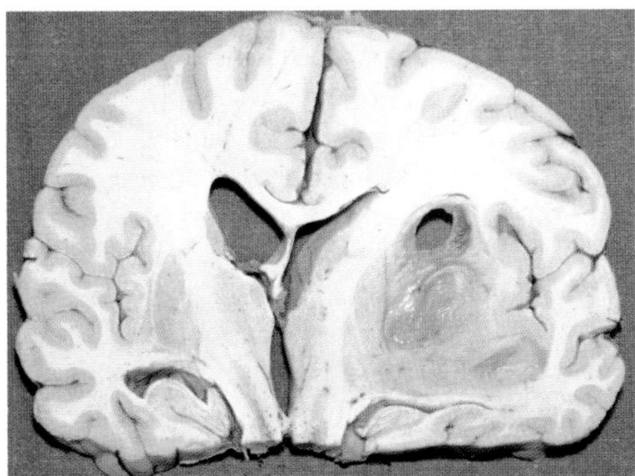

Figure 15.10 Astrocytoma. This large cystic astrocytoma is causing midline shift and ventricular compression.

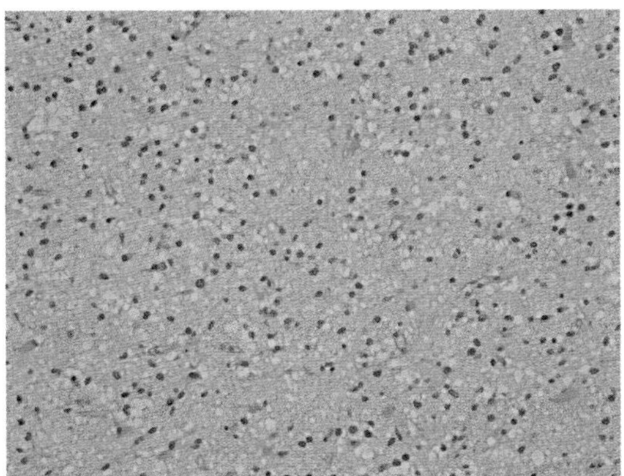

Figure 15.12 Diffuse astrocytoma. This fibrillary astrocytoma is hypercellular and has a dense fiber-forming stroma. H&E.

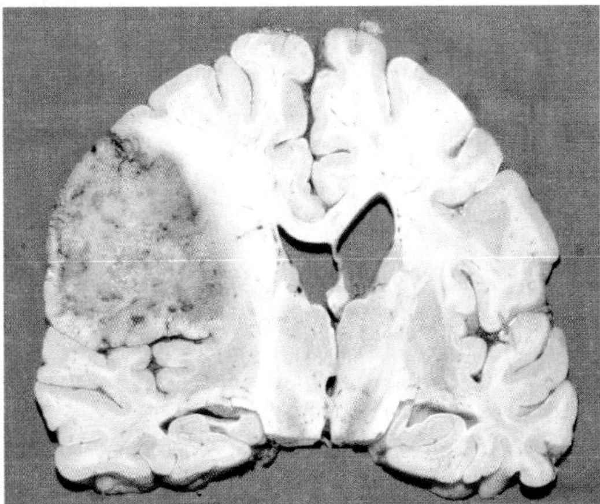

Figure 15.11 Glioblastoma. The necrotic component of the tumor is yellow. Although the tumor appears relatively well defined tumor cells diffusely infiltrate beyond the macroscopic edge of the tumor.

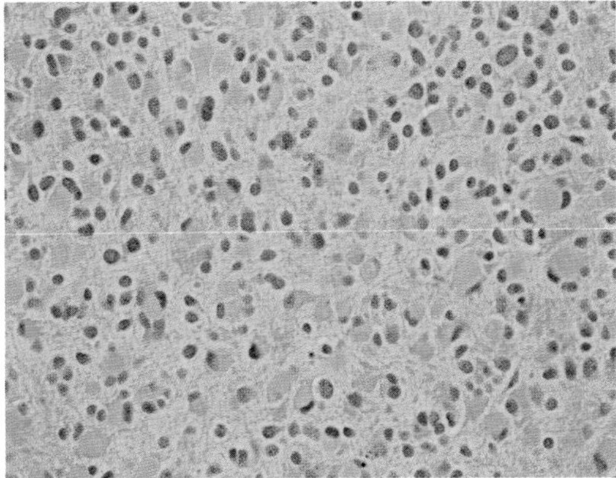

Figure 15.13 Gemistocytic astrocytoma. The tumor cells have abundant eosinophilic cytoplasm which displaces the nucleus. Occasional fibrils can be seen arising from the tumor cells. H&E.

name of glioblastoma multiforme acknowledged the wide range of histological appearances seen in glioblastomas.

Low-grade diffuse astrocytomas (WHO grade II)

These tumors are described as fibrillary, protoplasmic or gemistocytic. Fibrillary astrocytomas are composed of unevenly distributed, often loosely arranged, elongated cells, among which there is a characteristic fibrillary matrix produced by cellular processes (Fig. 15.12). Microcysts are common and there may be focal calcification. These tumors are strongly GFAP immunoreactive. Protoplasmic astrocytomas are uncommon. They may arise in gray matter and are composed of rather stellate cells with short processes and swollen cytoplasm separated by a matrix with few fibrils. Microcystic change is often prominent. GFAP immunoreactivity is variable but always at least focally positive. Gemistocytic astrocytomas are composed of large globoid or polygonal cells which have abundant homogeneous cytoplasm separated by glial fibrils (Fig. 15.13). They are strongly GFAP immunoreactive. The gemistocytic subtype is associated with a more rapid progression to anaplasia and glioblastoma.

Anaplastic astrocytoma (WHO grade III)

This tumor is one of increased cellularity and pleomorphism. The diagnosis requires demonstration of mitotic activity. In a stereotactic biopsy a single mitotic figure is important. In a large resection demonstration of a single mitotic figure is probably of less importance. There is neither necrosis nor microvascular proliferation.

Glioblastoma (WHO grade IV)

This is a highly cellular tumor with a very variable appearance. The tumor cells are poorly differentiated but usually fibrillary processes can be identified at least focally. An exception is the small-cell glioblastoma which is composed of small undifferentiated cells and may be difficult to differentiate from an anaplastic oligodendroglioma. EGFR amplification and 1p loss can be useful in differentiating these tumors. Multinucleated giant cells are not uncommon in glioblastomas. In some cases the tumor cells have an epithelioid architecture which may mimic carcinoma, and in very rare cases epithelial elements have been described. To allow the diagnosis to be made there must be microvascular proliferation and/or tumor necrosis. Microvascular proliferation is identified by thickened blood vessels with endothelial proliferation resulting in multi-layering (Fig. 15.14). A reticulin stain can be particularly useful in outlining blood vessels in cellular tumors. Tumor necrosis is often associated with pseudo-palisading; tumor cells align themselves around an area of necrosis (Fig. 15.15). Mitotic figures are usually, but not always, easy to find. Variants of glioblastoma include the *giant-cell glioblastoma* and the *gliosarcoma*. Macroscopically, the giant-cell glioblastoma is indistinguishable from glioblastoma but microscopically it is characterized by large numbers of multinucleated giant cells (Fig. 15.16). A gliosarcoma is macroscopically well defined and often feels firm. The neurosurgeon may be misled into thinking the tumor is a metastasis.

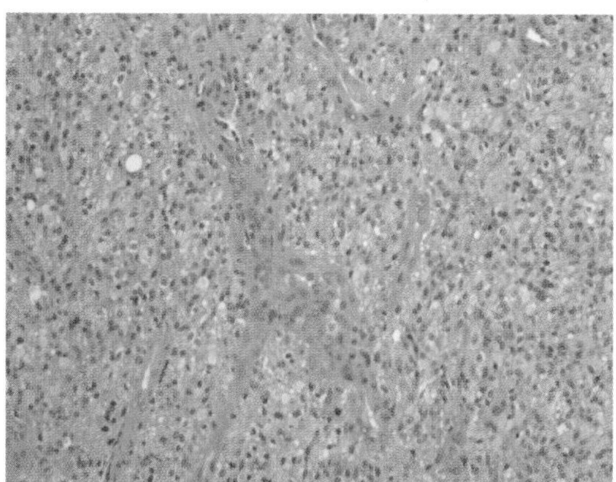

Figure 15.14 Glioblastoma. An important 'high-grade' feature is microvascular proliferation. The key feature is that of endothelial cell proliferation and stacking. H&E.

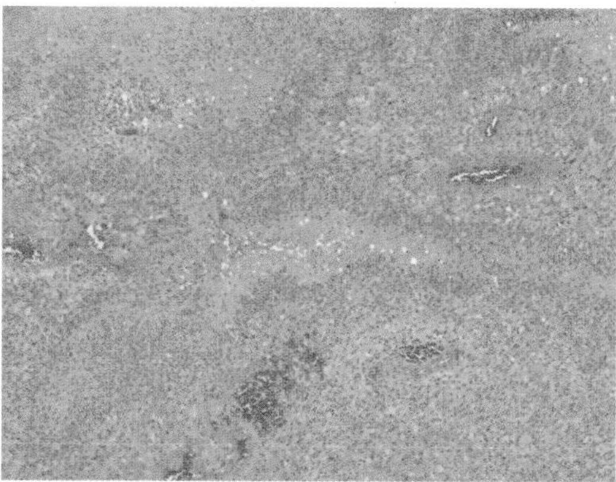

Figure 15.15 Glioblastoma. Tumor necrosis with pseudopalisading in an astrocytic tumor is indicative of a glioblastoma. There are ribbons of necrosis with increased tumor nuclei at the edge of the necrotic areas. H&E.

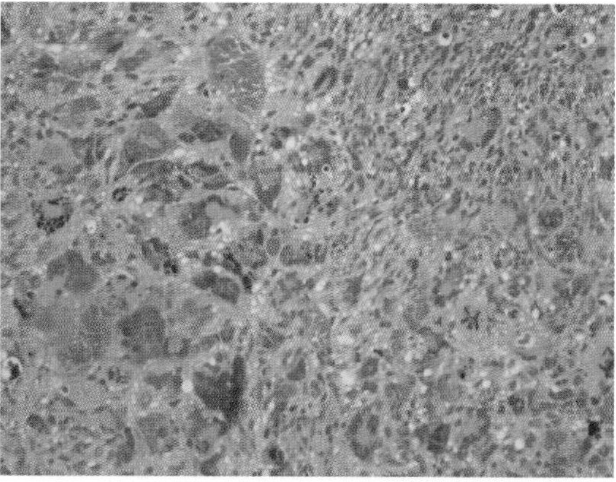

Figure 15.16 Giant-cell glioblastoma. While markedly pleomorphic and multinucleated cells may be seen in any glioblastoma, in giant-cell glioblastoma they are a prominent feature. Abnormal mitotic figures are easily identified. H&E.

Microscopically, a sarcomatous element is identified. In the commonest form this element has a fascicular architecture composed of malignant spindle cells producing abundant reticulin fibers. In rare cases the sarcomatous element may be heterologous, such as an osteosarcoma (Fig. 15.17). The sarcomatous element is negative for GFAP but immunoreactive for vimentin.

Specific astrocytic tumors

There are a number of astrocytic tumors which have specific clinico-pathological features and are considered as distinct entities.

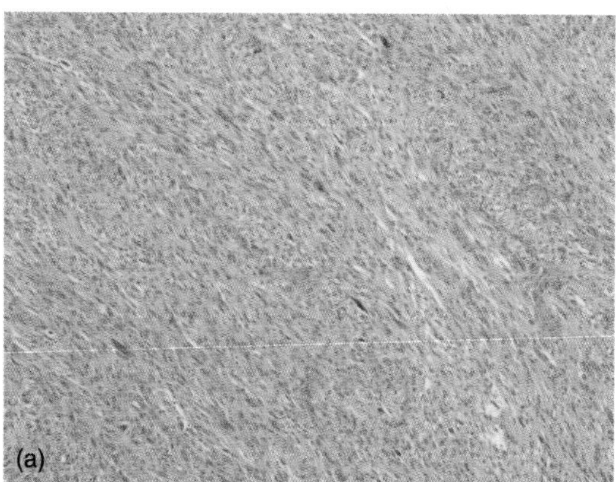

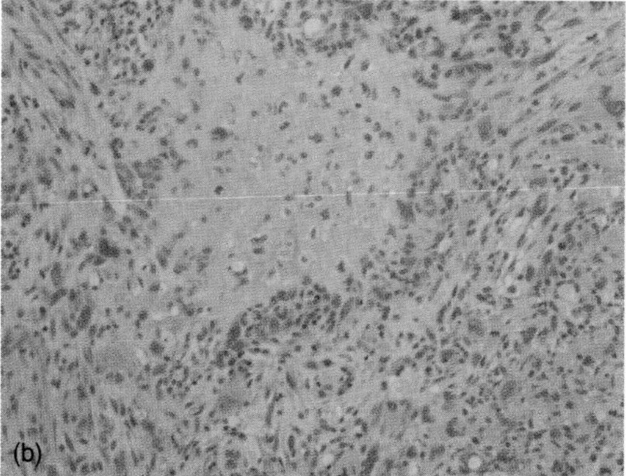

Figure 15.17 Gliosarcoma. (a) The commonest pattern of sarcomatous change resembles a fibrosarcoma, with spindle cells forming a fascicular architecture. Reticulin fibers can be demonstrated around malignant cells. (b) Rarely the sarcomatous element may take other forms, such as osteoid formation within the sarcomatous component of the tumor. (a) and (b) H&E.

Pilocytic astrocytoma (WHO grade I) This is a tumor seen predominantly in childhood classically associated with the cerebellum, optic tract or hypothalamus (Fig. 15.18). When it arises at other sites the normally good prognosis is more guarded. Macroscopically, in the cerebellum the tumor is typically cystic (Fig. 15.19). It may enhance on imaging, a feature usually associated with high grade gliomas. When the tumor arises in the optic nerve there is expansion of this structure. Histologically, the tumor shows a typically biphasic architecture; compact and microcystic (Fig. 15.20).

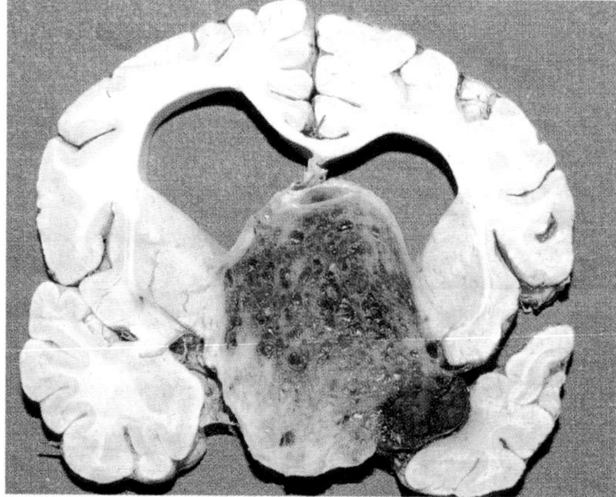

Figure 15.18 Pilocytic astrocytoma. This coronal section shows a hypothalamic pilocytic astrocytoma. The lesion is circumscribed and cystic spaces can be seen.

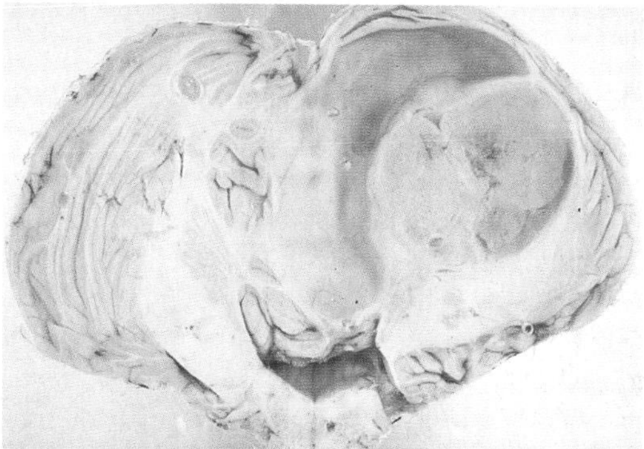

Figure 15.19 Pilocytic astrocytoma. A large cystic cerebellar pilocytic astrocytoma with a solid tumor nodule in the wall. The tumor is well demarcated from surrounding tissue.

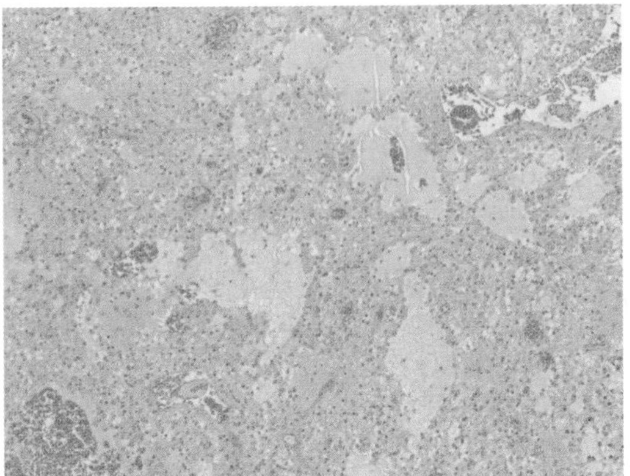

Figure 15.20 Pilocytic astrocytoma. The classic biphasic microscopic appearance of a pilocytic astrocytoma. There is a compact component and a microcystic component. H&E.

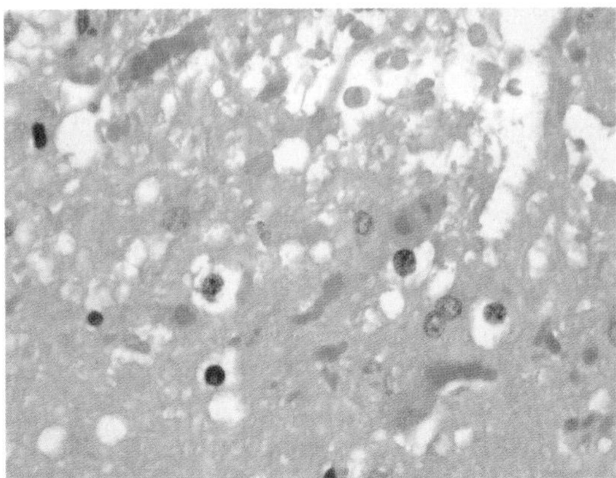

Figure 15.21 Pilocytic astrocytoma. Rosenthal fibers in a compact region of a pilocytic astrocytoma. The fibers are intensely eosinophilic but can be confused with stacks of red blood cells. H&E.

In the compact areas the cells are 'hair-like' (piloid) being elongated with long processes extending from each pole. Rosenthal fibers, aggregates of GFAP fibrils, which are structures required for the diagnosis to be made, are particularly prominent in compact areas (Fig. 15.21). Rosenthal fibers are not diagnostic of pilocytic astrocytomas as they may be seen in association with gliosis. Eosinophilic granular bodies may also be seen. There is microvascular proliferation but tumor necrosis and mitotic figures are not a feature. These tumors are potentially curable by complete surgical resection. Optic nerve pilocytic astrocytomas may be associated with neurofibromatosis type 1, and in this setting they may be bilateral.

Subependymal giant-cell astrocytoma (WHO grade I) These tumors are seen in the setting of tuberous sclerosis, a genetic syndrome produced by mutations in either the *TSC 1* (hamartin) or *TSC 2* (tuberin) genes. Macroscopically, the tumor is a nodular mass which lies in the wall of the lateral ventricle. Microscopically, the tumor is composed of cells with variable nuclear pleomorphism, abundant glassy cytoplasm and fibrillary processes (Fig. 15.22). Mitotic figures and tumor necrosis are not a feature. Immunohistochemically the tumor cells may express both glial and neuronal markers. Surgical excision is usually curative.

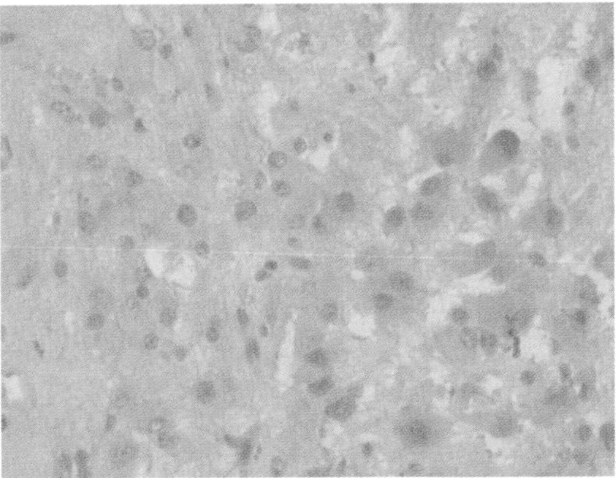

Figure 15.22 Subependymal giant cell astrocytoma. A population of cells within a subependymal giant cell astrocytoma have a ganglion cell-like appearance with abundant cytoplasm and a large pale nucleus. The stroma is fibrillary. H&E.

Superficial tumors

Both pleomorphic xanthoastrocytoma (PXA) (WHO grade II) and desmoplastic infantile ganglioglioma/astrocytoma (DIG) (WHO grade II) show a characteristic location, lying on the pial surface of the cerebral cortex (Fig. 15.23). DIG is only seen in infancy while PXA may also be seen in an older age group. Reticulin fiber deposition is prominent in both. PXA, microscopically, is composed of astrocytic cells with marked cellular pleomorphism and xanthomatous change in the cytoplasm (Fig. 15.24) but no mitotic

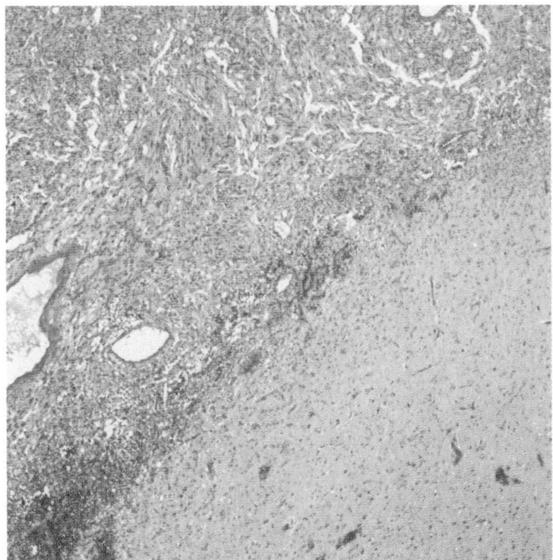

Figure 15.23 Pleomorphic xanthoastrocytoma. A low power photomicrograph shows the superficial location of a pleomorphic xanthoastrocytoma (PXA). The interface between tumor and cerebral cortex is clearly illustrated. H&E.

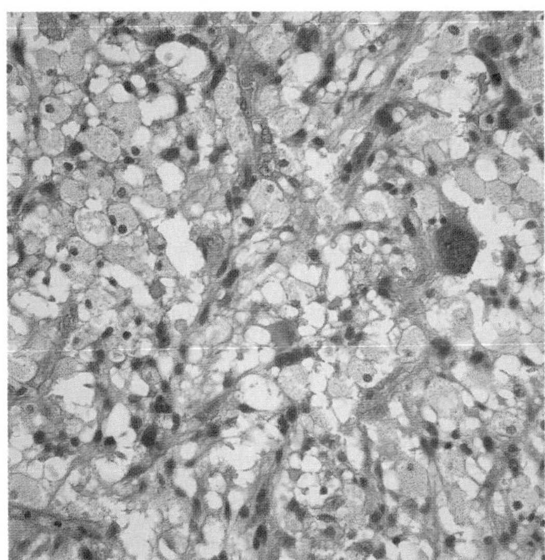

Figure 15.24 Pleomorphic xanthoastrocytoma. The proportion of xanthomatous cells in a PXA can vary greatly. In this example they are numerous. H&E.

activity or tumor necrosis, although anaplastic variants are now being described. Desmoplastic infantile astrocytoma is composed of spindle cells with little fibrillary matrix (Fig. 15.25), and the tumor

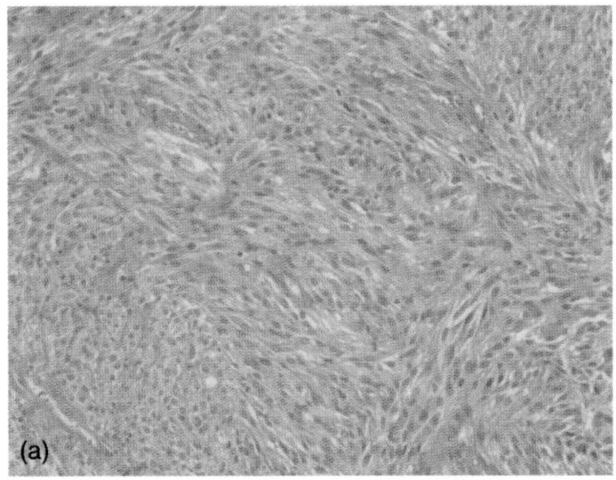

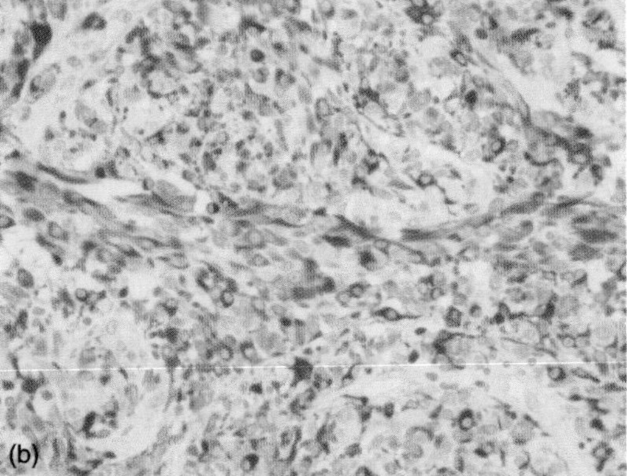

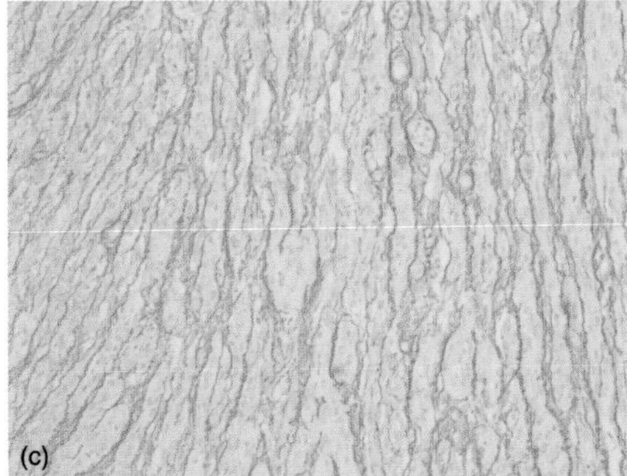

Figure 15.25 Desmoplastic infantile astrocytoma. (a) The tumor is composed of elongated astrocytic cells which in areas have a fascicular appearance. (b) The cells immunoreact strongly with GFAP. (c) Reticulin fibers are abundant in the stroma. (a) H&E. (b) Immunohistochemistry GFAP. (c) Reticulin.

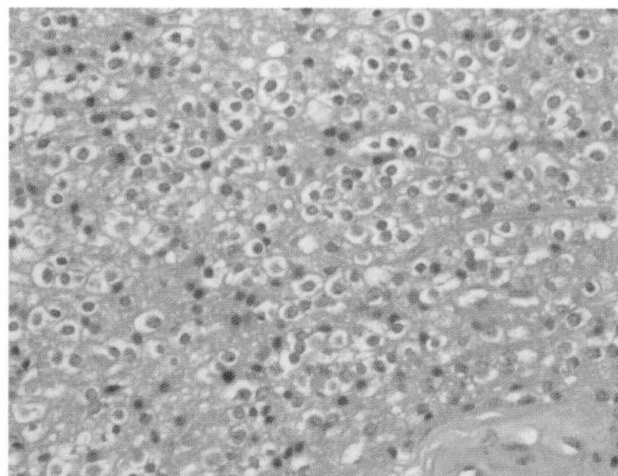

Figure 15.26 Oligodendroglioma. Cells with small round nuclei and perinuclear clearing (so called 'fried-egg' appearance) are typical of oligodendrogliomas. H&E.

cells immunoreact with GFAP. In the desmoplastic infantile ganglioglioma ganglion-like cells are also seen and immunoreact with neuronal markers.

Oligodendrogliomas

Oligodendrogliomas (WHO grade II) occur predominantly in the cerebral hemispheres particularly within the frontal lobes. They tend to be more sharply defined than astrocytomas. Calcification can be a prominent feature and may be obvious on imaging. Histologically, they are composed of compact masses of uniform cells with round nuclei and striking cytoplasmic clearing which gives a 'honeycomb' appearance (Fig. 15.26). This appearance is not pathognomic of oligodendrogliomas and may be seen in neurocytomas, dysembryoplastic neuroepithelial tumors and clear cell ependymomas. The stroma contains many thin-walled blood vessels. Small cells with an eccentric nucleus and eosinophilic cytoplasm may be seen; these 'mini-gemistocytes' will stain with GFAP whereas the typical oligodendroglioma cell is negative. Occasionally, a glioma may have both areas of definite astrocytoma and oligodendroglioma; in such cases the term oligo-astrocytoma should be applied. *Anaplastic oligodendroglioma* (WHO grade III) retains oligodendroglioma morphology but with increased cellular pleomorphism, mitotic activity and tumor necrosis. Small-cell glioblastomas may have a similar histological appearance. The concept of glioblastomas arising from oligodendrogliomas is controversial and currently no definite consensus has been agreed.

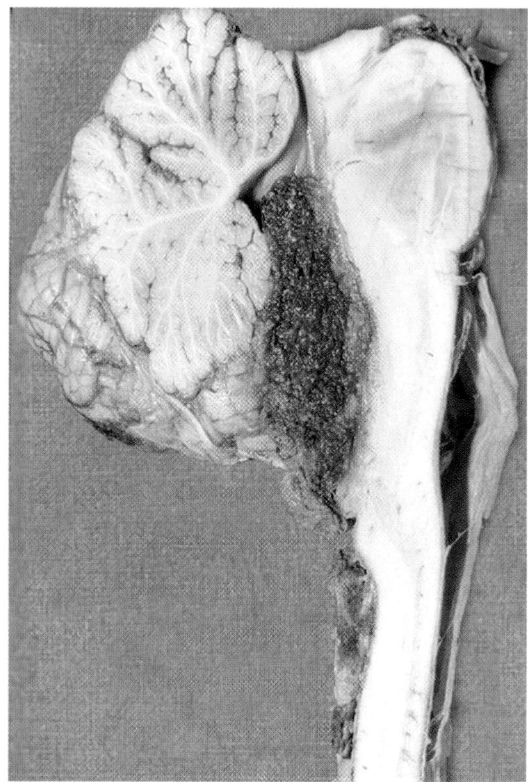

Figure 15.27 Ependymoma. An ependymoma arising in the fourth ventricle. The tumor fills the ventricle and superficially infiltrates surrounding parenchyma.

Ependymal tumors

This group of tumors occur more commonly in childhood and adolescence than in adult life. They arise in relation to any part of the ventricular system or spinal cord but they have a particular predilection for the fourth ventricle.

Ependymoma (WHO grade II)

These tumors extend into the ventricle but also diffusely infiltrate the adjacent tissue (Fig. 15.27). They can obstruct the flow of CSF resulting in the development of hydrocephalus. As they grow into

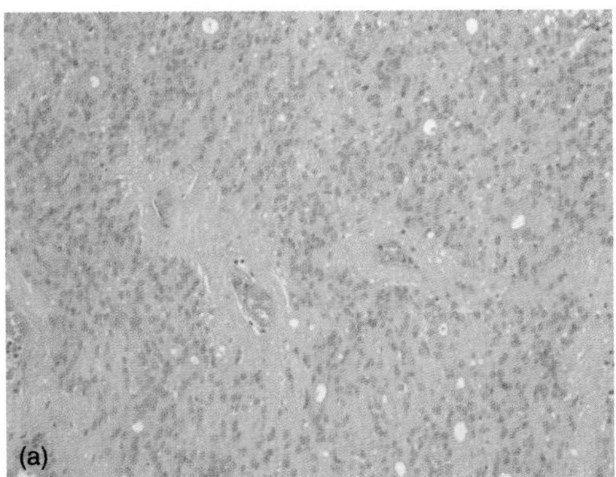

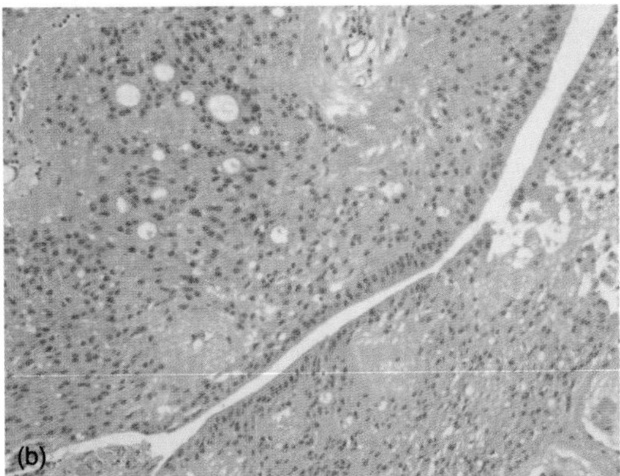

Figure 15.28 Ependymoma. (a) Perivascular pseudo-rosettes are a characteristic feature of ependymomas. The acellular region surrounding the blood vessels contains fine fibrillary processes which are GFAP immunoreactive. (b) Ependymal tubules are diagnostic of ependymoma, but not seen in all cases. In this example they are seen in both longitudinal and cross section. (a) and (b) H&E.

the ventricular cavity, meningeal gliomatosis is not infrequently associated with ependymomas. Microscopically, they are characterized by cells with small round nuclei and poorly defined cytoplasmic borders. They form fibrillary processes which are particularly prominent in relation to blood vessels producing perivascular pseudo-rosettes (Fig. 15.28a). Ependymal canals or tubules are diagnostic features (Fig. 15.28b). Several variants of ependymoma are recognized. *Cellular ependymomas* are hyper-cellular but without features of anaplasia. *Papillary ependymomas* have a papillary architecture but retain perivascular pseudo-rosettes. *Clear cell ependymomas* have a similar appearance to oligodendrogliomas and neurocytomas. *Tanycytic ependymomas* are usually seen in the spinal cord and are composed of spindle cells with a fascicular architecture. *Anaplastic ependymoma* (WHO grade III) is defined by the presence of mitotic activity, increased pleomorphism, microvascular proliferation and tumor necrosis.

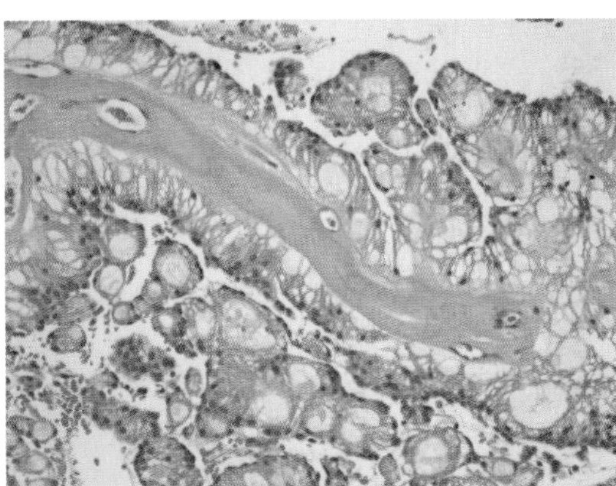

Figure 15.29 Myxopapillary ependymoma. These tumors, characteristically seen in the cauda equina, have papillae with fibrovascular cores around which tumor cells with fine fibrillary processes are arranged. H&E.

Myxopapillary ependymoma (WHO grade I)

These tumors arise in the region of the cauda equina. They are gelatinous tumors which ensheath the nerve roots of the cauda equina. They may erode local bone and present as a subcutaneous mass. Microscopically, these tumors have a papillary architecture with fine processes extending around hyalinized blood vessels (Fig. 15.29). The tumor cells are often large with vacuolated cytoplasm.

Subependymoma (WHO grade I)

This tumor lies deep to the ependymal lining of the ventricle, usually the lateral or fourth ventricles (Fig. 15.30). They protrude as smooth nodules into the ventricular lumen. Microscopically, there are small compact groups of ependymal cells with little pleomorphism separated by bands of astrocytic fibers. These tumors are very slow growing and may be an incidental finding at autopsy.

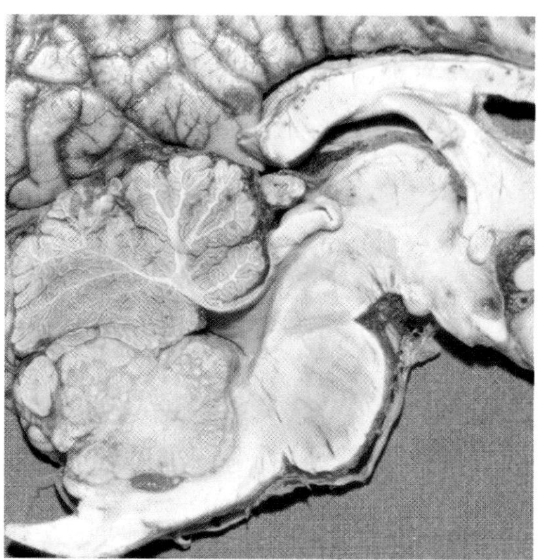

Figure 15.30 Subependymoma. A large nodular subependymoma lying between the cerebellum and brainstem. The tumor is circumscribed.

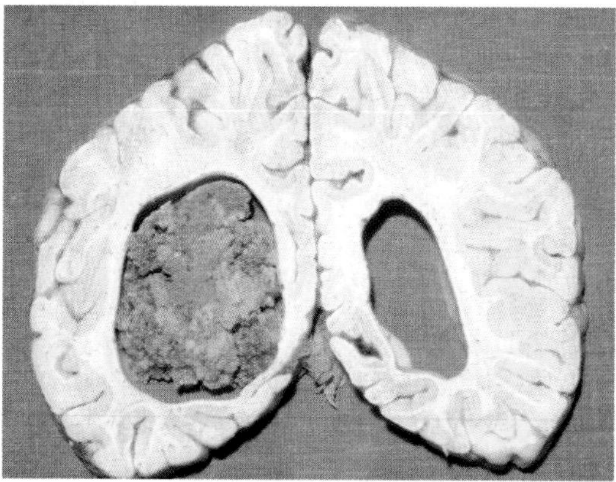

Figure 15.31 Choroid plexus papilloma. A typical finding in these tumors is the tumor filling the lateral ventricle. They are often very vascular at surgery.

Choroid plexus tumors

These tumors arise in childhood and range from *papillomas* (WHO grade I) to *carcinomas* (WHO grade III). They form bulky papillary masses which extend into the ventricle, most frequently the lateral ventricle (Fig. 15.31). They can produce hydrocephalus by obstruction of the CSF pathways. Microscopically, they range from papillae lined by a single cell layer (papilloma) (Fig. 15.32) to an epithelioid cohesive cellular mass (carcinoma) (Fig. 15.33). The carcinoma is associated with high grade features such as mitotic figures and tumor necrosis.

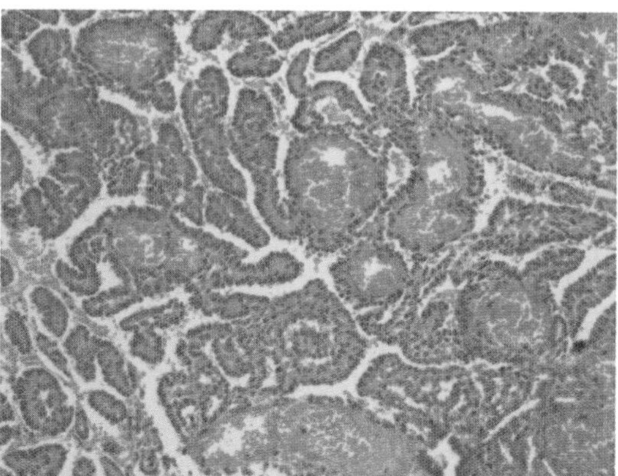

Figure 15.32 Choroid plexus papilloma. These low-grade tumors have an obvious papillary architecture and are lined by a simple cuboidal epithelium. H&E.

Glial tumors of uncertain origin

Gliomatosis cerebri (WHO grade III) is a diffusely infiltrating tumor which, by definition, involves more than two lobes. The tumor may be bilateral. Typically, there is no neoplastic mass but rather a diffuse expansion of tissue which is firm to touch. Microscopic examination shows increased cellularity within the white matter (Fig. 15.34) and diffuse infiltration of gray matter with preservation of neurons. There is usually considerable nuclear atypia of the diffusely infiltrating cells, but mitotic figures and other high-grade features are not seen.

Astroblastoma is a rare tumor which superficially resembles ependymal tumors. *Chordoid glioma of the third ventricle* (WHO grade II) is a bulky, relatively circumscribed tumor which grows into the third ventricle (Fig. 15.35). Microscopically, there are cords of epithelioid GFAP immunoreactive cells within a myxoid matrix (Fig. 15.36).

Neuronal and mixed neuronal–glial tumors

These are rare tumors. They tend to be slow growing although anaplastic variants are now being described

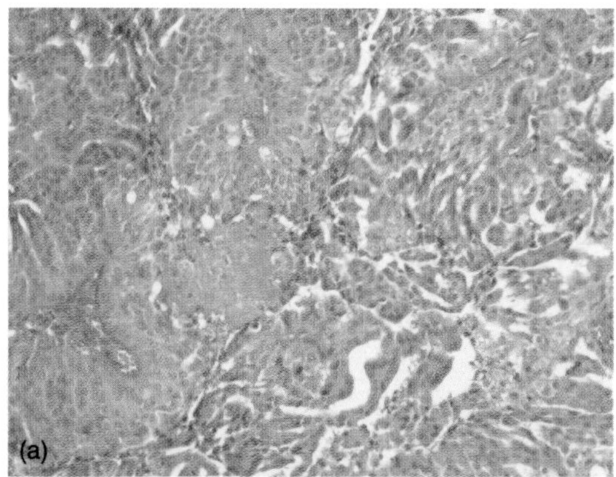

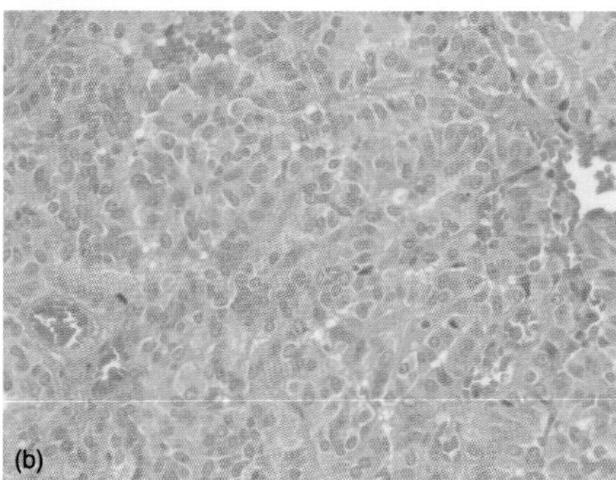

Figure 15.33 Choroid plexus carcinomas. (a) Papillary areas may be seen. (b) More commonly, however, they contain more solid epithelioid regions. Areas of necrosis are common and mitotic figures numerous. The epithelium lining the papillae is multilayered and pleomorphic. (a) and (b) H&E.

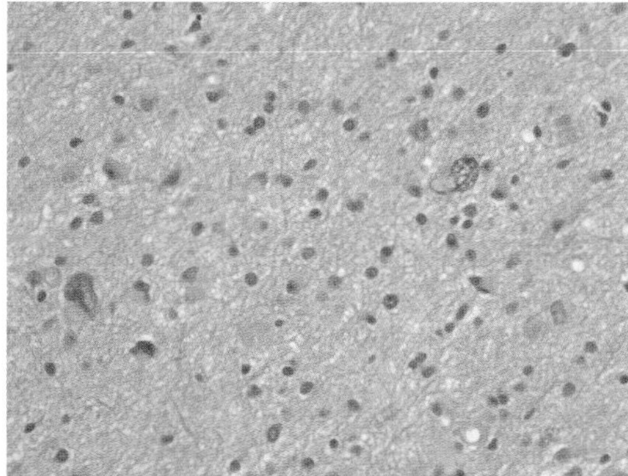

Figure 15.34 Gliomatosis cerebri. These uncommon tumors have no solid tumor focus but rather pleomorphic cells diffusely infiltrating the brain parenchyma. H&E.

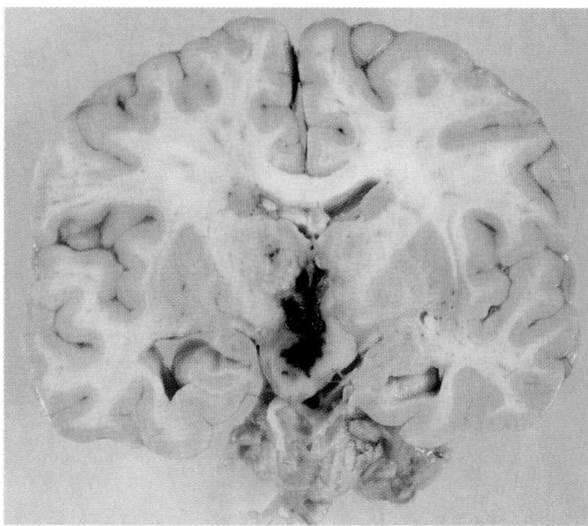

Figure 15.35 Chordoid glioma of the third ventricle. An area of hemorrhage within a chordoid glioma of the third ventricle. These recently described tumors are relatively well circumscribed with little involvement of surrounding tissues.

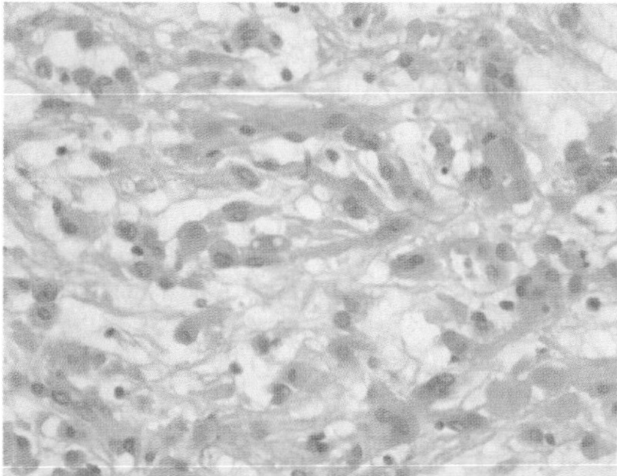

Figure 15.36 Chordoid gliomas of the third ventricle. Histologically, they are composed of epithelioid GFAP immunoreactive cells which have an architecture resembling chordomas. H&E.

for some. Intractable seizures are a common clinical presentation of these tumors, which are typically associated with the temporal lobes. A number of specific entities are currently described and outlined below. Mixed glio-neuronal tumors are increasingly being recognized, such as the papillary glio-neuronal tumor. These are not currently included in the WHO classification but are likely to be described in future revisions.

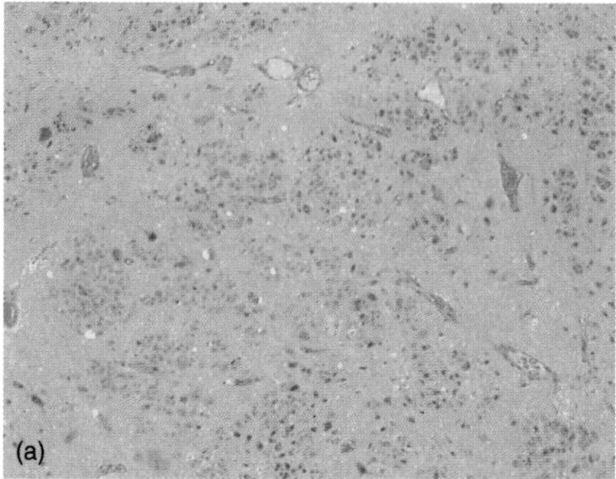

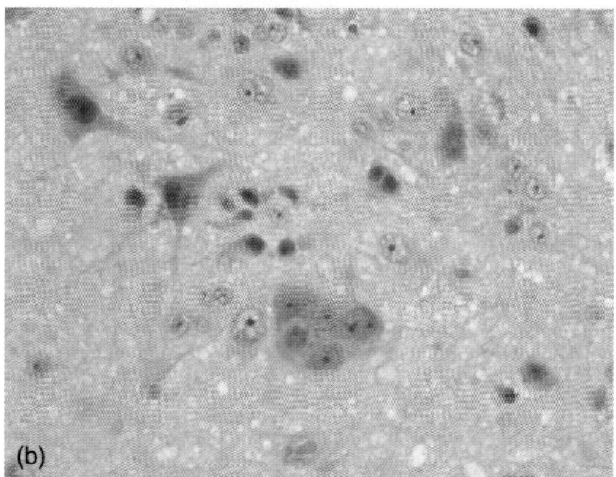

Figure 15.37 Gangliocytoma. These tumors are composed of groups of neuronal cells, ranging from neuroblast-like cells to mature ganglion-like cells. (b) Multinucleated cells may be seen but this does not imply malignancy. (a) and (b) H&E.

Gangliocytoma (WHO grade I) is a very slow growing tumor composed of groups of ganglion cells and smaller neuronal cells separated by fibrillary neuropil (Fig. 15.37a). Binucleate and multinucleate ganglion cells are often present (Fig. 15.37b).

Ganglioglioma (WHO grade II) has a similar appearance but the glial stroma is neoplastic resembling a low grade astrocytoma. They can be easily distinguished from astrocytomas by the presence of bizarre ganglion cells (Fig. 15.38). Granular bodies are common. Anaplastic variants have been described on the basis of mitotic activity and necrosis.

Dysembryoplastic neuroepithelial tumor (DNET) (WHO grade I) has a typical appearance radiologically, being intracortical and nodular (Fig. 15.39). Histologically, the tumors are microcystic and

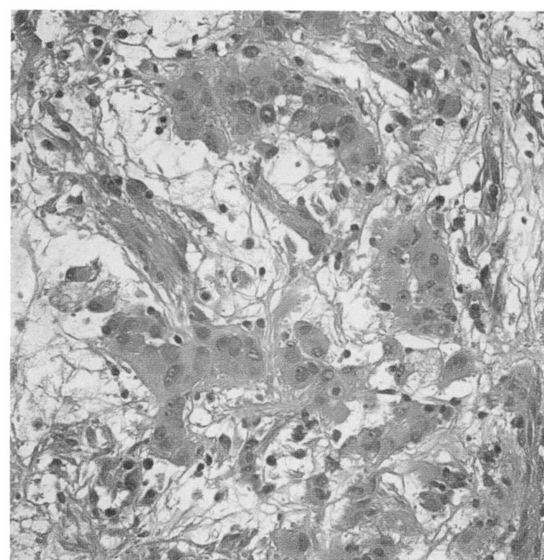

Figure 15.38 Ganglioglioma. These mixed tumors have both neuronal and glial components. The neuronal component is similar to gangliocytomas and immunoreacts with neuronal markers such as synaptophysin. The glial component forms fibrils and immunoreacts with GFAP. H&E.

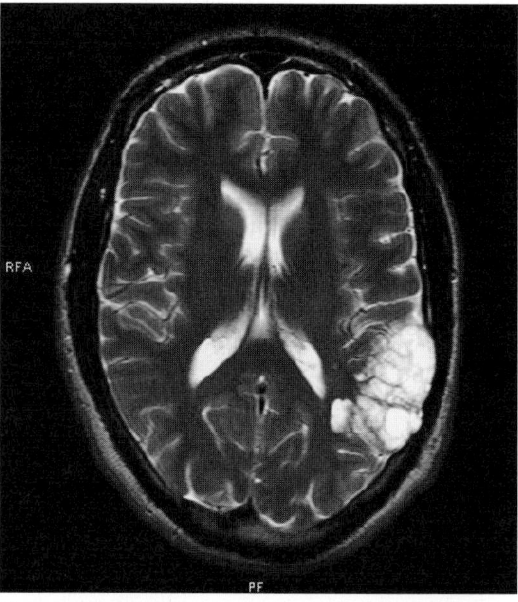

Figure 15.39 Dysembryoplastic neuroepithelial tumor. T2-weighted image of a dysembryoplastic neuroepithelial tumor (DNET). The tumor has a nodular architecture and an intracortical location.

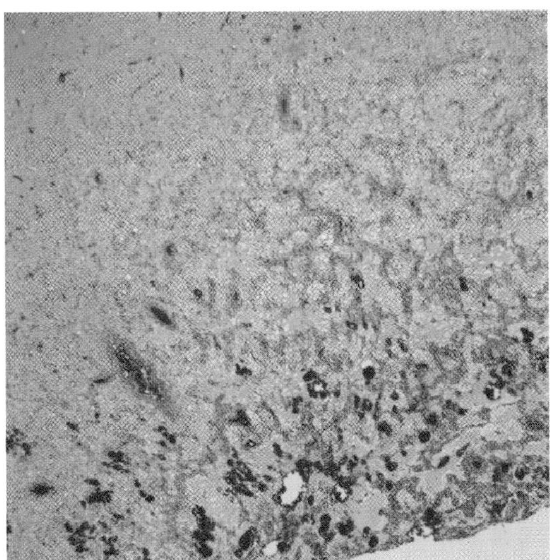

Figure 15.40 Dysembryoplastic neuroepithelial tumor. DNETs are confined to the cortex and do not involve underlying white matter. They have many microcysts within which 'floating' neurons may be seen. H&E.

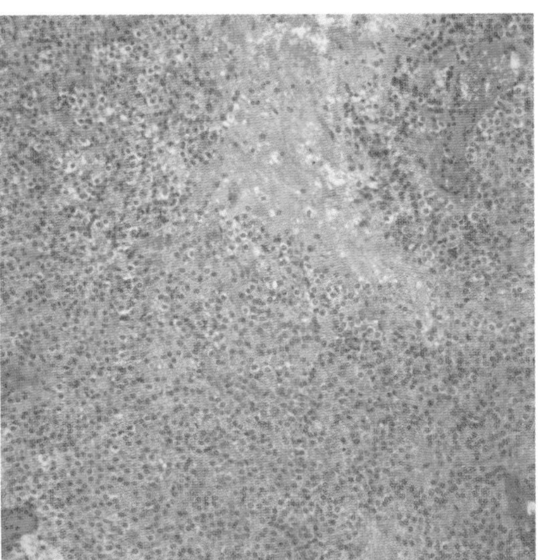

Figure 15.41 Central neurocytoma. These tumors superficially resemble oligodendrogliomas, with cells with small round nuclei. However, they do not have the dense capillary stroma associated with oligodendrogliomas and typically have acellular areas of neuropil within them. Synaptophysin immunohistochemistry is strongly positive. H&E.

composed of oligodendroglial-like cells with small numbers of mature ganglion cells (Fig. 15.40). Cortical dysplasia is usually present in the adjacent cortex and frequently there is calcification.

Central neurocytoma (WHO grade II) is seen most frequently in young adults. They are predominantly related to the ventricles, particularly the lateral ventricles, although intraparenchymal sites are described. Microscopically, they look very similar to oligodendrogliomas (Fig. 15.41). Immunohistochemistry will, however, reveal the neuronal nature of these tumors. *Cerebellar liponeurocytoma* is a neurocytic tumor seen in adults which arises in the cerebellum. The neurocytic component is mixed with mature adipocytes (Fig. 15.42).

Paraganglioma of the filum terminale is a tumor of extra-adrenal chromaffin tissues. The tumor has the same appearance as paragangliomas at other sites. They are composed of nests of neuroendocrine cells, often with granular cytoplasm, called 'zellballen' (Fig. 15.43). These nests will stain with neuroendocrine markers such as chromogranin and synaptophysin. Sustentacular cells lie between the cellular nests and immunoreact with S-100.

Pineal parenchymal tumors arise from the pineal gland and range from *pineocytomas* (WHO grade I) to *pineoblastomas* (WHO grade IV). They macroscopically expand the pineal region. Histologically, pineocytomas resemble normal pineal gland and have numerous confluent rosettes (Fig. 15.44). Pineoblastomas are poorly differentiated tumors with abundant mitotic and apoptotic activity. The cells have little discernable cytoplasm and hyperchromatic nuclei which may show moulding. Poorly formed rosettes may be seen. They often seed through the CSF and extra-neural metastases are described.

Embryonal tumors

Medulloblastoma

Medulloblastoma (WHO grade IV) is a primitive neuroectodermal tumor (PNET) of the posterior fossa. PNETs arising at other sites include retinoblastoma, pineoblastoma and supratentorial PNET. They are most commonly seen in childhood but can arise in adults, usually as the desmoplastic

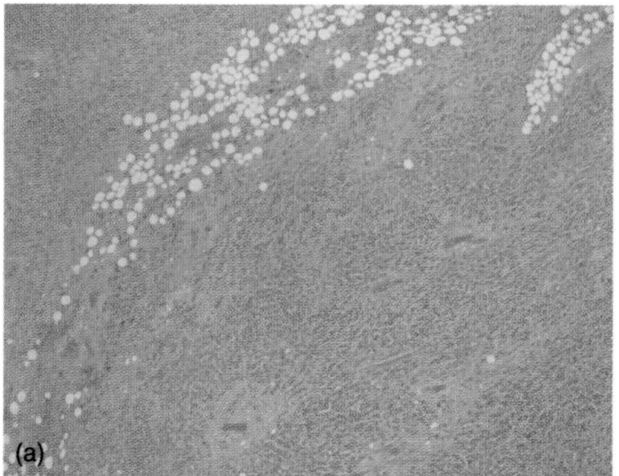

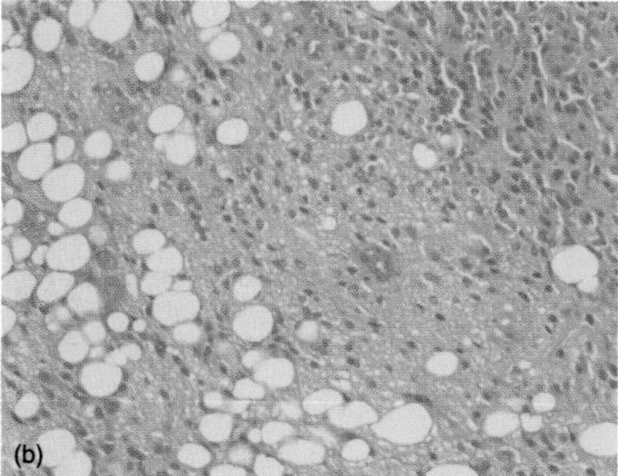

Figure 15.42 Cerebellar liponeurocytoma. (a) The tumor is composed predominantly of cells with small round nuclei. (b) Mature adipocytes are seen within the tumor. (a) and (b) H&E.

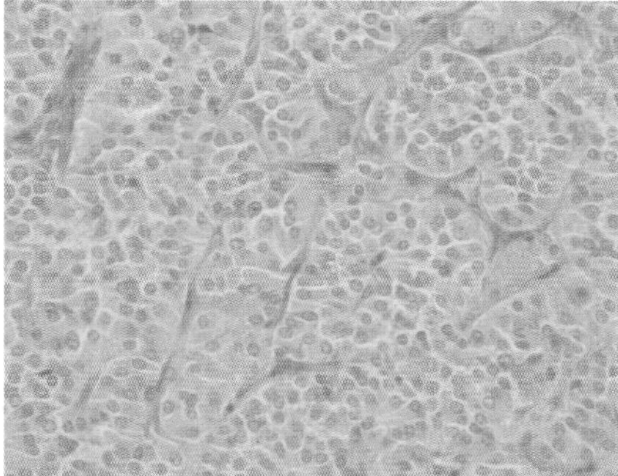

Figure 15.43 Paraganglioma of the filum terminale. The 'zellballen' are composed of cells with granular cytoplasm, and are separated by a vascular stroma. H&E.

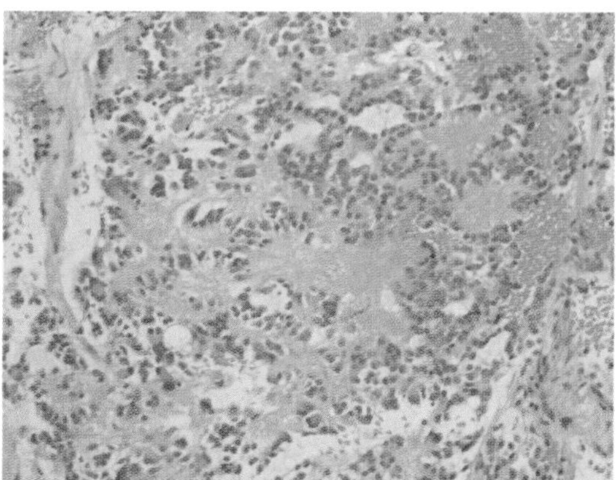

Figure 15.44 Pineocytoma. These tumors retain the overall architecture of the pineal gland with pineocytomatous rosettes. The tumor cells are small and show little pleomorphism. H&E.

variant. They are the commonest solid tumor of childhood.

In childhood the tumor typically arises in the midline of the cerebellum as a soft friable mass (Fig. 15.45a). Spread within the subarachnoid space is common and coating of the cerebellar surface may be seen (Fig. 15.45b). Due to the anatomical location of the tumor hydrocephalus may develop rapidly. Spinal imaging should be undertaken prior to surgery to investigate the possibility of CSF spread, and a CSF sample should be examined either preoperatively or at least several days post-operatively.

Histologically, the tumor is composed of sheets of small round cells with little discernable cytoplasm (Fig. 15.46). Neuroblastic rosettes may be seen. Mitotic figures and areas of tumor necrosis are easily identified. In the aggressive *large-cell variant* the nuclei are large with prominent nucleoli. In the desmoplastic variant the typical small cells are embedded within a reticulin-rich stroma and there are pale islands with no reticulin expression and evidence of cellular differentiation, both neuronal and glial. Rare medulloblastoma variants may show skeletal muscle differentiation (*medullomyoblastoma*) or melanin expression (*melanotic medulloblastoma*).

Other embryonal tumors

Ependymoblastoma, medulloepithelioma and *supratentorial PNET* are all rare, aggressive (WHO grade IV) tumors of infancy.

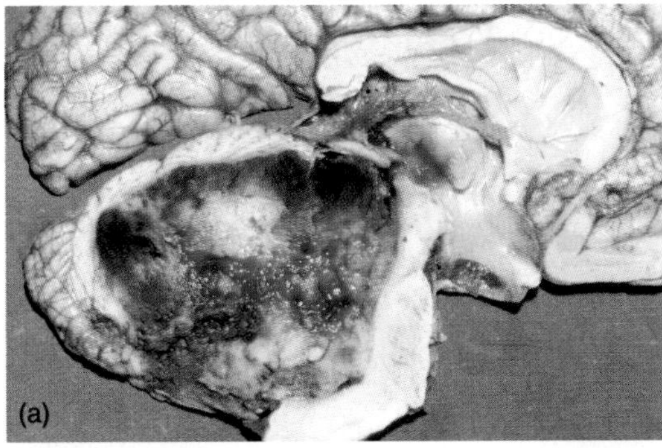

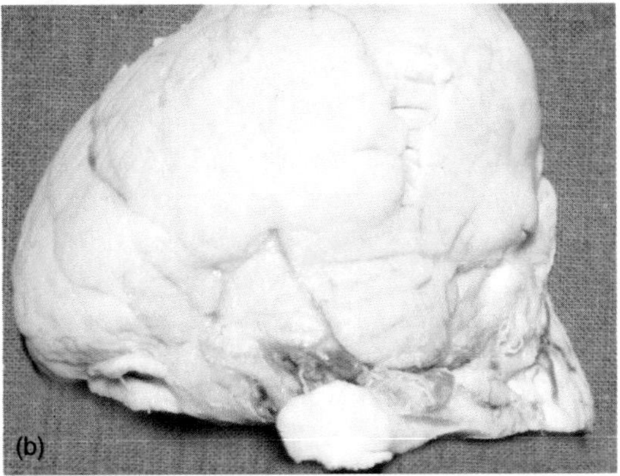

Figure 15.45 Medulloblastoma. (a) They usually arise in the midline of the cerebellum and infiltrate surrounding tissue. (b) They spread in the CSF and can cover the surface of the cerebellum.

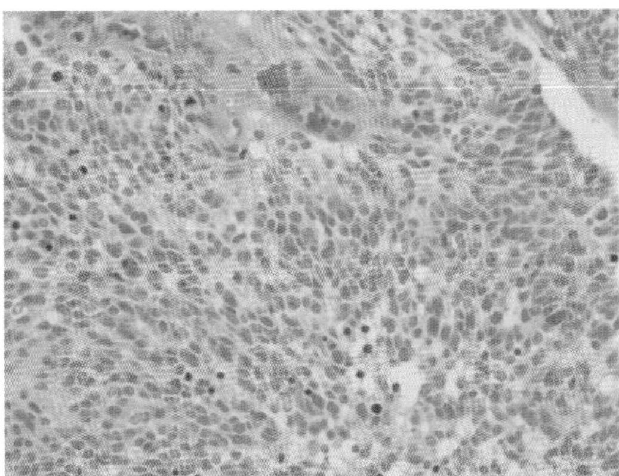

Figure 15.46 Medulloblastoma. Classical medulloblastomas are composed of pleomorphic cells with little discernable cytoplasm. Mitotic figures and apoptotic bodies are easily identified. Nuclear moulding is seen in areas. H&E.

Atypical teratoid/rhabdoid tumor (ATR) (WHO grade IV) is an aggressive tumor of childhood which is predominantly seen in the posterior fossa but may arise in the supratentorial compartment. Macroscopically, they diffusely infiltrate surrounding tissues and contain necrotic regions. Microscopically, they are pleomorphic but contain, at least in areas, cells with large pale nuclei and prominent nucleoli. These typical rhabdoid cells have abundant eosinophilic cytoplasm which displaces the nucleus (Fig. 15.47). Immunohistochemistry shows a range of phenotypic expression, often with epithelial (cytokeratin, EMA) and smooth muscle expression. GFAP and neuronal markers are variable. As with other rhabdoid tumors mutations of the *INI1/SNF5* gene on chromosome 22 are common.

TUMORS OF CRANIAL AND SPINAL NERVES

The commonest tumors of peripheral nerves are *schwannomas* and *neurofibromas* (both WHO grade I). They are both composed of schwann cells, the difference being that in schwannomas the tumor arises at the periphery of the nerve displacing the nerve bundle, while in neurofibroma the tumor arises within the nerve bundle resulting in expansion of the nerve from within.

Schwannomas (WHO grade I) are slow growing encapsulated tumors which can arise from any peripheral nerve but is most frequently encountered in relation to the VIIIth cranial nerve (vestibulocochlear nerve). Hearing loss is the commonest presentation. The tumor arises in the cerebello-pontine angle and may distort, but not invade, adjacent tissues (Fig. 15.48). Histologically, they show a biphasic architecture with compact areas composed of spindle cells with a fascicular architecture (Antoni A) and looser, less cellular areas (Antoni B) (Fig. 15.49). Palisading may be seen in Antoni A areas (Verocay bodies). Cystic degeneration is common and there may be evidence of previous hemorrhage. The blood vessel walls are often hyalinized.

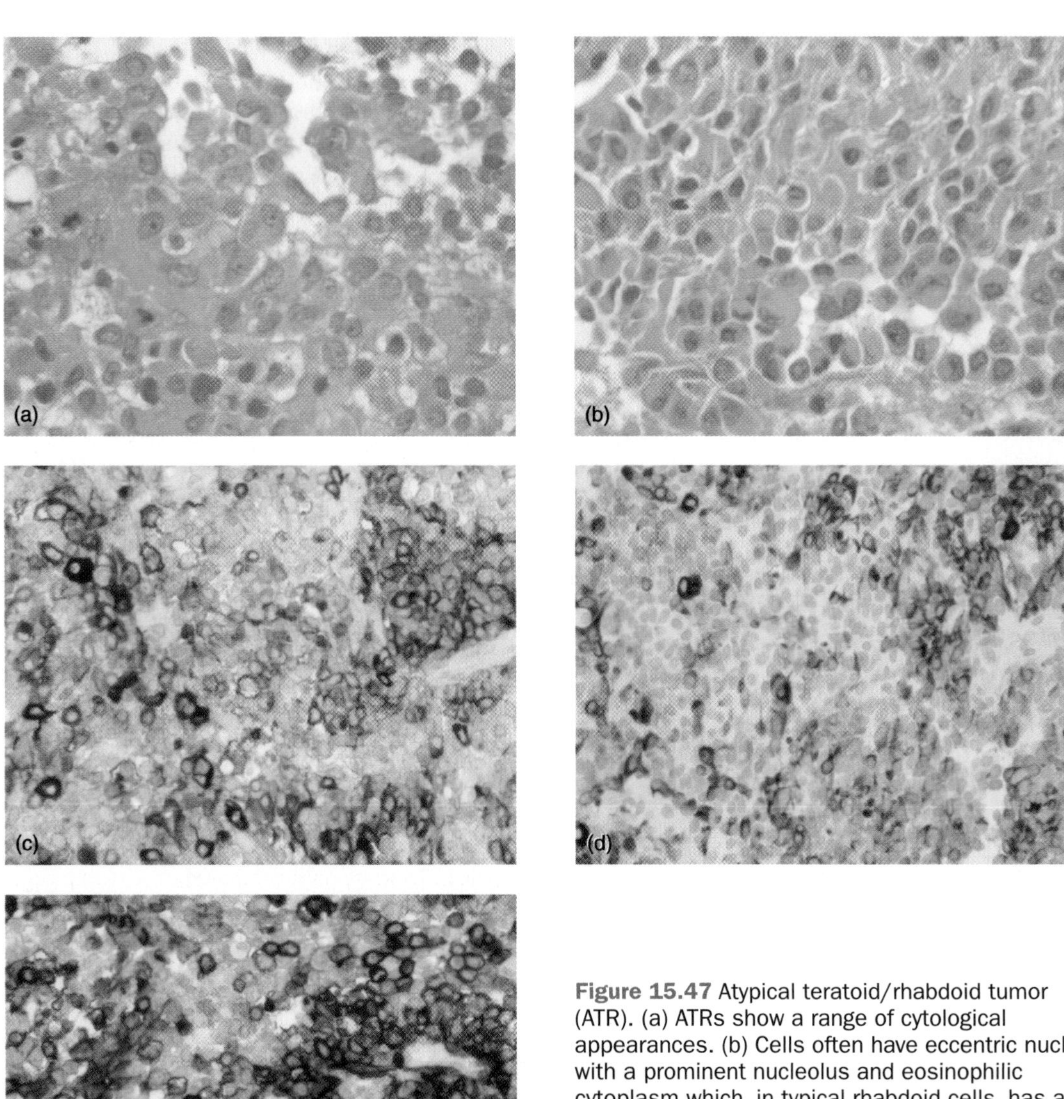

Figure 15.47 Atypical teratoid/rhabdoid tumor (ATR). (a) ATRs show a range of cytological appearances. (b) Cells often have eccentric nuclei with a prominent nucleolus and eosinophilic cytoplasm which, in typical rhabdoid cells, has a hyaline appearance. (c) EMA immunoreactivity is consistent. (d) There is also often at least focal cytokeratin expression. (e) GFAP expression is variable but usually at least focal. (a) and (b) H&E. (c) Immunohistochemistry EMA. (d) Immunohistochemistry pancytokeratin. (e) Immunohistochemistry GFAP.

Neurofibromas (WHO grade I)

These are common tumors of peripheral nerves but rarely involve cranial nerves. They are usually solitary but may involve adjacent nerves producing a plexiform neurofibroma which macroscopically is described as looking like 'a bag of worms'. They are pale tumors and usually have a mucoid texture on sectioning. Histologically, they are of low cellularity and have a pale stroma. The tumor cells are elongated and are often described as having twisting nuclei. As the tumor expands a nerve bundle from within, axons can be demonstrated within the tumor with neurofilament immunohistochemistry.

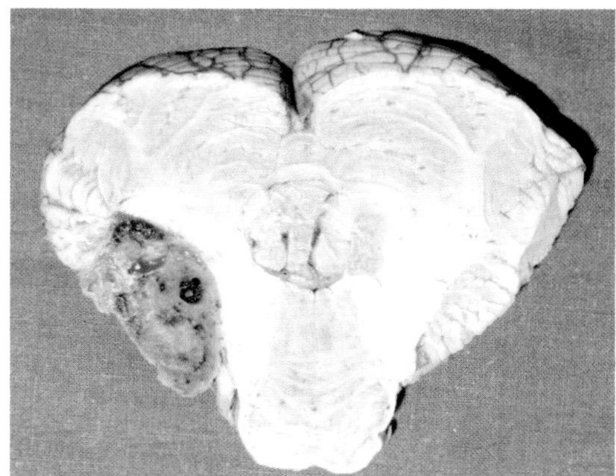

Figure 15.48 Schwannoma. The typical intracranial site of these tumors is the cerebello-pontine angle. There is local deformity but no infiltration of surrounding tissue.

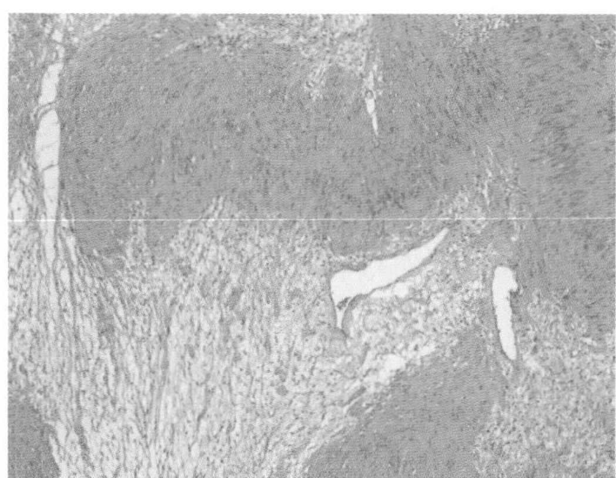

Figure 15.49 Schwannoma. The classical histological appearances of a schwannoma includes compact Antoni type A regions, with areas of nuclear palisading, and looser Antoni type B regions. H&E.

Malignant peripheral nerve sheath tumors

These are rare tumors which may arise from either schwannomas or neurofibromas, but are usually seen arising from neurofibromas in the setting of neurofibromatosis type 1. Macroscopically, they are non-encapsulated tumors which infiltrate surrounding tissues. Microscopically, they are sarcomatous and can show a variety of appearances from a fascicular tumor reminiscent of fibrosarcoma to a pleomorphic one with a range of phenotypic

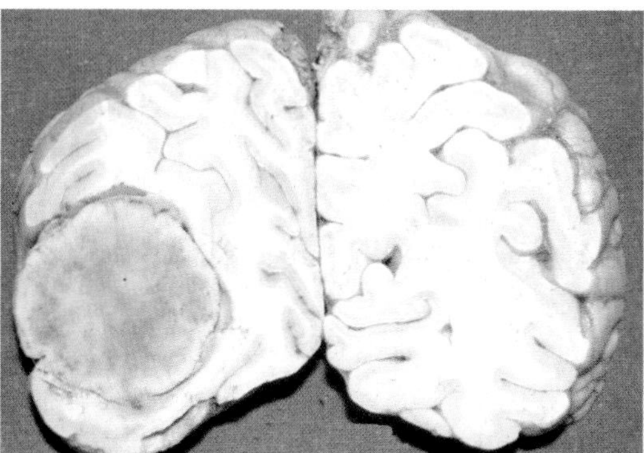

Figure 15.50 Meningioma. The tumor is sharply defined and with concave deformity of the underlying brain.

expression including skeletal muscle (Triton tumor). S-100 immunohistochemistry is usually at least focally positive and helpful in diagnosis. The epithelioid variant can be mistaken for carcinoma.

Neurofibromatosis

Neurofibromatosis is an autosomal dominant disease characterized by peripheral nerve tumors. In *neurofibromatosis type 1* neurofibromas are abundant and may be disfiguring. Plexiform neurofibromas are said to be pathognomic. In *neurofibromatosis type 2* bilateral acoustic schwannomas are typical.

TUMORS OF THE MENINGES

Tumors of meningothelial cells

Meningiomas are common, generally slowly growing tumors composed of neoplastic arachnoidal (meningothelial) cells. Macroscopically, they often form well-circumscribed masses which have a lobulated architecture (Fig. 15.50). Occasional tumors may grow in a more diffuse pattern over the dura, termed meningioma *en plaque* (Fig. 15.51). The majority are WHO grade I, reflecting their benign nature. However, atypical (WHO grade II) and anaplastic variants (WHO grade III) are recognized by a number of histological characteristics. *Benign meningiomas* (WHO grade I) follow a relatively slow

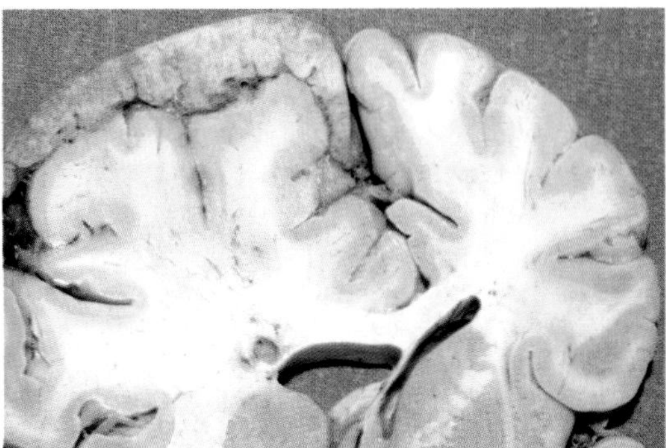

Figure 15.51 Meningioma *en plaque*. There is a sheet of tumor on the surface of the cerebral hemisphere.

Table 15.4 Variants of meningiomas currently described in the WHO classification

WHO grade	Variant
I	Meningothelial Transitional Fibroblastic Secretory Angiomatous Microcystic Psammomatous Lymphoplasmacyte-rich Metaplastic
II	Chordoid Clear cell Atypical
III	Papillary Rhabdoid Anaplastic (malignant)

clinical course, and have only occasional mitotic figures, although pleomorphic nuclei may be seen. A variety of architectural patterns are seen within this group (Table 15.4) and the tumor cells express EMA. It should be emphasized that it is the WHO grade and not the architectural pattern which is the important pathological information in determining management of the patient. The three most common architectural patterns are meningothelial, fibroblastic and transitional. The characteristic histological features of cellular whorls and psammoma bodies (round, calcified bodies) are seen most commonly in the transitional variant (Fig. 15.52). Fibroblastic meningiomas may resemble peripheral nerve sheath tumors such as schwannoma, but characteristic meningothelial cells are usually present, albeit only focally. Psammomatous meningiomas contain large numbers of psammoma bodies and may require a period of decalcification prior to tissue processing which may delay the reporting time. They characteristically occur in the thoracic spinal region of middle-aged women. Angiomatous meningiomas are highly vascular and can be confused histologically with a vascular malformation, though radiologically these are clearly distinct. Foci of meningothelial cells are always present in angiomatous meningiomas, although they may be sparse. Secretory meningiomas form intracellular lumina lined by cytokeratin immunoreactive cells. The lumina contain PAS-positive, CEA immunoreactive material.

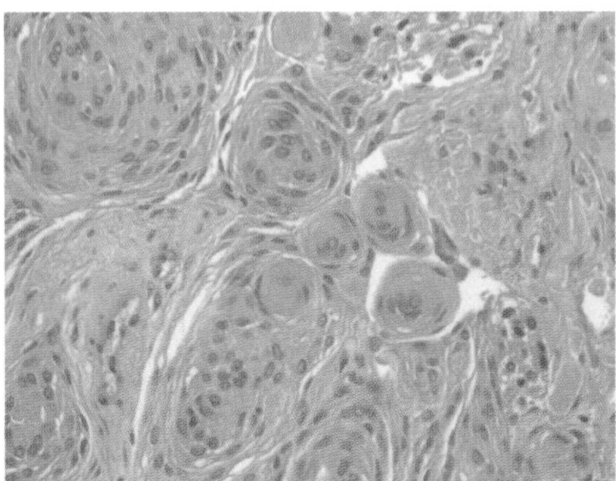

Figure 15.52 Meningioma. Cellular whorls are typical of the transitional meningiomas. H&E.

Two subtypes of WHO grade II meningiomas are recognized on the basis of their architectural pattern: clear cell and chordoid meningiomas. Chordoid meningiomas resemble chordomas, with trabeculae of epitheliod cells in a mucinous stroma.

Atypical meningioma (WHO grade II) is the term given to a meningioma with any architectural pattern, but with specific histological features. Of these features, a mitotic rate of at least four mitotic figures per ten high power fields is the most important, allowing a histological diagnosis of atypia in the absence of the other features (increased cellularity, small cells with high nucleus; cytoplasmic ratio, prominent nucleoli, sheet-like growth pattern, and 'geographic' necrosis). In the absence of this mitotic rate at least three of the other five features need to be present to allow a histological diagnosis of atypia. WHO grade II tumors have a higher incidence of recurrence, particularly following subtotal resection.

WHO grade III meningiomas are subclassified on the basis of their architectural pattern into papillary and rhabdoid subtypes. *Papillary meningiomas* are rare variants and are usually seen in children. They are defined by a perivascular pseudopapillary pattern. *Rhabdoid meningiomas* contain rhabdoid cells similar to those seen at other sites in the body. Rhabdoid cells have a specific microscopic appearance with eccentric nuclei, abundant globular eosinophilic cytoplasm and paranuclear inclusions, and show focal EMA immunoreactivity.

Anaplastic (malignant) meningiomas (WHO grade III) have obvious malignant cytology and/or a high mitotic rate (20 or more mitotic figures in ten high power fields). These tumors show a high incidence of local and brain invasion, recurrence and metastases.

Brain invasion is defined histologically as islands of neoplastic cells which have invaded through the pia to involve underlying cortical tissue, often producing a gliotic reaction. Brain invasion is not one of the criteria used for grading tumors in the WHO classification, but should always be commented upon in a pathological report, as brain invasion is associated with subtotal resection and a higher incidence of recurrence. Meningiomas of any grade may also infiltrate local tissues to extend into the soft tissues of the skull, including the orbit and pterygopalatine fossa. Such tumors are technically difficult to resect.

The likelihood of tumor recurrence is based on several features: the completeness of surgical resection (Simpson grade), the WHO grade based on the histological appearances, and the presence of brain invasion. Treatment decisions should take account of all these features.

Mesenchymal non-meningothelial tumors

Virtually every type of mesenchymal tumor has been described arising from the dura, ranging from benign fibroma and lipoma to malignant rhabdomyosarcoma and osteosarcoma. The commonest is *hemangiopericytoma* (WHO grade II). This is a cellular tumor composed of plump cells with poorly defined cytoplasmic boundaries and angular nuclei. The stroma is vascular and some blood vessels show a typical ‘stag-horn’ branching pattern (Fig. 15.53). Reticulin fibers are abundant. Mitotic figures and foci of tumor necrosis are easily identified. CD34 immunoreactivity is variable and the relationship between hemangiopericytomas and solitary fibrous tumors is uncertain. A histologically similar tumor is the *mesenchymal chondrosarcoma.* This can be differentiated from hemangiopericytoma by the presence of discrete chondroid nodules within the cellular sheets.

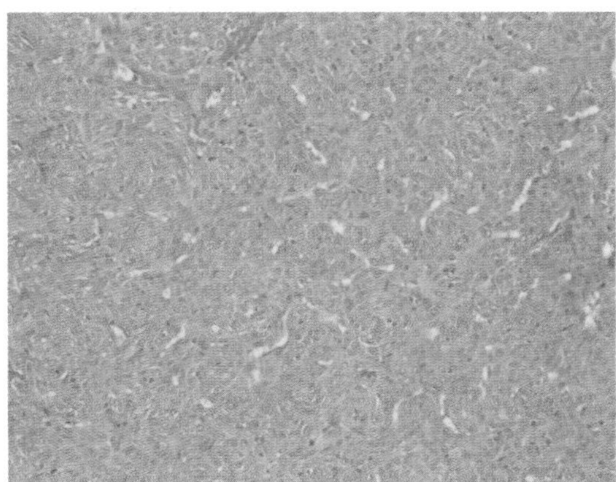

Figure 15.53 Hemangiopericytoma. This cellular tumor has prominent branching vascular spaces. H&E.

Solitary fibrous tumor is a rare benign tumor which appears similar to the more common pleural tumor. The tumor has a fascicular architecture and is composed of spindle cells which show strong CD34 immunoreactivity (Fig. 15.54). Malignant variants are described.

Primary melanocytic lesions can arise from melanocytes in the pia-arachnoid. They range from low grade melanocytomas through to the aggressive primary malignant melanoma. Diffuse meningeal melanosis can be associated with the genetic syndrome *neurocutaneous melanosis.*

TUMORS OF UNCERTAIN HISTOGENESIS

Hemangioblastomas (WHO grade I) are most commonly sporadic but may be part of the genetic

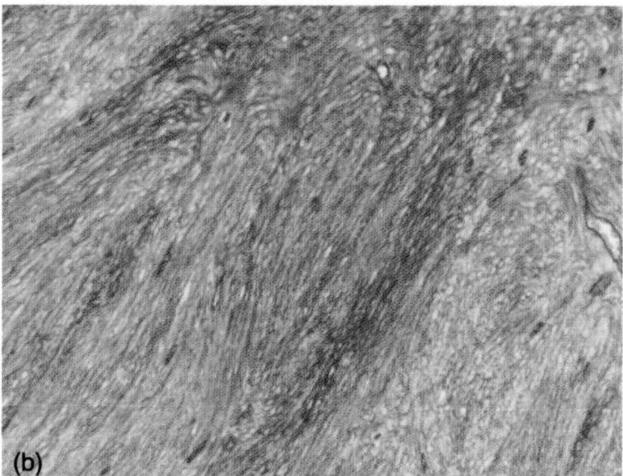

Figure 15.54 Solitary fibrous tumor. (a) The tumor is composed of sheets of spindle cells separated by bands of fibrous tissue. (b) There is strong CD34 immunoreactivity. (a) H&E. (b) Immunohistochemistry CD34.

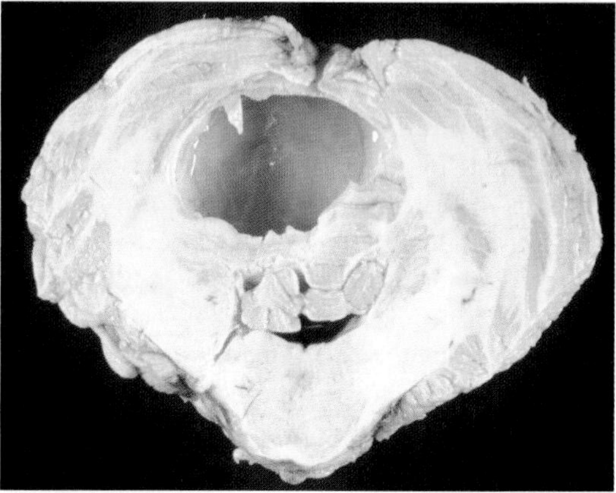

Figure 15.55 Hemangioblastoma. The cerebellum is the typical site for these tumors. They are often predominantly cystic with only a small nodule of tumor in the cyst wall.

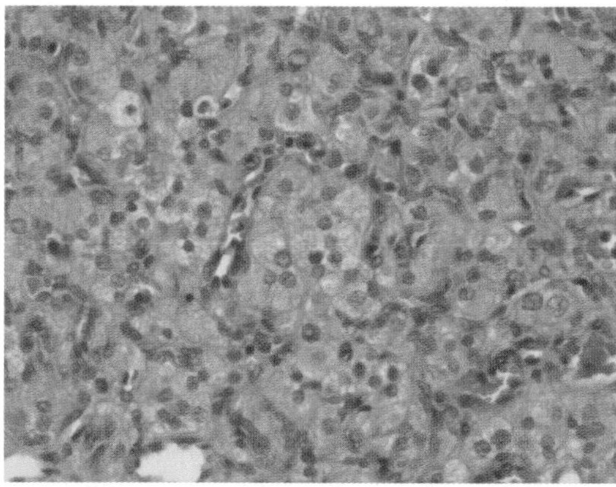

Figure 15.56 Hemangioblastoma. The tumor has a vascular stroma and large cells with pale foamy cytoplasm. H&E.

syndrome *Von Hippel–Lindau* (VHL) disease. When sporadic, these tumors occur in the cerebellum of adults. When part of VHL, the tumors may occur anywhere in the CNS although cerebellum remains the commonest site. In VHL they may be multiple. The tumor typically consists of a large cyst with a small mural nodule of solid tumor (Fig. 15.55) although rarely the tumor may be more solid. The histological appearances are of a highly vascular tumor composed of vascular channels of variable size, and a stroma composed of large polygonal cells that are usually distended with lipid (Fig. 15.56). Reticulin fibers are abundant within these tumors. The principal differential diagnosis, particularly in VHL patients, is metastatic clear cell carcinoma of the kidney. Immunohistochemistry may be helpful in that hemangioblastomas are usually negative for EMA and pan-cytokeratin. If uncertainty still exists ultrasound examination of the kidneys may be indicated.

HEMOPOIETIC NEOPLASMS

Hemopoietic neoplasms can involve the CNS as either primary disease (*primary CNS lymphoma, PCNSL*) or as part of a systemic disease. The commonest form of involvement is compression of the spinal cord by an extradural deposit of lymphoma,

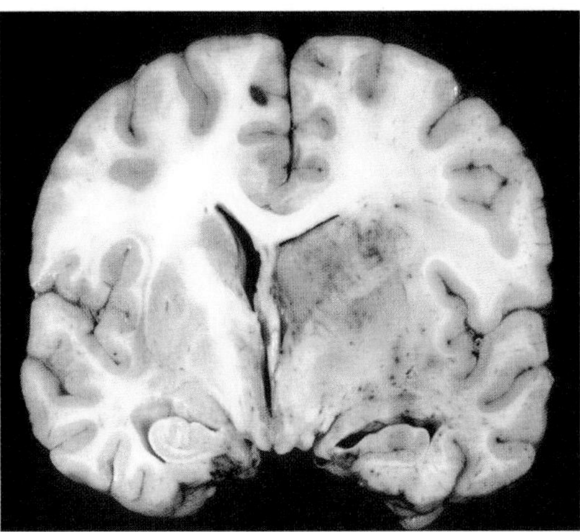

Figure 15.57 Lymphoma. The tumor is poorly defined. There is expansion of the basal ganglia on one side with ventricular compression and subfalcine herniation.

particularly plasma cell tumors. This neurological emergency can be a presenting feature of a systemic lymphoma. Both lymphoma and leukemia can present as an intracranial dural deposit which may mimic a meningioma. Acute leukemia in children may diffusely infiltrate the meninges and CSF monitoring is important in patients.

PCNSL is a rare neoplasm being seen in elderly patients or in individuals who are immunocompromised. PCNSL occurs commonly in the setting of acquired immunodeficiency syndrome (AIDS). PCNSL has a variable appearance macroscopically. It may solitary or multifocal; it may be a relatively well defined fleshy mass or a diffusely infiltrating poorly defined granular lesion (Fig. 15.57). The lesions are very sensitive to steroid therapy and may almost completely disappear radiologically after only a short course. This can make histological interpretation of steroid treated lesions very difficult.

Histological classification of lymphomas is based on either the Revised European-American classification of Lymphoid neoplasms (REAL) or on the current WHO classification. Neither classification system refers specifically to PCNSL. The majority of PCNSLs are diffuse large B-cell lymphomas. They are composed of large cells with prominent nucleoli which are predominantly perivascular but also infiltrate surrounding tissues. There is marked tissue necrosis associated with these tumors. The walls of blood vessels are expanded by malignant B-cells (Fig. 15.58), and this may be highlighted by a reticulin stain which shows an 'onion-skin' pattern. Other forms of mature B-cell neoplasms, including small lymphocytic lymphoma and follicular lymphoma, are described but are less common. Intravascular large B-cell lymphoma (angiotropic lymphoma) is a rare systemic B-cell lymphoma which involves the CNS in which malignant B-cells are seen within blood vessels resulting in vascular occlusion and infarction (Fig. 15.59). T-cell lymphomas are very uncommon and primary CNS Hodgkin's disease an extreme rarity. When assessing a T-cell infiltrate within a hemopoietic neoplasm it is important to remember that T-cells are common as part of a reactive response to B-cell lymphomas. By contrast any B-cells in the CNS should be treated with suspicion. B-cells very rarely contribute to a reactive process and when present in significant numbers are likely to indicate a B-cell lymphoma.

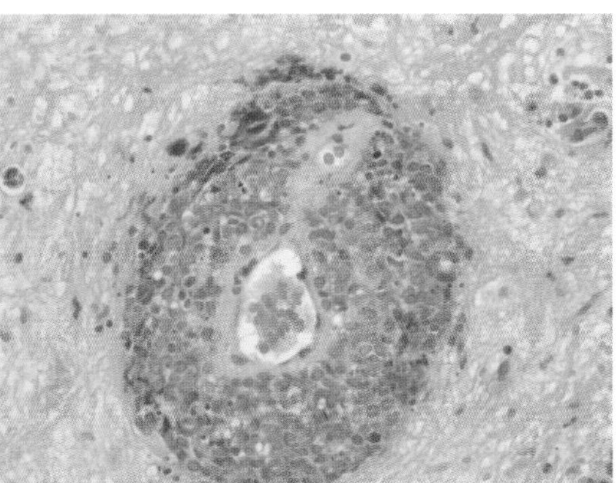

Figure 15.58 Lymphoma. Blood vessel walls are expanded by malignant lymphocytes. H&E.

Within the dura *extranodal marginal zone B-cell lymphomas* (MALT) may be seen. Other rare hemopoietic neoplasms which may involve the dura or brain parenchyma include *Langerhans cell tumors* and *Rosai–Dorfman disease.*

GERM CELL TUMORS

Germ cell tumors typically occur in young people and arise in the midline, pineal region, hypothalamic

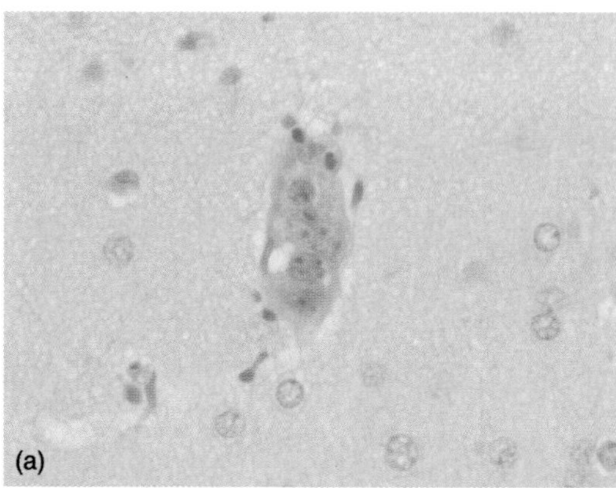

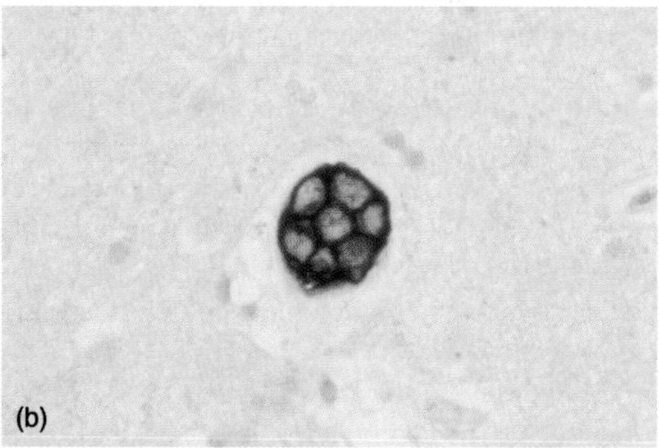

Figure 15.59 Intravascular large B-cell lymphoma. (a) Small blood vessels are plugged by pleomorphic tumor cells. (b) Immunohistochemistry reveals the B-lymphocytic lineage of the cells. (a) H&E. (b) Immunohistochemistry CD20.

region, and suprasellar region (Fig. 15.60). The commonest is the *germinoma* followed by *teratoma.* Teratomas may be mature or immature. *Yolk-sac tumors* and *choriocarcinomas* are uncommon in their pure forms although teratomas may contain focal elements. *Embryonal carcinomas* are also described within the CNS.

Germinomas are composed of large round cells with well defined cytoplasmic boundaries and a large nucleus often with a prominent nucleolus (Fig. 15.61). There is a prominent lymphocytic infiltrate surrounding the tumor cells. The tumor cells show at least focal placental alkaline phosphatase (PLAP) immunoreactivity. Increasingly, germ cell tumors are not biopsied as they can be diagnosed and monitored by assessment of germ cell markers (placental alkaline phosphatase [PLAP], α-fetoprotein, human chorionic gonadotrophin [hCG]) in the CSF. Germinomas respond well to therapy.

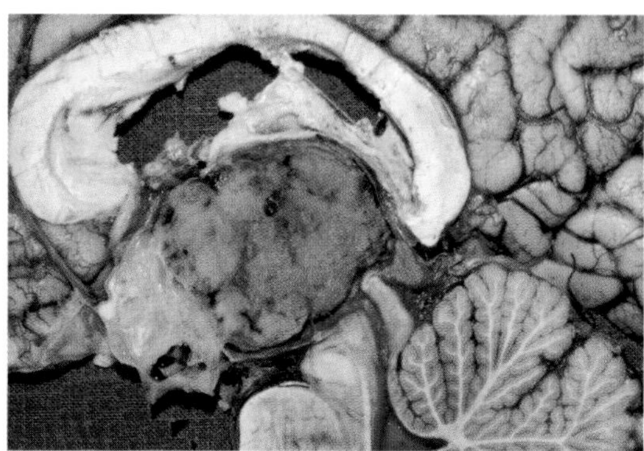

Figure 15.60 Germinoma. Germ cell tumors typically arise in the midline of the brain.

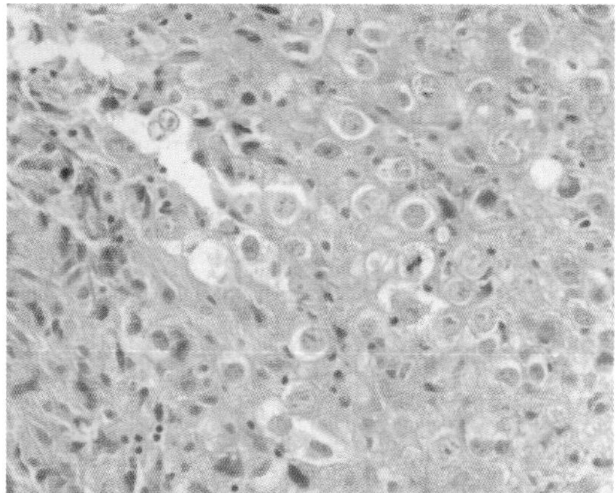

Figure 15.61 Germinoma. The malignant cells have large pale nuclei often with prominent nucleoli. H&E.

CYSTS AND TUMOR-LIKE LESIONS

A *Rathke's cleft cyst* is a lesion arising within the pituitary gland which often bulges upwards through the diaphragma sella. It is lined by low cuboidal epithelium and is basically an enlargement of the cleft that is normally found in the pituitary gland in lower primates and vertebrates between the anterior and intermediate lobes.

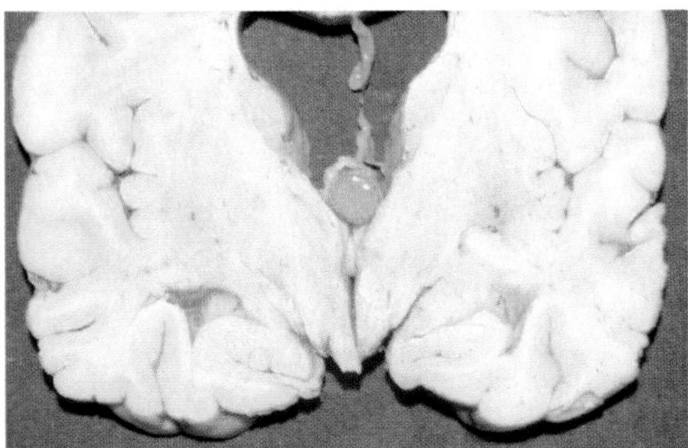

Figure 15.62 Colloid cyst. These cysts can obstruct at the foramen of Munro producing acute hydrocephalus.

Epidermoid and *dermoid cysts* are the same as similar cysts that occur elsewhere in the body. Epidermoid cysts are more common than dermoid cysts. They are seen most frequently in the cerebello-pontine angle but may arise within the brain, spine or bones of the skull. Dermoid cysts are seen in midline locations and are most common in the posterior fossa or lumbosacral spinal region. Rupture of these cysts releases keratin debris and produces an inflammatory response.

Colloid cysts occur in the third ventricle (Fig. 15.62). The lining epithelium is usually flat or cuboidal, but may be pseudo-stratified. PAS-positive cells are often present. Cilia are variable. A colloid cyst may have an intermittent ball-valve effect on the interventricular foramina which may be fatal as a result of acute hydrocephalus and raised intracranial pressure (ICP).

Enterogenous cysts are developmental abnormalities that occur within the vertebral canal. The cysts are most frequently lined by respiratory epithelium (Fig. 15.63) but gastrointestinal epithelium is also encountered.

Arachnoid cysts are collections of CSF enclosed within the pia-arachnoid. Their pathogenesis is not clear, but they may attain a considerable size without producing any increase in ICP. The commonest site is adjacent to a Sylvian fissure, when the typical features are a collection of fluid on the surface of the brain and considerable displacement of the insular opercula, such that the insula may be clearly seen (Fig. 15.64).

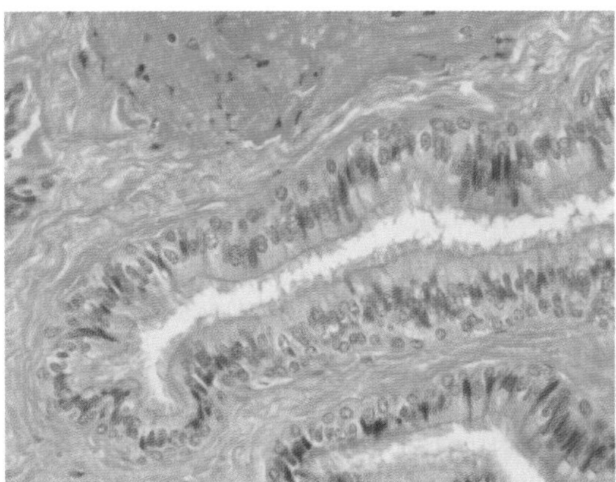

Figure 15.63 Enterogenous cyst. These cysts are lined by either respiratory or gastrointestinal-type epithelium. H&E.

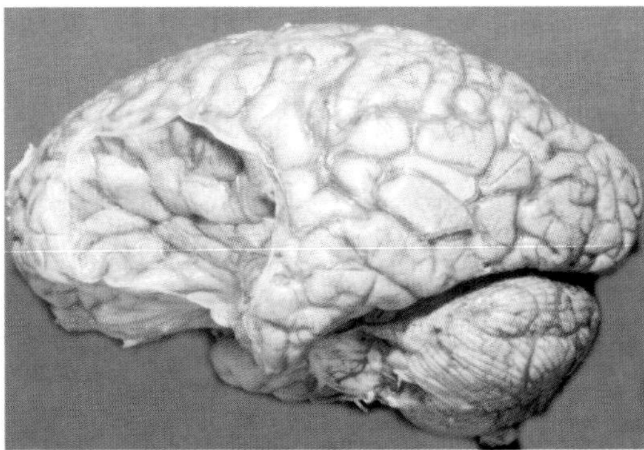

Figure 15.64 Arachnoid cyst. The cyst has produced considerable widening of the Sylvian fissure.

TUMORS OF THE SELLAR REGION

Tumors of the anterior gland

The tumors arising from the anterior gland are the pituitary adenomas and carcinomas. The normal cell population of the anterior gland includes somatotrophs (growth hormone [GH] producing), mammosomatotrophs (GH and prolactin [PRL] producing), lactotrophs (PRL producing), thyrotrophs (thyroid stimulating hormone [TSH] producing), corticotrophs (adrenocorticotrophic hormone [ACTH] producing) and gonadotrophs (luteinizing hormone

Table 15.5 Classification of pituitary adenomas based on an immunohistochemical profile

Adenoma type	Variants	Immunohistochemical profile	Clinical features
Endocrine hyperfunction			
PRL-cell	Sparsely granulated	PRL focal	Hypogonadism in males
	Densely granulated	PRL strong	Amenorrhea–galactorrhea in females
GH-cell	Sparsely granulated	GH focal	Acromegaly
	Densely granulated	GH strong	
Mixed GH-PRL cell		GH, PRL	Acromegaly and hyperprolactinemia
Mammosomatotroph adenoma		GH, PRL	Acromegaly and hyperprolactinemia
Acidophil stem-cell		PRL, GH	Hyperprolactinemia
Corticotroph adenoma	Sparsely granulated	ACTH focal	Cushing's disease
	Densely granulated	ACTH strong	Cushing's disease
Thyrotroph adenoma		TSH	Hyperthyroidism
Clinically non-functioning			
Gonadotroph adenoma		FSH, LH, α-subunit	Non-functioning sellar mass
Silent adenoma	Subtype 1	ACTH	Non-functioning sellar mass
	Subtype 2	ACTH	Non-functioning sellar mass
	Subtype 3	Any combination	Non-functioning sellar mass
Null-cell adenoma		Immunonegative	Non-functioning sellar mass
Oncocytoma		Immunonegative	Non-functioning sellar mass

PRL = prolactin; GH = growth hormone; ACTH = adrenocorticotrophic hormone; TSH = thyroid stimulating hormone; FSH = follicle stimulating hormone; LH = luteinizing hormone

[LH] and follicle stimulating hormone [FSH] producing). *Pituitary adenomas* are classified based on the hormones produced and their clinical symptoms (Table 15.5). They vary greatly in size from microadenomas no more than 1–2 mm in size to lesions of several centimeters in diameter (Fig. 15.65). They have two principal effects: hormonal and/or compressive. The former may take the form of increased production of hormone, as in acromegaly or Cushing's disease, or of a reduced secretion of hormones brought about by a non-functioning adenoma replacing the greater part of the anterior lobe. Compressive signs are usually secondary to a suprasellar expansion of the tumor, leading to involvement of the optic chiasm (hence the high incidence of defects in the visual fields) and the hypothalamus. The tumor may also extend laterally into the cavernous sinus.

Pituitary apoplexy refers to hemorrhage into a pre-existing adenoma. The classical presentation is of sudden onset of headache and acute visual deterioration.

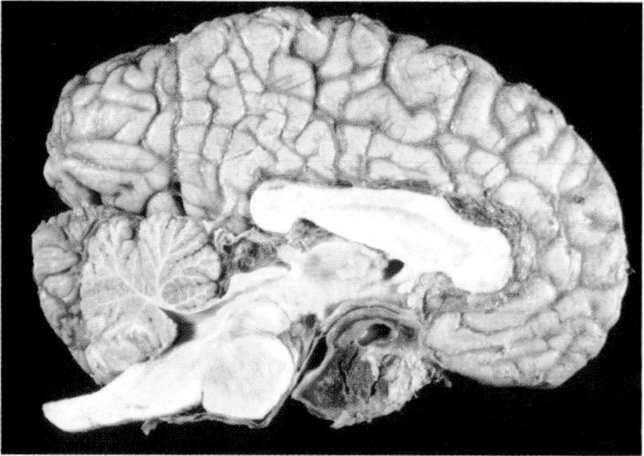

Figure 15.65 Pituitary adenoma. A macroadenoma with previous hemorrhage.

Histologically, adenomas show a range of appearances. They can show diffuse, lobular and trabecular architectural patterns. The tumor cells generally show little pleomorphism although GH cell adenomas can show marked pleomorphism (Fig. 15.66). The amount of cytoplasm tends to reflect the synthetic activity of the tumor cell. The stroma is often vascular and in prolactinomas amyloid deposition is common. Paranuclear fibrous bodies are seen in GH cell adenomas and Crooke's hyaline change, a perinuclear accumulation of cytokeratin microfilaments in non-neoplastic corticotroph cells, is seen in Cushing's disease. The cell of origin and pattern of hormone production is determined by immunohistochemistry. In some cases electron microscopy may be useful in providing information relating to the morphology of secretory vesicles.

Pituitary adenomas frequently show locally aggressive behavior, infiltrating surrounding structures. This behavior, however, does not indicate a carcinoma.

Pituitary carcinoma is clearly defined and rare. They are adenohypophyseal tumors which have associated craniospinal or systemic metastases. Like many other endocrine tumors it is not possible to predict aggressive behavior from the histological appearances.

Tumors of the neurohypophysis

Granular cell tumors (WHO grade I) are nodular masses of variable size composed of nests of large cells with abundant PAS-positive granular cytoplasm. They are often incidental findings at autopsy and symptomatic examples are rare.

Pituicytomas are gliomas derived from the glial elements of the neurohypophysis. They are solid tumors composed of elongated spindle cells with a fascicular architecture and show little mitotic activity (Fig. 15.67). Rosenthal fibers are not a feature.

Craniopharyngioma

This is a tumor arising in the region of the pituitary stalk from ectopic nests of squamous epithelium derived from Rathke's pouch, or from cells in the pars tuberalis of the pituitary gland that have undergone squamous metaplasia. It characteristically occurs as a suprasellar mass projecting upwards into the hypothalamus and the third

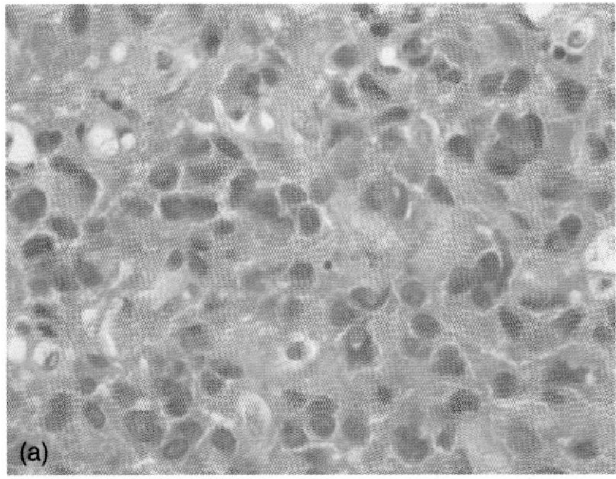

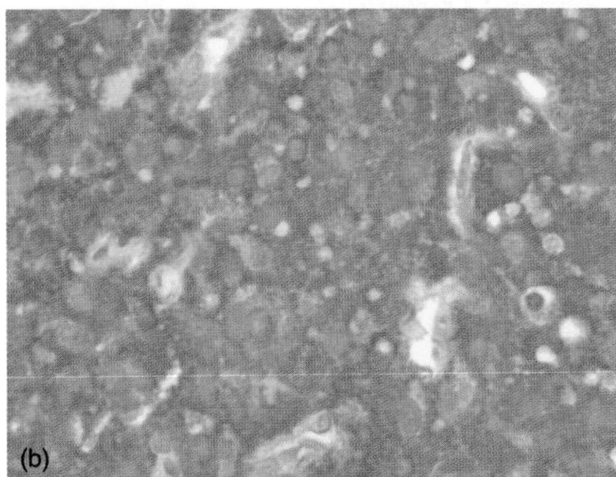

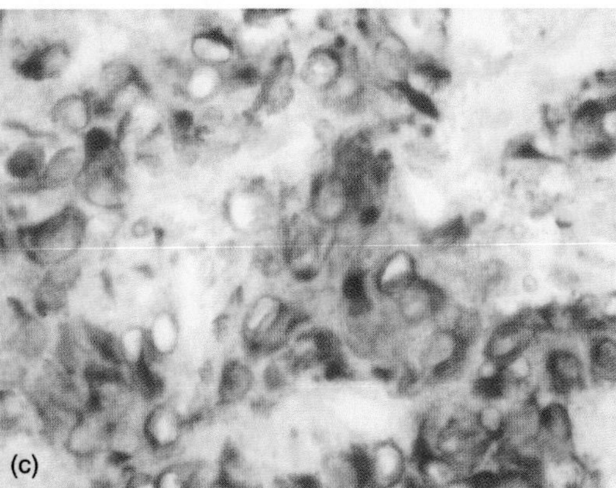

Figure 15.66 GH cell adenoma. (a) These adenomas often show moderate cellular pleomorphism. (b) There is abundant growth hormone in their cytoplasm. (c) Dense fibrous bodies can be demonstrated within the cytoplasm of some cells. (a) H&E. (b) Immunohistochemistry GH. (c) Immunohistochemistry pancytokeratin.

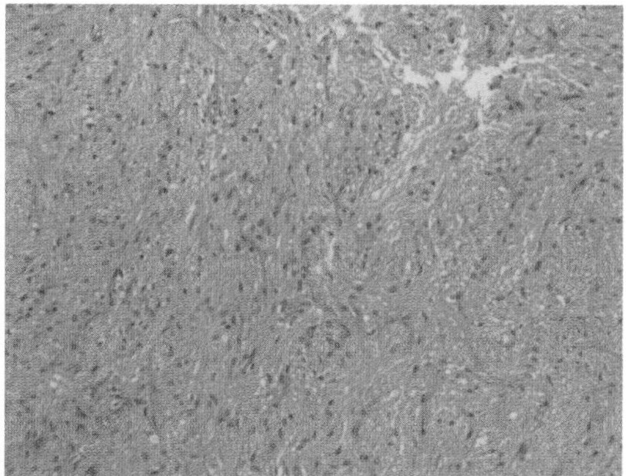

Figure 15.67 Pituicytoma. This low-grade glial tumor expands the pituitary stalk. H&E.

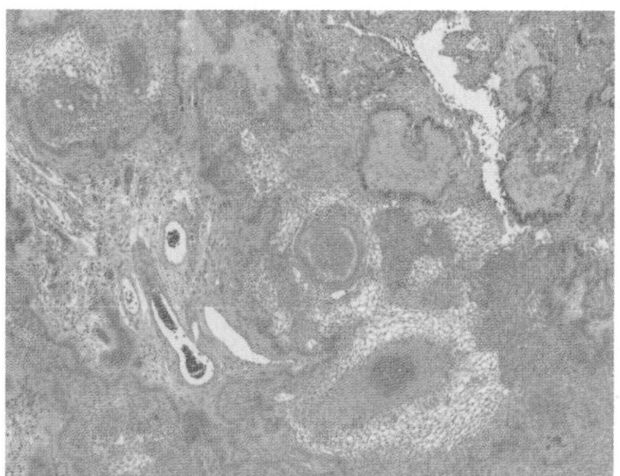

Figure 15.68 Craniopharyngioma. The tumor is composed of rather dissociated stratified squamous epithelium within which there are cystic spaces. H&E.

ventricle, and sometimes downwards into the pituitary fossa. The tumor is usually predominantly cystic and contains fluid which has the color and consistency of engine oil and contains cholesterol crystals which are visible on wet film preparations. The tumor is well encapsulated but microscopically it can extend into surrounding brain tissue. The solid parts of the tumor are composed of keratinizing stratified squamous epithelium which become separated by clear spaces producing an appearance similar to an adamantinoma (Fig. 15.68). There is nuclear palisading of the basal cells. Where cysts have ruptured there is a foreign body giant cell reaction and reactive astrocytosis in the adjacent brain. The cysts contain compact 'wet' keratin which may calcify. A rare variant is the *papillary craniopharyngioma* which is composed of stratified squamous epithelial pseudopapillae but lacks the 'wet' keratin and calcification.

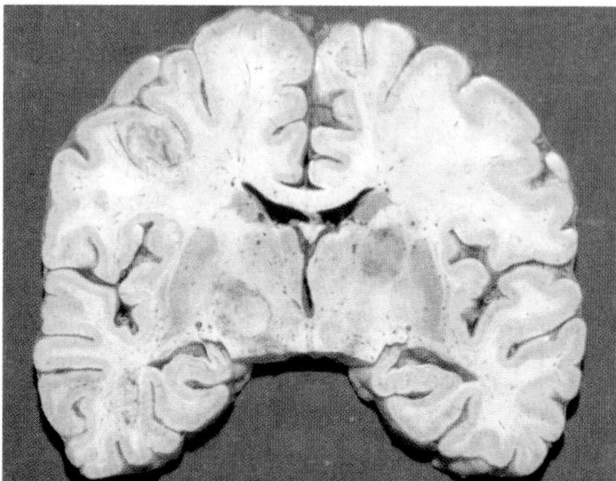

Figure 15.69 Metastases. Several discrete metastatic tumors are seen in this coronal section of brain.

METASTATIC TUMORS

Metastases can form either discrete lesions within the parenchyma or may diffusely infiltrate the subarachnoid space producing meningeal carcinomatosis. Metastases occur most frequently in the posterior frontal and parietal regions and in the cerebellum. They are characteristically multiple but patients may present with a solitary mass. Metastatic deposits are characteristically sharply defined from adjacent brain tissue (Fig. 15.69). They vary greatly in appearance although metastatic melanomas may be pigmented and are often hemorrhagic. Swelling in the adjacent brain is often marked producing shift and distortion. Within the spine, metastases tend to be extradural and cause compression. In meningeal carcinomatosis tumor cells normally enter the subarachnoid space via hematogenous spread through the choroid plexus. Macroscopically, the leptomeninges are usually opaque and may be thickened. Tumor nodules may be seen on nerve roots of the cauda equina which may become matted. In some cases, however, the macroscopic appearances may be unremarkable and the diffusely infiltrative nature of the tumor is only revealed microscopically. Therefore, at post mortem it is important to screen the brain from any patient with carcinoma and a history of neurological dysfunction.

Tumors in particular anatomical sites

There are several sites where tumors, whose type can only be established histologically, produce particular clinical syndromes.

Pineal region

Tumors in this region can infiltrate the tectal plate producing Parinaud syndrome, a characteristic paralysis of upward gaze and of convergence. They may also compress the aqueduct producing hydrocephalus. Tumors at this site include pineal parenchymal tumors, germ cell tumors, diffuse astrocytomas and meningiomas.

Cerebello-pontine angle

Tumors at this site typically cause disorders of hearing (deafness) and balance (vertigo). Acoustic schwannomas are the commonest but radiologically these may be mimicked by meningiomas and metastatic carcinomas. Epidermoid cysts, astrocytomas and hemangioblastomas may also arise at this site.

Spinal

Spinal tumors can be extradural or intradural, and intradural tumors may be extramedullary or intramedullary. All will result in cord compression with associated weakness and sensory disturbance. The commonest extradural tumors are metastatic carcinoma and lymphoma, including plasma cell tumors. Intradural extramedullary tumors are usually nerve sheath tumors (schwannoma, neurofibroma) or meningiomas. Intradural intramedullary tumors include astrocytic tumors and ependymomas, but metastatic lesions also occur.

Non-metastatic effects of malignancy

Paraneoplastic neurological syndromes are uncommon non-metastatic complications of malignancy that result in severely debilitating neurological abnormalities. These syndromes are recognized to have an autoimmune basis, and occasionally represent the presenting features of the underlying malignancy. They may involve the CNS, the peripheral nervous system (PNS), both CNS and PNS, or the neuromuscular junction. Clinical syndromes associated with these disorders include cerebellar degeneration, encephalomyelitis, sensory neuropathy, myasthenic syndrome, retinopathy and opsoclonus-myoclonus (Table 15.6). Western blotting analysis is used to identify the specificity of the autoantibodies present in either CSF or serum. The autopsy histological appearances of paraneoplastic syndromes are very variable; there may be no histological abnormality or a lymphocytic infiltrate with focal neuronal loss (see page 211).

Complications of treatments: Radiotherapy

Radiotherapy can induce changes within the tumor (large geographic areas of necrosis, fibrinoid necrosis of blood vessels) or within the adjacent normal brain. These may be acute or delayed late reactions occurring many years after radiotherapy. The acute effects are predominantly related to oedema and can be fatal due to raised intracranial pressure. The delayed effects are *focal radionecrosis* and *radiation leukoencephalopathy*. Focal radionecrosis consists of necrotic tissue (Fig. 15.70) within which hyalinized blood vessels are found (Fig. 15.71), some of which may show evidence of fibrinoid necrosis. The mass may act as a space-occupying mass and distinction from recurrent malignancy may be difficult radiologically. Radiation leukoencephalopathy is identified clinically by progressive cognitive decline with white matter lesions being seen on MRI. Histologically there are areas of demyelination (see page 181).

Table 15.6 Auto-antibodies currently recognized in paraneoplastic syndromes. The neurological syndromes and tumors indicated in the table are those most commonly associated with the given auto-antibody

Auto-antibody	Neurological syndrome	Tumors
Anti-Hu [ANNA-1] anti-neuronal nuclear antibody	Encephalomyelitis	SCLC
Anti-Yo [PCA1] anti-Purkinje cell cytoplasm antibody	Cerebellar degeneration	Ovary, breast
Anti-VGCC anti-Ca channel antibody	Lambert–Eaton myasthenic syndrome	SCLC
Anti-CV2 [CRMP5] anti-oligodendrocyte cytoplasm antibody	Cerebellar degeneration, encephalomyelitis, sensory neuropathy	SCLC
Anti-Ri [ANNA-2] anti-neuronal nuclear antibody	Brainstem encephalitis	Breast, SCLC
Anti-Ma2 [Ta]	Limbic encephalitis	Testicular germ cell tumors, lung
Anti-Tr	Cerebellar degeneration	Hodgkin's lymphoma
Anti-CAR anti-retinal nuclear antibody	Retinal dysfunction	SCLC
Anti-amphiphysin anti-neuronal synapses	Stiff-person syndrome	Breast, SCLC

SCLC = small-cell lung carcinoma.

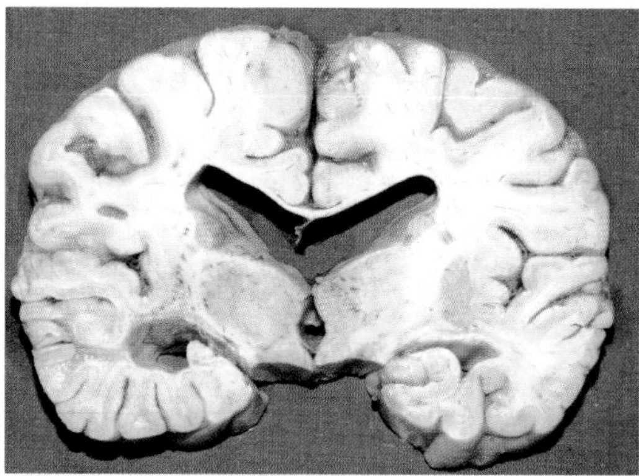

Figure 15.70 Radiation necrosis. There is generalized atrophy of the left cerebral hemisphere with focal cystic degeneration within the white matter.

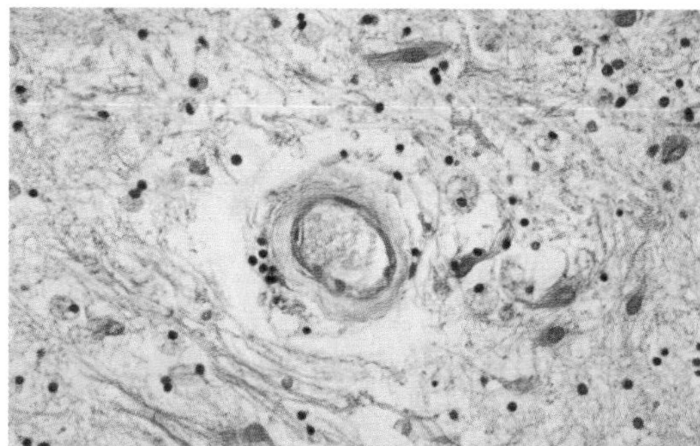

Figure 15.71 Radiation necrosis. The central blood vessel shows hyaline degeneration with reactive gliosis in the surrounding tissues. H&E.

CHAPTER 16

NEURODEGENERATIVE DISEASES, MOVEMENT DISORDERS AND SYSTEM DEGENERATIONS

James A R Nicoll

NEURODEGENERATIVE DISEASES

The neurodegenerative diseases (NDDs), although they each have distinct clinical and pathological features, have a number of features in common (Table 16.1). NDDs include important causes of dementia and disorders of movement. They pose a major challenge particularly to the developed countries in which the population profile is aging as a consequence of an increasing life expectancy and a decreasing birth rate. As inroads are made into the prevention and treatment of other major causes of mortality, such as cancers and vascular disease, the NDDs are likely to become more common in an aging population. Consequently, there is a degree of urgency in understanding the pathogenesis of NDDs in order to devise rational strategies for treatment or prevention.

Table 16.1 Features shared by neurodegenerative diseases

- Progressive – once the disease process has begun it continues relentlessly
- Fatal outcome
- Associated with aging
- Represent an increasing social and economic burden
- Degeneration of neurons – dysfunction and cell death
- Many of the diseases are characterized by abnormal accumulation of proteins in the CNS
- Causes still unknown for most disorders but increasing knowledge of genetic factors and to a lesser extent environmental factors such as toxins and transmissible agents
- Important role of rare familial cases in identifying key genes and proteins
- Therapy beginning to emerge based on understanding of the fundamental disease processes

Clinical features

Most of the NDDs present in either of the following two ways:

- *Specific neurological syndromes* due to dysfunction or cell death affecting a well-defined group of neurons sharing a common function, anatomy or neurotransmitter (e.g. depletion of motor neurons leading to muscle weakness and wasting in motor neuron disease; depletion of dopaminergic neurons in the substantia nigra

Table 16.2 Abnormal accumulation of proteins in the gray matter in neurodegenerative diseases

Disorder	Extracellular accumulation	Cytoplasmic accumulation	Intranuclear accumulation
'Normal' aging	(Aβ)	(Tau and ubiquitin)	
Motor neuron disease		Ubiquitin	
Huntington's disease			Polyglutamine (huntingtin) and ubiquitin
Parkinson's disease		α-synuclein and ubiquitin	
Multiple system atrophy		α-synuclein and ubiquitin	Polyglutamine
Alzheimer's disease	Aβ	Tau and ubiquitin	
Dementia with Lewy bodies		α-synuclein and ubiquitin	
Dementia pugilistica (boxers)	Aβ	Tau and ubiquitin	
Creutzfeldt–Jakob disease	PrP	Tau (rarely)	
Frontotemporal dementia		Tau and ubiquitin	
Corticobasal degeneration		Tau	
Progressive supranuclear palsy		Tau and ubiquitin	

leading to a disorder of movement in Parkinson's disease)

- *Dementia* due to widespread neuronal dysfunction or cell death (e.g. Alzheimer's disease, dementia with Lewy bodies)

It is important to recognize that, however convenient, this distinction is somewhat artificial and some disorders can be associated both with a specific neurological syndrome and dementia, such as Huntington's disease and Lewy body disease (i.e. Parkinson's disease and dementia with Lewy bodies). The NDDs which primarily cause specific neurological syndromes are dealt with in this chapter. The NDDs which primarily result in dementia are dealt with in Chapter 17.

Lack of a precise correlation between the pathology and the clinical features can occur and is a challenge for accurate classification of NDDs. For example, parkinsonian clinical features ('parkinsonism') can be associated with several different types of pathology affecting the basal ganglia in addition to idiopathic Parkinson's disease. Conversely, intraneuronal tau accumulation (i.e. tangles) is a feature of the pathology of many different NDDs.

Pathogenesis

Abnormal accumulation of proteins

Abnormal accumulation of proteins in the CNS is a common feature of NDDs (Table 16.2). The protein accumulation may occur in the extracellular space or in the intracellular compartment, either within the cytoplasm or within the nucleus. In many of these disorders histological diagnosis relies on demonstration of the accumulated protein by immunohistochemistry, for example, with antibodies to Aβ, tau, ubiquitin, α-synuclein or PrP. Proteins, particularly those in the extracellular space, may aggregate as amyloid fibrils with a β-pleated sheet structure and can be demonstrated with amyloid stains such as thioflavin S and Congo red. A classification of NDDs has been suggested based on the specific protein which accumulates (Table 16.3). In at least some NDDs there is evidence that the protein accumulation plays a major role in the initiation and perpetuation of the disease process (e.g. Creutzfeldt–Jakob disease, Alzheimer's disease). In others, it remains unclear whether the protein accumulation is causal or merely an epiphenomenon (e.g. Huntington's disease, Parkinson's disease).

Genetic factors

Genetic factors are of over-riding importance in some NDDs, such as Huntington's disease in which all cases have a genetic cause and occur either due to inheritance of a mutant gene or are due to a new mutation. In other NDDs the pattern is one in which most cases are sporadic, with no clear genetic or other cause, but with a small proportion of cases

Table 16.3 Classification of neurodegenerative diseases based on accumulated protein

β-amyloidopathies	Alzheimer's disease Cerebral amyloid angiopathy
Tauopathies	Frontotemporal dementia Progressive supranuclear palsy Corticobasal degeneration Tangle-only dementia Alzheimer's disease
Synucleinopathies	Parkinson's disease Dementia with Lewy bodies Multiple system atrophy
Polyglutamine tract disorders	Huntington's disease Spinocerebellar ataxia
Prion disorders (PrP)	Creutzfeldt–Jakob disease Gerstmann–Straussler–Scheinker disease Fatal familial insomnia Kuru

that are familial, inherited in an autosomal dominant fashion, or due to a specific point mutation. Study of such pedigrees has been of great importance in identifying key genes and their protein products, which have proved to be of relevance not only to the rare inherited versions of the disease but also to the more common sporadic forms. A genetic cause for an NDD results in challenging decisions in affected families, for pre-symptomatic individuals and for reproductive decisions including antenatal and preconception testing. Genetic counseling has an important role.

Oxidative stress

There is evidence that oxidative stress plays a role in causing neuronal injury in some NDDs. Toxic free radicals can cause damage to cells by peroxidation of lipid membranes, DNA damage and aiding protein aggregation. Some familial cases of motor neuron disease are due to point mutations in a superoxide dismutase gene (*SOD1*) which encodes an enzyme that has a role in detoxifying free radicals.

Programmed cell death

There is evidence that neuronal death in some NDDs may occur by apoptosis, which is a particular form of programmed cell death. Possible triggers for apoptosis include a toxic effect of an accumulated protein, cytokine production, energy failure and excitotoxicity.

Neuroinflammation

Activation and proliferation of microglia and astrocytes resulting in cytokine release is an almost ubiquitous feature of NDDs. Microglia can be identified by immunostaining for CD68, which is specific for lysosomes, or for MHC class II (CR3/43), and the astrocyte reaction can be identified by immunostaining for glial fibrillary acidic protein (GFAP). This glial reaction is usually assumed to be a secondary phenomenon but may play a role in perpetuating the disease process once it has begun.

Ubiquitin–proteasome system

Cells identify unwanted proteins for disposal within the cytoplasm by labeling them with ubiquitin. Intraneuronal ubiquitin accumulation is a feature of many of the NDDs. This may be a reflection of overload or failure of the ubiquitin–proteasome system. Because the presence of ubiquitin is not specific for any particular NDD it is not useful diagnostically, although ubiquitin immunohistochemistry can be a useful screen to determine whether neurodegenerative pathology is present in the CNS.

Mitochondrial failure

Mitochondria produce ATP which is needed to drive energy-requiring cellular reactions. Neurons are among the most highly energy demanding cells of the body. During the lifetime of an individual, mutations of mitochondrial DNA accumulate which may be associated with an age-related failure of ATP production. This age-related energy failure has been suggested to play a role in several NDDs, particularly in Parkinson's disease.

Therapy for neurodegenerative diseases

Understanding the pathogenesis leads to rational concepts for potential treatments or prevention of NDDs. The concept of disease-causing protein accumulation raises the possibility of interfering with protein accumulation by reducing production, preventing aggregation, disrupting or solubilizing protein aggregates and promoting elimination of the protein. This concept is particularly relevant to Alzheimer's disease (AD) and Creutzfeldt-Jakob disease (CJD). Other strategies currently under investigation include augmenting deficient neurotransmitters (dopamine in Parkinson's disease, acetyl choline in AD), immunization (AD, CJD and synucleinopathies), antioxidants (motor neuron disease), diet, environment, multivitamins, reducing neuroinflammation (AD), gene therapy (HD), cell transplantation (PD) and stem cell therapy.

SPECIFIC NEUROLOGICAL SYNDROMES DUE TO NEURODEGENERATION

Motor neuron disease (amyotrophic lateral sclerosis)

In motor neuron disease (MND), otherwise known as amyotrophic lateral sclerosis (ALS), the main target of the disease process is the lower motor neuron, located in the anterior horn of the spinal cord and in the brainstem motor nuclei (Table 16.4). The axons of the lower motor neurons project out through the anterior spinal roots and along the peripheral nerves, or along the cranial nerves, to innervate the skeletal muscles. There may also be involvement of upper motor neurons, the cells bodies of which are located in the primary motor cortex of the cerebrum, with axons that project along corticospinal or corticobulbar tracts to innervate lower motor neurons.

The clinical pattern of disease reflects the pattern of neuronal degeneration. Degeneration of the spinal lower motor neurons is associated with weakness, fasciculations and atrophy of limb muscles (progressive muscular atrophy). Involvement of motor neurons in the brainstem results in bulbar signs and symptoms such as wasting of the tongue, dysphagia and dysarthria (progressive bulbar palsy). Degeneration of upper motor neurons is associated with weakness and spasticity (primary lateral sclerosis). Although the clinical

Table 16.4 Diseases affecting motor neurons

Disease	Cause
Motor neuron disease (ALS)	Sporadic (90%) or autosomal dominant (10%)
Spinal muscular atrophy	Autosomal recessive
Hereditary spastic paraparesis	Autosomal dominant, recessive or X-linked
Hereditary progressive bulbar palsy	Autosomal recessive
Spinobulbar muscular atrophy	X-linked trinucleotide repeat disorder
Acute poliomyelitis	Enterovirus
Post-polio syndrome	Long term sequel to acute poliomyelitis
HTLV-1 associated myelopathy	HTLV-1
Paraneoplastic disease	Autoimmune
ALS–Parkinson–dementia complex of Guam	?Environmental toxin

ALS, amyotrophic lateral sclerosis.

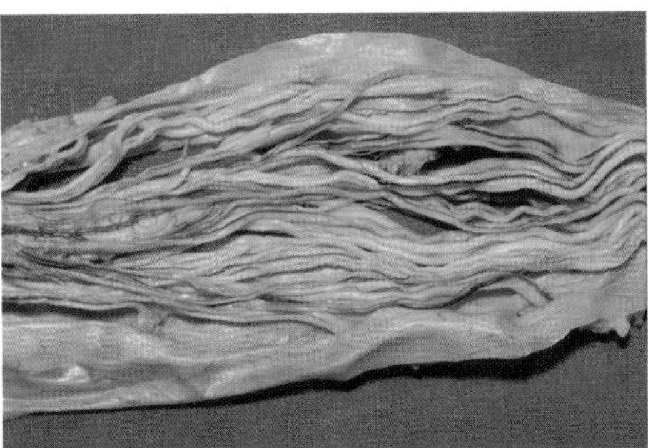

Figure 16.1 Motor neuron disease. There is atrophy and grey-brown discoloration of the anterior (motor) spinal roots compared to the posterior (sensory) spinal roots, reflecting depletion of motor neurons in the anterior horns of the spinal cord. This figure shows roots of the cauda equina with the conus medullaris at left.

presentation may reflect the predominant degeneration of one of the above groups of neurons, as the disease develops there is often evidence of involvement of other groups. It is increasingly recognized that frontal lobe dementia may be associated with MND. The terminal phase of MND is often characterized by failure of innervation of respiratory muscles and loss of reflexes protecting the airways leading to respiratory failure, aspiration and bronchopneumonia.

Most cases of MND are sporadic with no clear pattern of inheritance or other recognized cause. However, approximately 10% of MND is familial with autosomal dominant inheritance. Pedigrees have been identified in which there is a point mutation in the superoxide dismutase gene (*SOD1*), located on chromosome 21. Transgenic mice with *SOD1* point mutations develop degeneration of motor neurons as they age, providing a useful model of MND. A major role for *SOD1* is in the clearance of free radicals and this discovery led to interest that damage to neurons by free radicals may be of importance not only in familial MND but also in sporadic cases. However, more recent evidence raises the possibility that the mutation results in the production of a neurotoxic protein. Several other candidate genes are being explored. There is also evidence for damage to motor neurons by glutamate excitotoxicity and current therapy for MND is based at least in part on this concept.

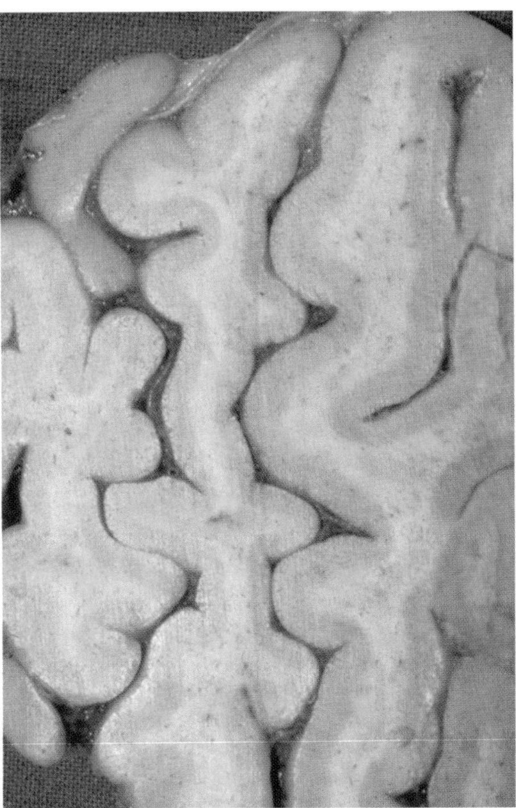

Figure 16.2 Motor neuron disease. This is a tangential section of the cerebrum showing the central sulcus running from top to bottom. There is selective atrophy of the primary motor cortex (precentral gyrus), which is to the left of the central sulcus in this image, compared to the primary sensory cortex (postcentral gyrus) to the right. Atrophy of the motor cortex is visible macroscopically only in cases with a long history of motor neuron disease.

At autopsy there is usually severe and widespread muscle wasting. Macroscopic examination may show atrophy and brown discoloration of the anterior (motor) spinal roots in comparison with the preserved posterior (sensory) roots (Fig. 16.1). The spinal cord itself rarely shows macroscopically detectable abnormalities, although there may be visible whitish-gray discoloration of the lateral columns on cut section of the spinal cord, reflecting corticospinal tract degeneration. Rarely, macroscopic atrophy of the pre-central gyrus may be detectable reflecting severe involvement of the primary motor cortex (Fig. 16.2). Macroscopic changes in MND are usually only visible at post mortem in patients with

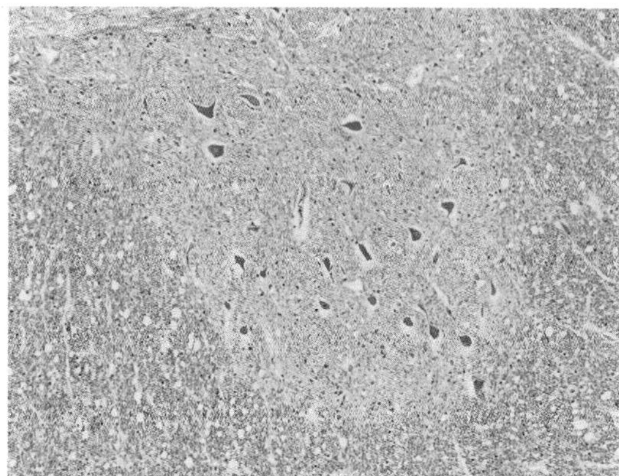

Figure 16.3 The anterior horn of the spinal cord in a control showing lower motor neurons for comparison with that in motor neuron disease in Figure 16.4. Luxol fast blue/cresyl violet.

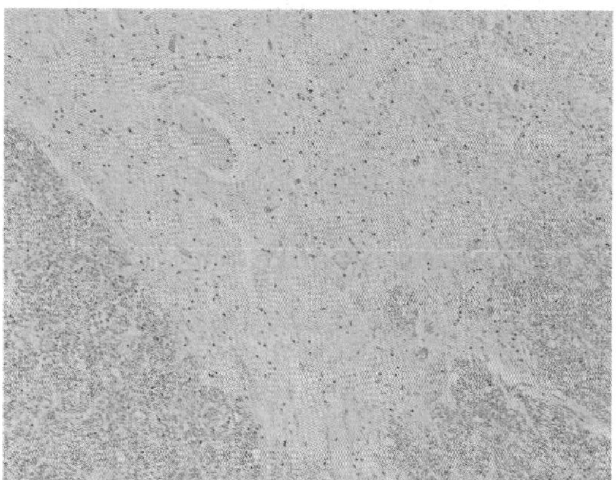

Figure 16.4 Motor neuron disease. Severe depletion of lower motor neurons in the anterior horn of the spinal cord. Luxol fast blue/cresyl violet.

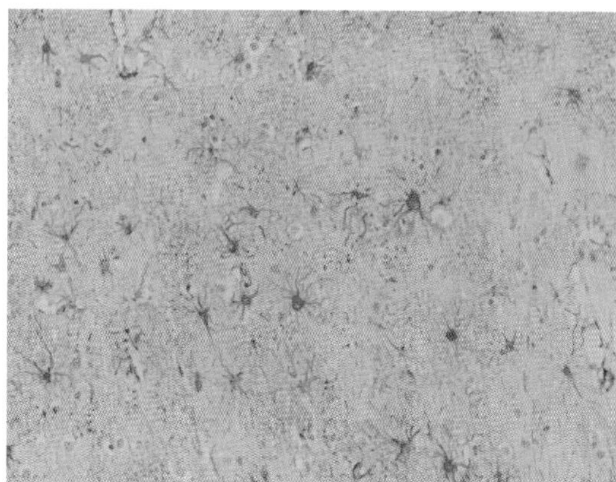

Figure 16.5 Motor neuron disease. In the primary motor cortex depletion of the large motor neurons is accompanied by gliosis. GFAP.

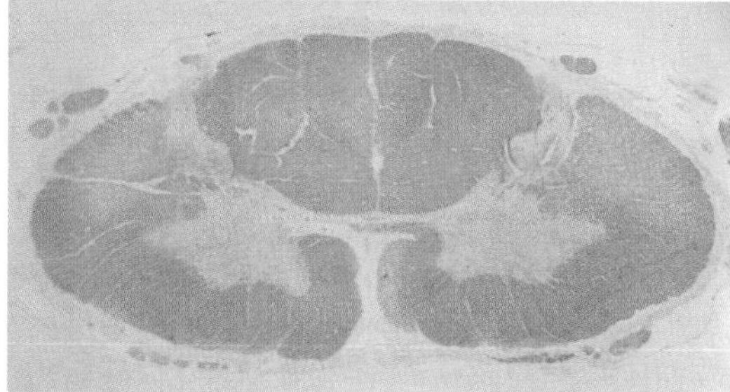

Figure 16.6 Motor neuron disease. Cases with longstanding loss of cortical motor neurons show degeneration of the corticospinal tracts, shown here by pallor on a myelin stain. Note the atrophy of the anterior spinal roots compared to the posterior roots. Luxol fast blue/cresyl violet.

a long history of the disease. Microscopic examination of the spinal cord shows bilateral atrophy of the anterior horns with loss of large motor neurons associated with reactive gliosis (Figs 16.3 and 16.4). In longstanding cases there may be almost complete loss of anterior horn cells although in patients with a relatively short survival the neuronal depletion may be subtle. Degeneration of axons of the motor neurons may be reflected by the presence of axonal swellings in the anterior horns, which can be demonstrated by silver stains or by immunostaining for neurofilament, and by a reduced density of axons in the anterior roots. Ubiquitin-containing tangle-like fibrillary inclusions may be present in the cytoplasm of residual anterior horn cells. There may be depletion of motor neurons in the brainstem nuclei (e.g. in the hypoglossal nucleus). Examination of skeletal muscle shows the changes of denervation. Microscopic examination of the precentral gyrus may show neuronal loss affecting the upper motor neurons (cells of Betz) with associated gliosis (Fig. 16.5). Histological blocks cut tangential to the surface of the cerebrum, and which include the gyri either side of the central sulcus are particularly useful in demonstrating these features. The upper motor neurons project from the primary motor cortex and descend through the corticobulbar and corticospinal tracts (lateral columns) to synapse with the lower motor neurons. Depletion of the upper motor neurons therefore results in loss of myelinated fibres in the corticospinal and corticobulbar tracts (Fig. 16.6).

Huntington's disease

The target for neurodegeneration in Huntington's disease (HD) is primarily the caudate nucleus. The consequence is a characteristic movement disorder known as chorea. Neurodegeneration may also be widespread throughout the cerebral cortex with associated effects on cognitive function.

Huntington's disease is familial with an autosomal dominant pattern of inheritance. The genetic abnormality is an increase in the number of trinucleotide repeats in the *Huntingtin* gene on chromosome 4. The *Huntingtin* gene in normal individuals has in the range of nine to around 37 CAG repeats. The presence of more than around 37 CAG repeats causes HD, and this forms the basis of the diagnostic test for HD. The number of repeats correlates with the severity of the disease and inversely with the age onset of the disease. The mutation is unstable with subsequent generations developing increasing numbers of trinucleotide repeats. This explains the long known phenomenon of anticipation in HD in which, as the disorder is passed from generation to generation, it tends to become earlier in age of onset and increased in severity. The trinucleotide CAG encodes the amino acid glutamine and consequently affected patients have increased numbers of glutamine amino acids (known as a polyglutamine tract) in the huntingtin protein. The abnormal huntingtin protein accumulates to form intranuclear inclusions, although it is not yet clear whether the protein aggregation is directly neurotoxic or merely an epiphenomenon of the disease process.

Macroscopic examination of the brain shows characteristic atrophy of the caudate nucleus (Fig. 16.7). More widespread atrophy involving the cerebral cortex and white matter may also be present. Histologically, there is pronounced neuronal loss and gliosis of the caudate nucleus (Fig. 16.8). The putamen and globus pallidus are often also affected. There is selective loss of neurons bearing spiny dendrites (spiny neurons). The intranuclear inclusions can be identified in neurons in the basal ganglia and cerebral cortex by immunohistochemistry with antibodies to ubiquitin or polyglutamine (Fig. 16.9). Disorders other than HD which can be associated with neuronal loss and gliosis in the basal ganglia

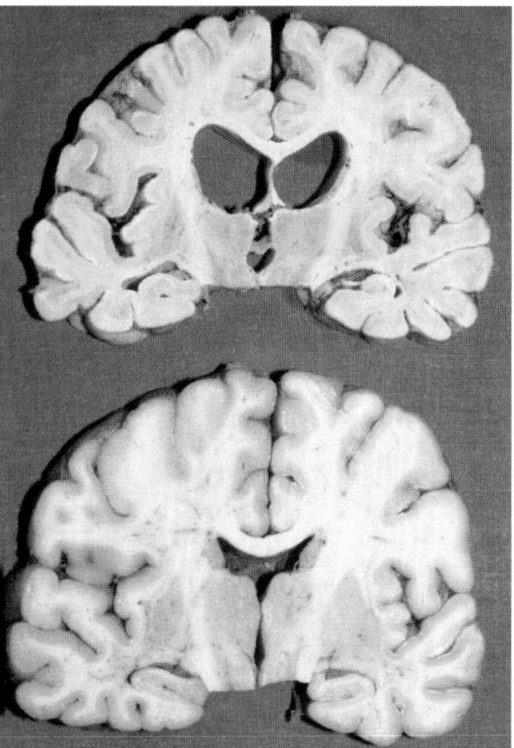

Figure 16.7 Huntington's disease (above) with a normal control (below). There is selective atrophy of the head of the caudate nucleus in Huntington's disease, giving the lateral wall of the lateral ventricle a concave profile. In this case there is also generalized widening of sulci reflecting cortical atrophy.

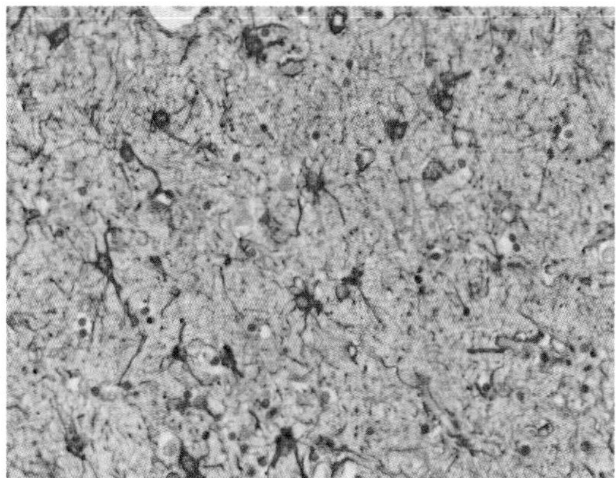

Figure 16.8 Huntington's disease. There is marked gliosis accompanying the neuronal loss in the caudate nucleus. GFAP immunohistochemistry.

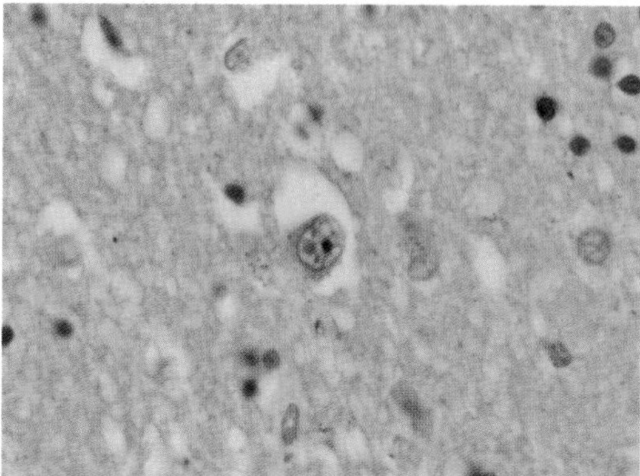

Figure 16.9 Huntington's disease. Intranuclear inclusions composed of aggregates of abnormal huntingtin protein can be demonstrated by immunohistochemistry for ubiquitin.

include multiple system atrophy and corticobasal degeneration.

Parkinson's disease

The major target of the neurodegenerative process in Parkinson's disease (PD) is the population of pigmented neurons of the substantia nigra in the midbrain. These neurons project to the corpus striatum where they supply the neurotransmitter dopamine. Loss of nigral neurons leads to the characteristic clinical features of PD with resting tremor, rigidity and bradykinesia. Dysphagia, autonomic dysfunction and dementia may occur in addition.

Loss of neurons in the substantia nigra results in a reduced dopaminergic input to the corpus striatum causing overactivity of neurons in the striatum, subthalamic nucleus and medial globus pallidus. Imaging of the dopaminergic system during life by PET or SPECT can distinguish idiopathic PD from other causes of parkinsonism (Table 16.5).

The prevalence of PD is approximately 1 in 1000. The pathogenesis is largely unknown but there is evidence of a role for genetic factors, environmental toxins, mitochondrial failure and toxic free radicals. A small percentage of PD is familial with an autosomal dominant pattern of inheritance. Mutations in several genes are now known to be capable of causing PD. Point mutations in the *PARK 1* gene, located on chromosome 4, cause autosomal dominant PD. *PARK 1* encodes α-synuclein, a synaptic

Table 16.5 Causes of parkinsonism and akinetic rigid movement disorders

Disorder	Cause
Parkinson's disease	Sporadic or familial
Drug-induced parkinsonism	Neuroleptic drugs Opiates contaminated with MPTP
Multiple system atrophy	
Progressive supranuclear palsy	
Corticobasal degeneration	
Arteriosclerotic pseudo-parkinsonism	Arteriosclerosis of basal ganglia
ALS–Parkinson–dementia complex of Guam	?Cycad nut toxicity
Post-encephalitic parkinsonism	Encephalitis lethargica ?virus
Dementia pugilistica	Repeated head trauma in boxers

ALS, amyotrophic lateral sclerosis.

protein, which is a major component of Lewy bodies. Transgenic mice with these *PARK 1* gene mutations develop a PD-like disease as they age. Other *PARK* genes result in either autosomal dominant or recessive patterns of inheritance.

There is some epidemiological and toxicological evidence of a role for environmental toxins in the etiology of PD. Exposure to MPTP, which may be present in synthetic opiates and in herbicides, can cause an acute Parkinson's-like disorder. MPTP is metabolized to MPP+ which is toxic to mitochondria, and mitochondria in the neurons of the substantia nigra appear particularly susceptible. The vast majority of PD, however, is sporadic with no clear genetic or environmental risk factors.

Macroscopically, the depletion of pigmented neurons in PD is reflected in pallor of the substantia nigra (Fig. 16.10). However, a substantia nigra that is macroscopically normally pigmented does not rule out PD. It is also important to appreciate that the substantia nigra is normally pale during adolescence and early adulthood and that the neuromelanin pigment accumulates progressively as part of the normal aging process. The locus coeruleus is the source of noradrenergic input to the cerebrum and in normal individuals appears as a dot-like area of pigmentation in the dorsolateral sector of the pons. In

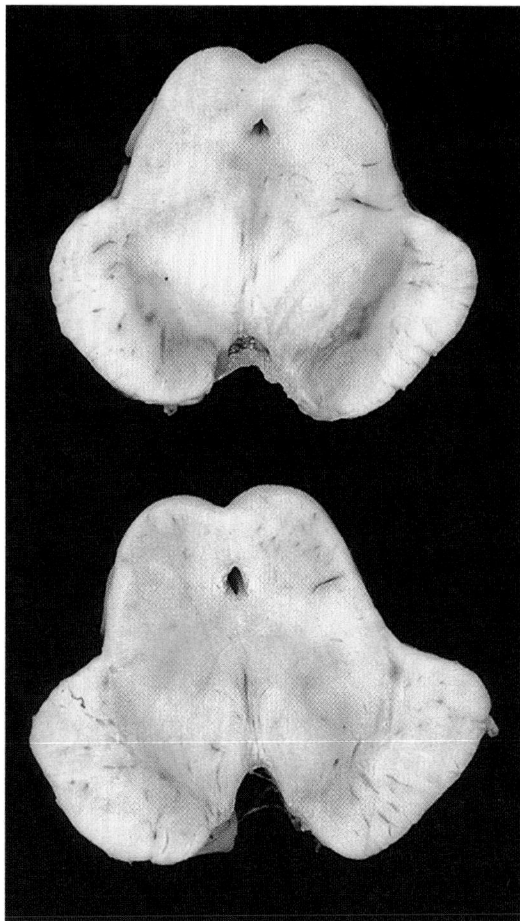

Figure 16.10 Parkinson's disease midbrain (below) and normal control (above). In Parkinson's disease there is pallor of the substantia nigra reflecting loss of dopaminergic pigmented neurons.

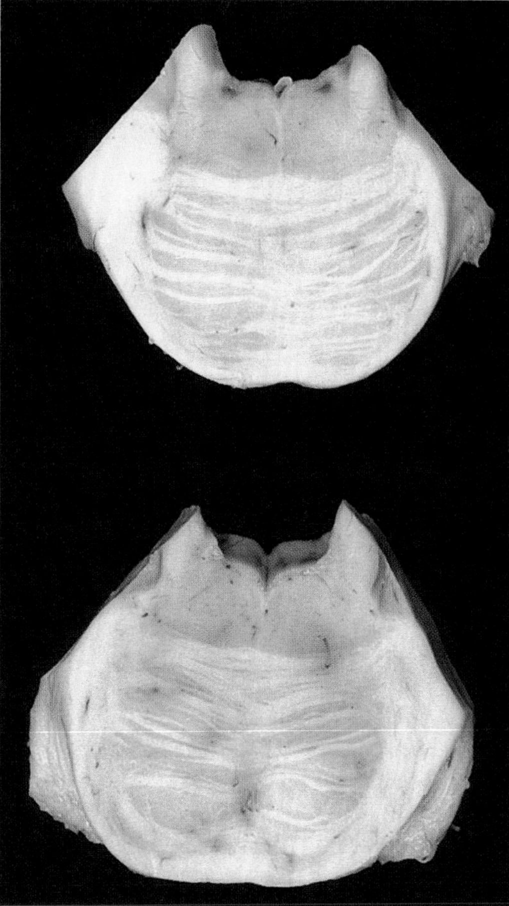

Figure 16.11 Parkinson's disease (below) and normal control (above) pons. In Parkinson's disease there is depigmentation of the locus coeruleus reflecting neuronal loss.

PD the locus coeruleus is often not visible because of loss of neurons (Fig. 16.11). The corpus striatum appears macroscopically normal.

Histologically, there is depletion of pigmented neurons in the substantia nigra. Extracellular neuromelanin pigment is often present in the form of small scattered granules, reflecting disintegration of nigral neurons, and neuromelanin may be located within macrophages. Lewy bodies are present in the cytoplasm of some remaining neurons (Fig. 16.12 and Table 16.6). Brainstem Lewy bodies are brightly eosinophilic, spherical, cytoplasmic inclusions which have a pale halo and on hematoxylin and eosin stained sections stand out clearly from the pigmented granules in the cytoplasm of the neurons. Lewy bodies can also be detected by immunostaining for ubiquitin and more specifically for α-synuclein. Ultrastucturally, Lewy bodies are composed of 7–20 nm intermediate filaments. Depletion of pigmented neurons and Lewy bodies are also detectable in the locus coeruleus and dorsal motor nucleus of vagus. The neuronal loss is accompanied by a reactive proliferation of astrocytes and microglia.

Cortical Lewy bodies are much harder to see on hematoxylin and eosin stained sections in the non-pigmented cortical neurons. Cortical Lewy bodies do not have a pale halo and are less clearly defined

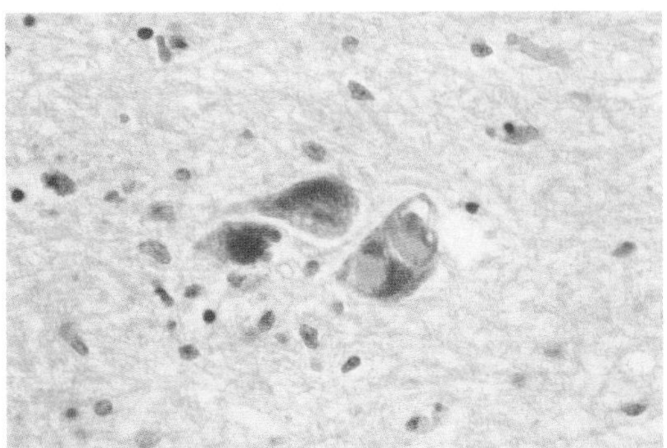

Figure 16.12 Parkinson's disease. There is depletion of pigmented neurons in the substantia nigra. One of the residual neurons in this field contains a Lewy body (center). There is scattered extracellular neuromelanin pigment representing the residue of dead neurons. H&E.

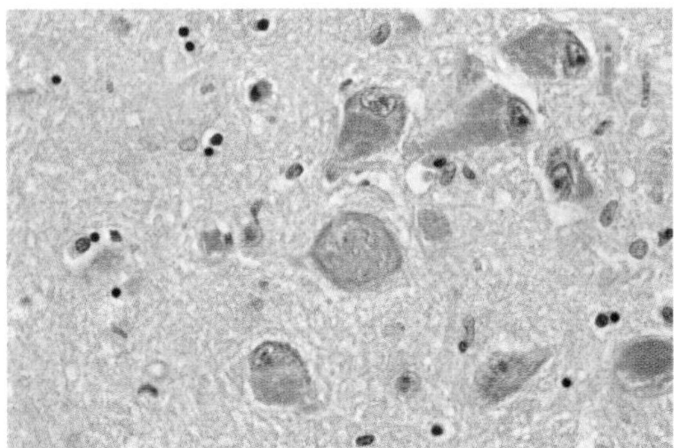

Figure 16.13 Progressive supranuclear palsy. Neurofibrillary tangles are present in brainstem neurons (center). H&E.

Table 16.6 Disorders associated with Lewy bodies

- Parkinson's disease
- Dementia with Lewy bodies
- Autonomic failure
- Dysphagia

structures. They are sometimes detectable in silver-stained sections, but are most reliably detected by α-synuclein or ubiquitin immunohistochemistry. Cortical Lewy bodies are a defining feature of dementia with Lewy bodies but they are also almost always present in patients with PD, even in the absence of dementia.

Current mainstream therapy for Parkinson's disease is based on enhancing the performance of the residual dopaminergic neurons rather than affecting the progressive neuronal degeneration. Pharmacological agents include levodopa, the amino acid precursor of dopamine, which acts by replenishing depleted striatal dopamine, and dopamine receptor agonists. Cholinergic agents, which influence the function of the reciprocal pathway from the striatum to the substantia nigra, are also used. Experimental therapies include surgical ablation of the globus pallidus and transplantation of dopamine-producing cells into the corpus striatum.

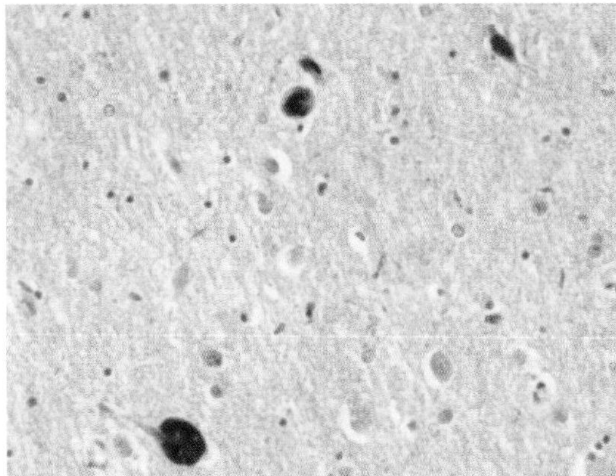

Figure 16.14 Progressive supranuclear palsy. Brainstem tangles. Tau immunohistochemistry.

Progressive supranuclear palsy

The key clinical features of progressive supranuclear palsy (PSP) are supranuclear gaze palsy (failure of upward gaze), axial rigidity and postural instability. Some patients have dementia in addition. The disease process is focused on the upper brainstem and basal ganglia. Macroscopic examination may show atrophy of the midbrain, pons and globus pallidus. Histologically, the affected areas show neuronal loss and reactive gliosis. There are intraneuronal tangles (Fig. 16.13) composed of tau protein (Fig. 16.14) and there is also accumulation of tau within glial cells. The brainstem tangles in PSP, which are readily detectable on hematoxylin and eosin stained sections, are somewhat different morphologically from the tangles in AD and appear

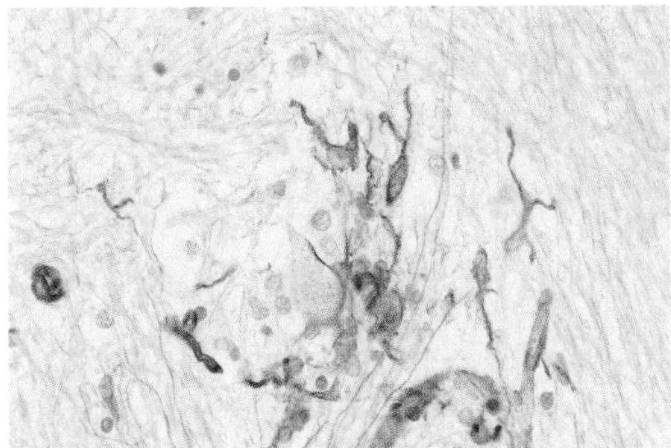

Figure 16.15 Progressive supranuclear palsy. Tufted astrocytes contain tau. Tau immunohistochemistry.

rectangular or globose in shape. Ultrastructurally, the tangles are composed of straight intermediate filaments. Tufted astrocytes, with multiple fine processes, are detectable in affected areas of gray matter in silver-stained sections or sections immunostained for tau (Fig. 16.15). Although not always present, tufted astrocytes have been suggested as being specific for PSP.

The accumulated tau in PSP is specifically the four-repeat tau isoform, which incorporates exon 10 of the tau gene. This differs from AD in which all six isoforms of tau are present in the tangles. There is evidence that polymorphisms in the tau gene may influence susceptibility to PSP. Brainstem tangles may be present in AD, but AD is distinguished histologically by the presence of abundant cortical plaques and tangles.

It is important to note that there is an imperfect relationship between the clinical and pathological features. Some patients with the clinical features of PSP have other neurodegenerative pathology such as corticobasal degeneration, frontotemporal dementia or AD. Conversely, some patients with the neuropathological features of PSP do not have the classical clinical features of the disease.

Corticobasal degeneration

Corticobasal degeneration (CBD) affects the cerebral cortex and basal ganglia. Clinical features include clumsiness, limb stiffness, myoclonus, alien limb, sensory disturbances and later dementia. Macroscopic examination of the brain may show cortical atrophy, particularly around the central (Rolandic)

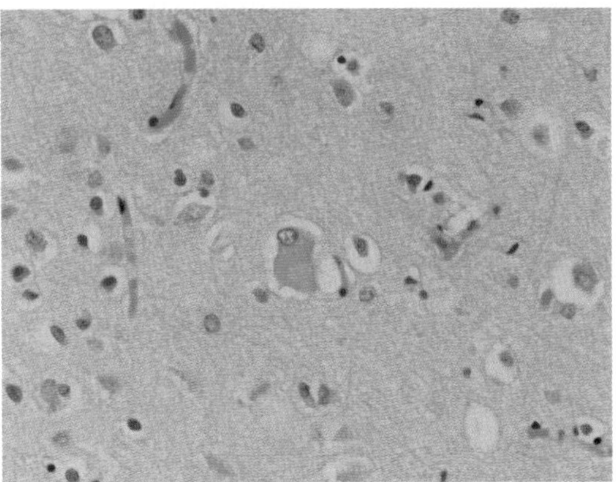

Figure 16.16 Corticobasal degeneration. A swollen or 'ballooned' cortical neuron. H&E.

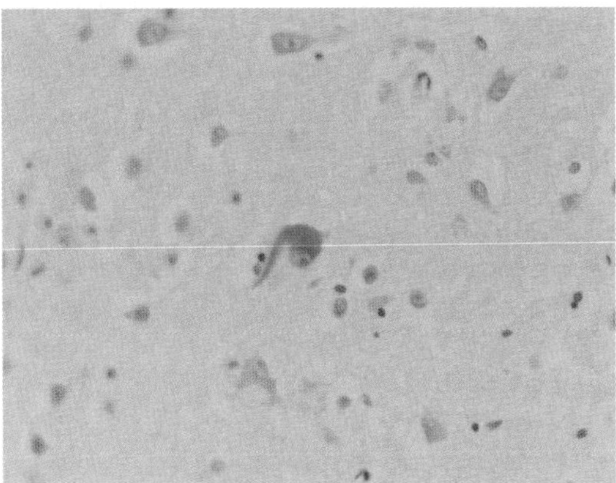

Figure 16.17 Corticobasal degeneration. The swollen cortical neurons contain $\alpha\beta$-crystallin. $\alpha\beta$-crystallin immunohistochemistry.

sulcus, and loss of pigment in substantia nigra. Microscopically (Figs 16.16–16.19) there is neuronal loss and gliosis in the affected areas. Tau accumulates within glial cells and neurons and there may be tau-immunoreactive threads. Ubiquitin accumulation is generally not a feature. Swollen neurons, most frequent in the peri-Rolandic cortex, are a characteristic feature and there may be superficial microvacuolation. On hematoxylin and eosin stained sections the tangles appear slightly basophilic like those of PSP. Astrocytic plaques, which are rings of thorn-like threads containing tau probably located in astrocyte processes, are a key feature of CBD. The tau protein which accumulates in CBD is the 4 repeat

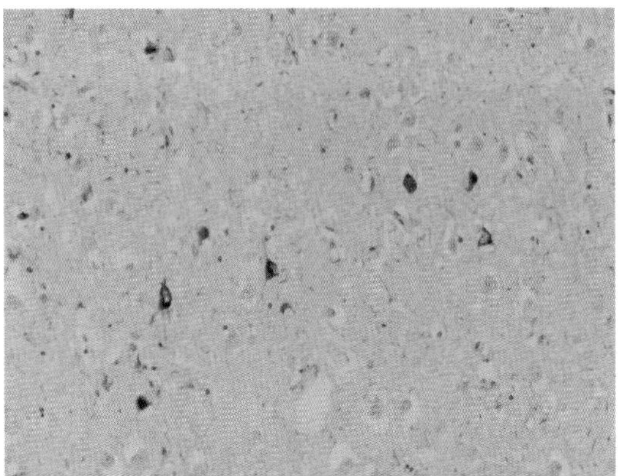

Figure 16.18 Corticobasal degeneration. Neurons in affected areas of cortex may contain tau-immunoreactive tangles. Neuropil threads are also present. Tau immunohistochemistry.

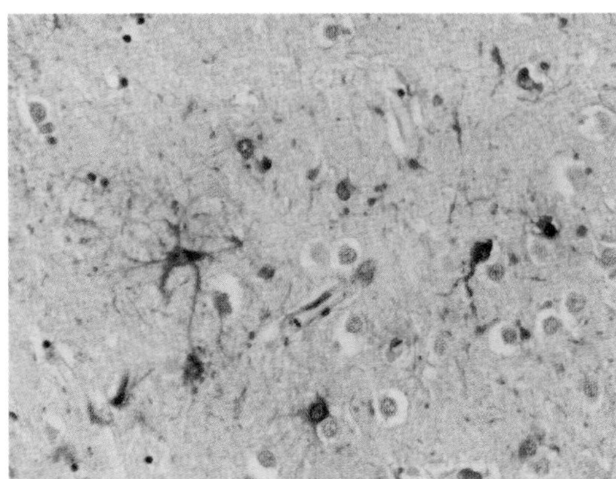

Figure 16.19 Corticobasal degeneration. Tau-containing glial cells are a prominent feature in the basal ganglia. Tau immunohistochemistry.

isoform, as in PSP. Most cases of CBD are sporadic, although some patients have *tau* gene mutations.

Multiple system atrophy

In multiple system atrophy (MSA) neuronal loss and gliosis affects specific ganglia and there is atrophy of their associated projection tracts (Table 16.7) (Figs 16.20–16.22). The clinical features of the disease reflect the macroscopic pattern of atrophy and the distribution of neuronal loss and gliosis. About 10% of parkinsonism is due to striatonigral degeneration involving neurons projecting from the striatum to the substantia nigra, the reciprocal of the dopaminergic nigrostriatal pathway which degenerates in Parkinson's disease. Although the clinical symptoms of striatonigral degeneration and Parkinson's disease may be similar, as striatonigral degeneration does

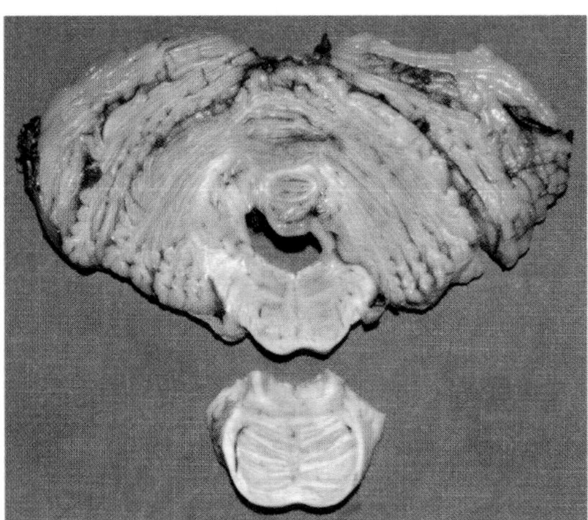

Figure 16.20 Multiple system atrophy (above) and normal control pons (below) demonstrating atrophy of the basis pontis and cerebellar peduncles in olivopontocerebellar atrophy.

Table 16.7 Multiple system atrophy

	Clinical symptoms	Distribution of neuronal loss and gliosis
Striatonigral degeneration	Parkinsonism	Putamen
Olivopontocerebellar atrophy	Cerebellar ataxia	Pontine nuclei, cerebellar Purkinje cells, atrophy of transverse pontine fibres and middle cerebellar peduncle
Shy–Drager syndrome	Autonomic failure	Intermediolateral column of the spinal cord

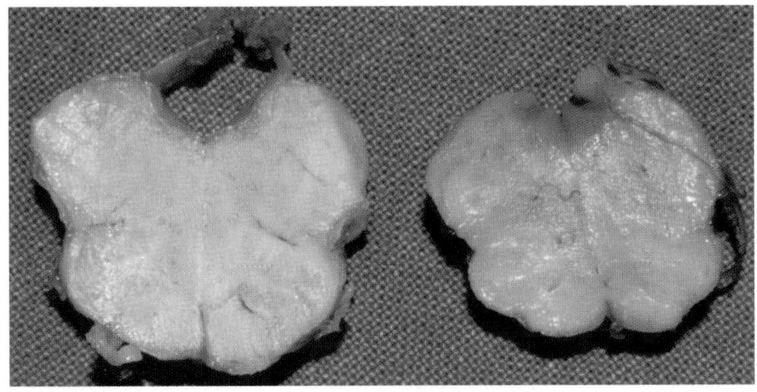

Figure 16.21 Multiple system atrophy (right) and normal control medulla (left) demonstrating atrophy and discoloration, including the inferior olivary nuclei (olivopontocerebellar atrophy).

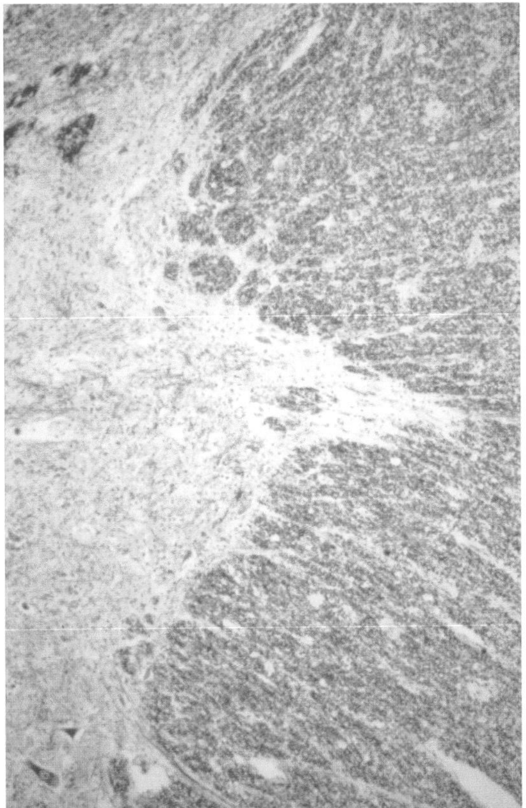

Figure 16.22 Shy Drager syndrome. There is loss of autonomic neurons in the intermediolateral column of the spinal cord. Luxol fast blue/cresyl violet.

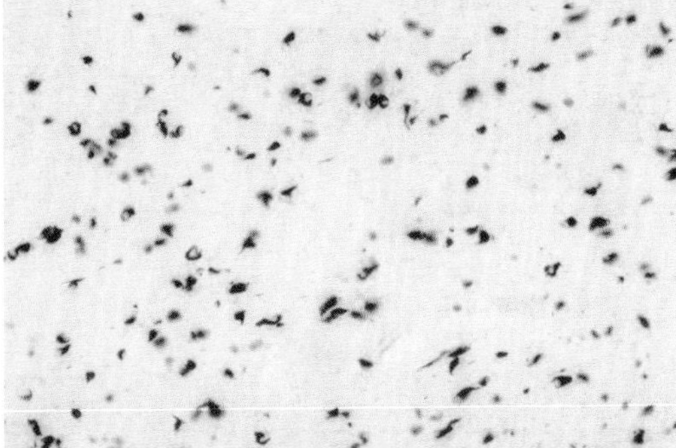

Figure 16.23 Multiple system atrophy. Glial cytoplasmic inclusions. Gallyas.

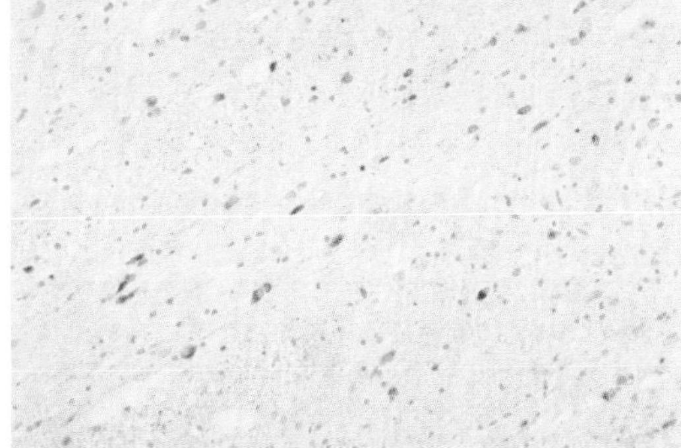

Figure 16.24 Multiple system atrophy. Glial cytoplasmic inclusions. Immunohistochemistry for α-synuclein.

not involve the dopaminergic pathway it is often resistant to dopamine therapy. The specific unifying feature of the various forms of MSA is the presence of glial cytoplasmic inclusions (GCIs) (Figs 16.23 and 16.24). GCIs are tangle-like aggregates of α-synuclein in the cytoplasm of glial cells, predominantly oligodendrocytes. There is variable immunostaining of the inclusions for tau and ubiquitin. GCIs may also be demonstrated by the Gallyas silver stain.

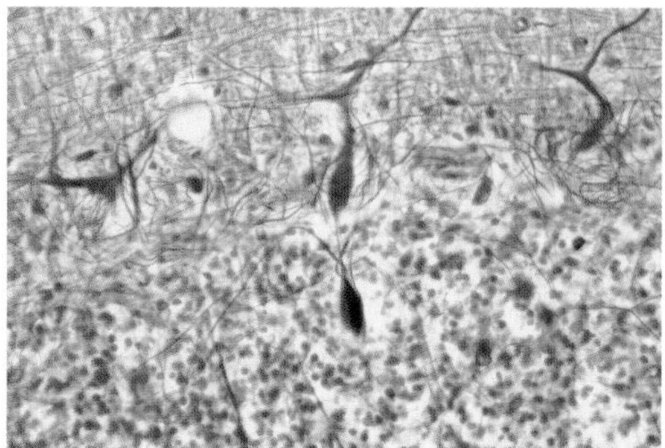

Figure 16.25 Cerebellar cortical degeneration. Purkinje cell with an axonal swelling ('torpedo'). Modified Bielschowsky.

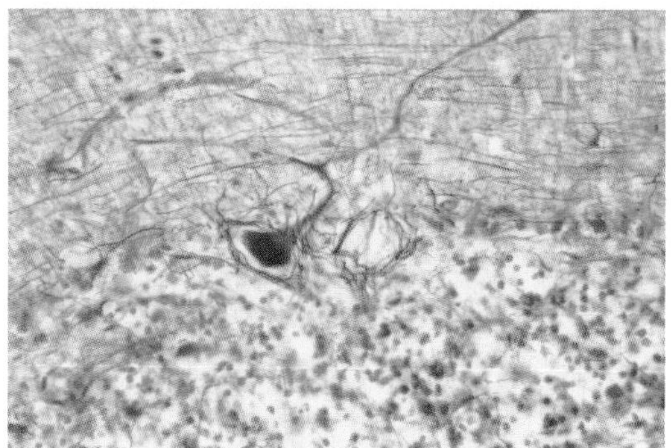

Figure 16.26 Cerebellar cortical degeneration. 'Empty basket' of residual neuronal processes marking the site of a degenerated Purkinje cell. A preserved Purkinje cell is present to the left. Modified Bielschowsky.

Cerebellar and spinocerebellar degenerations

Primary cerebellar cortical degeneration has, as its major features, cerebellar atrophy with prominent depletion of Purkinje cells (Figs 16.25 and 16.26). Residual clusters of neuronal processes mark the locations of degenerated Purkinje cells and are known as 'empty baskets'. Surviving Purkinje cells may have axonal swellings (torpedoes). There is proliferation of Bergmann astrocytes with their parallel processes in the molecular layer producing a pattern known as isomorphic gliosis (Fig. 16.27). There may be marked degeneration of cerebellar cortical granule cells.

Friedreich's ataxia, an autosomal recessive spinocerebellar degeneration, is the commonest form of hereditary ataxia. Onset occurs in childhood or adolescence with ataxia and sensory loss. There is degeneration of the dorsal columns, predominantly the gracile tracts, the gracile and cuneate nuclei, and the posterior roots. There is deficiency of the mitochondrial iron transport protein frataxin. Most cases of Friedreich's ataxia are associated with expansion of a GAA triplet repeat in the frataxin gene.

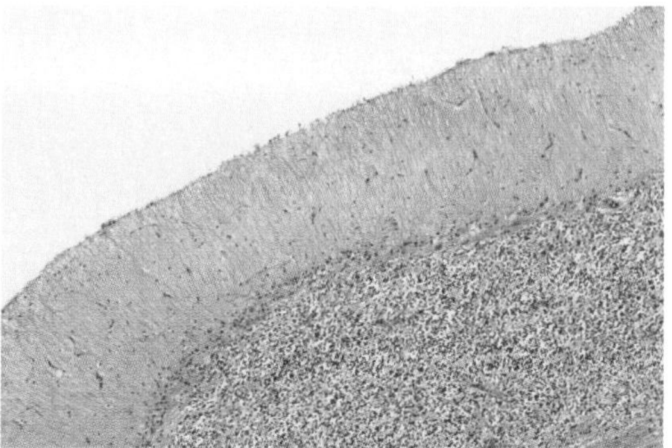

Figure 16.27 Cerebellar cortical degeneration. Proliferation of Bergmann astrocytes is associated with the presence of parallel glial processes in the molecular layer orientated perpendicular to the pial surface ('isomorphous gliosis'). PTAH.

Ataxia-telangiectasia is the commonest cause of ataxia in infants. There is mutation of a gene involved in control of the cell cycle and in DNA surveillance. Inheritance is autosomal recessive and clinical features include immunological deficiency, causing susceptibility to infections, and neoplasia. Neurodegeneration is widespread in the central nervous system and can involve the cerebral cortex, brainstem, cerebellum, spinal cord and sensory ganglia.

Spinocerebellar ataxia (SCA) has many autosomal dominant forms. The SCAs are trinucleotide repeat disorders and they are now classified by the gene which is mutated. The pathology includes atrophy of the cerebellum and associated afferent and efferent pathways and the neurodegeneration may also be much more widespread.

Dentatorubropallidoluysian atrophy (DRPLA) involves neuronal loss and gliosis in the dentate nucleus, red nucleus, globus pallidus and subthalamic nucleus. Clinical features include ataxia, chorea and dementia. DRPLA is a trinucleotide repeat disorder with expansion of CAG repeats in the atrophin-1 gene on chromosome 12.

CHAPTER 17

AGING AND DEMENTIA

James A R Nicoll

AGING

In aging the central nervous system faces a number of challenges to the homeostatic mechanisms which facilitate the maintenance of its structure and function (Table 17.1). Aging is usually associated with a slowly progressive decline in memory, cognitive function, reaction times and other functions. The precise cause of this decline is not known. In addition to the cumulative effects of a life time of events the neurodegenerative diseases (NDDs) are very common in the elderly. It has even been suggested that Alzheimer's disease (AD), which achieves a prevalence of close to 50% in those over 80–90 years of age, is an inevitable consequence of brain aging. An alternative view is that 'normal' aging is not associated with a decline in brain function, but that the studies documenting an age-related decline simply reflect inclusion of people in the early stages of NDDs such as AD. Currently, there is great interest in the clinical concept of age-related mild cognitive impairment (MCI) because it comprises a group at high-risk of progressing to dementia whether due to AD or other pathology. Patients with MCI therefore represent a target for preventative therapy to preserve cognitive function.

Table 17.1 Challenges to the central nervous system in aging

- Oxidative damage to macromolecules by toxic free radicals
- Reduction in trophic factors
- Programmed cell death
- Failure of protein degradation and elimination pathways
- Aging-associated mitochondrial DNA mutations
- Gliosis
- Neurodegenerative diseases
- Impairment of cardiac output
  - Myocardial disease
  - Cardiac arrhythmias
  - Cardiac valve disease
- Vascular disease
  - Hypertension
  - Atherosclerosis
  - Arteriosclerosis
  - Thrombosis and embolism
  - Hemorrhage
- Decline in respiratory function
- Decline in renal function
- Decline in hepatic function
- Diabetes
- Poor diet

Macroscopic changes in the aged brain include atrophy of gray and white matter. The frontal, parietal and temporal association cortex is usually affected, but there is relative sparing of the occipital cortex. Dilation of the lateral ventricles reflects atrophy of cerebral white matter. Although diffuse signal change in the cerebral white matter on MRI, termed leukoaraiosis, is very common in aging, the precise pathological correlate of this remains unclear. Age-related cerebral atrophy is typically associated with a loss of about 100g in brain weight in those over 60–70 years. In the basal ganglia there may be lacunes, which are greatly enlarged perivascular spaces or micro-infarcts, that can be large enough to be detectable macroscopically and on brain imaging *in vivo*. Thickening and opacification of the leptomeninges is common, particularly with a parasagittal distribution. The blood vessels of the Circle of Willis and the vertebrobasilar system are often affected by atherosclerosis.

Microscopically, arteriosclerosis is common particularly in the cerebral white matter and basal ganglia. Arteriosclerosis is reflected by collagenous thickening of the walls of small arteries and arterioles, with enlarged perivascular spaces which often contain a few hemosiderin-laden macrophages. There may be mineralization of small arteries and arterioles in the basal ganglia. Lipofuscin reflects accumulation of indigestible debris in neuronal lysosomes. There is hypertrophy and hyperplasia of astrocytes, detectable by immunohistochemistry for glial fibrillary acidic protein (GFAP) and associated with the accumulation of corpora amylacea. Microglia undergo hypertrophy, hyperplasia and immunological activation. Small dots of ubiquitin immunostaining are usually present throughout the gray and white matter. Diffuse Aβ plaques in the cerebral cortex, neurofibrillary tangles in the hippocampus and cerebral amyloid angiopathy are very prevalent, not only in those with overt cognitive dysfunction, but also in those with preserved cognition. In aging, pyramidal neurons in the hippocampus are susceptible to granulovacuolar degeneration and the formation of Hirano bodies, although the functional consequence of these features is unclear. At present there is little information on the pathological correlates of MCI. Until recently it was widely accepted that progressive loss of neurons was an inevitable consequence of the aging process. However, more sophisticated methods of quantification now suggest that neurons are well preserved in number. It is becoming appreciated that formation of new neurons (neurogenesis) occurs in adult life, and in the hippocampus is required for the formation of new memories. It is not known to what extent neurogenesis or synaptic plasticity is affected in aging.

DEMENTIA

Dementia reflects dysfunction and cell death affecting neurons distributed widely throughout the brain. Most cases of dementia result from forms of neurodegenerative disease (NDD), the basic principles of which have been described in the previous chapter. Alzheimer's disease is by far the commonest cause of dementia, being responsible for about 70% of cases and Dementia with Lewy bodies for a further 15%. Vascular pathology (vascular dementia) accounts for most of the remaining 15% of cases. There are many uncommon causes of dementia (Table 17.2).

Dementia is a common problem, affecting approximately 5% of the population over the age of 65 years and close to 50% of those over 85 years of age. Estimates suggest that 0.5 million individuals are affected by dementia in the United Kingdom, 8–16 million in Europe, and in the United States almost 5 million are affected by Alzheimer's disease alone. Dementia results in a high social and economic burden. The total financial cost of Alzheimer's disease in the United States alone is estimated at $100 billion dollars a year, mostly reflecting long-term care and loss of productivity of carers. Because of increasing life expectancy, in most parts of the world, the number of people affected by dementia is projected to increase dramatically over the coming decades. There is consequently an urgent need for effective treatment or, ideally, prevention of the disease processes which result in dementia.

Dementia can be defined as a progressive decline in multiple aspects of cognitive function, including memory, learning, attention span and executive function, in an individual of previously normal intellectual ability and alertness. The definition excludes an acute confusional state, impairment of consciousness, delirium or depression and also excludes mental impairment due to maldevelopment of the brain or due to a brain insult during development. The pathology is very widespread in the brain reflecting the impairment of multiple brain functions, but certain clinical patterns are recognized to correlate with the distribution of pathology (Table 17.3). The underlying disease processes

Table 17.2 Causes of dementia

Neurodegenerative diseases

- Alzheimer's disease (70%)
- Dementia with Lewy bodies (15%)
- Frontotemporal dementia
- Progressive supranuclear palsy
- Corticobasal degeneration
- Huntington's disease
- Dementia associated with motor neuron disease

Vascular diseases

- Multi-infarct dementia } (15%)
- Subcortical vascular dementia } (15%) (diffuse white matter arteriosclerosis)
- Vasculitis
- CADASIL
- Cerebral amyloid angiopathy

Infective/transmissible

- HIV/AIDS
- Neurosyphilis
- Tuberculosis
- Prion diseases (e.g. CJD)
- Progressive multifocal leukoencephalopathy

Toxic and metabolic

- Alcohol abuse
- Vitamin B_{12} deficiency
- Chronic drug abuse
- Folate deficiency
- Hepatic encephalopathy
- Uremic encephalopathy
- Hypothyroidism

Miscellaneous

- Traumatic brain injury
- Normal pressure hydrocephalus
- Multiple sclerosis
- Tumor
- Angiotropic lymphoma

Table 17.3 Clinical patterns of dysfunction correlate with the distribution of the pathology in the brain

Brain area	Dysfunction
Frontal	Disorders of behavior, mood, motivation, judgment, planning, reasoning, appetite and continence. Disinhibition
Temporal	Memory dysfunction
Parietal	Dysphasia and dyspraxia
Subcortical	Slowness of thought processes

evolve slowly over years or decades with a long preclinical phase. Most studies of the pathology of dementia have been based on patients seen in hospital and may not reflect the prevalent patterns of disease in the community. The relatively few large-scale community-based studies have shown a very marked burden of neurodegenerative pathology in the brains of aged but cognitively normal individuals. Clinical diagnostic criteria have been devised which careful clinico-pathological studies have shown to have a significant error rate, in the region of 10–20%. It is still the case that a definitive diagnosis of the cause of dementia can only made by microscopic examination of brain tissue. In the absence of specific therapy for most causes of dementia diagnostic biopsy is rarely justified. However, sometimes a biopsy is performed in order to confirm a clinical diagnosis of treatable pathology (e.g. cerebral vasculitis) and sometimes to confirm a presumptive diagnosis of Creutzfeldt–Jakob disease. There is now an urgent requirement for biomarkers to permit accurate diagnosis during the early stages of dementia for the validity of clinical trials of new disease-specific therapies.

Post mortem assessment of dementia

- Review the clinical history.
- Evaluate the clinical differential diagnosis.
- Consider the possibility of Creutzfeldt–Jakob disease which influences the autopsy procedure (see section on CJD autopsy on page 361, Table 17.9).
- Consider freezing samples of cerebral cortex for neurochemistry/genetics.
- Examine brain macroscopically after fixation in formalin.
- Select appropriate blocks for histology, e.g. frontal, temporal, parietal and occipital lobes, corpus striatum, thalamus, midbrain, pons, medulla and cerebellum.
- Stain with hematoxylin and eosin, Luxol fast blue and a silver stain (e.g. modified Bielschowsky) or thioflavin S.
- Immunohistochemistry for Aβ, tau, ubiquitin and α-synuclein as appropriate.

Histological stains for dementia pathology

Remarkably little abnormality can be seen in the cerebral cortex in AD or DLB in sections stained with hematoxylin and eosin and specific stains are required. Silver stains (e.g. modified Bielschowsky) are useful as they can demonstrate both plaques and tangles in addition to other inclusions such as Pick bodies and sometimes Lewy bodies. Modified thioflavin S demonstrates plaques, tangles and amyloid angiopathy but has to be visualized with ultraviolet light and tends to fade. Immunohistochemistry for Aβ, tau, ubiquitin and α-synuclein is used to demonstrate abnormal accumulation of those specific proteins.

A simple diagnostic approach to the histology

Are there abundant plaques and tangles in the temporal neocortex on silver or thioflavin S stained sections?

- Yes → *Diagnosis = Alzheimer's disease* (but also check for Lewy bodies and vascular pathology as indicated below because there may be mixed pathology).
- No → Are there Lewy bodies in the midbrain on hematoxylin and eosin stained sections?
- Yes → Perform immunohistochemistry for α-synuclein on sections of temporal and cingulate cortex and confirm the presence of cortical Lewy bodies. *Diagnosis = dementia with Lewy bodies.*
- No → Are there multiple widespread cortical infarcts?
- Yes → *Diagnosis = multi-infarct dementia.*
- No → Is there severe arteriosclerosis in the cerebral white matter and basal ganglia associated with degeneration of the white matter (hematoxylin and eosin, Luxol fast blue stained sections)?
- Yes → *Diagnosis = subcortical vascular dementia.*
- No → Re-evaluate clinical history. Was there really a progressive decline in cognitive function? Consider whether the cognitive dysfunction could have been due to a systemic abnormality (e.g. cardiac, respiratory, renal, hepatic or pancreatic disease, sepsis, alcohol abuse, drug abuse, toxins, deficiencies, etc.) or one of the rare causes of dementia (see Table 17.2).

Alzheimer's disease

Alzheimer's disease (AD) is progressive and inevitably fatal within about 5–15 years of onset unless an intercurrent illness intervenes. In AD the immediate cause of death is often a terminal infection such as bronchopneumonia. It has been suggested that AD is the third commonest cause of death in the developed world (after vascular disease and cancer). More than 95% of AD is sporadic without clear genetic or environmental causes. Approximately 1–2% of cases are familial with an autosomal dominant pattern of inheritance (Table 17.4). Clinically, progressive impairment of memory is an early and major feature of AD. Other cognitive deficits occur in language, in object recognition and in executive functioning. Behavioral symptoms such as agitation, depression, psychosis and wandering are common.

Macroscopic examination of the brain usually shows moderate or severe symmetrical cerebral atrophy (Figs 17.1 and 17.2). The atrophy affects the frontal, temporal and parietal lobes with relative sparing of the occipital lobes. Widening of sulci reflects loss of cortical gray matter. Ventricular dilation reflects loss of cerebral white matter. Correlating with memory failure as an important feature of AD, there may be relatively more pronounced atrophy of the medial temporal lobe structures including the hippocampi, medial temporal

Table 17.4 Genes and Alzheimer's disease

Autosomal dominant disease-causing point mutations	
• Amyloid precursor protein (APP; chromosome 21)	
• Presenilin 1 (*PSEN1*; chromosome 14)	
• Presenilin 2 (*PSEN2*; chromosome 1)	
• Down syndrome	Trisomy 21, i.e. *APP* gene triplication: all individuals > 40 years of age are affected
• Sporadic AD	
• Apolipoprotein E (*APOE*; chromosome 19)	
• Possession of *APOE* ϵ4 allele increases risk	
• Possession of *APOE* ϵ2 allele reduces risk	

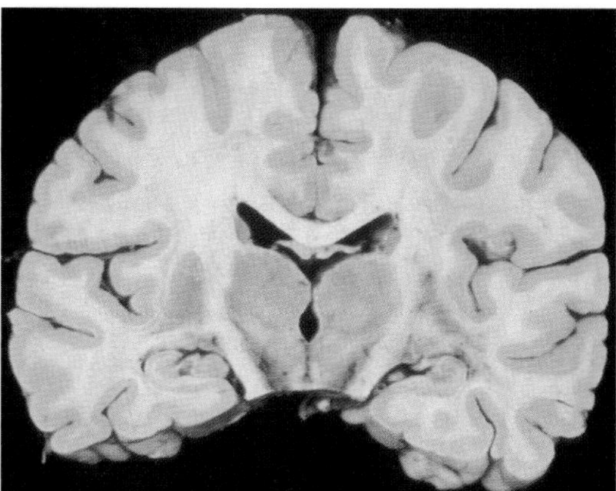

Figure 17.1 In 'normal' aging there is mild cerebral atrophy involving the frontal, parietal and temporal lobes, with relative sparing of the occipital lobes. In this coronal section there is slight widening of the sulci which reflects cortical atrophy and mild dilatation of the ventricles with rounding of the lateral angles of the lateral ventricles, reflecting atrophy of white matter.

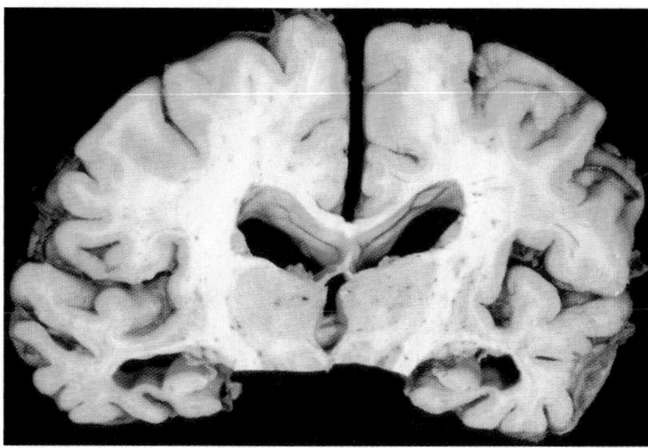

Figure 17.2 In Alzheimer's disease there is usually more severe atrophy than that seen in 'normal aging' (Fig. 17.1). There is widespread cortical atrophy, reflected by widening of the sulci. There is usually relative sparing of the occipital lobes. Severe atrophy of the medial part of the temporal lobes, as seen here, is typical. There is also white matter atrophy, reflected by the dilated lateral ventricles and thinned corpus callosum.

cortex and white matter. However, the severity of atrophy is very variable and in some cases the degree of atrophy may be no more than that accountable by the patient's age. The brain weight is usually reduced, in some cases markedly to below 1000 g, or may be normal. The substantia nigra is normally pigmented unless there is concomitant dementia with Lewy bodies. It should be noted that the macroscopic appearances are not specific for AD but can also be seen in a wide variety of neurodegenerative diseases. It follows that histological identification of the pathological features of AD, plaques and tangles in the cerebral neocortex, is required for a definite diagnosis (Table 17.5).

Table 17.5 Histopathological features of Alzheimer's disease

- Aβ accumulation: cortical plaques and cerebral amyloid angiopathy
- Tau accumulation: neurofibrillary tangles, plaque-associated dystrophic neurites and neuropil threads
- Loss of neurons and synapses

Plaques

The cerebral neocortex is densely peppered with plaques (Figs 17.3–17.7) which are protein aggregates composed predominantly of amyloid β-protein (Aβ) in association with other proteins. The Aβ protein accumulates in the extracellular space in the form of fibrillar amyloid or in non-amyloid form. Amyloid formed from Aβ has a β-pleated sheet configuration and stains with amyloid stains such as Congo red and thioflavin S. Plaques have a number of different morphological patterns including diffuse plaques, dense-cored plaques and neuritic plaques. Some investigators consider that neuritic plaques are of particular significance and their presence has been used as a major criterion in diagnostic protocols for AD. Neuritic plaques contain dystrophic neurites, which are irregularly thickened and tortuous neuronal processes containing hyperphosphorylated tau, and are often surrounded by microglia and astrocytes. In addition to the neocortex, plaques are present in the hippocampus, subiculum and entorhinal cortex. There is relative sparing of primary motor and sensory regions of the cerebral cortex. Relatively few plaques may be present in the basal ganglia and cerebellum and are usually exclusively diffuse, non-neuritic in type.

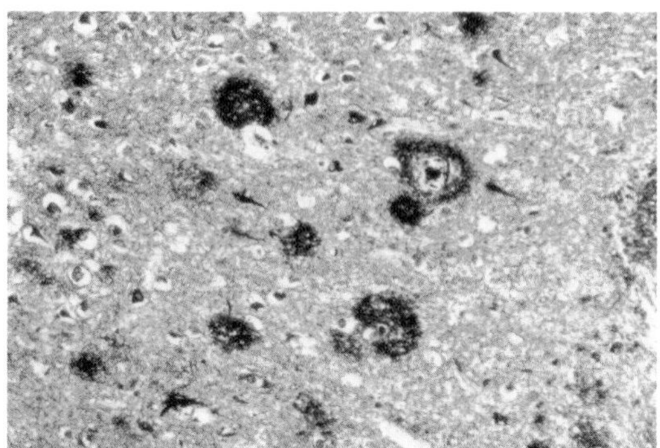

Figure 17.3 Alzheimer's disease. Silver stains such as modified Bielschowsky are useful for demonstrating the presence of both plaques and tangles in the cerebral cortex.

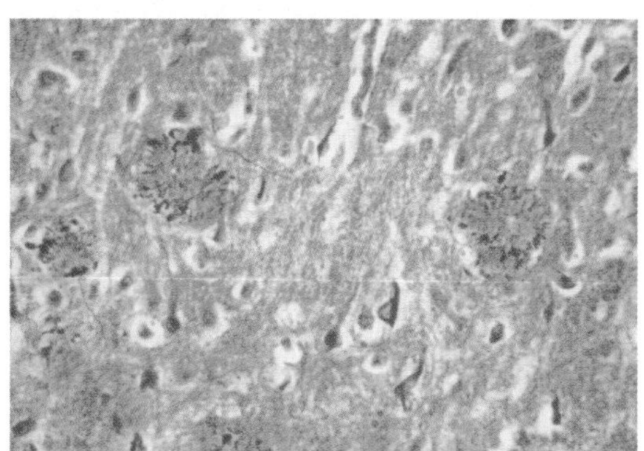

Figure 17.4 Alzheimer's disease. Plaques with prominent dystrophic neurites and tangles in the cerebral neocortex. Modified Bielschowsky.

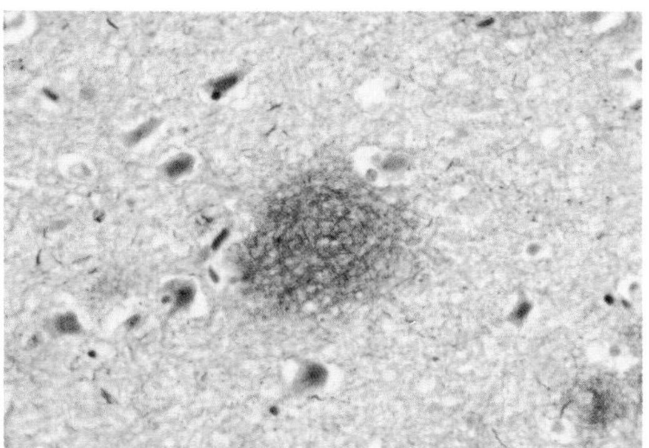

Figure 17.5 Alzheimer's disease. High-power view of a diffuse, non-neuritic plaque. Modified Bielschowsky.

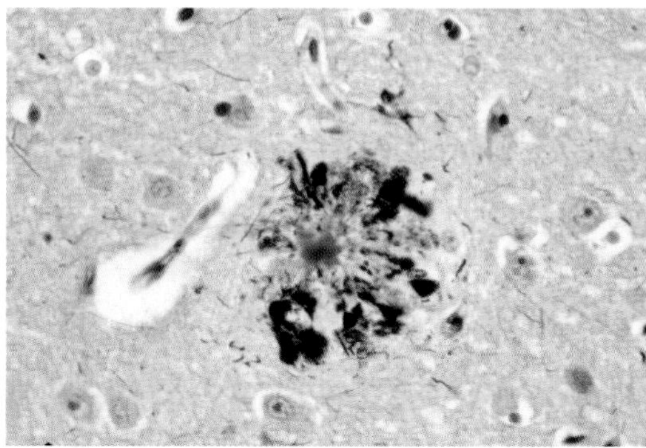

Figure 17.6 Alzheimer's disease. High-power view of a neuritic plaque with an amyloid core. Modified Bielschowsky.

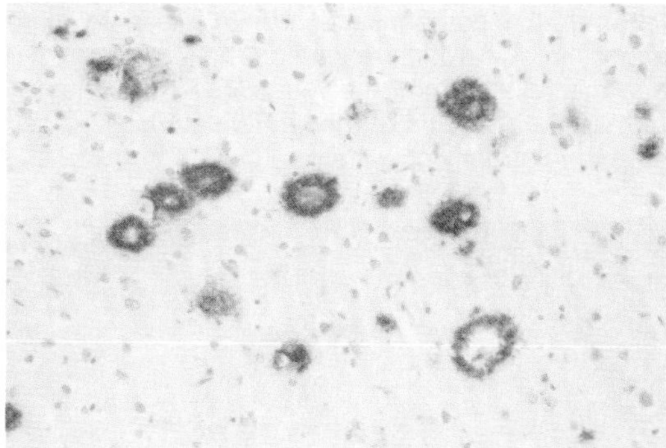

Figure 17.7 Alzheimer's disease. The major component of plaques is amyloid-β protein (Aβ). Immunohistochemistry for Aβ.

Neurofibrillary tangles

Tangles (Figs 17.8–17.12) are intraneuronal aggregates of filaments composed predominantly of the microtubule-associated protein tau. Ultrastructurally, the tau protein is arranged in the form of paired helical filaments (PHF-tau). Extracellular tangles can occur and presumably reflect the death of tangle-bearing neurons. Tangles can be demonstrated with silver stains, such as modified Bielschowsky, thioflavin S and by immunostaining for tau. Immunohistochemistry also demonstrates accumulation of tau in neurons which do not have tangles and this may represent a pre-tangle form of tau accumulation. A high proportion of tangles can also be identified in sections immunostained for ubiquitin,

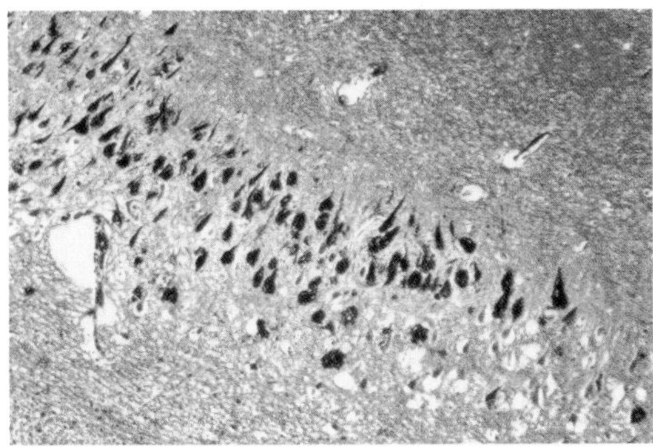

Figure 17.8 Alzheimer's disease. Abundant neurofibrillary tangles in the hippocampus. Modified Bielschowsky.

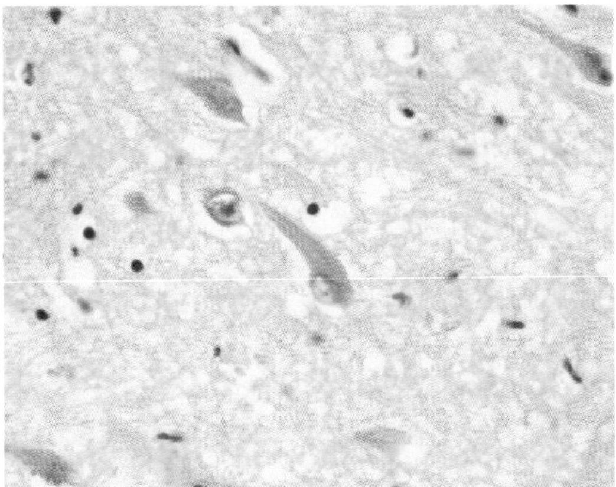

Figure 17.9 Alzheimer's disease. Tangles are discernible with difficulty on staining with H&E.

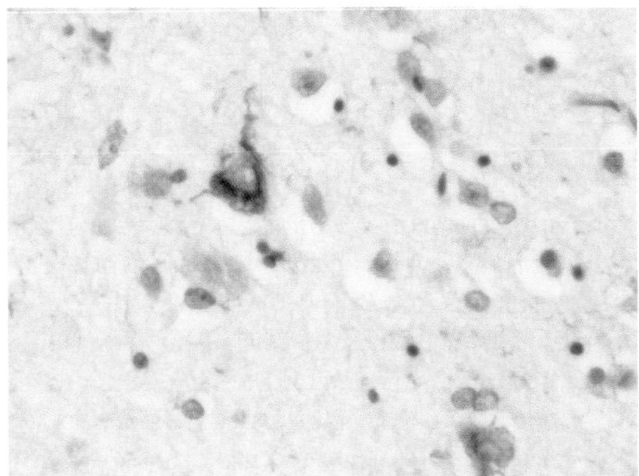

Figure 17.10 Alzheimer's disease. Tangles are composed predominantly of the microtubule-associated protein tau. Immunohistochemistry for tau.

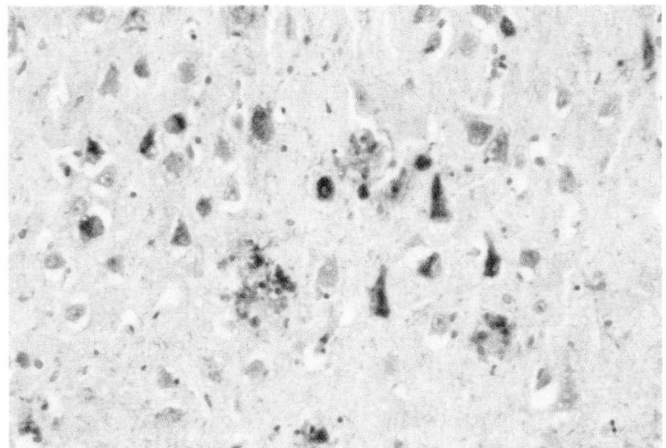

Figure 17.11 Alzheimer's disease. Lower power view of tau immunostaining showing tangles and plaque-associated dystrophic neurites in the cerebral neocortex.

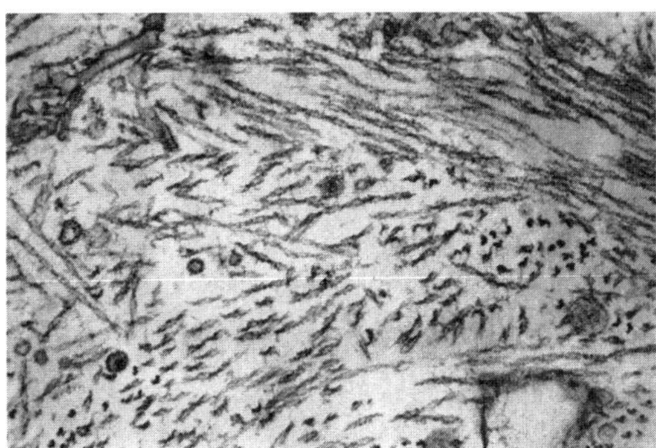

Figure 17.12 Alzheimer's disease. On electron microscopy tangles are composed of paired filaments twisted together in a helical fashion like rope (paired helical filaments).

although this method is not specific as ubiquitin is present in many other types of inclusion. On hematoxylin and eosin staining tangles have a faintly basophilic appearance but this is a very insensitive method of detection.

Neuropil threads

Neuropil threads (Fig. 17.13) are fine caliber neuronal processes which contain tau. They are scattered within the neuropil of the cerebral cortex and their density in AD is quite variable.

Loss of neurons and synapses

Quantitative studies have shown a 20–40% depletion of neurons and synapses in the cerebral cortex

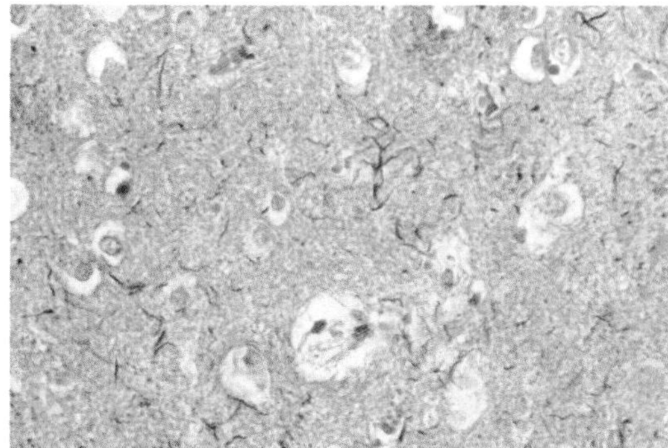

Figure 17.13 Alzheimer's disease. Neuropil threads in the cerebral cortex can be detected by silver stains, as shown here, or with tau immunohistochemistry. Modified Bielschowsky.

in AD. Some clinico-pathological studies have identified the severity of synaptic loss as the best correlate of the degree of dementia.

Cerebral amyloid angiopathy

Accumulation of Aβ in the walls of small arteries and arterioles in the cerebral cortex and overlying leptomeninges is termed cerebral amyloid angiopathy (CAA) (Figs 17.4–17.16). Blood vessels in the cerebellum may also be affected but those in cerebral white matter, basal ganglia and brainstem are spared. CAA is present in >90% of AD cases and is also common in elderly people who are cognitively intact. CAA is associated with destruction of smooth muscle cells in the walls of affected blood vessels. It is unclear whether or not this form of vascular pathology is associated with dysregulation of cerebral blood flow and may therefore contribute to the cognitive dysfunction.

Cholinergic dysfunction

There is evidence of cholinergic dysfunction in AD with a decrease in the concentration of the neurotransmitter acetylcholine (ACh) in the cerebral cortex and decreased activity of the enzyme which synthesizes ACh (choline acetyl transferase). The cortical cholinergic synapses are the projections of neurons located in the basal nucleus of Meynert, in the inferior part of the basal ganglia, in which there is profound neuronal loss in AD. This observation of cholinergic dysfunction forms the rationale for cholinergic therapy for AD. However, other neurotransmitter systems (e.g. noradrenergic, serotonergic and dopaminergic systems) are also variably affected in AD.

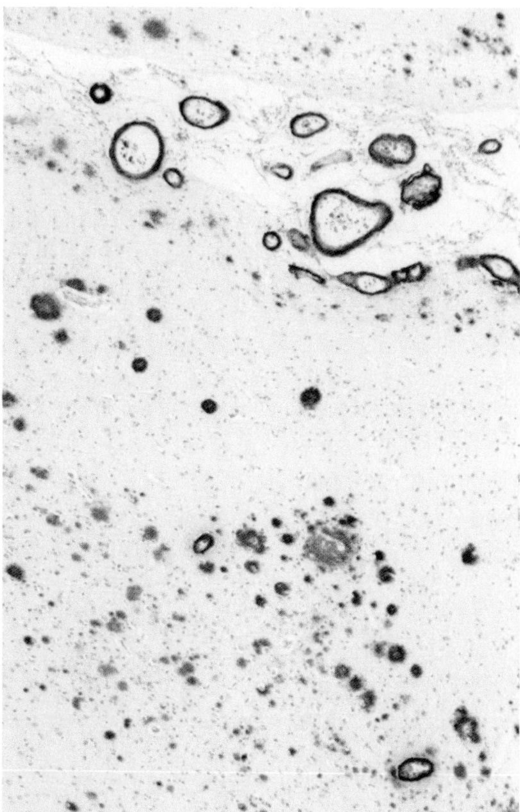

Figure 17.14 Alzheimer's disease. The severity of cerebral amyloid angiopathy (CAA) is variable. In this case there is severe CAA affecting small arteries and arterioles in the cerebral cortex, among the plaques, and in the overlying leptomeninges. Immunohistochemistry for Aβ.

Apolipoprotein E

Polymorphism of the apolipoprotein E gene (*APOE*) influences the risk of developing sporadic AD. This differs from the rare *PSEN1*, *PSEN2* and *APP* point mutations which are disease-causing mutations. There are three common *APOE* alleles designated ϵ2, ϵ3 and ϵ4. There is an increased frequency of the ϵ4 allele among patients with AD compared with non-demented groups indicating that possession of *APOE* ϵ4 is a risk factor for the development of the disease. Possession of *APOE* ϵ2 appears to be

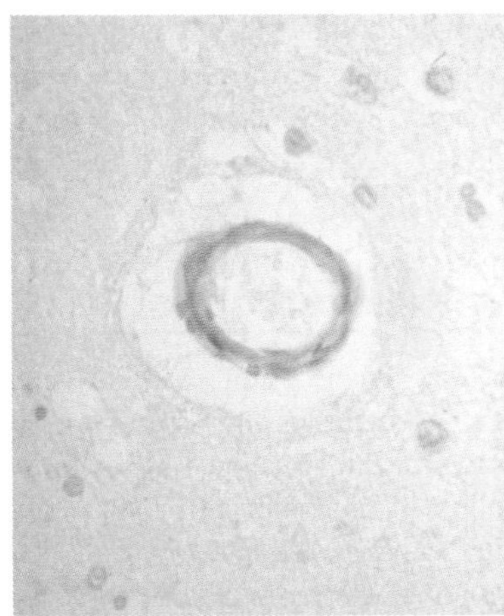

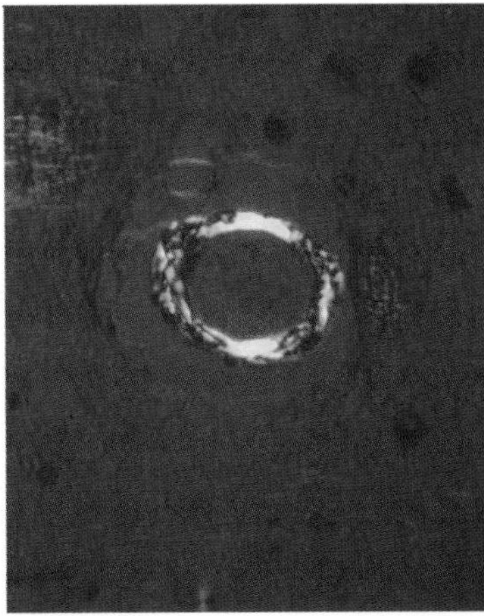

Figure 17.15 Alzheimer's disease. The Aβ in the walls of the blood vessels stains with Congo red (left) and shows apple-green birefringence in polarized light (right), confirming it as amyloid.

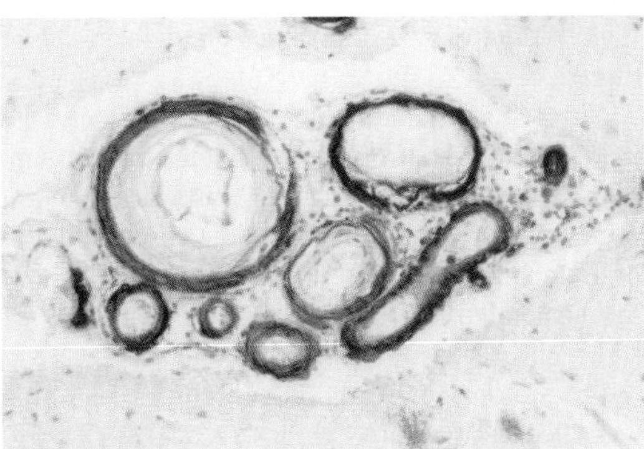

Figure 17.16 Alzheimer's disease. Severe CAA with accumulation of Aβ affecting the full circumference and full thickness of small arteries in the leptomeninges. Aβ immunohistochemistry.

Table 17.6 Evidence of a key role for Aβ protein in the pathogenesis of Alzheimer's disease (AD)

- Aβ accumulation is a consistent feature of AD
- Point mutations in the gene encoding APP, from which Aβ is derived, can cause AD
- AD-causing gene mutations (*APP*, *PSEN1* or *PSEN2*) are all associated with increased production of Aβ, especially the particularly fibrillogenic Aβ42
- AD is a consistent feature of Down syndrome beyond the age of 40 years. Presumably because three copies of the *APP* gene, located on chromosome 21, results in increased Aβ production
- *APOE* polymorphism, which modulates risk of sporadic AD, is associated with Aβ aggregation
- Transgenic mice with AD-causing gene mutations develop AD-like pathology

relatively protective. However, determination of *APOE* genotype has not proved helpful on an individual basis in predicting who will develop AD, or in AD diagnosis. The mechanism by which this genetic influence operates remains unclear, although apolipoprotein E appears to bind to Aβ and influence its aggregation. Also of potential relevance is the observation that apolipoprotein E is involved in the delivery of lipids to neurons for growth of neurites and synaptic maintenance.

The amyloid hypothesis

There is evidence to suggest that abnormal accumulation of Aβ plays a key role in initiating and perpetuating the neurotoxic events that culminate in dementia (Table 17.6). Amyloid precursor protein (APP) is a transmembrane protein of uncertain function. A 40–42 amino acid peptide known as amyloid β-protein (Aβ) is cleaved from APP by enzymes (β and γ secretases). Most Aβ in the brain is probably produced by neurons. The Aβ peptide is released into the extracellular space where, in aging and in AD, it aggregates to form plaques and accumulates in the blood vessel walls as CAA. The longer Aβ42 is particularly fibrillogenic and aggregates readily, possibly forming a nidus for subsequent accumulation of the less fibrillogenic Aβ40. Aβ42 is the major constituent of cortical plaques whereas Aβ40 forms the major contribution to CAA. Some studies suggest that the concentration of Aβ solubilized in extracellular space (soluble Aβ) correlates well with the severity of dementia. Recent studies have focused on oligomers of Aβ which appear to be synaptotoxic. It is presumed that the Aβ abnormalities cause tau aggregation, but the mechanism by which this occurs is unclear at present.

There is increasing evidence that there is a balance between production and elimination of Aβ in the brain. There is good evidence in familial AD (*PSEN1*, *PSEN2* and *APP* gene mutations) and in Down syndrome that increased production of the particularly fibrillogenic Aβ42 results in accumulation of Aβ. However, in the much more common sporadic AD there is little evidence for increased production of Aβ, and instead Aβ accumulation may be the result of decreased elimination. Recently, evidence has been provided for a number of different pathways for clearance of Aβ from the brain including local enzymatic degradation (e.g. by neprilysin and insulin degrading enzyme), glial cells, clearance across the blood–brain barrier mediated by LDL-receptor-related protein and clearance of Aβ by bulk flow of extracellular fluid along the perivascular drainage pathway. It is possible that one or more of these clearance mechanisms become impaired with aging leading to increased accumulation of Aβ within the brain and resulting in sporadic AD. This increasingly detailed understanding of the pathogenesis of AD is beginning to lead to new therapeutic or preventative strategies (Table 17.7). For example, recent studies have shown that peripheral immunisation with the Aβ protein can result in an immune response which clears amyloid plaques from the brain or prevents their appearance.

Table 17.7 Therapeutic strategies for Alzheimer's disease

- Boost cholinergic neurotransmission
  - Acetylcholinesterase inhibitors
- Reduce Aβ levels
  - Decrease production of Aβ (e.g. secretase inhibitors)
  - Increase elimination of Aβ (define and enhance normal clearance mechanisms)
  - Disrupt and solubilize amyloid plaques
- Anti-inflammatory agents (reduce microglial activation)
- Statins (mechanism of action currently unclear but possibly modulate production of Aβ)

Dementia with Lewy bodies

Dementia with Lewy bodies (DLB) is the second commonest neurodegenerative disease that causes dementia and is responsible for about 15% of cases. DLB has a number of characteristic clinical features by which it can be distinguished from AD including a fluctuating course, visual hallucinations and parkinsonian signs. The course may also be rapidly progressive, mimicking Creutzfeldt- Jakob disease.

Macroscopic examination of the brain often shows mild to moderate atrophy affecting the frontal, temporal and parietal lobes but with sparing of the occipital lobes. In the brainstem there is usually loss of pigment in the substantia nigra (Fig. 17.17) and locus coeruleus.

The characteristic neuropathological feature is the presence of Lewy bodies in cortical neurons, identified microscopically (Figs 17.18–17.21). Cortical Lewy bodies are difficult to detect using traditional stains such as hematoxylin and eosin or silver stains and consequently have only been recognized to be common in the last two decades. They are, however, readily detectable in sections immunostained for α-synuclein, which may also highlight fine caliber neuronal processes in the neuropil (Lewy neurites) (Fig. 17.22). Ubiquitin immunohistochemistry also demonstrates Lewy bodies but as it is less specific than α-synuclein immunohistochemistry it is less useful in practice. Lewy bodies are widely distributed throughout the cerebral cortex including in the cingulate gyrus and temporal cortex, particularly in the deeper layers, but their density is low.

A mixture of Lewy body pathology and Alzheimer pathology is common, which is to be expected because they are both common diseases. However, there is some evidence for a genuine overlap in the pathological entities of AD and DLB as some AD-causing APP gene mutations also produce Lewy bodies. DLB and Parkinson's disease are related in

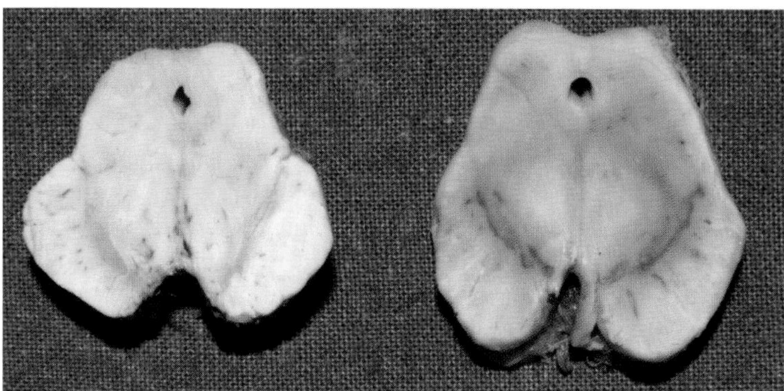

Figure 17.17 Midbrain in dementia with Lewy bodies (left) compared with a control (right). There is often pallor of the substantia nigra, as in Parkinson's disease, reflecting loss of pigmented neurons.

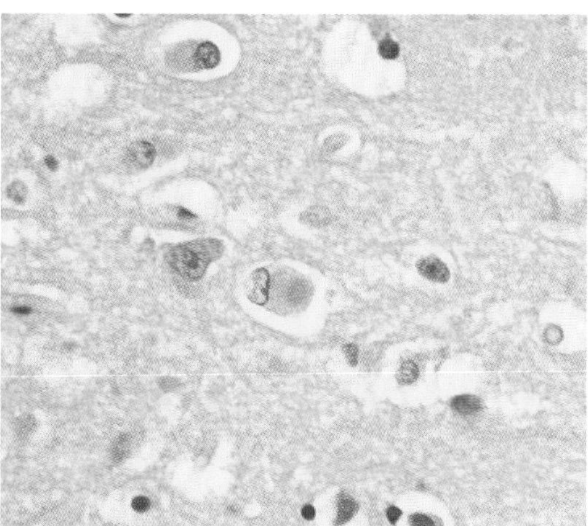

Figure 17.18 Dementia with Lewy bodies. Lewy bodies can be seen in cortical neurons with H&E staining, but they are more difficult to discern than nigral Lewy bodies. H&E.

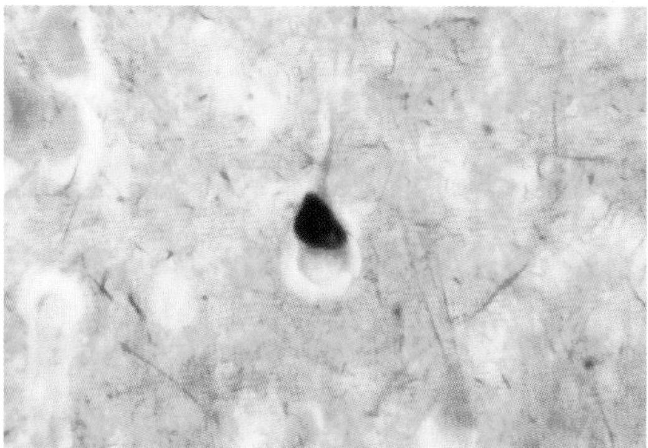

Figure 17.19 Dementia with Lewy bodies. Cortical Lewy bodies are sometimes clearly seen with silver stains. Modified Bielschowsky.

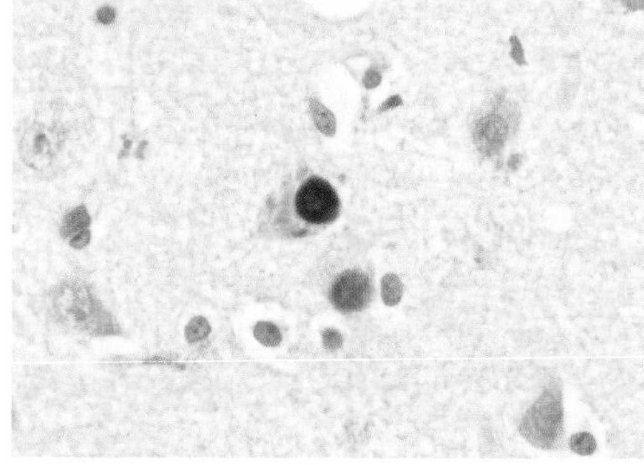

Figure 17.20 Dementia with Lewy bodies. Cortical Lewy bodies are most reliably and specifically demonstrated with α-synuclein immunohistochemistry.

Figure 17.21 Dementia with Lewy bodies. Even in the most severely affected regions, such as here in the cingulate gyrus, the density of cortical Lewy bodies is quite low. α-synuclein immunohistochemistry.

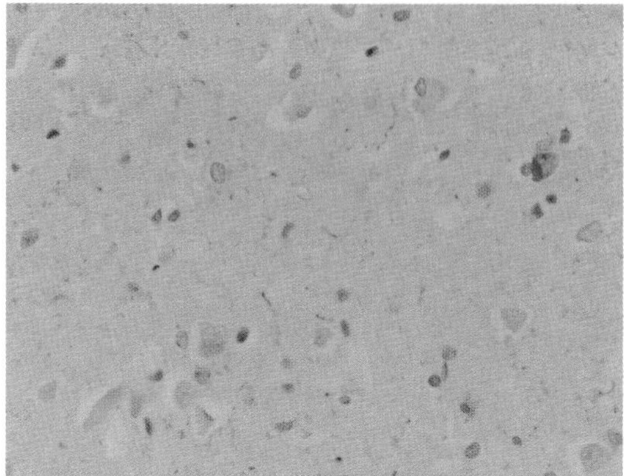

Figure 17.22 Dementia with Lewy bodies. In some cases α-synuclein immunoreactive Lewy neurites can be detected.

a manner which is not yet entirely clear. Patients with DLB may have dementia alone or accompanied by the motor features of parkinsonism either at presentation or at a later stage in the disease. Whichever clinical pattern occurs, all patients are found to have both cortical and nigral Lewy bodies at autopsy. Consequently, identifying Lewy bodies in a hematoxylin and eosin stained section of midbrain is a useful way of predicting their presence in the cortex of a patient with dementia and prompting α-synuclein immunohistochemistry on sections of cerebral cortex in order to confirm this. A striking feature of cortical Lewy bodies is low density at which they occur in the cortex (Fig. 17.21). This makes it hard to imagine that their presence alone is the cause of the cognitive dysfunction, instead it seems more likely that they represent a marker for an as yet uncharacterized disease process. The neuronal damage in the cortex is usually less severe than in AD and this may reflect the reversibility of some of the symptoms in DLB.

Vascular dementia

Vascular pathology is an important feature of the aging brain and commonly includes atherosclerosis, affecting the major arteries supplying the brain, and arteriosclerosis, affecting smaller blood vessels within the brain parenchyma. Consequently, ischemic damage to the brain in aging is common, often presenting with transient ischemic attacks or as a stroke. The contribution of age-related cerebrovascular disease to dementia is controversial and poorly understood. *In vivo* imaging shows diffuse signal changes in the cerebral white matter, termed leukoaraiosis, very commonly both in dementia and in cognitively normal aged people, which may reflect white matter damage due to small vessel disease. There are major variations in the proportion of cases of dementia estimated to have a vascular etiology depending, at least in part, whether the definition is clinical, radiological or pathological. In the last 20–30 years the estimated incidence of vascular dementia has fallen. It is not clear whether this is a genuine change due, for example, to the widespread use of anti-hypertensive therapy or whether it is due to better understanding of other contributions to dementia, particularly the recognition that dementia with Lewy bodies is common. Current studies generally estimate that about 15% of dementia has a vascular cause. Vascular dementia can be divided into multi-infarct dementia due to large vessel disease, and subcortical vascular dementia due to small vessel disease.

Multi-infarct dementia

Multi-infarct dementia is associated with multiple infarcts distributed widely throughout the cerebral hemispheres but affecting mainly the cerebral cortex (Fig. 17.23). Clinical features include focal neurological signs and a stepwise deterioration.

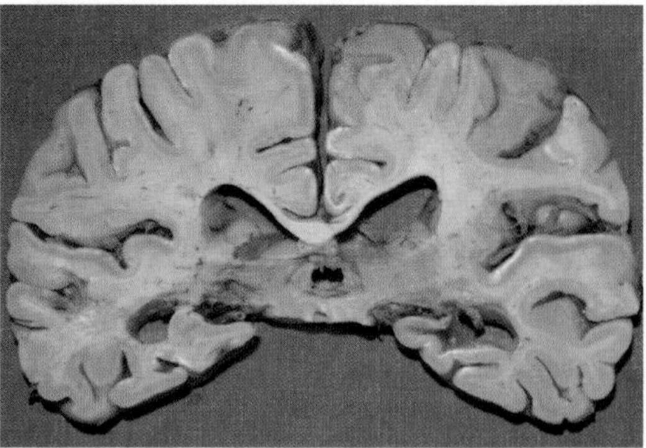

Figure 17.23 Multi-infarct dementia. Multiple infarcts are distributed through the cerebral hemispheres, in the absence of other pathological correlates of dementia.

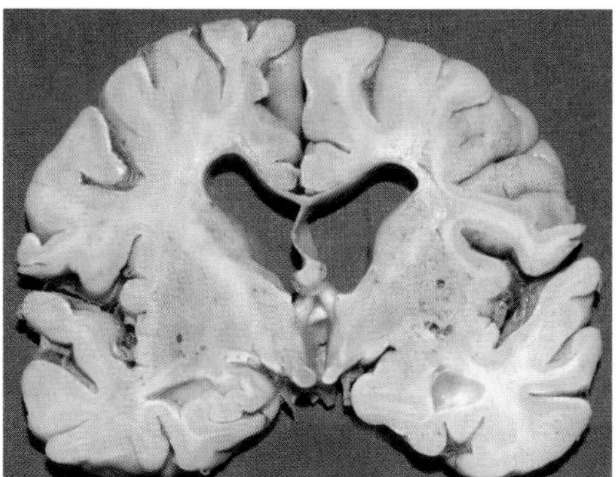

Figure 17.24 Subcortical vascular dementia. There is diffuse atrophy of the cerebral white matter associated with dilatation of the ventricles and thinning of the corpus callosum. Several lacunes are also visible in the basal ganglia.

The underlying pathology is usually atherosclerosis affecting the arteries supplying the brain and resulting in thromboembolic disease. Other potential sources of emboli include those associated with atrial fibrillation, myocardial infarction and cardiac valve disease. It has been suggested that the development of dementia correlates with loss of a critical volume of brain tissue (e.g. 50–100 mL) or that there may be specific brain regions, such as the thalamus and hippocampus, which if damaged by ischemia may lead to cognitive impairment. Brain damage due to an episode of hypoperfusion resulting in laminar cortical necrosis or hippocampal sclerosis may be excluded from the definition of dementia because it lacks a progressive course.

Subcortical vascular dementia

In subcortical vascular dementia there is widespread, diffuse ischemic degeneration of the cerebral white matter, and lacunes in the basal ganglia, associated with small blood vessel disease (Figs 17.24–17.26). The major form of vascular pathology is arteriosclerosis in which there is collagenous thickening of the walls of arterioles, frequently associated with enlargement of the perivascular spaces. Lesser degrees of this pathology are very common in aged cognitively normal individuals and presumably correspond to leukoaraiosis which is commonly identified by imaging *in vivo*. Lacunes are small cavitated lesions, a few millimeters in diameter, which can represent either small infarcts or greatly enlarged perivascular spaces. A severe form of subcortical vascular dementia is sometimes termed Binswanger's disease.

Figure 17.25 Subcortical vascular dementia. There is diffuse depletion of myelinated fibers in the cerebral white matter, reflected here by pallor on staining for myelin. Luxol fast blue/cresyl violet.

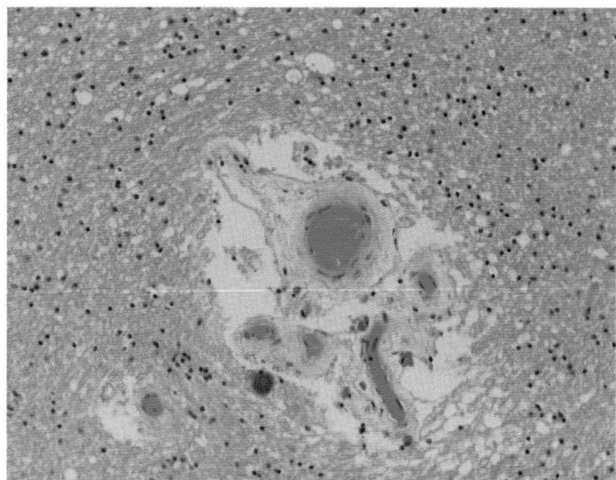

Figure 17.26 Subcortical vascular dementia. Arteriosclerosis affecting a blood vessel in the cerebral white matter is associated with an enlarged perivascular space, containing a few hemosiderin-laden macrophages, and degeneration of surrounding myelinated fibers. H&E.

CADASIL

Cerebral autosomal dominant arteriopathy with subcortical infarcts and leukoencephalopathy (CADASIL) is a familial form of vascular dementia associated with mutations in the notch 3 gene on chromosome 19 (Fig. 17.27). Affected patients have a specific vascular pathology affecting arteries and arterioles

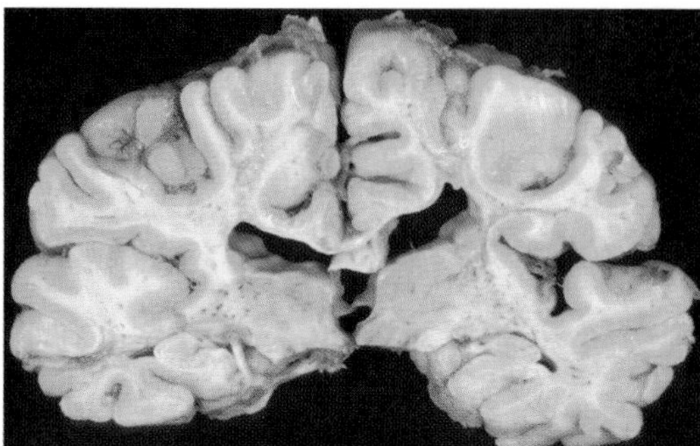

Figure 17.27 CADASIL. There is widespread diffuse or multifocal degeneration affecting mainly the cerebral white matter.

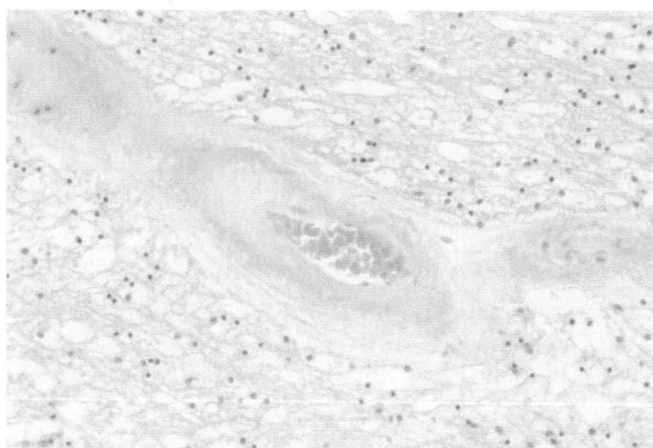

Figure 17.28 CADASIL. There is accumulation of eosinophilic material which has a granular texture in the media of affected blood vessels. H&E.

distributed widely throughout the central nervous system, particularly in the cerebral white matter and leptomeninges. The vascular pathology has a characteristic appearance with accumulation of eosinophilic granular material in the tunica media (Fig. 17.28). The ultrastructural appearance of the deposits gives rise to the term 'granular osmiophilic material' (GOM) (Figs 17.29 and 17.30). The vascular pathology is associated with multiple infarcts and widespread degeneration of cerebral white matter. Blood vessels outside the central nervous system can be affected and diagnosis is sometimes attempted by skin biopsy.

Vascular dementia and Alzheimer's disease

A diagnosis of pure vascular dementia clearly requires absence of other pathological substrates

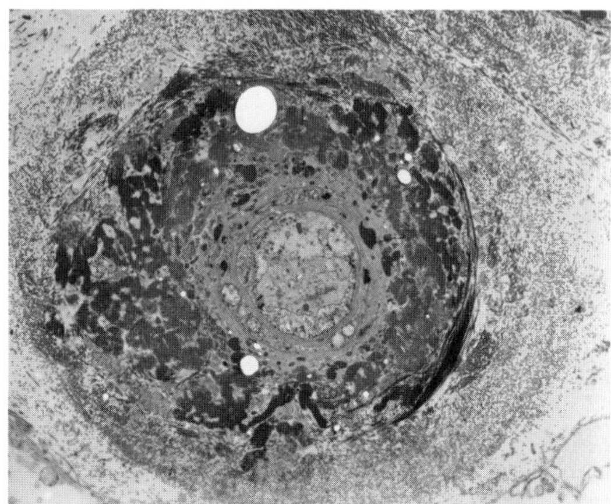

Figure 17.29 CADASIL. The accumulated matter in the media of affected blood vessels is termed 'granular osmiophilic material' (GOM) because of its ultrastructural appearance. Electron microscopy ×5000.

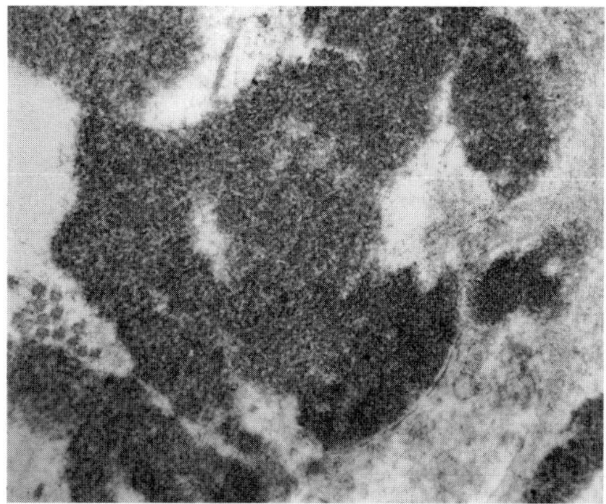

Figure 17.30 CADASIL. High-power electron microscope image of GOM. ×25 000.

for dementia such as Alzheimer's disease. However, cerebrovascular disease in the form of atherosclerosis, arteriosclerosis, infarcts and white matter degeneration are a common accompaniment to Alzheimer's disease. Cerebral amyloid angiopathy is also an almost ubiquitous feature of Alzheimer's disease. The extent to which these forms of vascular pathology contribute to the cognitive impairment in Alzheimer's disease is unclear. Interestingly, many of the risk factors for vascular disease have also been implicated in Alzheimer's disease, including hypertension, diabetes mellitus, cholesterol metabolism and *APOE* ε4. Although the precise mechanism remains unclear it is emerging that controlling vascular risk factors, for example with antihypertensive therapy and statins, appears to protect against the development of dementia in aging.

Frontotemporal dementia

Frontotemporal dementia (FTD) is a group of disorders in which there is relatively selective and prominent involvement of the frontal and temporal lobes (Fig. 17.31). The clinical features particularly reflect frontal lobe involvement (see Table 17.3) and memory is preserved, at least initially, unlike in Alzheimer's disease. The affected regions show neuronal loss and gliosis (Fig. 17.32). Tau accumulation in neurons and glial cells is a prominent feature (Fig. 17.33). The classification of these disorders is evolving as our understanding, particularly of genetic factors, improves. The following are some of the main subtypes that are currently recognized.

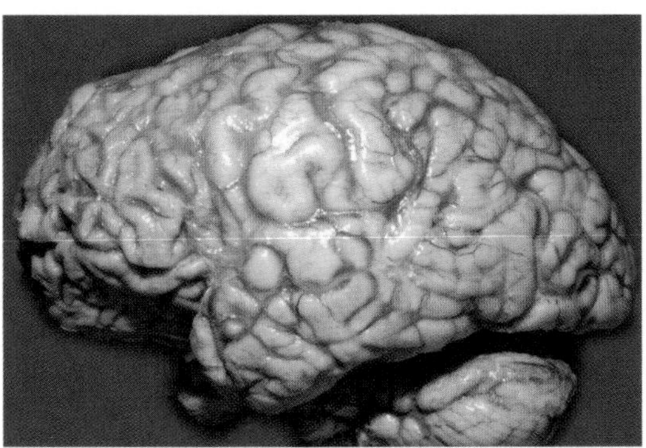

Figure 17.31 Frontotemporal dementia (FTD). In FTD there is relatively severe atrophy of the frontal and/or temporal lobes.

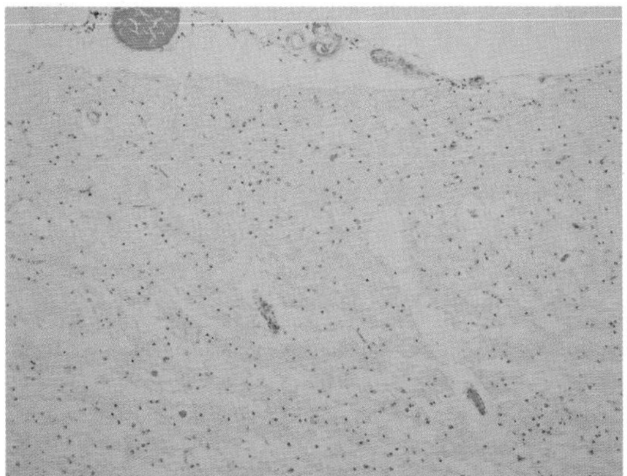

Figure 17.32 Frontotemporal dementia. In the affected areas of cortex there is severe neuronal and synaptic loss with associated gliosis. H&E.

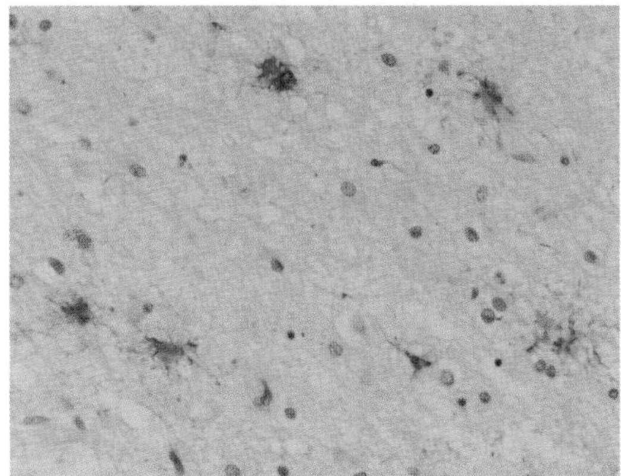

Figure 17.33 Frontotemporal dementia. There is tau immunoreactivity of glial cells and to a lesser extent also of neurons. Immunohistochemistry for tau.

Pick's disease

Clinical features include behavioral disorders, disinhibition and language impairment. Macroscopically, there is very severe atrophy involving the frontal and temporal lobes which may be asymmetric. There may be relative sparing of the posterior part of the superior temporal gyrus. The characteristic histological feature is the presence of spherical neuronal intracytoplasmic inclusions (Pick bodies) which can be detected on hematoxylin and eosin or silver stained sections and by immunohistochemistry for neurofilament, tau and ubiquitin. Swollen neurons (Pick cells) may also be present.

Frontotemporal dementia with parkinsonism linked to chromosome 17 (FTDP-17)

This form of frontotemporal dementia is due to mutation of the tau gene and is inherited as an autosomal dominant trait. Increasingly, familial Pick's disease is being reassigned as FTDP-17 when tau mutations are identified.

Others

There is pathological overlap of FTD with corticobasal degeneration and progressive supranuclear palsy. When dementia occurs in these tau-related disorders it tends to have a frontotemporal pattern. Frontotemporal dementia can also occur in association with motor neuron disease.

Prion diseases: Creutzfeldt–Jakob disease

The prion diseases, also known as spongiform encephalopathies, occur in several different forms (Table 17.8). The least rare is Creutzfeldt–Jakob disease (CJD), occurring throughout the world with an incidence of approximately one case per million of the population per year. Clinically, it is characterized by a rapidly progressive dementia, with typically 6–12 months from onset to the time of death, myoclonus and characteristic EEG changes late in the disease. CJD is a particularly intriguing disease process in that it can be inherited as an autosomal dominant trait, be acquired by transmission or occur sporadically. Transmission of CJD from person to person is extremely uncommon, requiring parenteral inoculation of affected tissue and therefore most cases are iatrogenic. When acquired by transmission the incubation period in humans ranges from several years to decades. Prion disorders can be studied by experimental transmission of affected human tissue to experimental animals and between experimental animals. Although the clinical suspicion of CJD may be strong, a definite diagnosis still requires histological recognition of the characteristic features. Diagnosis can be made by brain biopsy but is more usually made at autopsy (Table 17.9).

The characteristic histological features of CJD are microscopic vacuolation of gray matter (Fig. 17.34), giving rise to the term spongiform encephalopathy, and extracellular accumulation of a protein known as protease resistant peptide (PrP) (Figs 17.35 and 17.36). Spongiform change characteristically takes the form of sharply circumscribed small vacuoles in otherwise well preserved neuropil. It can be challenging to distinguish spongiform change from artefactual vacuolation associated with post mortem autolysis, fixation and processing, though artefact usually produces pericellular and perivascular vacuolation. Spongiform change may also be difficult to distinguish from neuropil degeneration seen in other neurodegenerative diseases, particularly in Alzheimer's disease and dementia with Lewy bodies. Microvacuolation in other neurodegenerative diseases is known as status spongiosus and reflects severe loss of neurons and synapses. Immunohistochemistry for PrP is required for confirmation of the diagnosis of CJD. PrP accumulates in the extracellular space with several different patterns including, diffuse synaptic, perivacuolar or pericellular, and plaque-like. The distribution of spongiform change and PrP accumulation is variable and may be very extensive throughout the cortical gray matter, basal ganglia and gray matter of the brainstem and cerebellum or alternatively may be restricted and multifocal. There is neuronal loss and synaptic loss accompanied by proliferation and hypertrophy of astrocytes and microglia. In contrast to other transmissible disorders lymphocyte infiltration is not a feature.

Table 17.8 Human prion diseases

• Creutzfeldt–Jakob disease (CJD) – Sporadic CJD – Iatrogenic CJD: cadaveric pituitary-derived hormones (historic), neurosurgical instruments, dural grafts, corneal grafts – Familial CJD: *PrP* gene point mutations – Variant CJD: oral ingestion of BSE contaminated meat, blood transfusion from an affected person	
• Gerstmann–Straussler–Scheinker disease	*PrP* gene point mutations, prominent involvement of cerebellum
• Fatal familial insomnia	*PrP* gene point mutations, prominent involvement of thalamus
• Kuru	Oral or parenteral transmission from Kuru-infected human tissue (Papua New Guinea – historic)

Table 17.9 The autopsy in a case of suspected Creutzfeldt–Jakob disease

- Because of the potentially transmissible nature of the disease a post mortem examination in a patient suspected of having CJD needs careful consideration
- It should be performed as a high-risk procedure in an appropriate post mortem facility and by appropriately experienced staff
- Our usual practice is to take small samples for histology from the intact fresh brain from the cortex of the frontal lobe, temporal lobe and cerebellum. Following fixation in formalin, the tissue samples are incubated in formic acid and processed for histology. Corresponding samples are frozen and the remainder of the brain is fixed intact in formalin
- Sections of the three small paraffin blocks are stained with hematoxylin & eosin to assess the presence of spongiform change and immunostained for PrP to detect abnormal PrP accumulation
- If the diagnosis of CJD is confirmed then it may be appropriate to refer the case to a specialist center for registration and further study. Following the outbreak of spongiform encephalopathy in cattle (bovine spongiform encephalopathy) many countries now have a national register for CJD
- If the preliminary histology indicates that the dementia was not due to CJD then the remainder of the formalin-fixed brain can be dissected and sampled for histology in the usual way (see beginning of this chapter)
- An unusual feature of spongiform encephalopathy is resistance of the affected tissue to routine sterilization and decontamination procedures. Transmissibility is not inactivated by formalin fixation or by conventional autoclaving. Tissue samples for histology can be treated by incubation in concentrate formic acid for 1 h. Instruments and surfaces can be decontaminated using sodium hydroxide or sodium hypochlorite. Autoclaving at 134–137°C for 18 min is effective

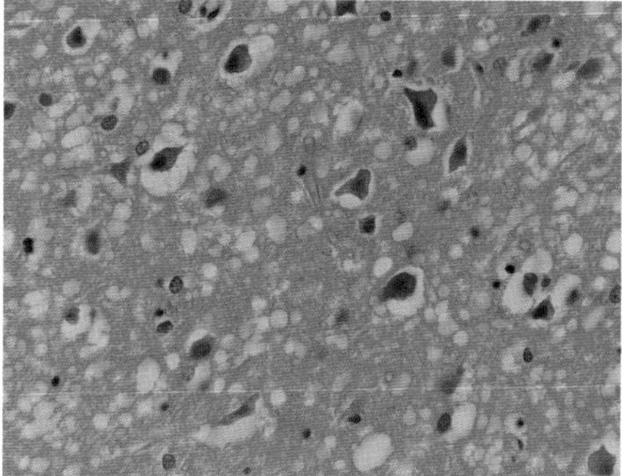

Figure 17.34 Sporadic CJD. Spongiform change: in the gray matter there are multiple well-demarcated vacuoles in otherwise well-preserved neuropil. H&E.

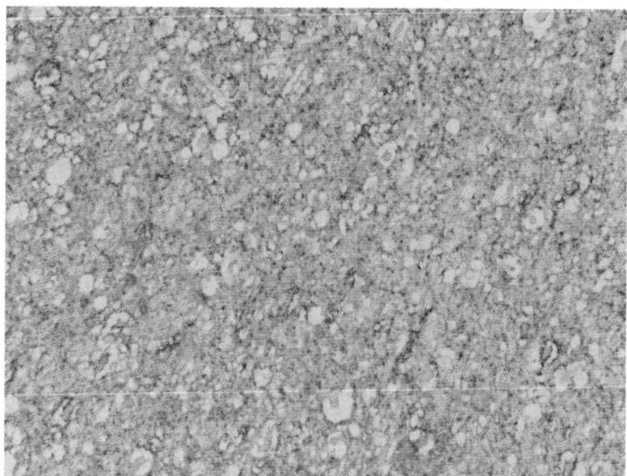

Figure 17.35 Sporadic CJD. Accumulation of PrP occurs in several different patterns in affected gray matter. This Figure shows a diffuse granular pattern of staining – the so-called 'synaptic pattern'. PrP immunohistochemistry.

The prion hypothesis

PrP is a normal cellular transmembrane protein (PrP^c) of uncertain function. Prion disease is due to an abnormal form of the protein (PrP^{sc}) which has a tendency to aggregate, accumulating in the extracellular space and causing spongiform change. Both PrP^c and PrP^{sc} appear to have a similar amino acid sequence but a different three-dimensional structure or conformation. PrP accumulation can be due to:

- Catalytic conversion of host PrP^c to PrP^{sc} by inoculated PrP^{sc} (explaining transmissibility of CJD)

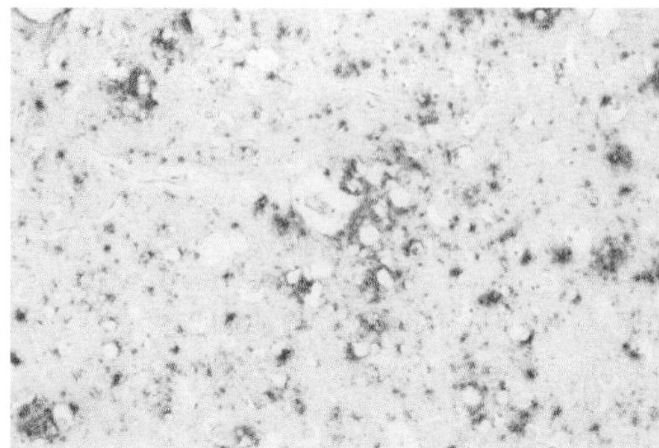

Figure 17.36 Sporadic CJD. In this case the accumulated PrP is forming more discrete foci resembling plaques or cell outlines. PrP immunohistochemistry.

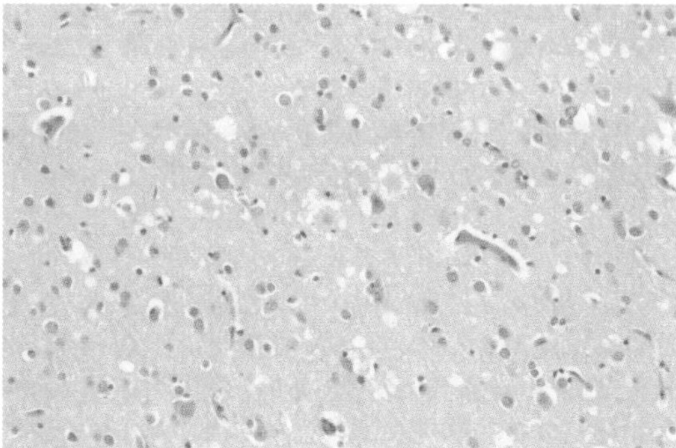

Figure 17.37 Variant CJD. A characteristic feature is the presence of 'florid' plaques composed of a discrete amyloid core surrounded by a ring of vacuoles. H&E.

- Host PrP^c which has an abnormal amino acid sequence rendering it susceptible to take up the abnormal conformation of PrP^{sc} (explaining CJD due to inherited PrP point mutations)
- Very rarely, PrP^c converts to PrP^{sc} as a chance event (explaining sporadic CJD)

There is a common polymorphism of the PrP gene at codon 129, which may encode methionine or valine, giving three genotypes (MM, MV and VV). This polymorphism has an important influence on disease susceptibility and on the pathological pattern of disease. Codon 129 homozygotes (MM and VV) appear to be relatively susceptible to spongiform encephalopathy whereas codon 129 heterozygotes (MV) are relatively protected.

Variant CJD

In the late 1980s and early 1990s there was an epidemic of prion disease in cattle in the United Kingdom known as bovine spongiform encephalopathy (BSE). Although it is still not certain, this probably arose due to the recycling of infected bovine meat in cattle feed. As a consequence, PrP^{sc} is presumed to have been ingested by a large proportion of the population of the UK. Several years after the peak of the BSE epidemic a new variant of CJD (vCJD) was identified in the United Kingdom. Initially, this affected younger patients than is typical for CJD and with a relatively prolonged time course. Histologically, the distinctive feature of vCJD is the presence of 'florid' plaques which take the form of plaques of PrP surrounded by a ring of microvacuoles (Figs 17.37–17.40). Florid plaques occur mainly in the cerebral cortex and cerebellar cortex. The thalamus is also severely affected by the pathology and altered signal on MRI in the thalamus is proving a useful diagnostic aid *in vivo*. vCJD differs from other forms of CJD in that there is accumulation of PrP^{sc} in systemic lymphatic tissues including lymph nodes, tonsil and spleen. On western blotting the PrP in vCJD has a pattern equivalent to that seen in BSE, both aiding in the diagnosis of vCJD and providing confirmation vCJD has origins in BSE. Although vCJD has currently affected relatively few individuals with approximately 150 cases in the UK to date, and

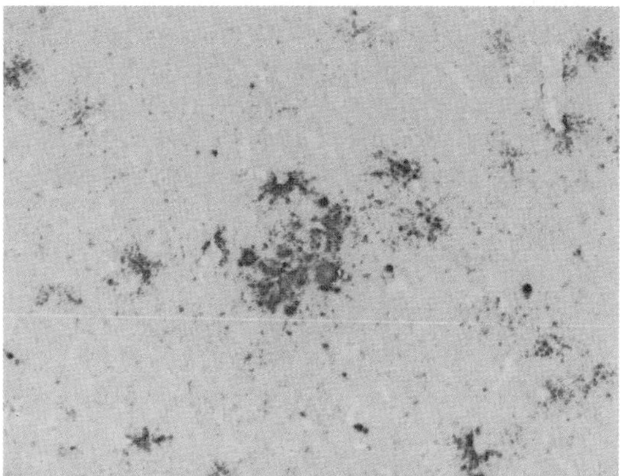

Figure 17.38 Variant CJD. Plaques of PrP in the cerebral cortex. PrP immunohistochemistry.

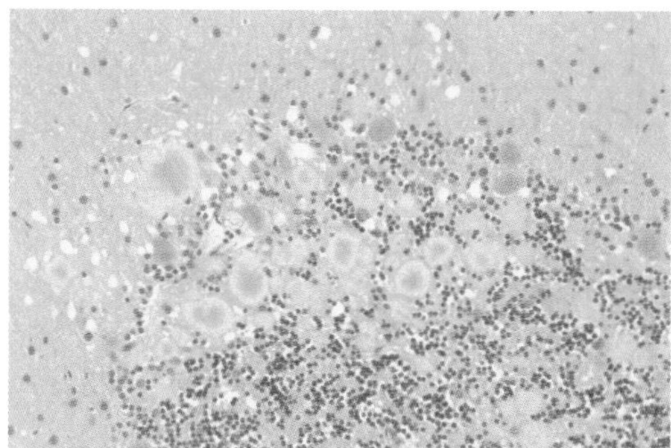

Figure 17.39 Variant CJD. Plaques are frequent in the cerebellum. H&E.

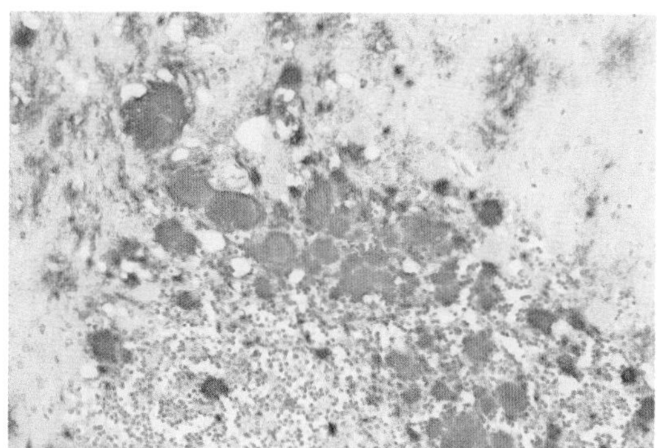

Figure 17.40 Variant CJD. Cerebellar plaques. PrP immunohistochemistry.

smaller numbers in other countries, it has provoked a great deal of interest in relation to disease pathogenesis, public health and animal husbandry. There has been major expenditure in the UK, initially for the culling of affected or potentially affected cattle, and subsequently for alteration in the re-use of surgical instruments and for altered sourcing and handling of blood products for transfusion in an attempt to reduce the risk of iatrogenic transmission.

CHAPTER 18

SKELETAL MUSCLE AND PERIPHERAL NERVE

Susan Robinson

NORMAL ANATOMY

Skeletal muscle is composed of bundles of longitudinally orientated muscle fibers. Each bundle is surrounded by connective tissue known as the perimysium. The endomysium is the fibrous tissue separating individual fibers within each fascicle: normally it is virtually invisible on light microscopy, but increases when there is fiber destruction. The connective tissue enclosing all fascicles is called the epimysium. Each fascicle consists of longitudinally arranged muscle fibers. The different components of muscle are shown in Fig. 18.1.

Epimysium
Fascicle with perimysium
Individual muscle fibres

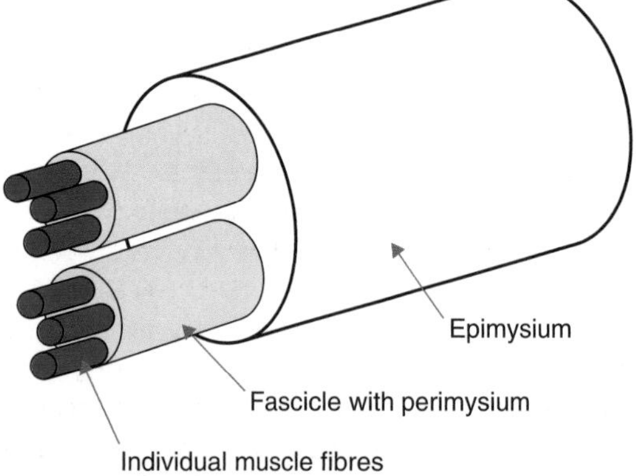

Figure 18.1 Diagram of muscle showing the relationship and orientation of the different components.

The muscle fiber membrane is termed the sarcolemma, and the cytoplasm the sarcoplasm. A network of proteins forms the contractile apparatus, the skeleton being seen on electron microscopy (Fig. 18.2).

NEUROPHYSIOLOGY

An understanding of basic neurophysiological terms is helpful to the pathologist in approaching a clinical question in an informed manner. Not all patients referred for nerve or muscle biopsy have had a prior electrophysiological assessment but a

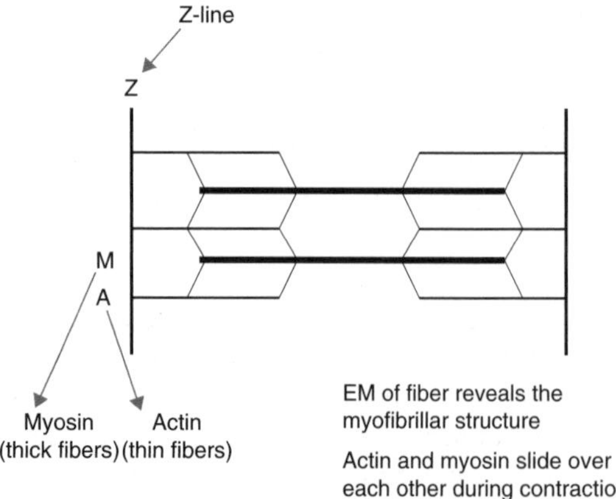

Figure 18.2 Diagram of the contractile proteins actin and myosin in relation to the Z-line seen on electron microscopy (EM).

considerable number will have been evaluated by these techniques. Neurophysiology is neither highly specific nor sensitive. Indeed, if this were the case, biopsy would be obsolete.

Nerve conduction studies

These measure the speed and strength of an electrical impulse along a sensory or motor nerve. A bipolar stimulator is placed proximally (motor conduction) or distally (sensory conduction) and recordings are made at a measured point further along the nerve under study. The sensory nerve action potential (SNAP) and compound motor action potential (CMAP) thus derived can be displayed on an oscilloscope screen. Latency and conduction velocity depend upon intact myelin whereas the waveform of the SNAP or CMAP depends upon the number of functioning axons within the nerve. Slowing of conduction is indicative of a demyelinating neuropathy such as Guillain–Barré syndrome (GBS) or chronic inflammatory demyelinating polyneuropathy (CIDP) while axonal loss is a feature of conditions such as uremia or neoplasia-related (paraneoplastic) neuropathy.

Conduction studies can also be used to study proximal nerve function such as that of the proximal plexuses or nerve roots. Here the antidromic spread of a stimulus up the anterior horn cell and back down again is recorded. The electrophysiological signature of this round trip is the 'F-wave latency' (a marker for proximal disease) while the 'H reflex' more accurately tests the whole reflex arc involving the anterior horn cells.

Needle electromyography

A needle-recording electrode is used to sample muscle activity in a number of selected muscles and recordings made at insertion, rest and after voluntary contraction. This allows objective assessment of five parameters: insertional activity, spontaneous activity motor unit configuration, motor unit recruitment and interference pattern. From these observations the neurophysiologist can comment on motor function from the anterior horn cell to the muscle itself. Electromyography (EMG) studies have their limitations and may be normal in conditions such as McArdle syndrome. Normal investigation does not negate biopsy when muscle disease is presumed. EMG findings can be specific for certain conditions and are an integral part of international criteria applied to the diagnosis of motor neuron disease.

Tests of the neuromuscular junction

Using the standard nerve conduction set-up a series of supramaximal stimulations are applied to a peripheral motor nerve. This is termed 'repetitive stimulation'. The CMAP is measured and normally should maintain its amplitude throughout. In disorders that affect the neuromuscular junction the CMAP is abnormal. In post-synaptic disease (e.g. myasthenia gravis), this diminishes (or decrements) while in pre-synaptic disorders (e.g. Lambert–Eaton syndrome), it increments. The neuromuscular junction can be further investigated by single-fiber EMG studies. These record potentials generated by a single muscle fiber. The interval between stimulus and response is measured on several occasions and where variable, as in neuromuscular junction disease, it is referred to as 'jitter'.

GENERAL PRINCIPLES OF MUSCLE BIOPSY

Clinical information and discussion within a multidisciplinary team are essential: there is very little pathognomonic morphology. A proforma is very helpful for the referring physician to complete when requesting a pathological opinion. Optimal clinical information to be gathered before the biopsy includes the information included in Table 18.1.

Creatine kinase (CK), also known as phosphocreatine kinase or creatine phosphokinase (CPK), catalyses the conversion of creatine to phosphocreatine, consuming adenosine triphosphate (ATP) and generating adenosine diphosphate (ADP). Elevation of CK is an indication of damage to muscle. The normal range of creatine kinase is 24–195 U/L.

Table 18.1 Clinico-pathological correlation

Patient characteristic	Specific features	Examples
Age		Congenital myopathies Congenital muscular dystrophy
Sex		Dystrophinopathies
Family history		Dystrophies
Distribution of weakness	Proximal	Polymyositis
	Distal	Inclusion body myositis
	Symmetrical	
Focal signs	Swallowing	Oculopharyngeal dystrophy
	EOM involvement	Myasthenia gravis
Cramps		Metabolic disorders
Time course	Episodic	
	Congenital	
	Fatigability	Myasthenia gravis
	Precipitating events	Anesthesia
Systemic events	Connective tissue disease	Myositis
	Vasculitis	
	Neoplasms	Dermatomyositis Myasthenia gravis
	Central nervous system	Laminin α2-deficient congenital muscular dystrophy
	Cardiac (ECG, ECHO)	Emery–Driefuss muscular dystrophy Myotonic dystrophy
	Skin	Dermatomyositis
Creatine kinase	High	Inclusion body myositis
	Very high	Duchenne muscular dystrophy Rhabdomyolysis
Drugs	Steroids, statins, etc.	

EOM, external ocular muscles.

Quadriceps is usually biopsied but it is important to choose a diseased muscle. End-stage atrophic muscle will not yield diagnostic material; the muscle is frequently replaced by fat and fibrous tissue. The pathologist should be aware that there are different complements of fiber types in different muscles which can be important in overall interpretation: quadriceps has approximately twice as many type II fibers as type I, while gastrocnemius and deltoid are predominantly type I. EMG needle sites cause damage and should be avoided as biopsy sites.

There are two major biopsy techniques: needle and open. There is considerable variation between centers in choice. Regardless, muscle pathology partly involves enzyme histochemistry so it is imperative to keep the tissue fresh and prevent drying. It is important that the specimen is brought to the laboratory directly for transverse orientation and freezing. The specimen should not be fixed in formalin or transported in saline. Part of the muscle is stored frozen, part is frozen and stained and part may be fixed in gluteraldehyde for electron microscopy. If the biopsy is small, formalin fixation for paraffin embedding is unnecessary. Routine morphometry probably adds little in adults but it is valuable for measuring fiber diameters in infants (objectivity is very difficult in infants without this). An eyepiece graticule is adequate.

Stains vary depending on the clinical history. It is best to discuss panel selection with the local

Table 18.2 Common stains

Stain	Use	Example of use
Hematoxylin and eosin	General purpose stain	
Periodic acid–Schiff	Glycogen	
PAS diastase	Sarcolemmal stain	
Sudan black	Lipid	
Gomori trichrome	Ragged red fibers, nemaline rods	
Reduced nicotinamide adenine dinucleotide–tetrazolium reductase (NADH-Tr)	Architecture	Myofibrillar architecture, cores Ring fibers are highlighted by NADH-Tr in myotonic dystrophies In denervation, targets are well demonstrated
Cytochrome oxidase	Mitochondrial pathway	Mitochondrial activity
Succinic dehydrogenase	Mitochondrial pathway	Mitochondrial activity
Acid phosphatase	Detects macrophages, lysosomal activity, lipofuscin	Necrosis Lysosomal disorders Acid phosphatase detects lysosomal activity and so is positive in areas of necrosis and acid maltase deficiency
Myophosphorylase		Absent in McArdle's
Adenosine triphosphatase (ATPases pH 4.3, 4.6, 9.4)	Fiber typing	Grouping
Expression of HLA-ABC		Upregulated in untreated myositis

muscle physicians. A very comprehensive baseline on frozen section is provided in Table 18.2, which lists the common stains.

Stored muscle is kept indefinitely, ideally in liquid nitrogen. This is very useful and frequently used as medical advances occur. It is possible to go back to fresh frozen tissue to investigate the patient further as frozen tissue may also be required for blotting, for genetics and to be available for enzyme assay.

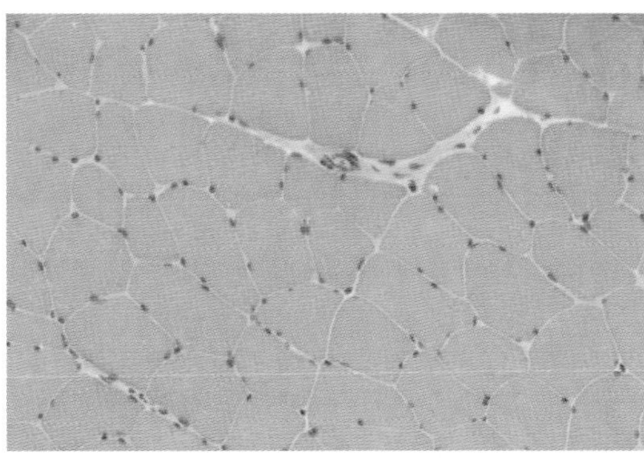

Figure 18.3 Normal muscle demonstrating closely packed, evenly sized fibers. H&E.

THE HISTOLOGICAL EXAMINATION

When interpreting muscle histology the morphological changes should be taken in conjunction with all other available information. Figure 18.3 shows the closely packed, evenly sized fibers in normal muscle.

It is important to note fiber size and shape and interpret these in context. Fiber diameter increases with childhood maturation: neonates have an average diameter of 12 μm; at 10 years the average is 40 μm; and adults have an average diameter between 40 and 80 μm (Table 18.3). Excess variability within the normal range is pathological.

The distribution of atrophic fibers is important: whether random or grouped, as in reinnervation, or perifascicular, as in dermatomyositis. The number and location of nuclei is notable. Nuclei are usually peripheral. Internal nucleation does not normally exceed 3% of all fibers. There is an increase in internal nucleation in some conditions such as dystrophies, centronuclear myopathy and myotonic

Table 18.3 Change of muscle fiber diameter with increasing age

Age	Mean fiber diameter (μm)
Birth	12
3 months	17
3 years	20
10 years	40
Adult	40–80

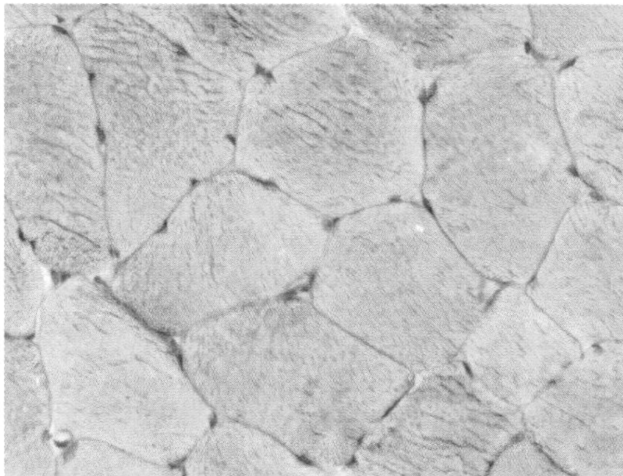

Figure 18.4 Normal muscle stained for glycogen. PAS.

dystrophy. Fibrosis, necrosis and regeneration are all indicative of destruction. Inflammation is notable, but may be the cause of the pathology as in myositis or the result of muscle damage, for example in dystrophies. Inclusions, vacuoles and blood vessels may all aid diagnosis.

Glycogen and lipid are stained for, but expected abnormalities may not be seen in practice (Figs 18.4 and 18.5). These are non-specific indicators of pathology. The enzyme stains are very useful in muscle pathology and are direct indicators of muscle function. Cytochrome oxidase and succinic dehydrogenase indicate oxidase activity well. Oxidative activity must be interpreted in the knowledge of the patient's age: there is some decrease in activity with age. A combination of stains is useful for demonstrating certain features. For example, central cores running the length of fibers are seen on electron microscopy, but there is an absence of staining which is well demonstrated in Gomori trichrome (Fig. 18.6), nicotinamide adenine dinucleotide-tetrazolium reductase (NADH-Tr) (Fig. 18.7), cytochrome oxidase and succinic dehydrogenase.

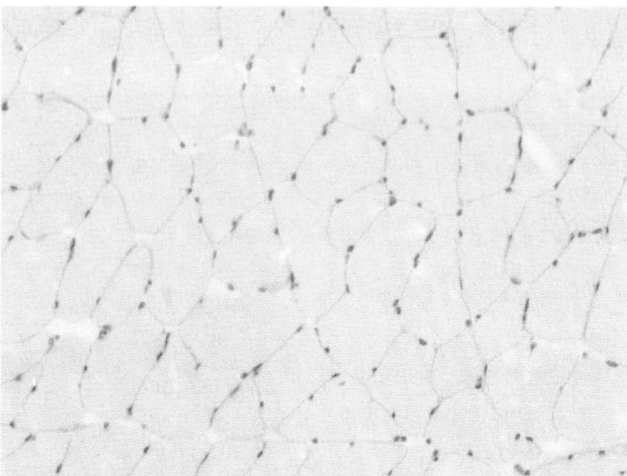

Figure 18.5 Normal muscle architecture. PASD.

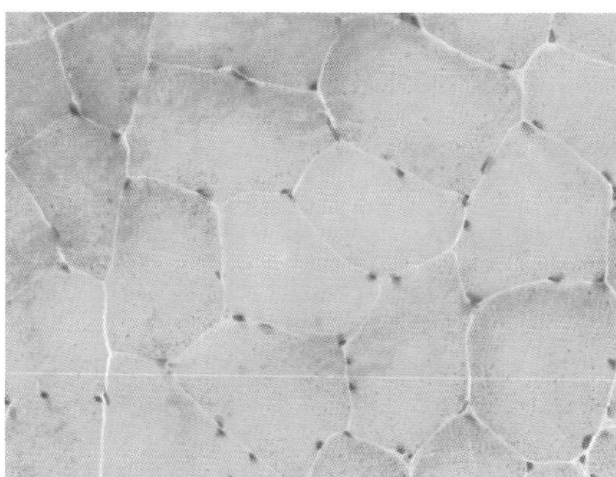

Figure 18.6 Normal muscle. Gomori trichrome.

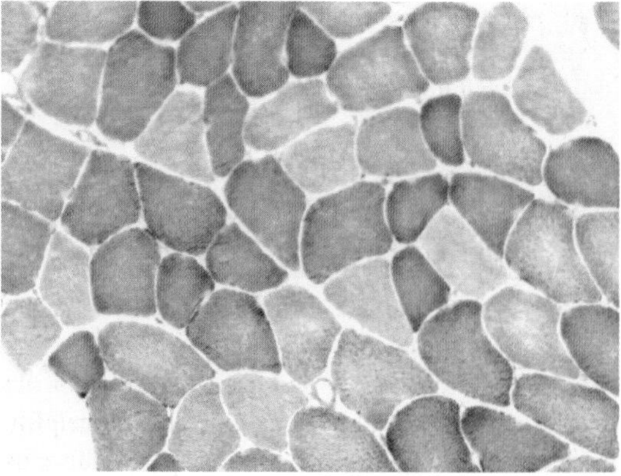

Figure 18.7 Normal muscle. NADH-Tr.

The main enzyme used for fiber typing is adenosine triphosphatase (ATPase) (Fig. 18.8 and Table 18.4). This differentiates the fiber types by exploiting different reactions with changes in pH. The normal

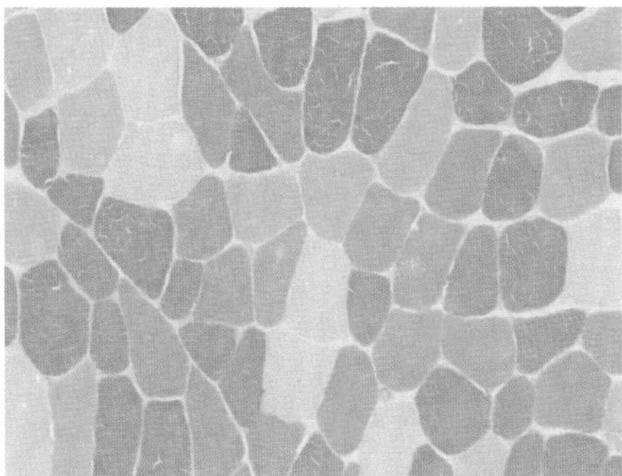

Figure 18.8 Normal ATPase at pH 4.6 indicating type 1 (dark), 2A (light), 2B (intermediate).

Table 18.4 Fiber type staining with ATPases

	Type 1	Type 2A	Type 2B	Type 2C
AT pH 4.3	+++	–	–	++
AT pH 4.6	+++	0	++	++
AT pH 9.4	+	+++	+++	+++

Table 18.5 Changes on electron microscopy

Feature on electron microscopy	Disease association
Abnormal mitochondria, including paracrystalline inclusions	Mitochondrial dysfunction – primary or secondary
Nemaline rods	Nemaline myopathy
Filamentous inclusions	Inclusion body myositis
Central cores	Central core disease

fiber type arrangement is a mosaic pattern: no fiber is next to a fiber of the same type. Changes in this pattern are very important because grouping of fiber type is indicative of reinnervation in neurogenic disorders. Type-specific abnormalities may be helpful.

Subsequent panels depend on history but most frequently involve a variety of structural proteins in potential dystrophies.

Electron microscopy may determine the nature of changes seen, such as areas with absence of staining or better defined structures such as inclusions (Table 18.5).

Table 18.6 Classification of myopathies

Destructive myopathies	Relatively non-destructive myopathies
Dystrophies	Congenital myopathies
Myositis	Myotonias
Some toxins	Metabolic myopathies
	Endocrine myopathies
	Ion channel and neuromuscular junction disorders

CLASSIFICATION OF MUSCLE DISORDERS

Broadly, there are two main groups of pathology, those primarily affecting muscle, termed myopathic myopathies, and those secondary to proximal motor nerve damage, termed neurogenic myopathies. The changes seen in reinnervation are unequivocal in the diagnosis of neurogenic pathology.

Myopathic disorders can be further subdivided in different ways; however, there are always overlaps, which can lead to confusion. One way is to group all destructive myopathies together. This grouping could include dystrophies, myositis and some toxic disorders (Table 18.6). Destructive myopathies result in fibrosis. Relatively non-destructive disorders include congenital myopathies, myotonias, metabolic and endocrine myopathies, ion channel and neuromuscular junction disorders.

INFLAMMATORY MYOSITIS

The more common myositic disorders comprise polymyositis, dermatomyositis and inclusion body myositis. These are destructive myopathies. In terms of diagnosis the presence of inflammatory cells does not necessarily equate to myositis: for example, such cells can be seen in dystrophies.

Polymyositis

Polymyositis presents with proximal symmetrical weakness and myalgia, usually in adults. The serum CK is high. There may be more systemic manifestations such as heart and lung pathology,

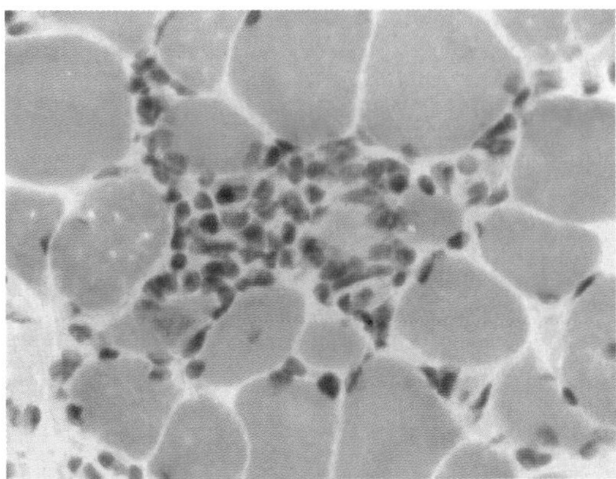

Figure 18.9 Necrotic muscle fiber being engulfed by macrophages. H&E.

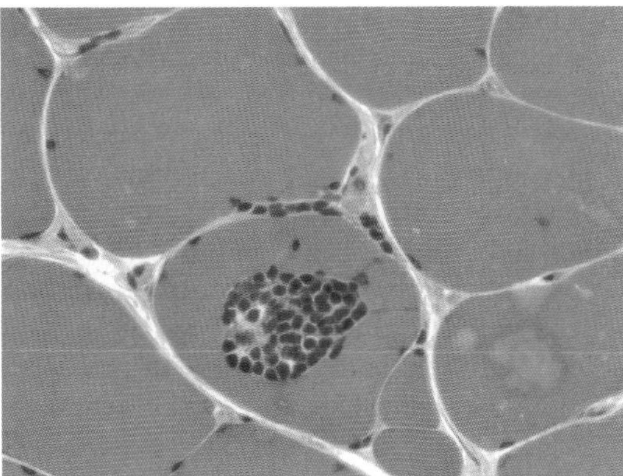

Figure 18.10 Segmental necrosis of a fiber. H&E.

including myocarditis and interstitial lung disease. In some patients the anti-Jo antibody is detected. There is a possible increased incidence in malignancy, although there is some debate about this. Potential underlying causes of polymyositis include drugs, classically D-penicillamine, and collagen vascular diseases. Figures 18.9 to 18.13 show changes often seen in polymyositis.

The muscle shows random scattered atrophy with necrosis, regeneration and fibrosis. Endomysial T-cells are present and there is HLA–ABC upregulation.

Dermatomyositis

Dermatomyositis also causes proximal symmetrical weakness and pain. There is an associated heliotrophic facial rash, vasculitic lesions such as nailfold infarcts, and widespread systemic

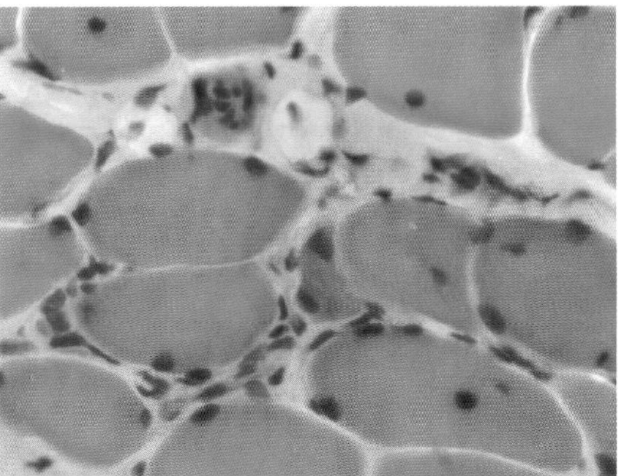

Figure 18.11 The blue fiber is regenerating. H&E.

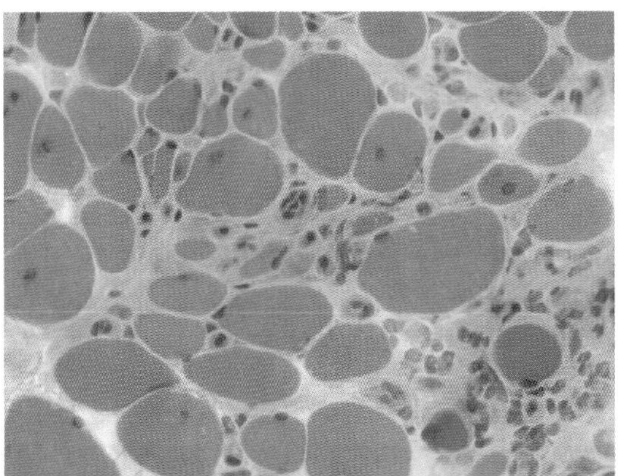

Figure 18.12 Fibrosis indicating a destructive process separating the fibers. H&E.

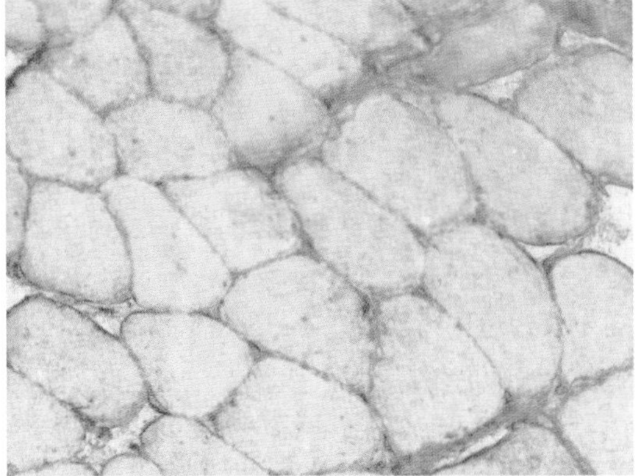

Figure 18.13 Upregulation of HLA-ABC in myositis. Immunohistochemistry.

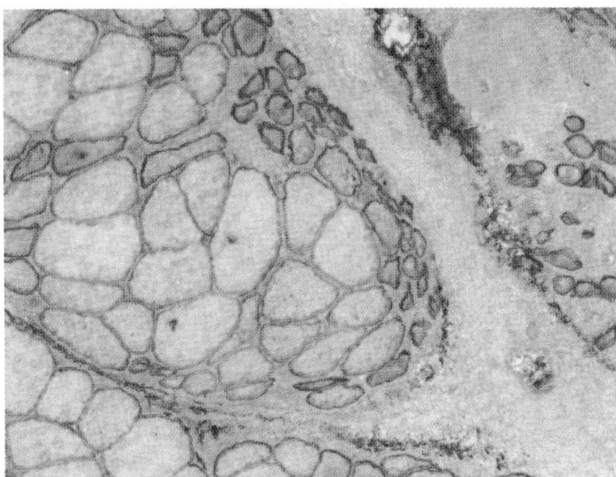

Figure 18.14 Perifascicular fiber atrophy in dermatomyositis. Immunohistochemistry.

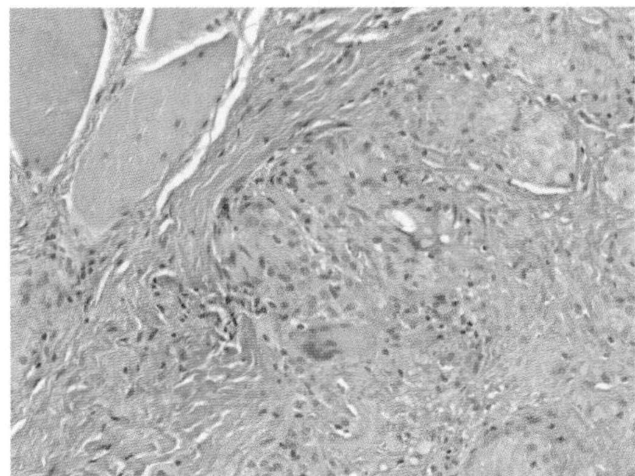

Figure 18.15 A large sarcoid granuloma within muscle. H&E.

symptoms including, for instance, myocarditis. Two age peaks are seen, one in childhood and the other in late middle age. Here there is a well-established relationship to malignancy, ovarian carcinoma being the most common. Serum CK is high at around 50 000 IU. The postulated mechanism of damage is vasculitis. The muscle shows destructive features with characteristic perifascicular atrophy (Fig. 18.14). A perimysial perivascular vasculitis may be seen.

Inclusion body myositis

Inclusion body myositis presents as an insidious asymmetrical distal weakness in the late middle-aged, more frequently in men. It is often been misdiagnosed as polymyositis and is referred because the patient fails to improve with immunosuppression: an appropriate treatment for polymyositis but not inclusion body myositis. Serum CK is not as high as polymyositis, typically less than 10 000 IU. The disease can cause dysphagia. There is no increased incidence in malignancy. The etiology is unknown. Like polymyositis there are destructive features with a random scattered atrophy and a CD8+ T-cell infiltrate; however, blue-rimmed vacuoles are seen. The vacuoles contain filamentous material and are 15–21 μm in length. Frequently, there are secondary mitochondrial abnormalities and the finding of ragged red fibers is not unexpected.

Viral myositis

Viral myositis tends to manifest as a myalgia such as in influenza. Coxsackie B is myotrophic and can lead to necrosis. Human immunodeficiency virus (HIV) and human T-cell lymphotropic virus 1 (HTLV-1) cause a polymyositic picture.

Bacterial myositis

Muscle is relatively resistant to bacteria but abscesses may form secondary to inoculation; for example, in intravenous drug abusers.

Nematode and protozoal infections

Nematodes cause worldwide pathology: *Trichinella* can migrate to muscle from infected, poorly cooked pork and incite an eosinophilic reaction. Protozoa such as *Toxoplasma* can accumulate in muscle fibers, as can trypanosomes.

Granumolmatous myositis

The most common granulomatous inflammatory disorder is sarcoidosis. The picture is that of systemic sarcoid and a destructive myositis in which granulomata are seen (Fig. 18.15).

DYSTROPHIES

These are genetically determined, chronic progressive destructive myopathies leading to increasing weakness and frequently a raised serum CK. Many

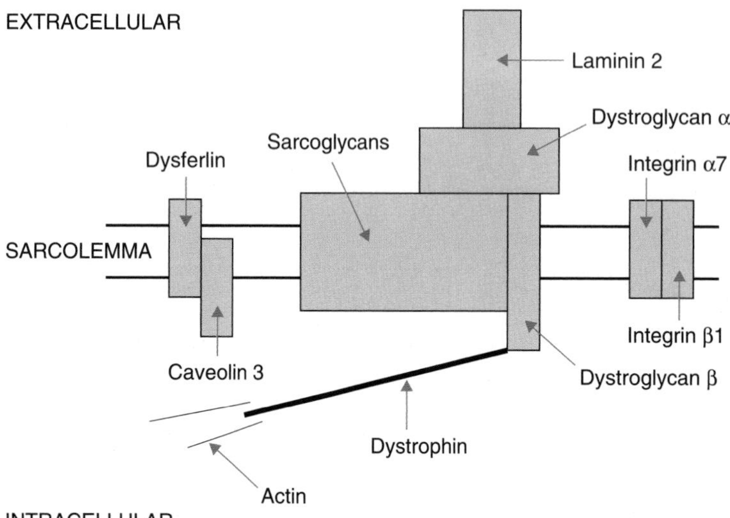

Figure 18.16 Sarcolemmal (membrane) proteins in relation to the extracellular matrix and sarcoplasm.

are multisystem disorders reflecting the wide expression of the proteins involved; however, the protein is typically an important skeletal muscle component leading to symptomatic muscle disease. Autosomal and X-linked inheritance are seen, and female carriers occasionally have muscle weakness due to skewed X-inactivation. An increasing number of dystrophies is being recognized.

Where there is active destruction there is often an inflammatory component. Later on, less-specialized connective tissue replaces muscle so that fibrosis and adipose tissue form with loss of the normal muscle architecture. The morphological changes may be very subtle in infants even in severe dystrophies because accumulated damage has not yet had the time to occur (Fig. 18.16).

Extensive immunohistochemical panels are required for diagnosis of dystrophies and secondary protein losses are very common; this leads to difficulties in interpretation. Western blotting and genetics are important in ultimate diagnosis.

Dystrophinopathies: The Xp21 dystrophies Duchenne and Becker

Dystrophin is the largest sarcolemmal-associated protein and provides an anchor for intracellular proteins, and indirectly to the extracellular matrix. A defect in one of the dystrophin-associated proteins frequently leads to secondary abnormalities in other structural proteins compounding the pathology. This has a clinical impact but must also be borne in mind by the pathologist interpreting the investigations. *Dystrophin* is normally expressed in different tissues resulting in the potential for a multisystem disorder.

There are two major disorders resulting from mutations in the *dystrophin gene* situated on Xp21: Duchenne muscular dystrophy, which is usually caused by a frame-shift deletion; and Becker muscular dystrophy, often caused by an in-frame deletion. The effect of the different mutations results in variable quantities of the protein dystrophin, with a total loss in Duchenne muscular dystrophy, but a reduction in Becker muscular dystrophy. It is the quantity of dystrophin that leads to the clinical symptoms and presentations. Becker is milder, presents later and has a slower rate of progression.

Duchenne muscular dystrophy is a severe, progressive destructive myopathy affecting 1/3500 liveborn males (Figs 18.17 and 18.18). Fiber destruction leads to high CK in the blood. Infants may be floppy, later developing a waddling gait, combined with the Gower's maneuver, using their hands to climb up their body when attempting standing. Calf muscles are hypertrophic. As the disease progresses there is a loss of ability to walk around 12 years of age. Eventually, the respiratory muscles are affected. Intelligence is characteristically lower, often with

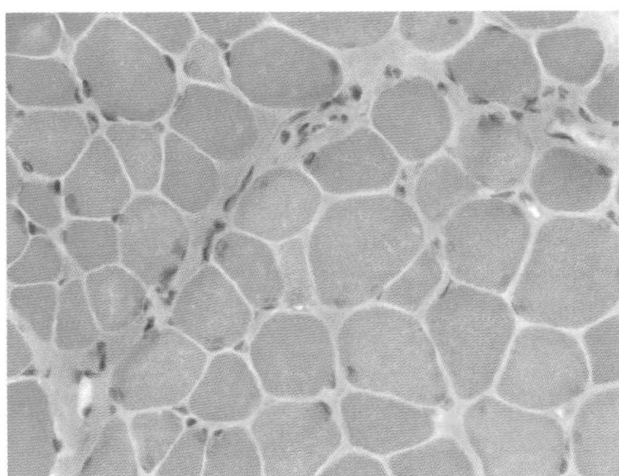

Figure 18.17 Duchenne muscular dystrophy in a 2-year-old. H&E.

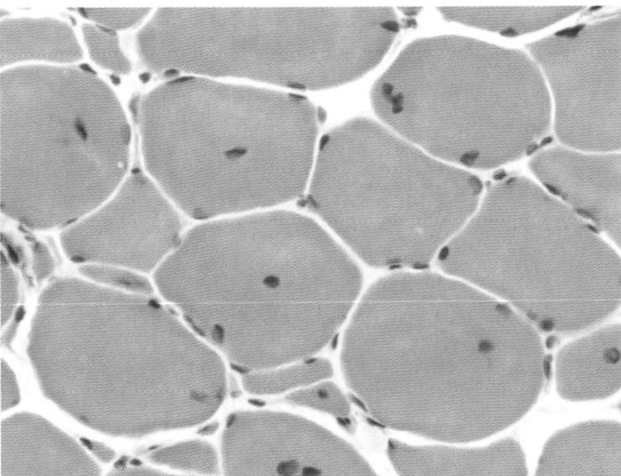

Figure 18.18 Duchenne muscular dystrophy in a 6-year-old. H&E.

learning difficulties, when compared with unaffected siblings. Cardiomyopathy may be a serious problem manifesting as disordered heart rhythm.

In Becker muscular dystrophy the history is as for Duchenne but much milder: there are fewer symptoms and rate of progression is slower, whilst affected boys are older. Indeed, in some patients, the symptoms do not become manifest until middle age. Becker muscular dystrophy affects 1/17 500 live-born males. Again, cardiomyopathy may be a serious problem.

Biopsy changes

These increase with age and accruing damage. There is a marked variation in fiber size with both atrophic and hypertrophic fibers. Fiber necrosis and regeneration are present. Endomysial fibrosis and

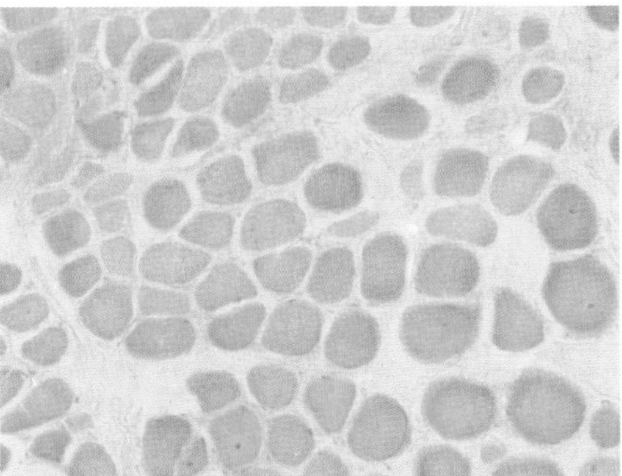

Figure 18.19 Duchenne muscular dystrophy showing total loss of dystrophin 2. Immunohistochemistry.

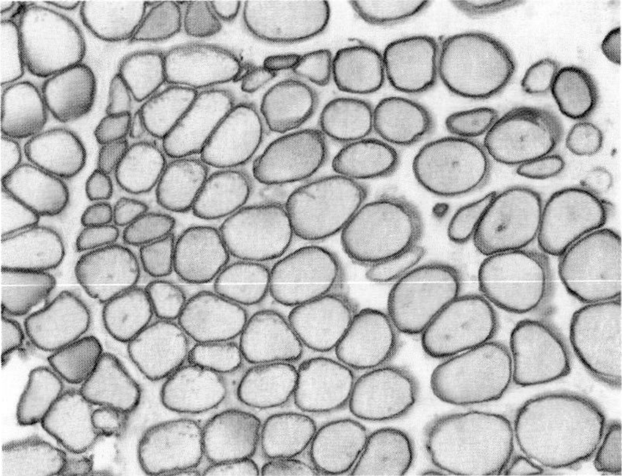

Figure 18.20 Duchenne muscular dystrophy normal spectrin control. Immunohistochemistry.

adipose replacement are seen. Staining using antibodies to the dystrophin protein shows a total loss in Duchenne muscular dystrophy (Fig. 18.19), and a variable reduction in Becker muscular dystrophy. Care must be taken to use three different antibodies (dystrophins 1, 2 and 3) covering a large part of the dystrophin protein in conjunction with antibodies to spectrin and urotrophin to determine the integrity of the sarcolemma (Figs 18.20 and 18.21). It is possible in Becker muscular dystrophy to have a total loss of one epitope.

Female carriers

Occasionally the disease is manifest ('manifesting carriers') in women. This occurs when the embryological inactivation of one X-chromosome in

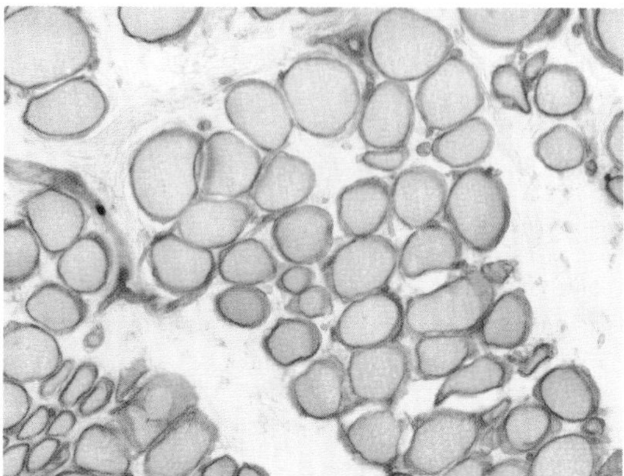

Figure 18.21 Duchenne muscular dystrophy utrophin upregulation.

many nuclei results in a high percentage of affected nuclei remaining.

Emery–Dreifuss disease

Emerin and lamin A/C are among the proteins embedded in the inner nuclear membrane. The functions of these are poorly understood. Two dystrophies are described: an X-linked deficiency of emerin termed X-linked Emery–Dreifuss muscular dystrophy, and an autosomal dominant deficiency of lamin A/C confusingly called autosomal dominant Emery–Dreifuss muscular dystrophy. In both, there are early limb contractures, a slowly progressive humero-peroneal wasting and weakness. Myocardial disease can result in sudden death. Dystrophic changes are seen on biopsy. Emerin staining is negative in the X-linked form, but this is not the case with loss of lamin A/C where emerin staining is normal.

The limb-girdle muscular dystrophies

Limb-girdle muscular dystrophies (LGMDs) form a heterogeneous group of mainly recessive autosomal conditions. They usually develop in adulthood. The serum CK varies with the underlying condition.

The classic nomenclature is confusing; however, the dominant dystrophies are LGMD-1, whereas the recessive are LGMD-2, with letters from 'A' onwards indicating the clinical disease pattern. As protein deficiencies are increasingly identified the diseases are being labeled this way, e.g. LGMD-2B is dysferlinopathy.

Table 18.7 Classification of sarcoglycan-opathies

Protein	Site of mutation	Inheritance and subtype of LGMD
α-sarcoglycan	17q21	Recessive LGMD-2D
β-sarcoglycan	4q12	Recessive LGMD-2E
γ-sarcoglycan	13q12	Recessive LGMD-2C
δ-sarcoglycan	5q33–34	Recessive LGMD-2F

Sarcoglycanopathies

The classification of sarcoglycanopathies is given in Table 18.7. The sarcoglycans are situated within the skeletal muscle sarcolemmal membrane. α-, β-, γ-, and δ-sarcoglycan are each associated with an auto-somal recessive limb-girdle dystrophy. They are closely related physically with dystrophin; thus, a defect in one sarcoglycan can lead to a secondary dystrophin loss as reflected in immunohistochemistry. The sarcoglycans form a linked protein complex, the loss of one leading to a severe loss of the others. ζ-sarcoglycan is not associated with a limb-girdle dystrophy and ϵ-sarcoglycan has a very low expression in normal skeletal muscle.

α-sarcoglycanopathy is the most common, although all are rare. α-sarcoglycan is also known as adhalin.

There is a very wide variation in limb-girdle weakness depending on the amount of protein lost and there may be a cardiomyopathy. There is a high serum CK. Biopsies morphologically resemble other dystrophies.

Dysferlinopathies 2p13.3 recessive LGMD-2B

Clinically, autosomal recessive mutations in the *dysferlin* gene at 2p13 manifest as two disorders: Miyoshi myopathy and LGMD type 2B. These are distal myopathies: in the leg, gastrocnemius is especially affected. Very rarely, both forms are described in the same family. Both result in dysferlin protein deficiency. There is a typical dystrophic picture and serum CK is high.

Caveolinopathies 3p25 dominant LGMD-1C

Here there may be no dystrophic changes in muscle but the serum CK is elevated and the patient complains of muscle cramps. Weakness is usually proximal, while muscle rippling can be elicited on percussion.

Calpainopathy 15q15 recessive LGMD-2A

Calpain-3 deficiency results in a myopathy varying from a clinical picture of muscle with normal strength but a raised CK to a severe dystrophy and weakness. There are different disease patterns: scapular, pelvic and trunk to a proximal limb-girdle picture. Toe walking is common in infants and quadriceps may be spared.

Other dystrophies

Facioscapulohumeral dystrophy 4q35 dominant

Facioscapulohumeral dystrophy is associated with a characteristic reduction in size of a DNA fragment at the telomere of 4q35. The size of the deletion determines the severity of the disease and the age of onset. When severe it may be congenital, associated with epilepsy, cognitive impairment and cardiac conduction defects; in its mild form it is asymptomatic. The face is often initially involved with progression to arms and legs. Scapular winging is seen. There is no extraocular involvement. Disease progression is often slow with long survival. In the early stages a heavy CD8+ T-cell inflammatory infiltrate of the muscle is common.

Oculopharyngeal dystrophy

This dystrophy manifests as a proximal myopathy with external ophthalmoplegia and dysphagia. CK is normal or mildly elevated. Patients are usually over 45 years of age. An autosomal dominant defect at 14q11.2–q13 affects the polyadenylate binding protein nuclear (*PABN*) gene. This is a GCG repeat disorder, longer repeats resulting in more severe and earlier-onset disease. Histologically, there are intranuclear inclusions composed of 8.5 μm filaments. Vaculoes can be seen within the fiber cytoplasm.

Merosin (laminin α2) deficient congenital muscular dystrophy 6q22 recessive

This is the most common of the rare congenital muscular dystrophies due to laminin α2 deficiency. Clinically, babies are floppy with a high serum CK. There are diffuse periventricular white matter brain changes on cranial MRI. Prolonged prenatal laminin α5 persistence occurs which is functionally poor. Neonatal disorders can have a striking inflammatory cell infiltrate; laminin α2 deficiency may be misdiagnosed as infantile polymyositis. With severe disease patients die in their second to third decade due to respiratory failure.

CONGENITAL MYOPATHIES

Centronuclear/myotubular myopathy

This often refers to a severe congenital myopathy, genetically characterized by X-linked inheritance with myotubularin loss. *In utero* there is polyhydramnious with weak fetal movements, and when born, babies are globally weak. The respiration is poor and they rapidly become ventilator dependent. The prognosis is very poor; death often occurs at around 5 months. Milder, later onset autosomal forms exist which present with a limb-girdle distribution of weakness. Biopsies show type 1 predominance and type 1 atrophy, while the type 1 fibers also have a single central nucleus.

Nemaline rod myopathy

This congenital myopathy is distinctive with nemaline rod accumulation in muscle fibers. The most common mutation involves 1q42.1 resulting in abnormal α-actin. Occasionally, other proteins are abnormal: α-tropomyosin 3, nebulin, β-tropomyosin or troponin T1. The myopathy causes

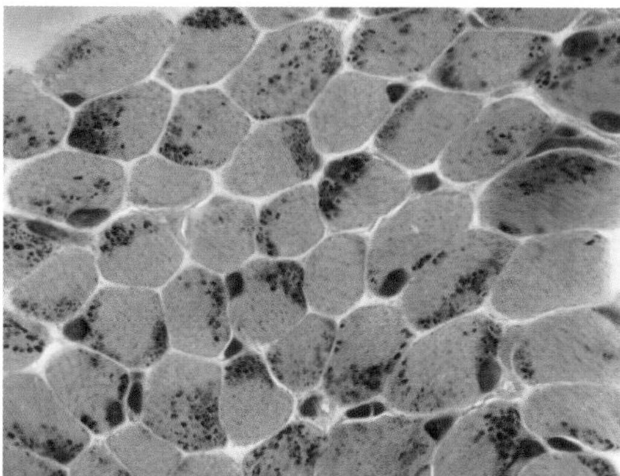

Figure 18.22 Nemaline rods in the muscle fibers. Gomori trichrome.

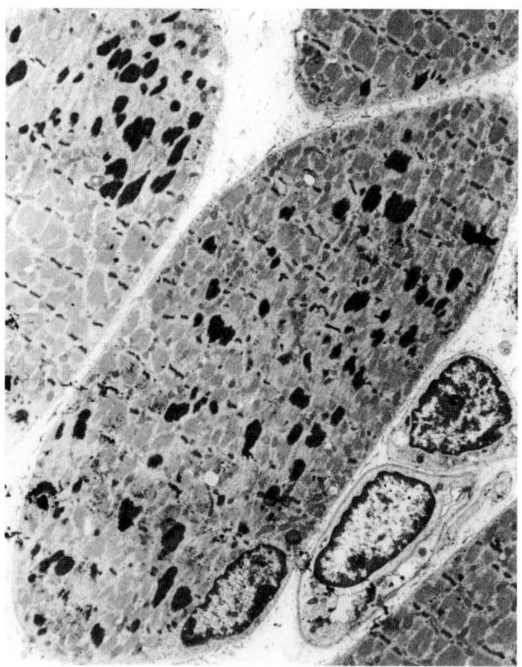

Figure 18.23 Nemaline rods. Electron microscopy ×3500.

respiratory failure and hypotonia. Death is due to respiratory failure. Histologically, red-colored rods are seen in the fiber cytoplasm in the Gomori trichrome stain (Fig. 18.22). These rods are composed of thin filaments. They are more common in type 1 fibers and there is no relation between the numbers of rods and disease severity (Fig. 18.23).

Central core disease

Most cases of central core disease are attributable to a dominant mutation at 19q13.1 involving the *ryanodine receptor gene*. The resultant protein is normally responsible for calcium transport. In itself it is a non-progressive or a slowly progressive disorder that can ultimately result in a limb-girdle picture. A notable clinical feature is the predisposition to malignant hyperthermia with halothane anesthesia. It is important to comment on this risk in the pathological report and ensure that the patient is informed. The patient's family may also be at risk. Non-anesthetic-related sudden death can also occur.

Malignant hyperthermia manifests as calcium-induced muscle contraction, tachycardia, lactic acidosis and hyperthermia. Muscle necrosis occurs with consequent CK and myoglobin release into blood and subsequently urine, sometimes precipitating acute renal failure. Morphologically, cores are seen extending the entire length of the muscle fiber.

Minicore disease

Here the cores do not extend the length of the muscle fibers. Although not in general associated with malignant hyperthermia, there are a few reported overlap cases. This is a genetically heterogeneous group with mutations identified in the *ryanodine receptor gene, selenoprotein N1 gene* and short-chain acyl-CoA dehydrogenase activity.

The onset is often with axial weakness, a scoliosis and respiratory insufficiency. Arthrogryposis and ophthalmoplegia are common.

CONGENITAL FIBER-TYPE DISPROPORTION

Here type 1 fibers are hypotrophic, while type 2 are normal. Many cast doubt on this condition being a distinct entity. No characteristic genetic defect has been found, nor a defined clinical syndrome, and a variety of identified conditions can cause differences in fiber sizes; for example, centronuclear, nemaline rod and minicore myopathies.

METABOLIC DISEASES: GLYCOGENOSES AND LIPID DISORDERS

Histochemistry can only to a degree be helpful here; to prove a serious disorder direct enzyme assay is required, with genetics if possible.

Glycogenoses

Myophosphorylase deficiency

Principal among the group of disorders known as glycogenoses is myophosphorylase deficiency or McArdle's disease. In teenage/early-adult onset disorder there are glycogen-containing vacuoles. Myophosphorylase staining is negative. Exercise intolerance is noted, especially after brief intense exercise. Thence follows a 'second wind' after a short break. Cramps are also a feature. CK is elevated at rest. The ischemic lactate test shows a 'flat curve', the serum lactate failing to rise after anerobic exercise. This finding characterizes all glycolytic pathway metabolic muscle disorders.

Acid maltase deficiency (acid α-1,4-glucosidase)

Acid maltase (acid α-1,4-glucosidase) deficiency (Pompe disease) is also notable. This glycogen storage disease affects 1/50 000 live births. Many mutations have been identified and the level of the resultant enzyme activity correlates well with age of onset and disease severity. Severe, infantile disease results in hypotonia, with prominent cardiac and liver involvement. Respiratory distress occurs and death ensues within a few months of birth. Glycogen accumulates in most tissues. In adult-onset acid maltase deficiency fatigability, cramps and muscle weakness are seen. Biopsy shows membrane-bound vacuoles containing glycogen and also shows increased acid phosphatase staining indicative of lysosomal activity.

Phosphofructokinase deficiency

Phosphofructokinase deficiency (Tarui's disease) can result from many different mutations in the gene coding for phosphofructokinase. This can result in an adult-onset myopathy that results in cramps, exercise intolerance and hemolytic anemia. Biopsy shows vacuoles of polysaccharide, in this instance not digested by diastase. Myophosphorylase is negative.

Lipid disorders

Mitochondrial oxidative metabolism of lipids is a major source of energy production for skeletal muscle. Cramps and myoglobinuria are classically induced by exercise. These disorders may be associated with cardiomyopathy and sudden death. Biochemical analysis and genetics are important in diagnosis.

Carnitine is required as part of the enzyme carnitine palmitoyltransferase that transports fatty acids into mitochondria. Therefore, deficiencies in carnitine itself or mutations in the gene coding for this enzyme result in fatty acid disorders.

Systemic carnitine disorders can occur where there is reduced protein synthesis, such as malnutrition and organ failure. Carnitine can be lost because of reduced renal reabsorption due to loss or dysfunction of the transporter enzyme, carnitine transporter. In mutations of the gene coding for this enzyme systemic illness in infancy is notable, manifest as hypoglycemia, encephalopathy, myopathy, cardiomyopathy and hepatomegaly.

Carnitine palmitoyltransferase 2 deficiency reduces fatty acid Co-A transport into mitochondria. This usually presents in young adults who reveal a history of cramps and repeated myoglobinuria after exercise.

MITOCHONDRIAL DISORDERS

This is a heterogeneous group, the pathology of which can manifest in any organ; however, skeletal muscle, the heart and the brain are frequently involved because of their high oxidative requirements. Disorders in this group can be sporadic, inherited or secondary.

The DNA coding for the mitochondrial proteins is derived from two sources: mitochondrial (mtDNA) and nuclear (nDNA). There are many disorders in this group, some resulting from large deletions, others from point mutations, and different mutations can cause the same clinical syndromes under certain circumstances. mtDNA is maternally derived resulting in non-Mendelian inheritance; nDNA undergoes the typical Mendelian route.

Critical to the understanding of these disorders is the concept of heteroplasmy. Each fiber contains many mitochondria. It is possible for some mitochondria to be abnormal while adjacent mitochondria are normal. The number of abnormal mitochondria will determine the muscle fiber's overall ultimate oxidative capacity. In addition, adjacent fibers can have different percentages of functioning mitochondria. Should function be below a threshold level, symptoms will result and anerobic respiration results in lactate production. Fibers homoplasmic for abnormal mitochondria will have no respiratory function at all. Further, heteroplasmy may be skewed in that the mutation load may only surpass the symptomatic threshold in one tissue leading to an atypical clinical presentation.

The muscle biopsy may be abnormal in a mitochondrial disorder. Simple stains for glycogen and lipid can sometimes show non-specific changes indicating poor metabolic function. Modified Gomori trichrome may reveal ragged red fibers that are aggregates of mitochondria (Fig. 18.24). The histochemical stains are more helpful. Cytochrome oxidase is often negative, while succinic dehydrogenase is the most sensitive stain and may show increased staining (Figs 18.25 and 18.26). These patterns are not pathognomonic and variations may be seen. The diagnostic requirement for electron microscopy is questionable; however, abnormal mitochondria are often bizarre and may have paracrystalline inclusions (Figs 18.27 and 18.28). If a mitochondrial disorder is suspected then regardless of the biopsy results muscle is usually sent to national reference centers for mitochondrial enzyme assay and genetic analysis.

Myoclonic epilepsy with ragged red fibers (MERRF)

This is a disorder resulting from a point mutation *A8344G* in mtDNA in 80% of patients.

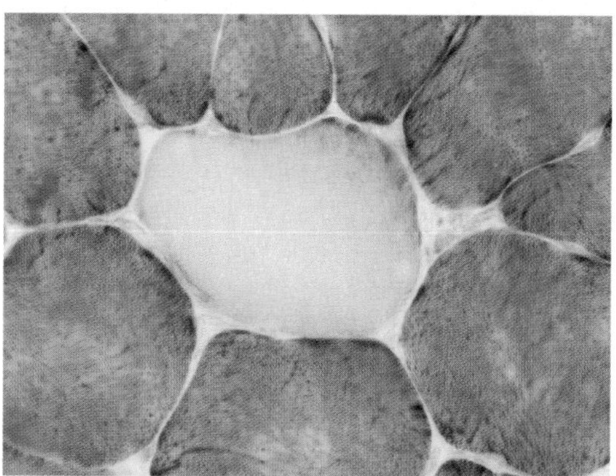

Figure 18.25 Cytochrome oxidase-negative fiber. COX histochemistry.

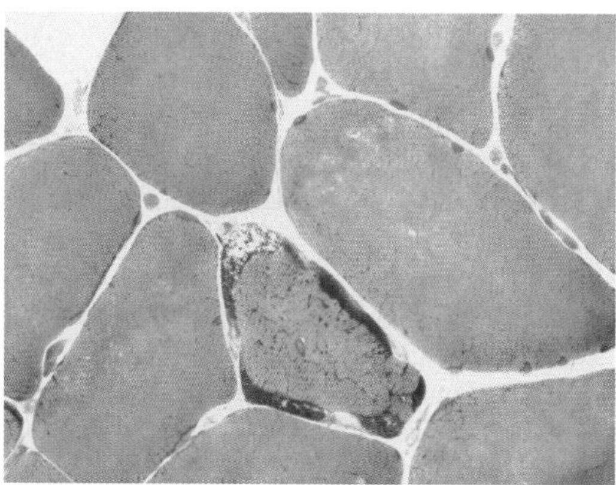

Figure 18.24 Ragged red fibers. Gomori trichrome.

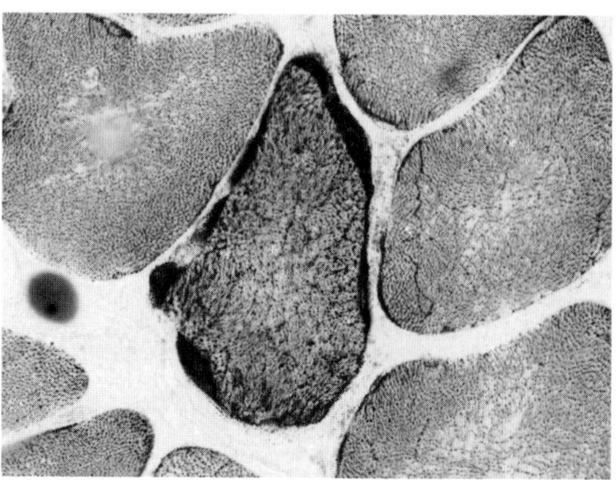

Figure 18.26 Succinic dehydrogenase-positive fiber. SDH histochemistry.

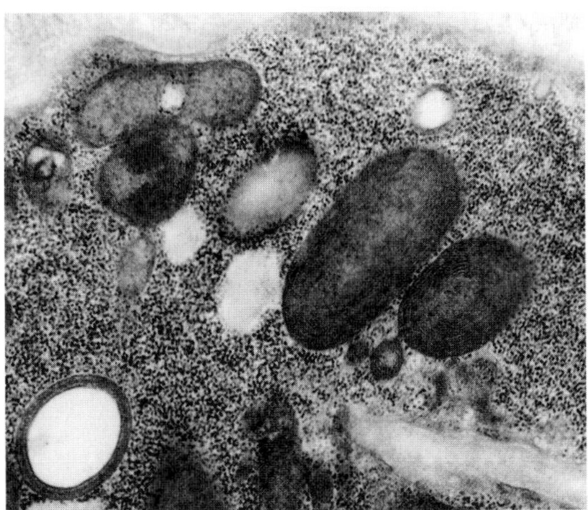

Figure 18.27 Abnormal mitochondria. Electron microscopy ×50 000.

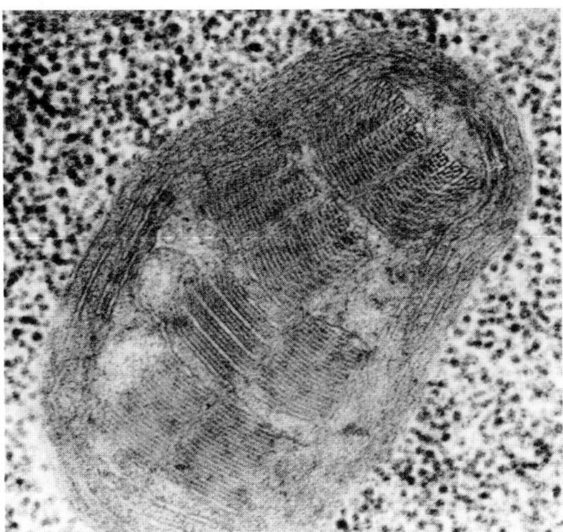

Figure 18.28 Paracrystalline inclusions in a mitochondrion. Electron microscopy ×120 000.

Manifestations due to central nervous system involvement include myoclonic epilepsy and ataxia, while there is also skeletal muscle weakness.

Mitochondrial encephalomyopathy like symptoms with lactic acidosis and stroke (MELAS)

This is another disorder due to point mutations, this time mtDNA *A3243G*. Patients here may present with migraine-like attacks. Blood vessels in the brain show abnormal levels of succinic dehydrogenase (in frozen section). It is this vascular pathology that causes the strokes. Cardiomyopathy is seen in approximately 15% of patients. Muscle fibers display mitochondrial pathology as may the blood vessels in the muscle biopsy.

Kearns–Sayre syndrome

This is an example of mitochondrial disorder caused by a large mtDNA deletion. There is a large number of features, including external ophthalmoplegia, dysphagia, weakness, ataxia, dementia, cardiac and endocrine abnormalities.

Of secondary disorders, ragged red fibers are often seen in inclusion body myositis, while the drug azidothymidine (AZT, zidovudine) classically affects mitochondria.

ION CHANNEL DISORDERS

Calcium, potassium and sodium channel disorders can cause myopathies. Periodic weakness and myotonia are the 'hallmark' clinical features. Importantly, these patients, also, may develop malignant hyperthermia after anesthesia.

The disorders are attributable to mutations in the nucleic acid coding for the subunits forming the channels in the sarcolemma. Although among the non-destructive myopathies, this is a relative term because repeated attacks result in cumulative muscle damage. There may be vacuolation and accumulation of T-tubules during and just after paralytic episodes. One of the calcium channel proteins, ryanodine receptor 1, is associated with central core disease when abnormal. Occasionally, cardiac abnormalities are present in channelopathies manifesting as arrhythmias.

MYOTONIC DYSTROPHY

Myotonic dystrophy type 1 (DM1) is the most common form involving 98% of patients. The gene for myotonic dystrophy protein kinase (*DMPK*) on 19q13.3 contains abnormal CTG repeats. There is an autosomal dominant pattern of inheritance. The larger the triplet repeat number the more severe the disease and the earlier the onset. There is

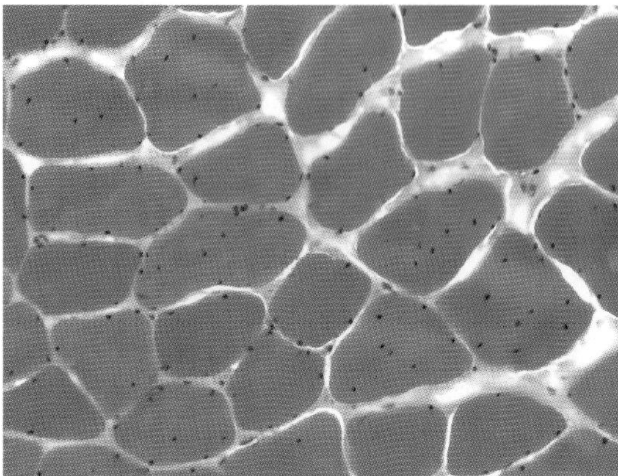

Figure 18.29 Multiple internal nuclei in muscle fibers in a case of myotonic dystrophy. H&E.

genetic anticipation, meaning the CTG repeat number increases through generations, resulting in succeeding offspring being more severely affected at a younger age.

There is myotonia and weakness of muscles, the latter affecting the face and limbs. There is no ophthalmoplegia. Approximately 20% are cognitively impaired and subcortical white matter changes are seen on MRI. Frontal balding and cataracts are seen, while hypogonadism and insulin resistance are also features. Respiratory function can be compromised. Cardiac arrhythmias occur leading to an increased risk of sudden death. The cardiorespiratory problems can lead to difficulties with anesthesia.

Muscle biopsy shows selective type 1 atrophy and type 1 predominance. Ring fibers are present and there are many internal nuclei within muscle fibers (Fig. 18.29).

Myotonic dystrophy type 2 (DM2) is much less common. It is also known as proximal myotonic myopathy (PROMM). This is a dominant disorder affecting the gene for zinc finger protein 9 on chromosome 3q21. Clinical symptoms are very similar to type 1.

MOTOR END-PLATE MYOPATHIES

Myasthenia gravis

Myasthenia gravis has a bimodal age of onset: in the third decade with a female predominance, and in the seventh decade with a male predominance. The presenting symptoms are ocular in 50% of cases with ptosis and diplopia, respectively, due to extraocular muscle or levator palpebrae weakness. The pupils are normal. Limb, facial and bulbar weakness also are seen. Respiratory failure may occur. The characteristic diagnostic feature is that of muscle fatigability.

The disease is caused by IgG antibodies against the α-1 subunit of the acetylcholine receptor on the neuromuscular junction.

The antibodies may be seen as part of a paraneoplastic syndrome secondary to a thymoma. Thirty percent of patients with thymoma have myasthenia gravis and 15% of myasthenic patients have thymomas.

The tensilon (edrophonium HCl) test is useful in diagnosis. Here edrophonium inhibits acetylcholinesterase, which prolongs action of acetylcholine at the neuromuscular junction. It is not specific for myasthenia gravis. Electrophysiology (single-fiber electromyography) is supportive and mediastinal imaging by magnetic resonance or computerized tomography may show thymoma.

Lambert–Eaton syndrome

This is a paraneoplastic myasthenic syndrome most often associated with small-cell carcinoma of the lung or lymphoma. This is a presynaptic disorder with IgG antibodies against calcium channels. The presence in serum of voltage-gated calcium channel antibodies (VGCCA) is diagnostic.

OTHER CONDITIONS

Toxic myopathies, including drugs

A large number of toxins affect muscle; many different mechanisms are seen. Alcohol can cause acute necrosis, corticosteroids frequently are associated with type 2 atrophy, D-penicillamine is the classic example for polymyositis, although statin myotoxicity can manifest with similar pathology. Azidothymidine is often associated with secondary mitochondrial abnormalities. Among the more exotic causes of toxic myopathies are some snake venoms that may cause rhabdomyolysis. A drug history is crucial in interpretation of muscle pathology.

Disuse

Disuse of muscle regardless of the cause results in atrophy, the type 2 fibers being preferentially affected.

Endocrine

Skeletal muscle may be involved in thyroid disease. In hypothyroidism this can manifest as weakness, myalgia and cramps with a raised creatine kinase. Myxedema may occur. Occasionally, rhabdomyolysis develops. In hyperthyroidism weakness with fasciculation may be present. A thyroid 'crisis' may trigger rhabdomyolysis.

Cushing's disease causes similar features to corticosteroid therapy, namely type 2 atrophy. Acromegaly leads to muscle hypertrophy.

Muscle in neurogenic disease

Muscle undergoes a variety of changes in neurogenic disease. Here, the primary pathology is not in the muscle itself but in the motor peripheral nervous system supplying it. Denervation results in fibers undergoing atrophy, which may be so marked as to largely obscure the fiber cytoplasm, leaving only nuclei.

Reinnervation results in healthy motor units supplying denervated fibers and this results in loss of the normal checkerboard pattern seen on fiber typing, i.e. grouping. Figures 18.30 to 18.36 show the changes leading to grouping.

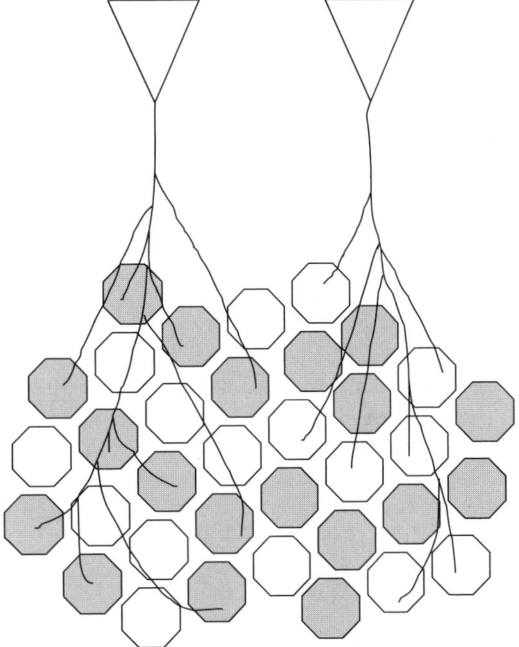

Figure 18.30 Different but adjacent neurons supplying fast and slow fibers, respectively (normal checkerboard pattern).

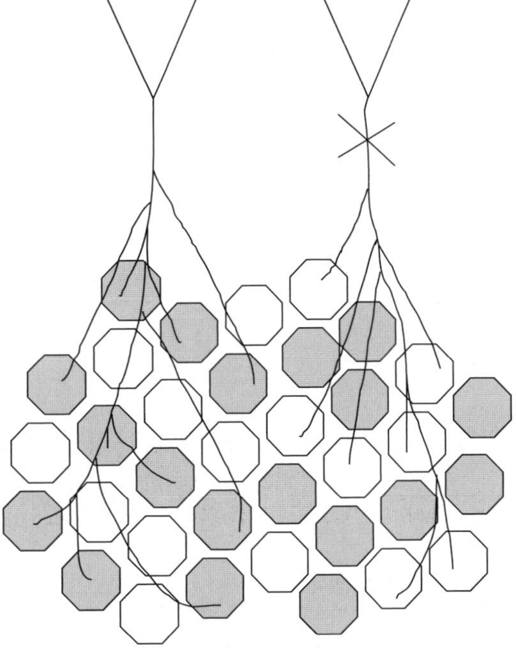

Figure 18.31 Transection of one neuron.

ANTERIOR HORN CELL DISORDERS

Spinal muscular atrophy (SMA)

Spinal muscular atrophy is caused by an abnormality in the survival motor neuron 1 (*SMN 1*)-gene on chromosome 5 at q12.2–q13. The mutation is recessive. The disease incidence is 1 in 6000 to 10 000 births. The protein SMN 1 is normally expressed at high levels in the brain and spinal cord during development. Protein deletion causes loss of motor neurons. In muscle, the same

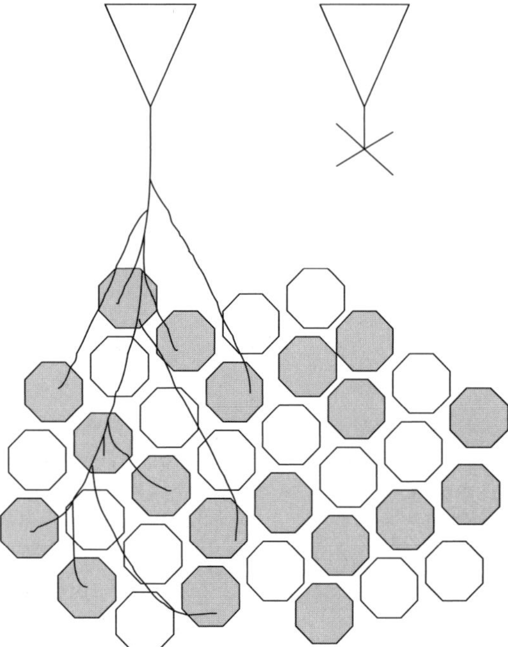

Figure 18.32 Axonal input from dead neuron is lost.

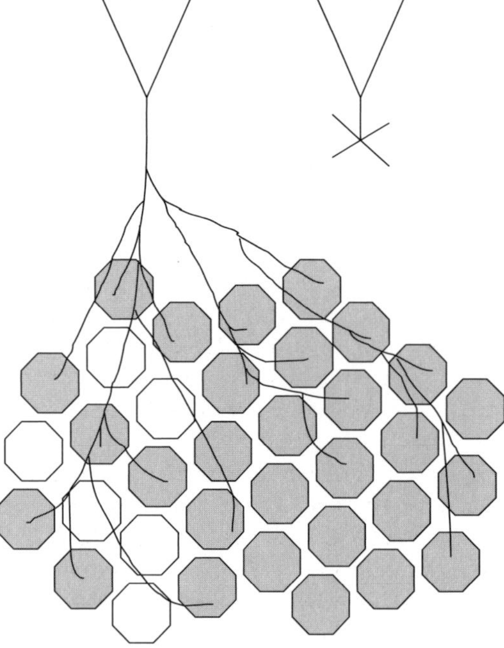

Figure 18.33 Adjacent neuron sends axons to the adjacent fibers resulting in fiber type conversion (groups are seen).

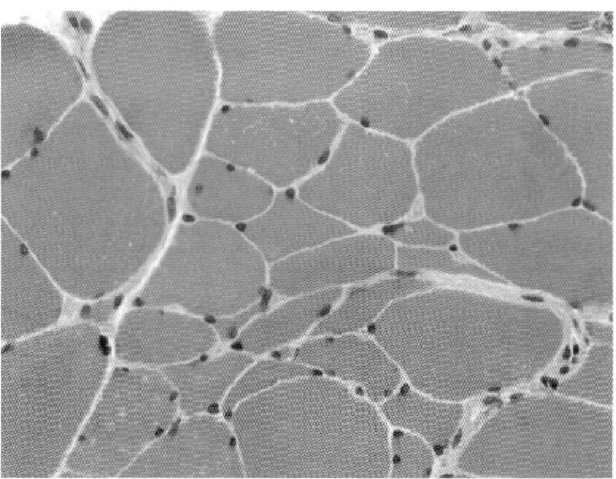

Figure 18.34 Angular fibers in neurogenic atrophy. H&E.

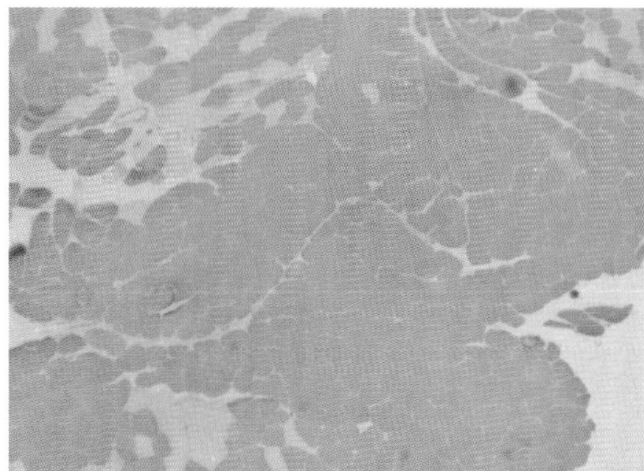

Figure 18.35 Fiber type grouping. ATPase 4.6.

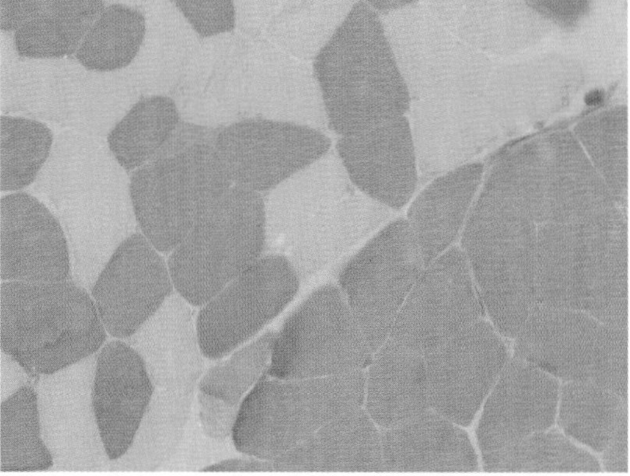

Figure 18.36 One fascicle demonstrating grouping and the adjacent fascicle with a normal checker-board pattern. ATPase 4.6.

protein is concentrated at neuromuscular junctions. Three clinical forms are seen: congenital SMA 5q with arthrogryposis, Werdnig–Hoffmann disease and Kugelberg–Welander disease.

Poliovirus and other enteroviruses

Here the virus infects anterior horn cells in the spinal cord leading to loss of motor nerves and consequent neurogenic atrophy.

Motor neuron disease

This neurodegenerative disease, occasionally associated with superoxide dismutase (*SOD1*) gene mutation, results in loss of anterior horn cells causing a secondary neurogenic atrophy.

NERVE BIOPSY

A peripheral nerve is composed of nerve fibers running in fascicles set within connective tissue. Around each fascicle is the perineurium. The epineurium is the connective tissue outwith the perineurium (Figs 18.37 to 18.39).

A nerve biopsy is a destructive procedure and is not entered into unless an answer to a specific question is sought. As with muscle, it is imperative to have good clinico-pathological correlation. A comprehensive clinical history is very helpful and should cover family, occupational, drug history, disease development and systemic illness. Results of additional investigations, such as electrophysiology, are vital.

The sural nerve, which is a purely sensory nerve, is usually chosen. If a motor nerve is required the musculocutaneous nerve is sampled, along with the underlying muscle. In diffuse pathologies fascicular biopsies may be performed, but these are unsuitable if the pathology is patchy.

The nerve has to be handled very gently to prevent artefacts that can mimic pathology. To facilitate maximum investigations part of the nerve is fixed in formalin for routine paraffin histology, part in glutaraldehyde for both plastic sections and electron microscopy, and part frozen. Plastic sections

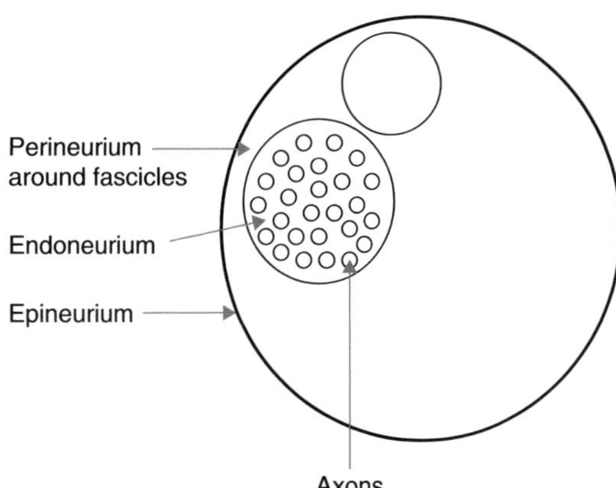

Figure 18.37 Transection of a peripheral nerve indicating relationship of axons, fascicles and connective tissue compartments.

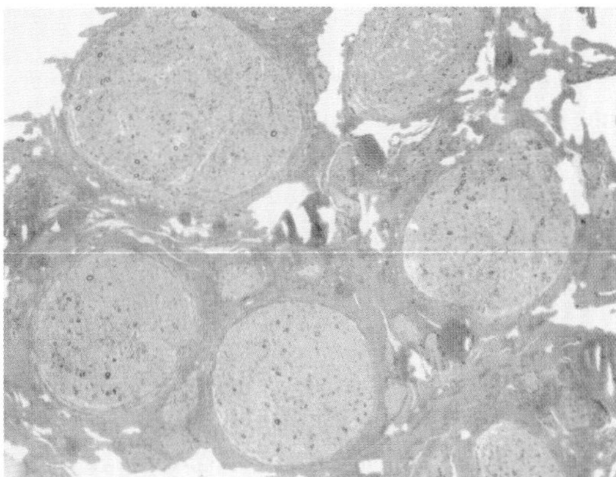

Figure 18.38 A transverse section of nerve illustrating the fascicular architecture. Resin.

are essential for examination of the endoneurium. Electron microscopy is useful to examine unmyelinated fibers and the myelin. Fiber teasing is carried out after osmification in some laboratories and is very helpful to differentiate demyelination from axonal degeneration.

Morphometry has little use in routine practice, but if facilities are present it is most useful in pediatric practice. Useful indices addressed by morphometry include the ratio of myelinated to unmyelinated fibers, the 'g'-ratio (which is the diameter of the axon compared to the diameter of the fiber), the sizes of unmyelinated, small and large myelinated fibers and fiber density. Large myelinated fibers average 9–12 μm in diameter while small myelinated fibers

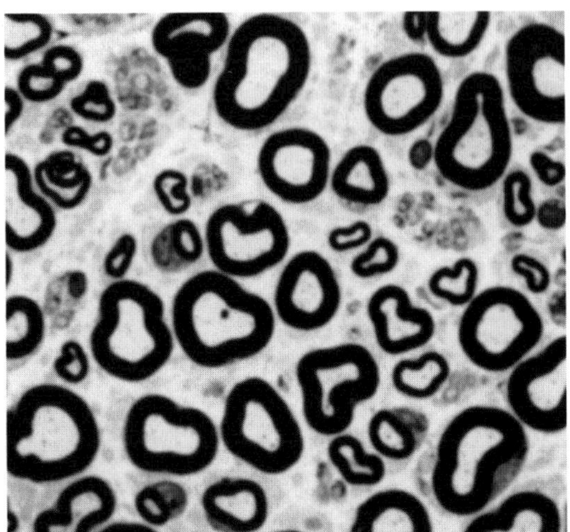

Figure 18.39 Large and small myelinated fibers. Resin.

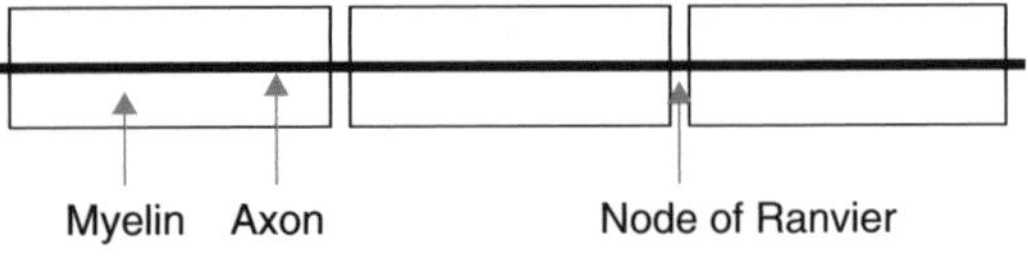

Figure 18.40 Normal myelinated axon.

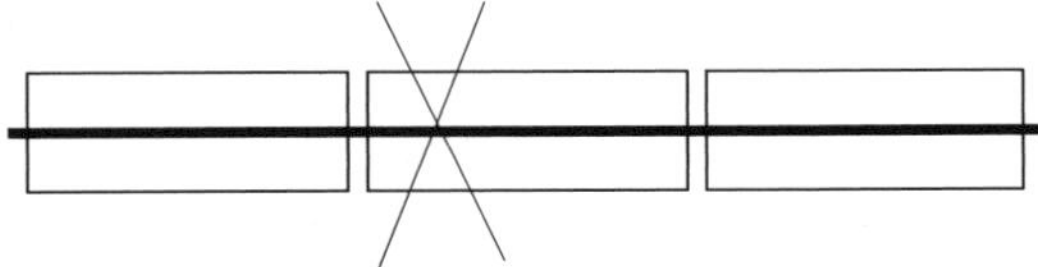

Figure 18.41 Transected myelinated axon.

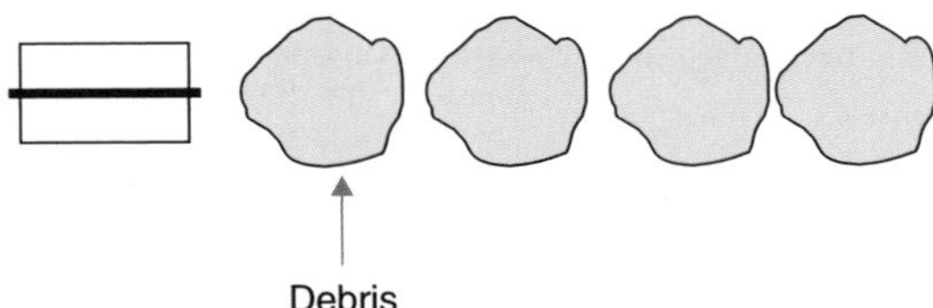

Figure 18.42 Distal degeneration of the myelinated axon.

average 3–5 μm. Unmyelinated fibers have an average diameter of 1.5 μm. Fiber density decreases with age, but there are 7000–10 000 myelinated fibers/mm^2 of endoneurium and 20 000–35 000 unmyelinated fibers/mm^2 of endoneurium in the sural nerve of an average 25-year-old person.

Teased fibers are particularly helpful for assessing internodal lengths. An internode is the length between two nodes of Ranvier serviced by one Schwann cell. Teasing is useful because, after demyelination, Schwann cells proliferate and potentially lead to remyelination. The resulting remyelinated area has a shorter internodal length.

REACTIONS TO INJURY AND DISEASE

Morphological changes in nerve take into account the epineurium, perineurium and endoneurium. It is important to examine the blood vessels at different levels throughout the biopsy. Granulomata, usually due to sarcoid, may be seen. Amyloidosis should be excluded. Assessment of the fascicles to determine if pathology is irregular or diffuse is helpful. Inflammation and vasculitis often result in patchy pathology. It may be helpful to look for preferential loss of large fibers or small myelinated fibers (Figs 18.40 to 18.50).

Axonal degeneration

Axonal pathology has a number of pathological pictures, including ‘dying back’ and Wallerian degeneration.

Dying back is a symmetrical process affecting the longest axons first. *Wallerian degeneration* is the acute pathology distal to axonotomy. Once degeneration has occurred and macrophages phagocytosed debris, then the myelinated axon regenerates and sprouting is seen extending down through bands of Büngner (Figs 18.43 to 18.50).

Axonal degeneration may be due to disorders of the perikaryon. These are not distinctive in biopsy transverse section but may involve specific types of axons (Fig. 18.47).

Features such as axonal swellings due to neurofilament accumulation and collagen pockets may be seen in axonal degeneration and very occasionally help point to the underlying cause (Fig. 18.48).

The actual changes seen depend on the time after onset of pathology. Initially, myelin ovoids are seen which represent the remaining myelin surrounding the degenerating axon. Phagocytosis then ensues with influx of macrophages. If regeneration occurs axonal sprouts appear (Fig. 18.49).

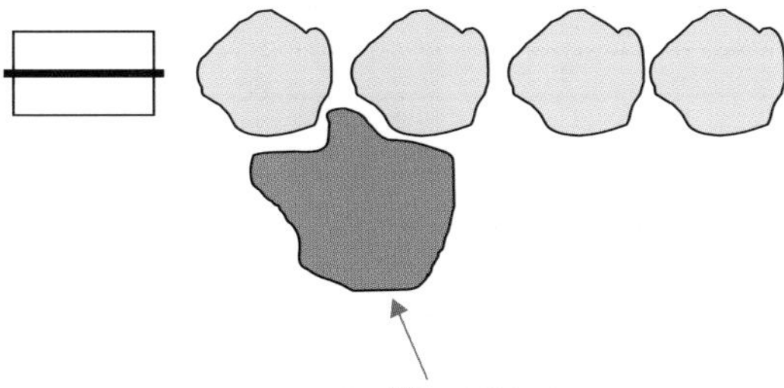

Figure 18.43 Macrophage phagocytosis of debris.

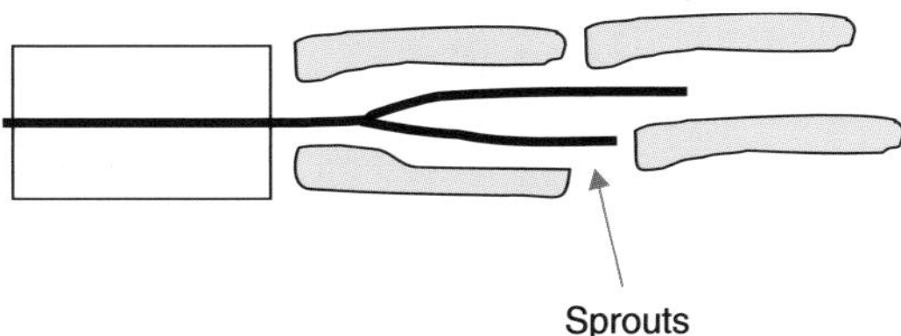

Figure 18.44 Axonal regeneration (sprouting).

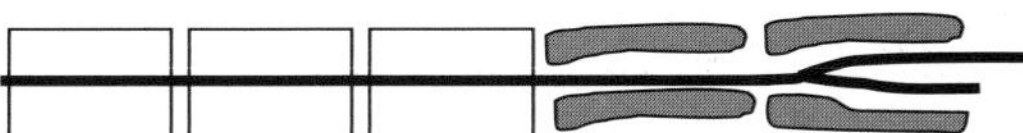

Figure 18.45 Further growth.

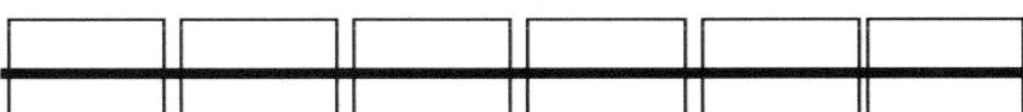

Figure 18.46 Regeneration.

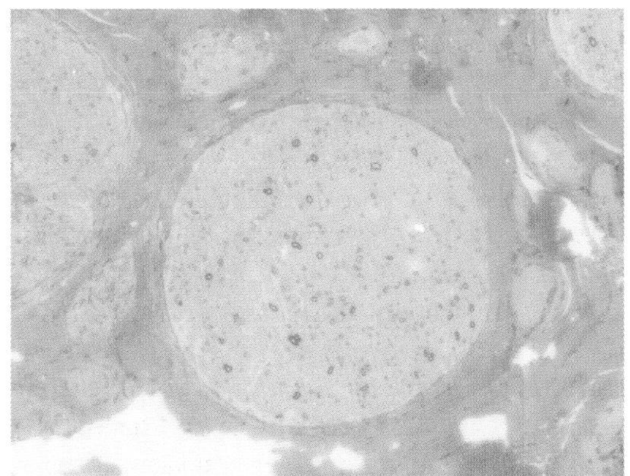

Figure 18.47 Loss of myelinated axons. Resin.

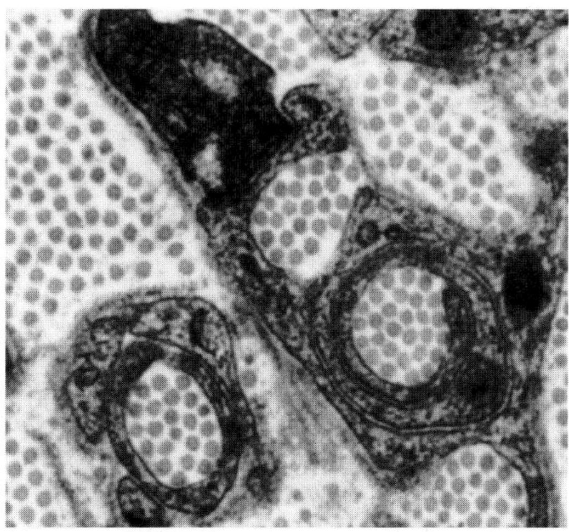

Figure 18.48 Collagen pockets associated with unmyelinated fiber loss. Electron microscopy ×15 000.

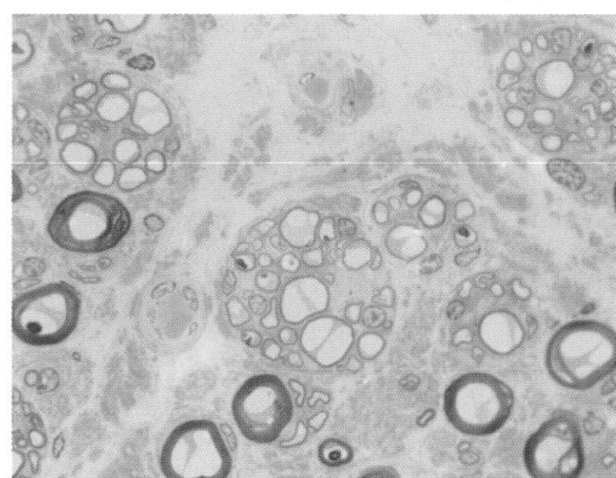

Figure 18.49 Axonal sprouts. Resin.

Remyelination

This may only occur over extremely short lengths of demyelination. The resulting myelin coat will be thin. Repeated demyelination with attempts at remyelination results in Schwann cell onion bulbs. Figures 18.51 to 18.55 illustrate the change.

Certain diagnostically helpful features may be seen, e.g. tomaculae are folds in myelin giving the fiber a swollen appearance. These occur in certain conditions, e.g. hereditary neuropathy with liability to pressure palsies. An examination of

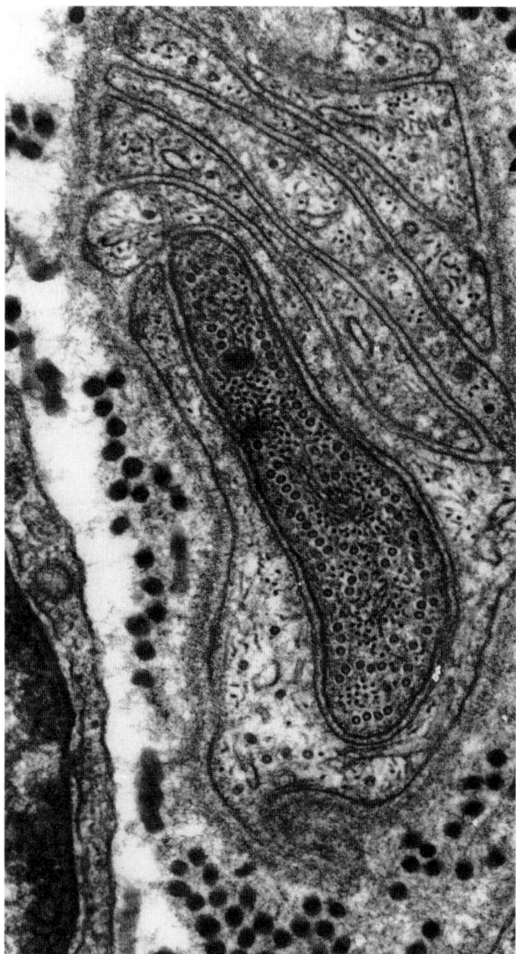

Figure 18.50 Schwann cell banding in response to axonal degeneration. Electron microscopy ×45 000.

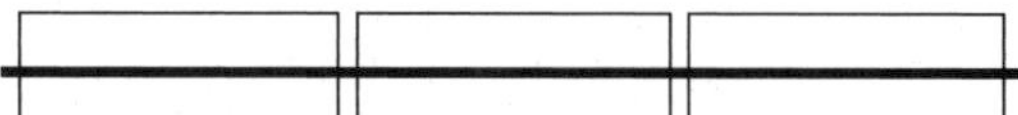

Figure 18.51 Normal myelinated nerve.

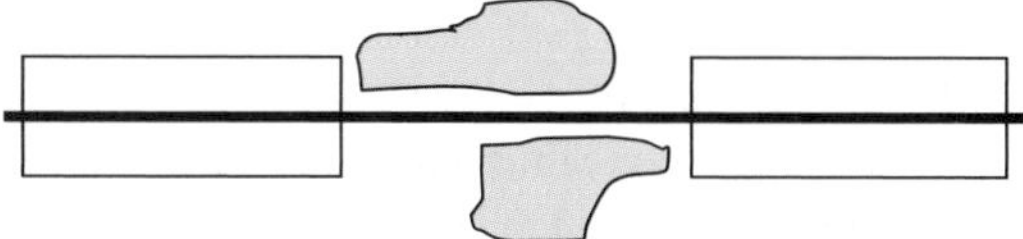

Figure 18.52 Focal demyelination.

myelin periodicity may help determine the etiology of the myelin pathology. *Primary dysmyelination* occurs where myelin is not formed or is poorly formed.

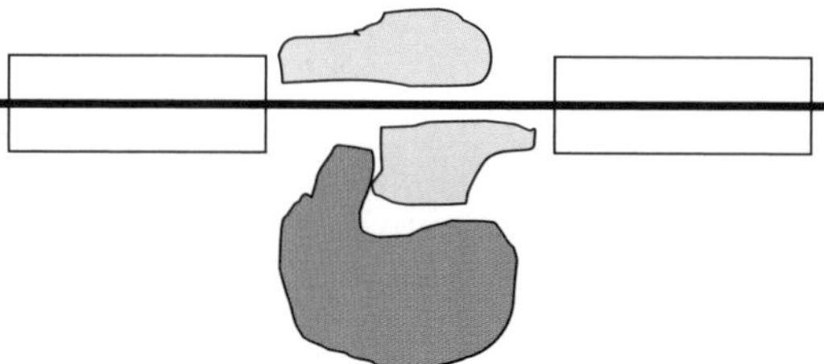

Figure 18.53 Macrophage phagocytosis.

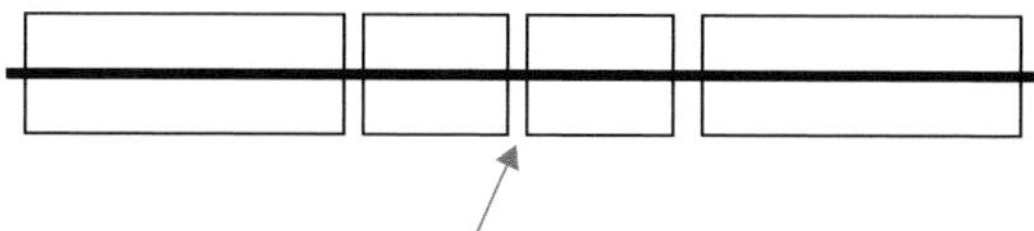

Figure 18.54 Remyelinated short segment with decreased internodal length.

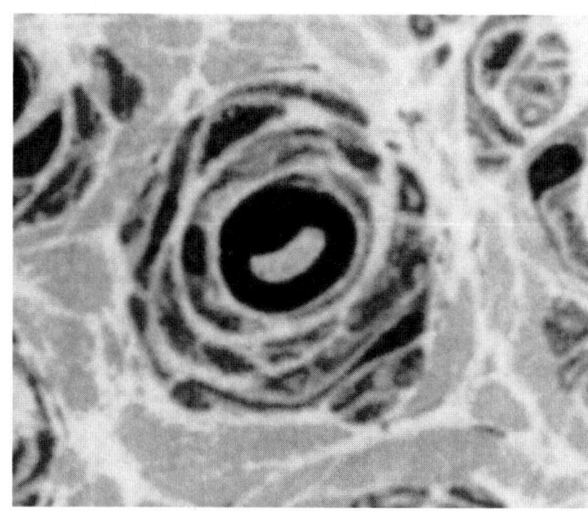

Figure 18.55 Schwann cells around an axon forming an onion bulb. Resin.

VASCULITIS

Diagnosing systemic or peripheral-nerve-confined vasculitis is one of the major reasons for performing a nerve biopsy (Fig. 18.56). Typically, the presentation is that of a mononeuritis multiplex characterized by asymmetric and patchy peripheral nerve involvement. In addition there may be systemic symptoms attributable to the specific underlying vasculitic disorder e.g. Churg–Strauss syndrome.

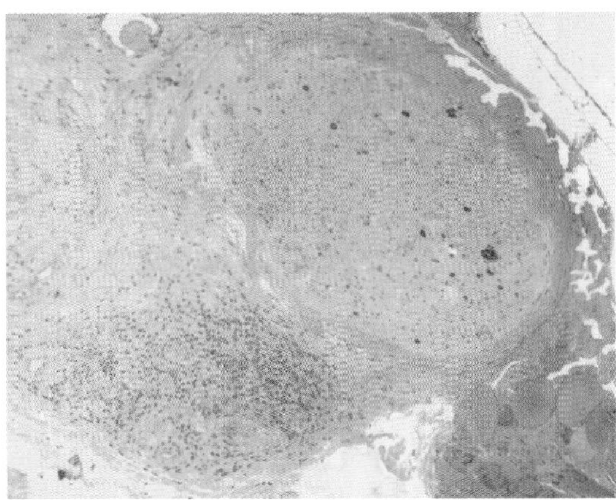

Figure 18.56 Axonal degeneration (right) secondary to small vessel vasculitis (left). Resin.

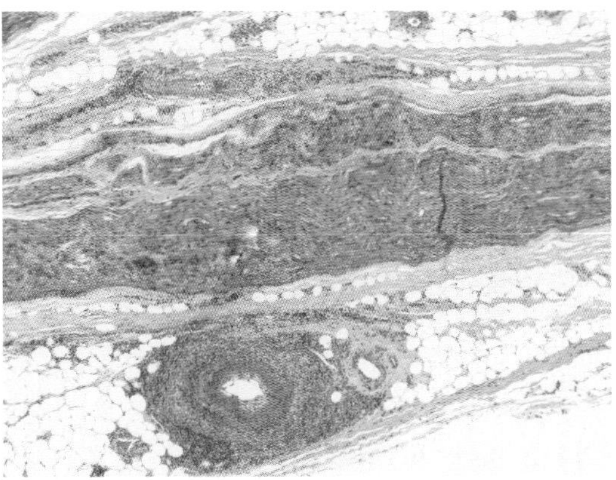

Figure 18.57 Polyarteritis nodosa. H&E.

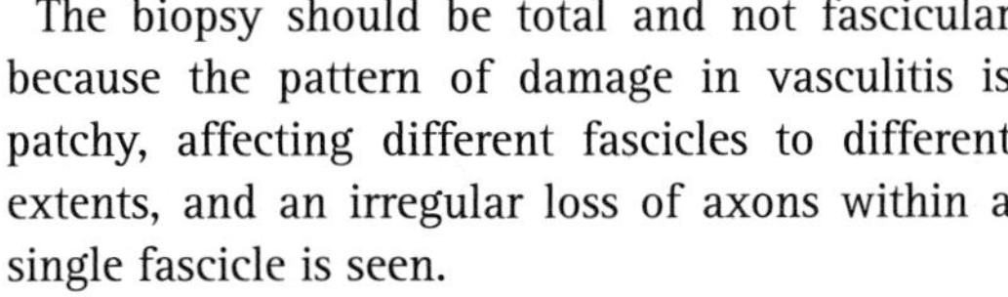

The biopsy should be total and not fascicular because the pattern of damage in vasculitis is patchy, affecting different fascicles to different extents, and an irregular loss of axons within a single fascicle is seen.

The pathology of vasculitis reflects the underlying condition: a necrotizing vasculitis involving medium-sized blood vessels is seen in polyarteritis nodosa (Figs 18.57 to 18.59), Churg–Strauss and Wegener's granulomatosis; and a small blood vessel vasculitis is seen in many disorders, e.g. systemic lupus erythematosis (SLE), and HIV. In Churg–Strauss eosinophils are seen, while in Wegener's there are granulomata with a positive c-antineutrophil cytoplasmic antibody (c-ANCA).

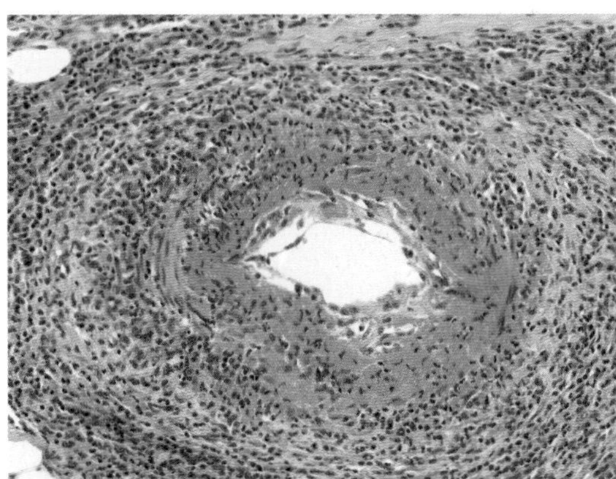

Figure 18.58 Polyarteritis nodosa (high power of Fig. 18.57). H&E.

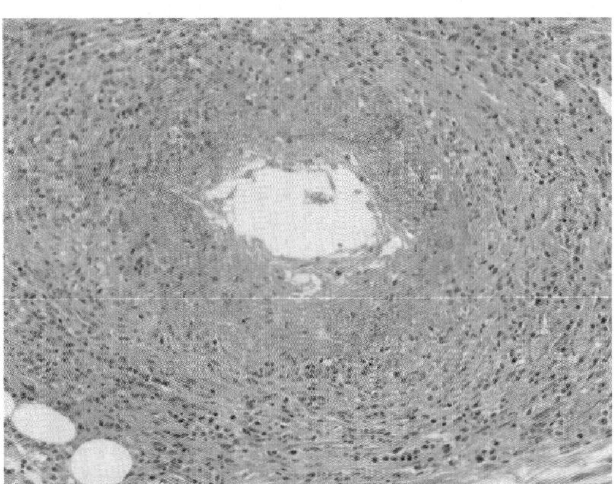

Figure 18.59 Polyarteritis nodosa. MSB.

GUILLAIN–BARRÉ SYNDROME AND CHRONIC IMMUNE DEMYELINATING POLYNEUROPATHY

Guillain–Barré syndrome (GBS) refers to an acute disease, whilst chronic inflammatory demyelinating polyneuropathy (CIDP) refers to a more chronic disorder.

GBS is the commonest cause of acute neuromuscular paralysis with an incidence of 2 per 100 000. It is a mixture of conditions: acute inflammatory demyelinating polyradiculopathy (AIDP), acute motor axonal neuropathy (AMAN), acute motor–sensory axonal neuropathy (AMSAN) and the Miller–Fisher syndrome. In the UK 90% have the AIDP subtype.

This is a severe inflammatory polyneuropathy with a mortality of 5–10%. Ventilation is required in up to 20% although most recover over a long period of time.

There is a definite relationship with HIV, cytomegalovirus, *Campylobacter jejuni*, Epstein–Barr virus, *Mycoplasma pneumoniae* and *Hemophilus influenzae*. All these have ganglioside-like epitopes as the postulated mechanism initiating an autoimmune response. *Campylobacter jejuni* infection precedes in 26% of patients in the UK.

Diagnosis is confirmed by typical neurophysiological findings on nerve conduction studies (NCSs) and an elevated CSF protein with no cellular reaction. Antiganglioside antibodies are occasionally detected.

A sural nerve biopsy may not reveal inflammation because the pathological lesions are mainly proximal. Nerve biopsy is not usually necessary for diagnosis but may help exclude other possible differential diagnoses. The pathology is of segmental demyelination secondary to a T-cell infiltrate. Treatment is by immunotherapy.

OTHER CAUSES OF NEUROPATHY

Neoplasia

Peripheral nerve biopsy can occasionally show infiltration by tumour e.g. in non-Hodgkin's lymphoma. This is not a commonly detected feature in life but is found more often at autopsy. More often the nerve is involved in paraneoplastic pathology associated with a tumor, prior to tumour development or associated with a monoclonal gammopathy.

Paraproteinemias can lead to deposition of proteins, e.g. amyloid light chains, or IgM myelin-associated glycoprotein antibodies (anti-MAG antibodies) as in Waldenstrom's macroglobulinemia. IgM anti-MAG pathology leads to demyelination by deposition within myelin, seen as widened myelin lamellae on electron microscopy.

Table 18.8 Toxic neuropathies

Toxin	Predominant neuropathy
Amiodarone	Demyelination
Chloroquine	Demyelination
Isoniazid	Axonal
Metronidazole	Axonal
Cispatin	Axonal
Vincristine	Axonal
Organophosphorus toxins	Axonal and inhibition of anticholinesterase
Hexanes	Axonal
Arsenic	Axonal

Diabetes

Twenty-five years after the onset of diabetes 50% of patients have a symptomatic neuropathy. The risk of neuropathy increases with poor glycemic control. Various neuropathies are seen. The most common is a symmetrical sensorimotor neuropathy preferentially involving small myelinated fibers. An autonomic neuropathy affects 30% of patients. Diabetes is the most common cause of autonomic neuropathy in developed countries. Mononeuropathies involving single nerves occur, e.g. a III cranial nerve palsy, carpal tunnel syndrome.

Toxic neuropathies

Axonal loss is a manifestation of many drugs and toxins. These should be excluded by clinical history; occupational history and illicit drug use are highly relevant. Among substances causing axonal loss are: acrylamides, alcohol, arsenic, gold, hexacarbons, lead, organophosphates, phenytoin, statins and chemotherapeutic agents (Table 18.8). Demyelination can be seen with other substances such as tacrolimus, chloroquine, perhexiline and procainamide.

Amyloidosis

Neuropathies can be seen in both acquired and familial amyloidoses. Typically, there is a small fiber sensory loss, carpal tunnel syndrome or autonomic neuropathy. The protein is deposited as β-pleated sheets that are insoluble.

Acquired amyloidosis may occur with paraproteinemias if light chains are formed: light chains cause the AL type. The nerve biopsy shows axonal degeneration with amyloid deposition.

Uremic neuropathy

Sixty-five percent of patients with chronic renal failure have distal symmetrical axonal degeneration.

Acquired immune deficiency disorder (AIDS)

A variety of pathologies can be seen including chronic inflammatory demyelinating polyneuropathy, involvement of dorsal root ganglia in late disease, vasculitis and iatrogenic toxic neuropathies. Neuropathies due to secondary infections may also occur.

CHAPTER 19

THE ORBIT

Fiona Roberts

ANATOMY

Bony orbit

The orbit functions to protect, support, and maximize function of the eye. The bony orbit separates the orbital contents from the intracranial fossa and the paranasal sinuses. The superior wall is separated from the frontal lobe of the brain by a thin bony plate, which can be easily penetrated by a sharp object passing into the orbit. Anteriorly the frontal sinus may be the source of an inflammatory process extending into the orbit. The lacrimal fossa is located in the anterolateral bony orbit, and erosion of the bone indicates a potentially malignant extension of a tumor of the lacrimal gland. The inferior orbital wall is easily penetrated by neoplasms arising in the maxillary sinus. Similarly, the medial wall, formed by the thin ethmoid bones, may be affected when a tumor arises in the nasal cavity or the paranasal sinuses. The lower aspect of the medial wall contains the lacrimal fossa which surrounds the lacrimal sac and may be eroded by extension of inflammatory or neoplastic processes. There are several apertures in the orbital bone that allow the passage of blood vessels and nerves. These include the narrow optic foramen or canal, situated at the apex of the orbit, through which pass the optic nerve, the ophthalmic artery and sympathetic nerve fibers. The superior orbital fissure transmits the sensory nerve (V) and the motor nerves (III, IV and VI) to the extraocular muscles, which enter the orbit in close relation with the superior ophthalmic vein. It is in this region that a space-occupying lesion can cause most damage to the blood vessels and nerves. The infraorbital sulcus crosses the floor of the orbit and carries the infraorbital artery, infraorbital vein, and infraorbital nerve from the infraorbital fissure to the infraorbital foramen. Clinically, the infraorbital foramen provides a route of spread for infection or maxillary tumors to the orbit and the skull base.

The extraocular muscles

Six extraocular striated muscles are present in the orbit. The four rectus muscles originate at the annulus of Zinn, a fibrous tendon that encircles the optic foramen and inserts into the episclera anterior to the equator of the globe. The aponeuroses of the four muscles unite to form a conical capsule (Tenon's) which ensheathes the globe and the fat that surrounds the optic nerve and closely related nerves and blood vessels. Unlike the rectus muscles, the superior and inferior oblique muscles originate separately from the posterior orbital wall. The superior oblique first passes through the trochlea, the only cartilagenous structure in the orbit, and then redirects to attach to the posterolateral episclera of the globe. The inferior oblique muscle inserts into the back of the globe on the temporal side just below the midline.

Connective tissue planes

Tenon's capsule is surrounded by orbital fat and allows smooth movement of the globe within the orbit. Anteriorly the capsule fuses with the septum derived from the periosteum of the orbital rim and this orbital septum separates the stroma of the conjunctiva from the orbital fat. The septum is condensed in the horizontal plane to form the medial and lateral orbital ligaments. If the septum or ligaments are divided, the eye and extraocular muscles are no longer stabilized, resulting in abnormal eye movement.

Eyelids

The eyelids form the anterior boundary of the orbit and serve to protect the anterior surface of the eye.

CLINICO-PATHOLOGICAL BACKGROUND

The most common clinical symptoms and signs of orbital pathology include disturbance in ocular motility, visual loss and proptosis. Secondary space-occupying effects may occur also due to the rigid confines of the bony orbital wall. For example compression of orbital veins leads to massive transudation and tissue edema of the conjunctiva and lids whereas arterial compression may result in ischemia of the retina and optic nerve. Extreme proptosis may lead to corneal exposure and ulceration with secondary endophthalmitis.

Modern imaging techniques, including computed tomograpy (CT) and magnetic resonance imaging (MRI) have improved clinical diagnostic accuracy such that some conditions, e.g. dysthyroid orbitopathy are rarely biopsied. Nonetheless, the orbit is the site of a wide variety of diseases ranging from inflammatory lesions to highly malignant tumors requiring accurate histological diagnosis. In terms of specimens submitted to pathology the most common entities in adults include vascular tumors, non-Hodgkin's lymphoma, chronic idiopathic orbital inflammation and malignant tumors of the periorbital and lacrimal gland. In children most orbital pathology is represented by cysts, vascular lesions and malignant tumors.

ORBITAL INFLAMMATIONS

Infectious orbital inflammation

Bacterial infection

Acute bacterial infection of the orbit may be blood-borne or secondary to spread from adjacent sinuses. Clinically, orbital cellulitis usually presents with abrupt onset of pain, eyelid edema and conjunctival hyperemia. It is unlikely that tissue will be submitted for histopathological examination. *Hemophilus influenzae* is the commonest causative organism in young children. Other common pathogens include *Streptococcus pneumoniae* and *Staphylococcus aureus* although anaerobic organisms may also cause infection. Tuberculosis can occur as an isolated orbital or lacrimal gland mass.

Fungal infection

Aspergillosis

Infection is caused by *Aspergillus* species usually as a complication of infection via the nasal cavity or the paranasal sinuses. Most patients are immunocompetent although orbital disease occasionally occurs in the immunocompromised. Histopathological examination reveals a granulomatous reaction with numerous multinucleated giant cells and fibrosis. The septate, branching hyphae may be identified on H&E or with PAS and methenamine silver stains.

Mucormycosis

Mucormycosis, also known as phycomycosis, is a group of infections caused by *Rhizopus*, *Absidia* and *Mucor* species. Infection usually occurs in patients with poorly controlled diabetes or other conditions associated with immunosuppression. The causative organisms are ubiquitous and are normally non-invasive, non-pathogenic, opportunistic organisms in the upper respiratory tract. Clinical signs of early infection included sinusitis, pharyngitis, nasal discharge and orbital pain. As the disease evolves a characteristic eschar may be seen in the nose or mouth.

Histopathological examination of biopsy specimens reveals extensive infarction of tissue with large, non-septate, branching hyphae within the tissues and within the walls and lumina of blood vessels, which are frequently thrombosed (Fig. 19.1). The fungal hyphae are readily visible on H&E but PAS and methenamine silver stains may assist in their identification. In addition to antifungal therapy and stabilizing diabetic control, the management may include wide surgical debridement and orbital exenteration may be performed for advancing mucormycosis. Despite treatment the disease is fatal in over 50% of cases.

Parasitic infections

Parasitic infections are rare. Hydatid cysts due to *Echinococcus granulosus* may form a mass lesion in the orbit. Microfilaria (e.g. onchocerciasis and loiasis) have rarely been observed in the orbit.

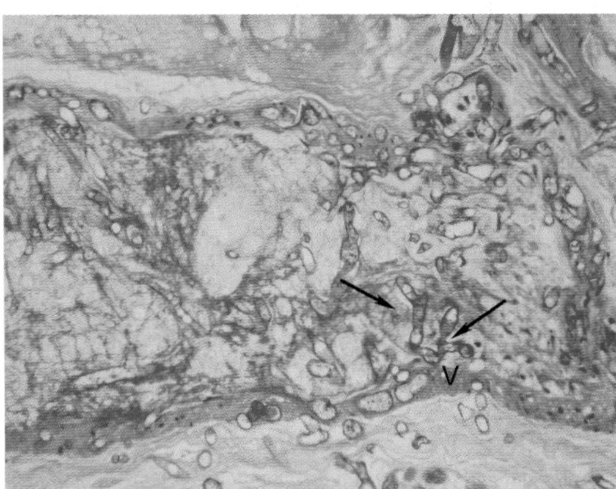

Figure 19.1 Mucormycosis. Large, non-septate, branching hyphae (arrows) have invaded through the wall of a blood vessel (v) within orbital fat. There is ischemic infarction of the surrounding tissues. H&E.

Non-infectious orbital inflammation

Dysthyroid orbitopathy

Dysthyroid orbitopathy affects the extraocular muscles. It is most commonly associated with hyperthyroidism but may be seen in hypothyroidism. Women are affected three times more often than men. Clinically, the patient usually shows proptosis with eyelid retraction associated with conjunctival redness or edema. The diagnosis is usually made on CT scan or MRI which show enlargement of the rectus muscles with sparing of the muscle tendons and orbital fat. On the rare occasion when biopsy is performed histopathological examination reveals muscle fibers separated by ground substance and characteristic clusters of lymphocytes known as 'lymphorrhages' (Fig. 19.2). At later stages in the disease there is replacement fibrosis.

Wegener's granulomatosis

In Wegener's granulomatosis orbital involvement may occur as part of the generalized systemic disease or its limited form. Generalized disease classically presents with renal, lung, upper respiratory tract and paranasal sinus involvement. The limited forms manifest by upper respiratory and lung disease without kidney involvement. Clinically, the

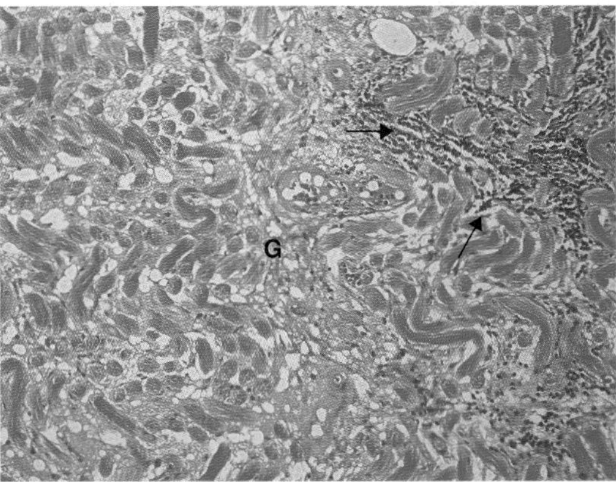

Figure 19.2 Endocrine exophthalmos. The extraocular muscle fibers are separated by ground substance (G) and there are 'lymphorrhages' (arrows). H&E.

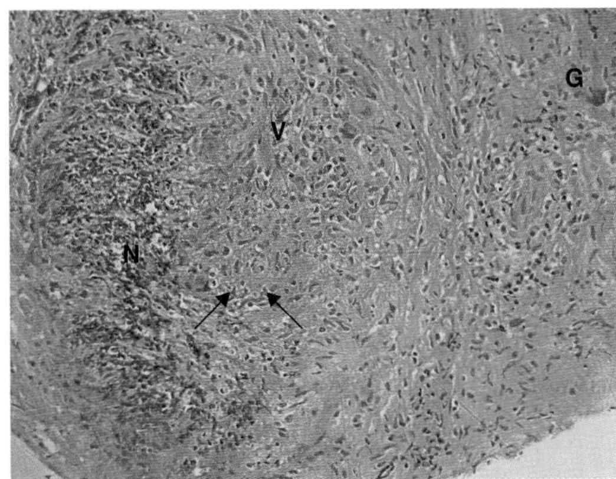

Figure 19.3 Wegener's granulomatosis. An orbital biopsy showing classical features of Wegener's granulomatosis with destruction of a small blood vessel (V) by granulomatous inflammation (arrows) and areas of necrosis (N). There is also a characteristic 'smudged' giant cell (G). H&E.

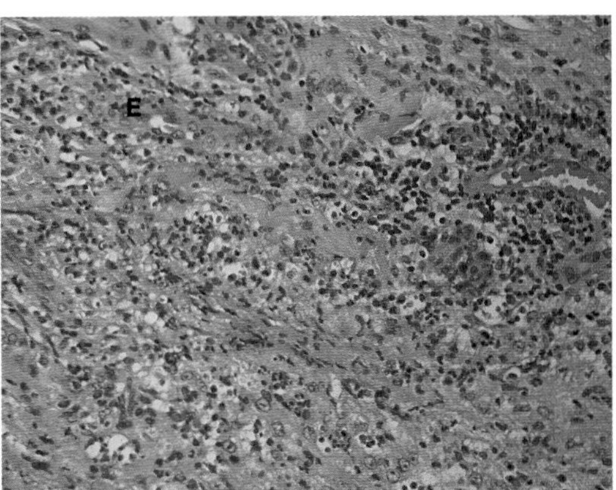

Figure 19.4 Wegener's granulomatosis. The orbital tissues contain a dense mixed inflammatory cell infiltrate including prominent eosinophils. The endothelial cells (E) are swollen but there is no definite vasculitis. H&E.

presenting symptom is usually proptosis accompanied by pain and erythema of the eyelids. Bilateral involvement is not uncommon. Other ocular complications of Wegener's granulomatosis may also be identified most commonly including scleritis and corneoscleral ulceration. Serology for c-ANCA is positive in over 90% of patients with generalized Wegener's granulomatosis but in only 60% of those with the limited form.

The classical histological picture is of a small-vessel vasculitis with necrosis and granulomatous inflammation (Fig. 19.3). Giant cells are seldom seen but when present the nuclear chromatin frequently appears smudged. The classical triad of features has been demonstrated in just over 50% of orbital biopsies from patients with proven Wegener's granulomatosis. Therefore in the appropriate clinical context biopsies showing a mixed inflammatory infiltrate with evidence of necrosis but no vasculitis should not be interpreted as non-specific (Fig. 19.4).

Sarcoidosis

This multisystem disease may involve the orbit as an inflammatory mass although the lacrimal gland is more frequently involved. An elevated serum angiotensin-converting enzyme is strongly suggestive of the clinical diagnosis. Histological examination reveals the presence of non-caseating granulomas in the orbital fat (Fig. 19.5).

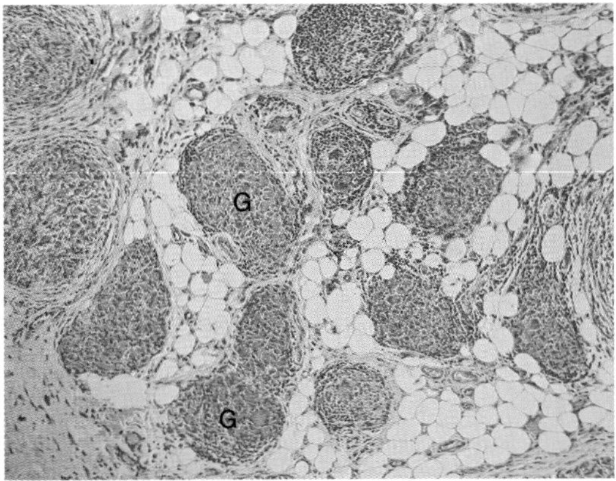

Figure 19.5 Orbital sarcoidosis. The orbital fat contains numerous well-formed epithelioid granulomas (G). Some to these are surrounded by fibrous tissue and others by a cuff of small lymphocytes. H&E (Courtesy of Emeritus Professor W.R. Lee, University of Glasgow).

Idiopathic orbital inflammation

Idiopathic orbital inflammation (formerly inflammatory pseudotumor) is a non-granulomatous inflammatory process within the orbit for which

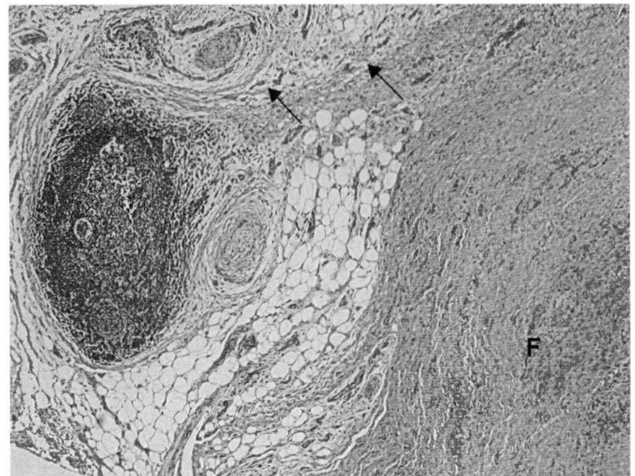

Figure 19.6 Idiopathic orbital inflammation. At an early stage there is edema (arrows) and patchy fibrosis (F) of orbital tissues with scattered inflammatory cells in addition to a lymphoid follicle (L). H&E.

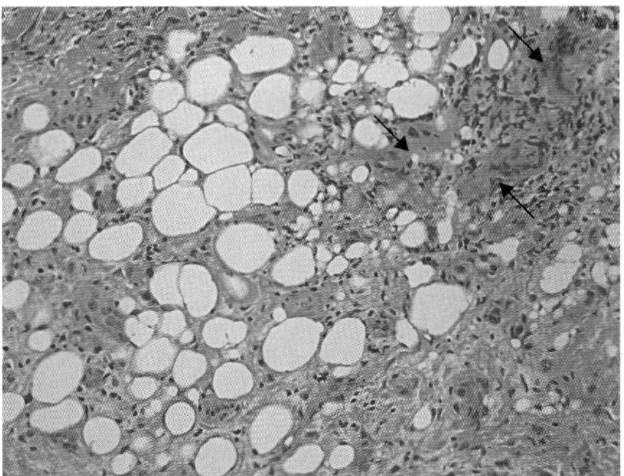

Figure 19.7 Idiopathic orbital inflammation. A lipogranulomatous reaction with disrupted adipocytes, histiocytes and occasionally multinucleated giant cells (arrows) may be seen at the edge of the main lesion. H&E.

there is no recognized local cause or any underlying systemic disease. The clinical presentation usually includes proptosis, pain, chemosis and restriction of eye movements. The disease may be unilateral or bilateral and the onset may be acute or slowly progressive. It is recognized that similar clinical features may occur due to a local orbital lesion such as infection or a ruptured dermoid cyst, or may develop as part of a systemic disease such as Wegener's granulomatosis or the collagen vascular diseases. A secondary cause should therefore be excluded by appropriate clinical investigations. In most instances the diagnosis is based on a combination of clinical and MRI findings and biopsy is reserved for patients with multiple recurrences or those unresponsive to therapy.

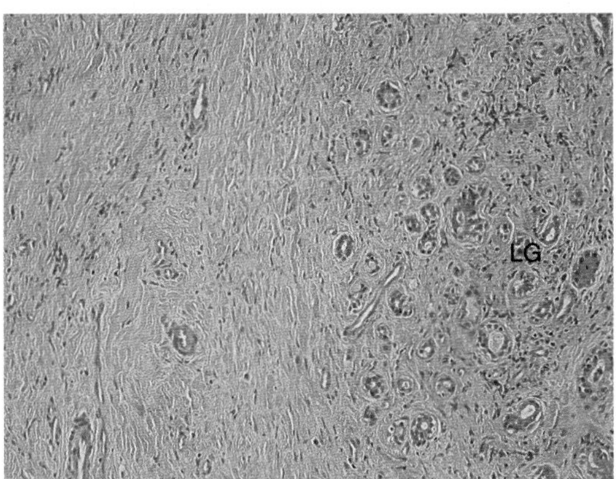

Figure 19.8 Idiopathic orbital inflammation. In this late-stage lesion the lacrimal gland (LG) is surrounded by dense fibrous tissue leading to atrophy of the secretory acini. H&E.

This is one of the most difficult areas in diagnostic orbital pathology. In early lesions there is edema of orbital tissues and an inflammatory infiltrate composed predominantly of lymphocytes and plasma cells with smaller numbers of eosinophils and plasma cells. Lymphoid follicles may be present (Fig. 19.6). As the disease progresses collagen is laid down and the collections of inflammatory cells may be separated by fibrous tissue. When there is involvement of orbital fat there may be a lipogranulomatous reaction at the edge of the lesion (Fig. 19.7). Involvement of extraocular muscle (orbital myositis) may lead to atrophy of muscle fibers. Similarly involvement of the lacrimal gland (dacryoadenitis) may lead to atrophy of secretory acini in the lacrimal gland (Fig. 19.8). Necrosis, however, is not usually a feature. Most cases show a dramatic response to corticosteroid therapy unless the lesion has extensive fibrosis. Other immunosuppressive agents, such as azathioprine, or low-dose radiotherapy may be used in patients who fail to respond to steroids.

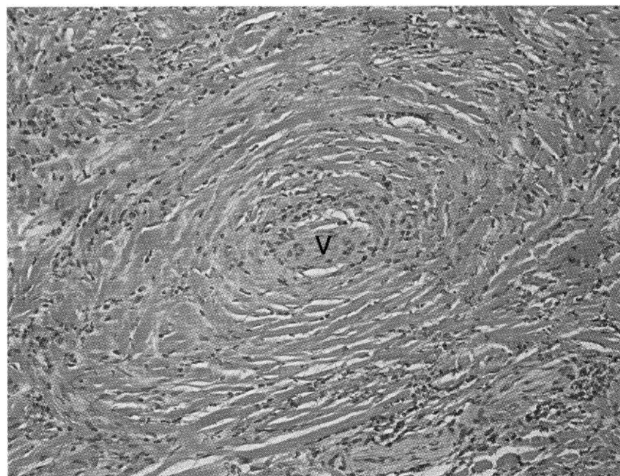

Figure 19.9 Idiopathic sclerosing inflammation. The lesion consists of densely hyalinized collagen bundles that replace the orbital tissues. The collagen may be deposited in concentric whorls around blood vessels (V). H&E.

Orbital apical syndrome (Tolosa–Hunt syndrome)

Orbital apical syndrome may be caused by a similar non-specific inflammatory reaction in the apex of the orbit and in the optic nerve sheath leading to compression effects on nerves and blood vessels. Clinically, the patient presents initially with retrobulbar pain followed by extraocular motility dysfunction and ultimately visual loss. There is usually a good response to steroids. Other lesions affecting the apex of the orbit may cause a similar clinical picture.

Idiopathic sclerosing inflammation

This is a distinct form of orbital inflammation characterized by a slow and relentless fibrosing process with progressive involvement of orbital structures. Biopsy shows relatively sparse chronic inflammation and densely hyalinized collagenous bundles replacing the orbital tissues (Fig. 19.9). Inflammatory cells are often scattered throughout the lesion rather than in aggregates and eosinophils are frequently seen. A prominent feature is whorls of concentrically deposited collagen often in relation to blood vessels. The histological appearances are similar to other sclerosing processes including retroperitoneal fibrosis. It should be noted that some pathologists consider that sclerosing orbital inflammation represents the late stages of idiopathic orbital inflammation where fibrosis predominates rather than a separate process *ab initio*. Without treatment the disease may be relentlessly progressive and can result in exenteration due to corneal exposure. Treatment with corticosteroids and radiotherapy is usually less successful than for non-sclerosing orbital inflammation.

Multifocal fibrosclerosis

Multifocal fibrosclerosis describes the association of idiopathic sclerosing orbital inflammation with similar processes occurring at other sites including retroperitoneal fibrosis, sclerosing cholangitis, sclerosing mediastinitis and Riedel's thyroiditis. Multifocal fibrosclerosis is rare but occurs in around 15% of patients with retroperitoneal fibrosis. With appropriate treatment (corticosteroid or antimetabolite therapy) the prognosis is relatively good.

TUMORS OF THE ORBIT

Vascular lesions

Capillary hemangioma

Capillary hemangioma is usually located in the eyelid in childhood but can also occur in the orbit. These lesions show gradual enlargement for 1–2 years and then undergo gradual regression. Histological examination reveals small vascular channels with a lobulated growth pattern that can infiltrate all the orbital structures (Fig. 19.10). Treatment is only required if the lesion interferes with vision and there is a danger of amblyopia.

Cavernous hemangioma

Cavernous hemangioma is a tumor that occurs in adults. These lesions are usually retrobulbar in location, resulting in axial proptosis, although they may occur in other locations. They can be reliably diagnosed by CT scans or MRI and may require treatment for compressive symptoms. The excised lesion has a spongy cut surface. Histological examination reveals thick-walled blood vessels with intervening fibrous

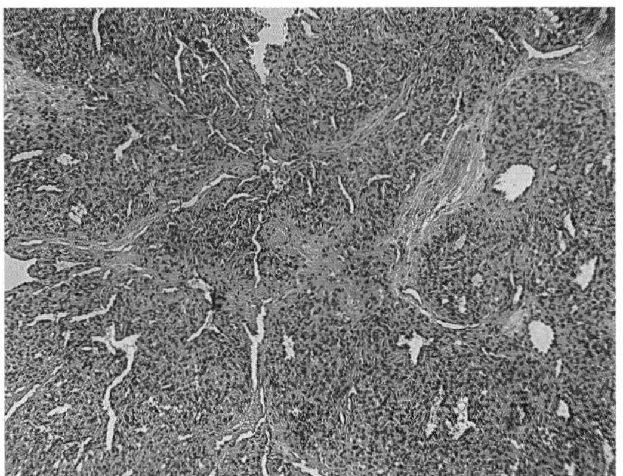

Figure 19.10 Capillary hemangioma. The lesion is composed of lobules of capillaries separated by fibrous septa. The amount of fibrous tissue increases as the lesion regresses. H&E.

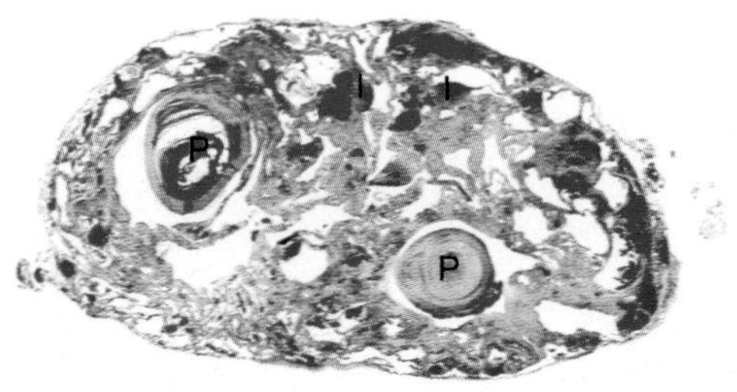

Figure 19.11 Cavernous hemangioma. The lesion is well-circumscribed and is composed of large cavernous spaces separated by thick fibrous septa. Inflammatory cells (I) are present as a consequence of bleeding into the walls. Thrombosis within vascular spaces has resulted in the formation of phleboliths (P). H&E.

septae that often contain inflammatory cells and hemosiderin laden macrophages as a consequence of previous hemorrhage (Fig. 19.11). Thrombosis of blood vessels may occur and may undergo dystrophic calcification with the formation of phleboliths.

Epithelioid hemangioma (angiolymphoid hyperplasia with eosinophilia)

Epithelioid hemangioma is a benign vascular lesion most commonly occurring in the scalp, preauricular region, forehead and eyelids of adults. However, it may form a localized orbital mass. Histological examination reveals an ill-defined mass consisting of numerous blood vessels lined by prominent endothelial cells, follicular lymphoid hyperplasia and numerous eosinophils. The epithelioid endothelial cells are usually immunoreactive with CD31 and factor VIII-related antigen. Many cases are also immunoreactive for CD34. Local excision is the treatment of choice but recurrences are not infrequent. It remains controversial as to whether epithelioid hemangioma is a reactive lesion or a true benign neoplasm.

Lymphangiomas

Lymphangiomas occur in the eyelids, conjunctiva and orbit where they may be defined as a choristoma. They may cause slowly progressive proptosis and eyelid swelling and usually become symptomatic in the teenage years. However, a fluctuating course is common. Hemorrhage into the lesion may cause fulminant proptosis. Upper respiratory tract infections may also cause lymphangiomas to enlarge due to hyperplasia of lymphoid tissue present in the lesion. Histological examination shows an unencapsulated tumor that diffusely infiltrates the orbital tissues and is composed of lymphatic channels of varying caliber. Secondary hemorrhage and inflammatory changes are also commonly seen. Complete surgical excision is impractical but surgical debulking may be required in some cases.

Angiosarcoma

Primary angiosarcoma of the orbit is rare.

Fibrohistiocytic tumors

Fibrous histiocytoma

Benign fibrous histiocytoma of the orbit is considered to be relatively common. It usually presents in middle-aged individuals with signs and symptoms of an orbital mass, which have progressed over 1–2 years. Histopathological examination

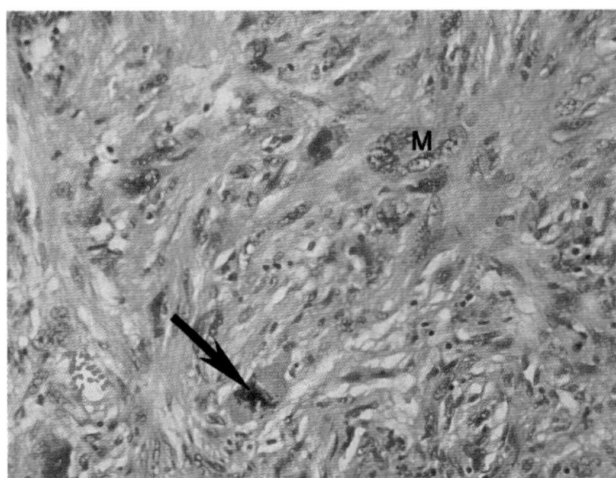

Figure 19.12 Malignant fibrous histiocytoma. The tumor is composed of pleomorphic spindle cells with occasional multinucleated giant cells (M) and frequent mitotic figures (arrow). H&E.

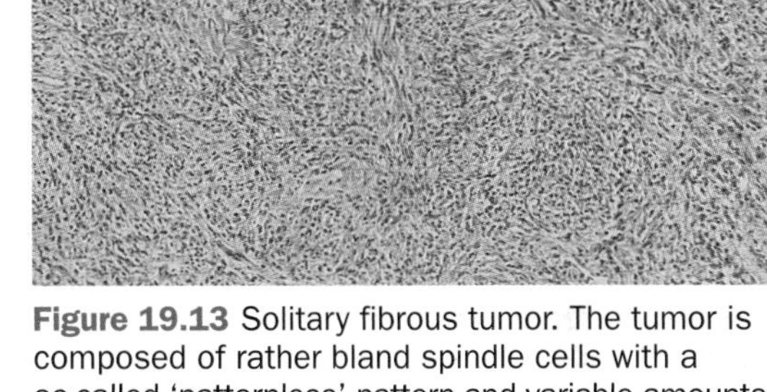

Figure 19.13 Solitary fibrous tumor. The tumor is composed of rather bland spindle cells with a so-called 'patternless' pattern and variable amounts of collagen. H&E.

reveals a tumor composed of fibroblasts often with areas showing a storiform pattern. Foamy histiocytes may be present within the lesion. It is probable that with modern immunohistochemistry some of these lesions may be reclassified as solitary fibrous tumor.

Malignant fibrous histiocytoma

Malignant fibrous histiocytoma is a high-grade sarcoma that may rarely present as a primary tumor in the orbit (Fig. 19.12).

Solitary fibrous tumor

Solitary fibrous tumor (SFT) of the orbit was first described in 1994 and although initially considered to be an extremely rare tumor it is now apparent that this was due to under-recognition of this entity. The tumor usually presents in middle-aged adults as unilateral proptosis but may also occur in children. Imaging shows a well-delineated mass.

Histopathological examination reveals alternating hypocellular and hypercellular areas separated by hyalinized collagen. The more cellular areas are composed of bland spindle cells with a so-called 'patternless' pattern (Fig. 19.13). There may be areas with a prominent branching hemangiopericytoma-like vascular pattern. Myxoid change and areas of fibrosis may be present. The majority of SFTs show immunoreactivity for CD34, CD99 and Bcl-2. A few tumors are also positive for epithelial membrane antigen and smooth muscle actin. SFTs are cytogenetically heterogeneous. Surgical excision is the treatment of choice. Local recurrences of SFT are possible and usually follow an incomplete initial excision. Recurrent tumors in the orbit have shown a tendency to infiltrate the surrounding tissues and the bone, rendering complete secondary excision more difficult. Recurrent orbital SFT also has the potential for malignant transformation. One case of malignant transformation has been reported.

Hemangiopericytoma

Hemangiopericytoma was historically considered to be a tumor derived from pericytes. They are now considered to represent a group of lesions that have in common the presence of a thin-walled branching vascular pattern and show considerable histological overlap with solitary fibrous tumor. As such, similar to SFT, hemangiopericytoma usually presents in middle-aged adults as a painless, unilateral proptosis. In contrast to SFT hemangiopericytoma shows an evenly distributed cellularity with a prominent branching vascular pattern (Fig. 19.14). The immunohistochemical profile is similar to SFT in

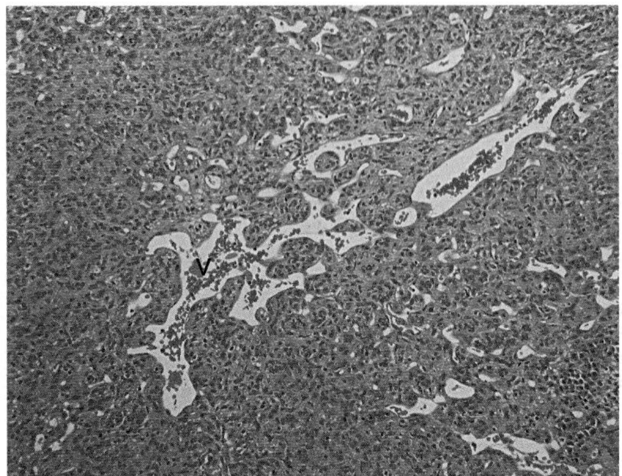

Figure 19.14 Hemangiopericytoma. These tumors are of more uniform cellularity than solitary fibrous tumor with a prominent branching or staghorn vascular pattern (V). H&E.

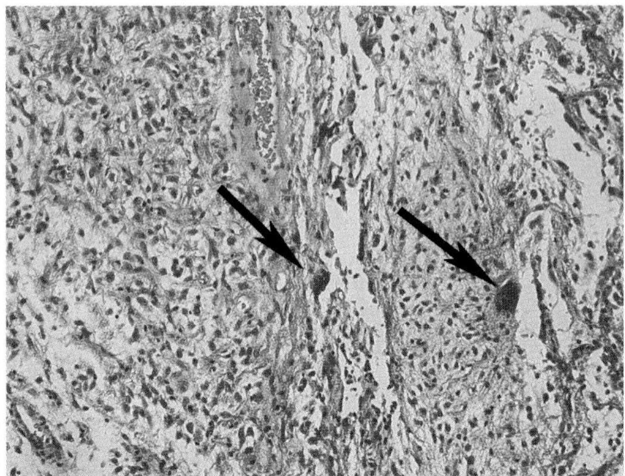

Figure 19.15 Giant cell angiofibroma. The tumor is composed of bland spindle-shaped cells which is this area lie within a myxoid stroma. There are scattered multinucleated giant cells (arrows) lining pseudovascular spaces. H&E.

most cases. The majority of hemangiopericytomas (70%) will pursue a benign clinical course but a significant number will behave in a malignant fashion. The prognosis is difficult to predict but the presence of four or more mitoses per high-power field and large size are worrying features. Similar tumors have been described in the meninges and extension from an intracranial lesion should be considered in the differential diagnosis. Complete local excision is the treatment of choice and recurrence is common following piecemeal removal. Proton beam therapy has been used in the treatment of recurrent lesions.

Giant cell angiofibroma

Giant cell angiofibroma is a distinctive benign neoplasm that most often involves the orbital region and eyelids of middle-aged adults. Clinically, it presents as a slow-growing orbital mass and may be painful. On imaging it is usually well circumscribed. Histological examination reveals areas similar to solitary fibrous tumor as well as multinucleated giant stromal cells, often lining pseudovascular spaces (Fig. 19.15). The immunohistochemical profile is again similar to SFT. These tumors pursue a benign course and recurrences after excision are exceptional.

There is considerable histological and immunohistochemical overlap between solitary fibrous tumor, hemangiopericytoma and giant cell angiofibroma supporting the view that these tumors are closely related. Indeed they are thought by some authors to represent morphological variations of a single entity.

Myogenic tumors

Rhabdomyosarcoma

Rhabdomyosarcoma is the most common orbital malignancy of childhood. It generally occurs in the first two decades of life and usually presents with rapidly progressive proptosis and displacement of the eye. If clinical suspicions are high then a prompt biopsy should be performed to confirm the diagnosis and the patient treated with a combination of chemotherapy and radiotherapy. With this regimen the survival of children with rhabdomyosarcoma has dramatically improved. On macroscopic examination these tumors consist of tan-coloured fleshy tissue. On histopathological examination rhabdomyosarcoma can be divided into three subtypes.

Embryonal rhabdomyosarcoma is the most common type in the orbit. It consists of small ovoid to spindle-shaped cells with hyperchromatic nuclei often arranged in alternating cellular and myxoid

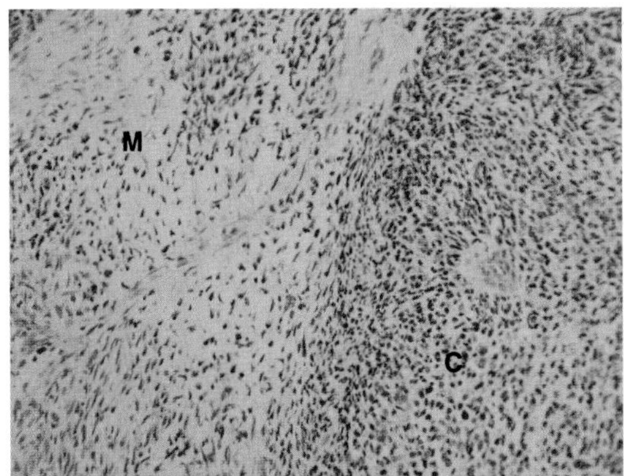

Figure 19.16 Embryonal rhabdomyosarcoma. The tumor is composed of undifferentiated, hyperchromatic cells with alternating cellular (C) and myxoid (M) areas. H&E. (Courtesy of Emeritus Professor W.R. Lee, University of Glasgow.)

areas (Fig. 19.16). Occasional larger round or tadpole-shaped cells may be identified. Cytoplasmic cross-striations can be seen, with difficulty, in a small number of cases and the diagnosis now rests on immunohistochemical confirmation with MyoD1 in combination with muscle-specific actin, myoglobin and desmin. Cytogenetic studies have found both numerical and structural chromosomal changes including gains of chromosomes 2, 8 and 13 and rearrangements of 1p11–q11 and 12q13 in some cases. Molecular analysis has shown allelic loss in chromosomal region 11p14 in the majority of cases.

Alveolar rhabdomyosarcoma is the second most common histological variant. This tends to occur in slightly older children and the inferior orbit is more likely to be involved. On histological examination the tumor is divided into alvelolar spaces by fibrous septae and the rhabdomyoblasts within the 'alveoli' are often discohesive (Fig. 19.17). Cytogenetic studies have shown a t(2;13)(q35;q14) in the majority of cases with a t(1;13)(p36;q14) in a smaller subset of cases.

Pleomorphic rhabdomyosarcoma is rare in the orbit and usually occurs in adults. These tumors consist of large pleomorphic cells often with copious eosinophilic cytoplasm.

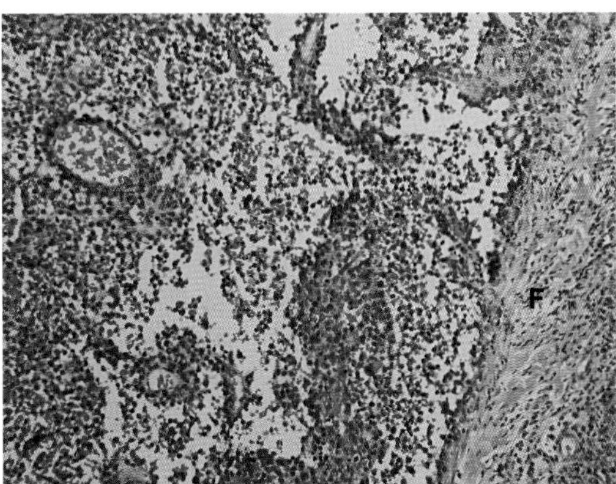

Figure 19.17 Alveolar rhabdomyosarcoma. The tumor cells are discohesive and are separated by fibrous septae (F). H&E.

Lipomatous tumors

Orbital lipomas are considered to be relatively rare but this may reflect underdiagnosis due to the difficulty of distinguishing a lipoma from excised orbital fat. Variants of lipoma including spindle cell and pleomorphic lipoma of the orbit have been described.

Primary liposarcoma rarely involves the orbit. The tumors are usually well differentiated although dedifferentiated liposarcoma has been described.

Neural tumors

Neurofibroma

Three types of neurofibroma may occur within the orbit. *Solitary neurofibromas* are the most common and the least likely to be associated with neurofibromatosis type 1 (NF 1) compared with other subtypes. Histopathological examination reveals wavy bundles of Schwann cells with variable amounts of fibrous and myxoid stroma. Residual axons can usually be identified with immunohistochemical stains for S-100 or neurofilaments. Solitary neurofibroma, unless associated with NF 1 tends to occur in the third to fifth decades of life. Symptoms and signs are generally those of an orbital mass lesion. Surgical excision is the treatment of choice. In some instances, debulking surgery may be performed because complete surgical removal is not possible.

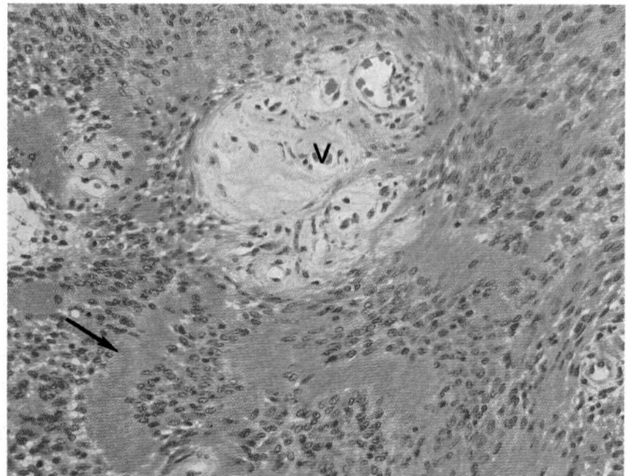

Figure 19.18 Schwannoma. In Antoni A areas there is pallisading of nuclei forming areas of relative acellularity (arrow), also called Verocay bodies. Thick-walled blood vessels (V) are common in schwannomas particularly at a late stage. H&E.

Plexiform neurofibromas only occur in patients with NF 1. Histopathological examination reveals massive expansion of several adjacent nerves by Schwann cells and fibroblasts with entrapped axons. Each abnormal nerve bundle is surrounded by a perineurium.

Diffuse neurofibromas may be associated with NF 1. Histopathological examination reveals a non-circumscribed proliferation of peripheral nerve sheath elements that permeates orbital fat and extraocular muscles.

Schwannoma

Schwannoma may originate from any sensory nerves of the orbit. Like solitary neurofibroma the symptoms are usually those associated with a slow-growing orbital mass. Treatment is by surgical excision. Histopathological examination reveals an encapsulated lesion consisting of varying proportions of solid cellular tissue (Antoni A pattern) and looser myxoid tissue (Antoni B pattern). In Antoni A areas there may be pallisading of nuclei, a pattern known as Verocay bodies (Fig. 19.18). Thick-walled blood vessels with evidence of previous hemorrhage and atypical nuclei may occur as degenerative changes. Occasionally, a schwannoma may contain melanin pigment and the differential diagnosis of extraocular extension of a spindle cell melanoma should be considered. Immunohistochemical staining for S-100 is usually strongly positive but staining for melan A is negative.

Malignant peripheral nerve sheath tumors

Malignant peripheral nerve sheath tumors are rare in the orbit. Most arise *de novo* without prior evidence of a neurofibroma or schwannoma. On histopathological examination they may be composed of pleomorphic spindle or epithelioid cells. Staining for S-100 may be weak or patchy and strong diffuse staining should cast doubt on this diagnosis.

Lymphoid tumors

The tissues behind the orbital septum contain neither lymphatics nor lymphoid tissue. Lymphocytes may be found in the conjunctiva, the lacrimal gland and lacrimal drainage system, however. The orbit may be the site of extranodal lymphoid proliferations or may be involved as part of systemic disease. Orbital lymphoid tumors are relatively common representing approximately 10% of biopsy-proven tumors. Lymphoid tumors of the orbit generally have a long history of slowly progressive proptosis and mild motility disorders without additional overt inflammatory clinical signs. Patients are usually over 50 years and tumors are uncommon in childhood except in areas where Burkitt's lymphoma is endemic.

Prior to the widespread availability of immunohistochemistry and molecular technique the classification of orbital lymphoid neoplasms was confusing and controversial. It is now accepted that the majority of lymphoid proliferations can be classified as benign (reactive lymphoid hyperplasia) or malignant (lymphoma).

Benign lymphoid hyperplasia

A similar process to reactive follicular hyperplasia of lymph nodes may form a tumor mass within the orbit. There are well-formed follicles of varying size and shape with a surrounding mantle of mature lymphocytes (Fig. 19.19). There should be scanty fibrous stroma distinguishing this process

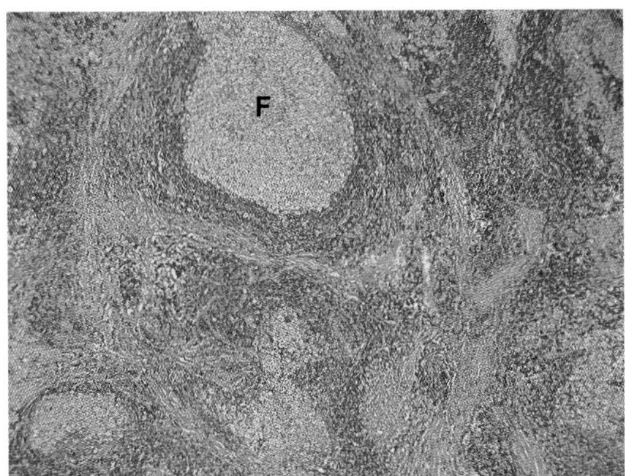

Figure 19.19 Benign lymphoid hyperplasia. In benign lymphoid hyperplasia the mass is composed of well-formed lymphoid follicles (F) surrounded by uniform small lymphocytes. H&E.

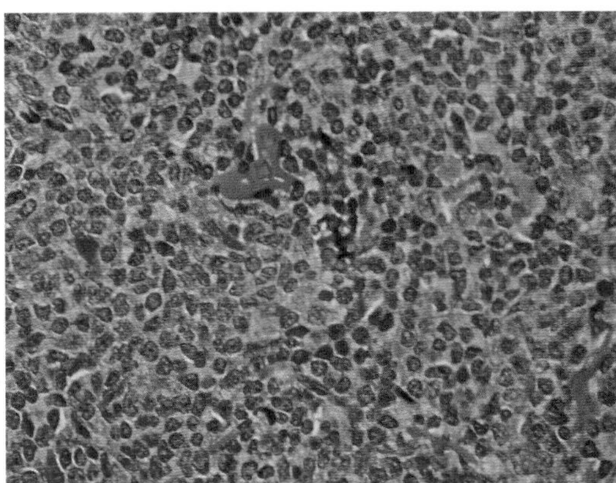

Figure 19.20 Extranodal zone lymphoma of the orbit. This orbital mass is composed of sheets of small to medium-sized lymphoid cells with irregular nuclei. H&E.

from idiopathic orbital inflammation where lymphoid follicles may be a feature. Immunohistochemistry may be helpful in differentiating benign lymphoid hyperplasia from lymphoma. In particular, the follicles in benign lymphoid hyperplasia are negative for antibodies to Bcl-2 in contrast to follicular lymphoma.

Lymphoma

Lymphomas of the ocular adnexa include lesions of the conjunctiva, eyelids, lacrimal gland and orbit. Those situated in the conjunctiva are associated with a lower incidence of systemic disease (20%) compared with those of the orbit (35%), lacrimal gland (40%) or eyelid (67%). The WHO classification of tumors of hemopoietic and lymphoid tissues is the most suitable for subdividing orbital lymphomas. A full description of this is beyond the scope of this chapter but the most common subtypes are described.

Extranodal marginal zone lymphoma

Extranodal marginal zone lymphoma (EMZL) is the most common type of orbital lymphoma and is a low-grade B-cell lymphoma composed of centrocyte like cells, cells resembling monocytoid cells and scattered large blast-like cells (Fig. 19.20). Plasma cell differentiation including Dutcher bodies may be identified in a proportion of cases and may cause diagnostic confusion with lymphoplasmacytic lymphoma. In problematic cases lymphoplasmacytic lymphoma can usually be excluded clinically since the majority of patients will have a monoclonal IgM serum paraprotein (Waldenstrom macroglobulinemia). The usual immunohistochemical profile of EMZL is CD20+, CD79a+, CD5− and CD10−. Negative staining for CD10 and cyclin D1 helps distinguish EMZL from other small B-cell lymphomas. There is little information on the cytogenetics of orbital EMZL. At other sites cytogenetic abnormalities such as trisomy 3 and t(11;18)(q21;q21) occur in a proportion of cases. Unlike other EMZL no epithelial component can be identified. Although these usually demonstrate an indolent course they may recur at extranodal sites and blastic transformation with a correspondingly aggressive clinical course has been described.

Follicular lymphoma

The appearance of follicular lymphoma in the orbit is identical to its nodal counterpart consisting of centrocytes and centroblasts, which commonly demonstrate a follicular pattern (Fig. 19.21). In around 80% of cases it represents part of systemic disease but rarely may be isolated at this site. Follicular lymphoma may be graded according to the number of centroblasts in 10 neoplastic follicles. This is expressed per ×40 high-power field (hpf) where grade 1, 2 and 3 cases have 0–5 centroblasts

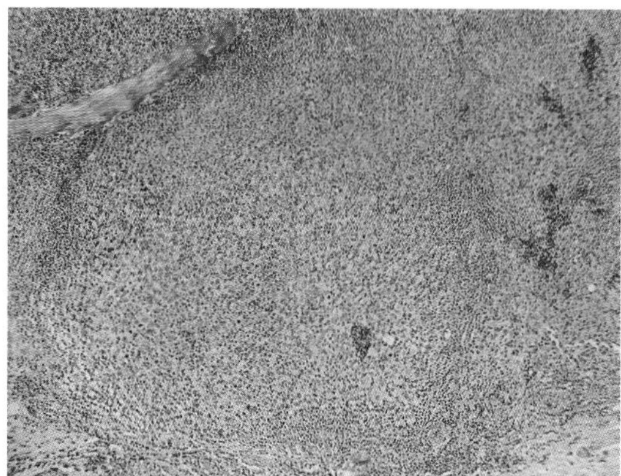

Figure 19.21 Follicular lymphoma. This orbital mass is composed of lymphocytes arranged in a nodular pattern. The pseudofollicles are composed of irregular-shaped centrocyte-like cells.

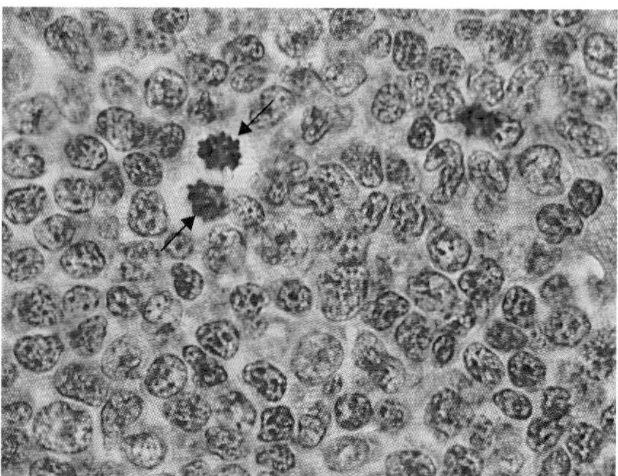

Figure 19.22 Diffuse large B-cell lymphoma. This orbital mass is composed of sheets of large, irregular lymphoid cells and mitotic figures are easily identified (arrows). H&E.

per hpf, 6–15 centroblasts per hpf and >15 centroblasts per hpf, respectively. The usual immunohistochemical profile of follicular lymphoma is CD20+, CD79a+, CD5− and CD10+. The tumor cells may also express Bcl-2 and Bcl-6. A prominent meshwork of follicular dendritic cells may be identified in follicular areas with CD21 and CD23. The most common cytogenetic abnormality is t(14;18)(q32;q21), which involves rearrangement of the *BCL2* gene. The rare isolated orbital lesions may be treated by radiotherapy but chemotherapy is usually required for those with systemic disease.

Diffuse large B-cell lymphoma

Diffuse large B-cell lymphoma (DLBCL) is uncommon and around 40% of cases are associated with systemic disease. The histology is similar to other sites and consists of a diffuse proliferation of large neoplastic lymphoid cells (Fig. 19.22). Diffuse large B-cell lymphomas express pan-B markers such as CD20 and CD79a. There is variable expression of CD5, CD10, Bcl-2 and Bcl-6. The proliferation fraction, as assessed by immunohistochemical staining for Ki-67, is usually high (>40%). A few DLBCL show the t(14;18) translocation usually found in follicular lymphoma but most cases exhibit complex cytogenetic abnormalities. These lymphomas tend to pursue an aggressive clinical course.

Other lymphomas

Many other lymphomas may uncommonly involve the orbit including mantle cell lymphoma, B-cell chronic lymphocytic leukemia, Burkitt's lymphoma, peripheral T-cell lymphoma and natural killer cell lymphoma. Leukemic infiltration of the orbit may also occur. In particular, granulocytic sarcoma can present as an isolated orbital mass in an otherwise healthy child.

MISCELLANEOUS TUMORS AND TUMOR-LIKE CONDITIONS

Other sarcomas

Alveolar soft part sarcoma is a rare sarcoma, of disputed histogenesis, that may arise in the orbit of children and young adults. Histopathological examination reveals polygonal cells with granular eosinophilic cytoplasm separated by a fine connective tissue framework to give an alveolar pattern. Tumors showing a more sheet-like pattern without the prominent connective tissue framework are more common in children and appear to carry a more favorable prognosis (Fig. 19.23). Characteristic intracytoplasmic crystals are seen with PAS

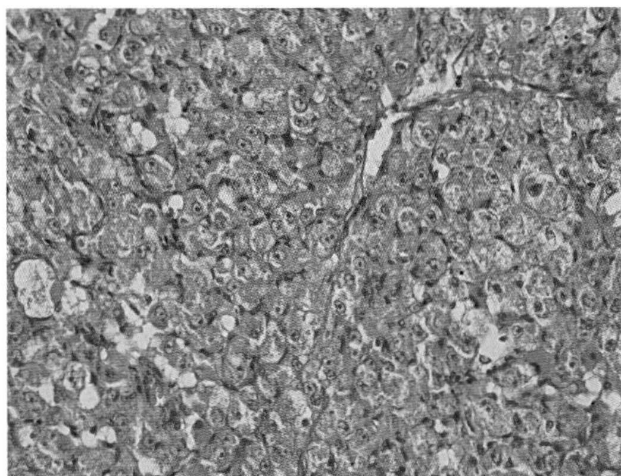

Figure 19.23 Alveolar soft part sarcoma. The tumor is composed of relatively uniform sheets of large polygonal tumor cells with abundant, granular, eosinophilic cytoplasm. H&E.

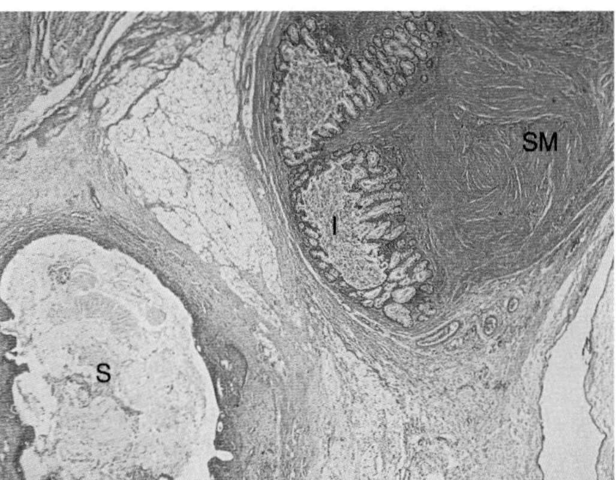

Figure 19.24 Orbital teratoma. The tumor is composed of cystic spaces lying within the orbital fat behind the eye. The cysts are lined by squamous (S) and intestinal (I) epithelium. There is also a proliferation of smooth muscle (SM). (Courtesy of Emeritus Professor W.R. Lee, University of Glasgow.)

stain. About 25% of cases show positive staining for MyoD1 and desmin may also be positive. Cytogenetic studies have shown a t(X;17)(p11.2;q25) in the majority of cases.

Other malignant sarcomas that rarely occur in the orbit include epithelioid sarcoma, synovial sarcoma, leiomyosarcoma, mesenchymal chondrosarcoma and PNET.

Teratoma

Orbital teratomas are rare congenital tumors thought to arise from misdirected germ cells. Clinically, they usually present with pronounced congenital proptosis often with marked conjunctival chemosis and eyelid swelling. The tumor contains elements of the three embryonic germ layers. Histopathological examination may therefore show cystic spaces lined by squamous, intestinal or respiratory epithelium whilst the stroma contains a variety of mesodermal tissues such as fat, cartilage and fibrous tissue (Fig. 19.24). Most orbital teratomas are benign and surgical removal with preservation of the eye, when possible, is curative.

Sinus histiocytosis with massive lymphadenopathy

Sinus histiocytosis with massive lymphadenopathy is a rare systemic condition, also known as Rosai–Dorfman disease that has a predilection for African children but has also been described in adults. It usually produces massive generalized, but particularly cervical, lymphadenopathy but it may involve the orbit as an extranodal site producing unilateral or bilateral proptosis. Histological examination reveals sheets of histiocytes with interspersed small lymphocytes. Lymphophagocytosis may be observed. The histiocytic cells stain with S-100 and CD68. The orbital lesions respond well to steroid therapy or low-dose radiotherapy.

Erdheim–Chester disease

Erdheim–Chester disease is a rare systemic histiocytosis that affects multiple organ systems including lung, kidney, heart, bones and retroperitoneum. Orbital involvement has been described and is characterized by xanthelasma of the eyelids and bilateral proptosis. Histopathological examination reveals sheets of foamy histiocytes, a mild lymphocytic infiltrate and a marked degree of fibrosis. Touton-like giant cells may be scattered throughout the lesion. Immunoreactivity for CD68 and negative staining for S-100 and CD1a differentiates Erdheim–Chester disease from sinus histiocytosis, described above, and Langerhans cell histiocytosis.

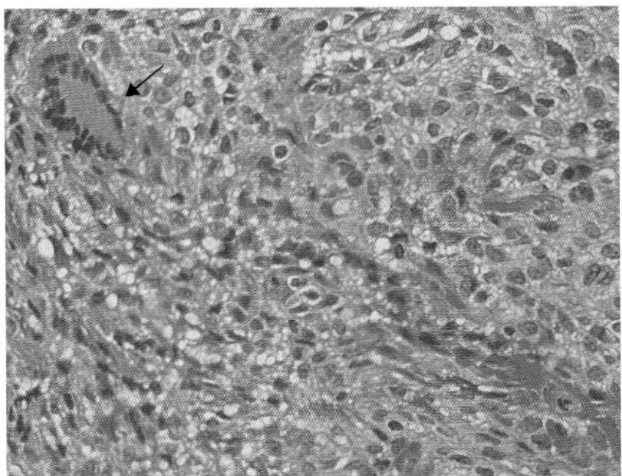

Figure 19.25 Juvenile xanthogranuloma. The tumor is composed of sheets of histiocytes with occasional multinucleated Touton-type giant cells (arrow). H&E.

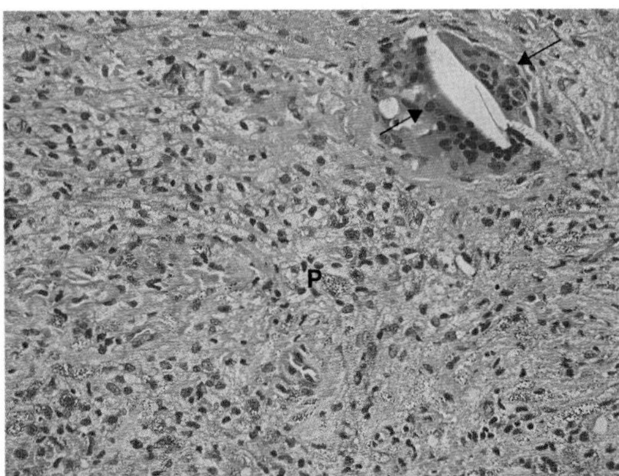

Figure 19.26 Hematic cyst. The wall of a hematic cyst consists of fibrous tissue with numerous macrophages, many containing iron pigment (p) and cholesterol clefts surrounded by foreign body giant cells (arrows). H&E.

Juvenile xanthogranuloma

This histiocytic proliferation usually occurs in the eyelids or iris but may present as an orbital mass. Histological examination reveals a proliferation of histiocytes, some with foamy cytoplasm. In addition there are usually Touton-like giant cells and a variable infiltrate of lymphocytes and eosinophils (Fig. 19.25).

Nodular fasciitis

Nodular fasciitis is a reactive inflammatory process that tends to occur in young patients as a rapidly growing mass. Histopathological examination reveals a proliferation of fibroblasts often with myxoid areas showing a 'tissue culture' appearance. Mitotic figures may be numerous but nuclear hyperchromasia and pleomorphism are absent. Scattered inflammatory cells and focal hemorrhage may be evident. These myofibroblastic proliferations are typically positive for smooth muscle actin and negative for desmin, cytokeratins and S-100. Local excision is curative.

Amyloid

Localized amyloid deposits may rarely occur in the orbit and in the lacrimal gland. Clinically, they are indistinguishable from many other orbital masses without biopsy. Histological examination reveals nodules of acellular eosinophilic material. Deposition around orbital fat cells and in the walls of blood vessels may also be seen. There may be an inflammatory reaction including foreign body giant cells. Amyloid may be confirmed with Congo or Sirius red stain and additionally by immunohistochemistry for amyloid components or electron microscopy.

Cystic lesions

Hematic cyst

A spontaneous or post-traumatic orbital hematoma may form a tumor-like mass with bony erosion. These are usually situated beneath the periosteum of the frontal bone. Histological examination reveals an organizing hematoma usually with secondary inflammatory changes including cholesterol granulomas, fibrosis and prominent iron deposition (Fig. 19.26).

Mucocele

In adults with chronic paranasal sinus inflammation a cystic evagination of the mucosa may protrude into the orbit. On histological examination the cyst is often lined by flattened epithelium but respiratory epithelium may be identified (Fig. 19.27). There is usually secondary inflammation, hemorrhage and fibrosis within the cyst wall.

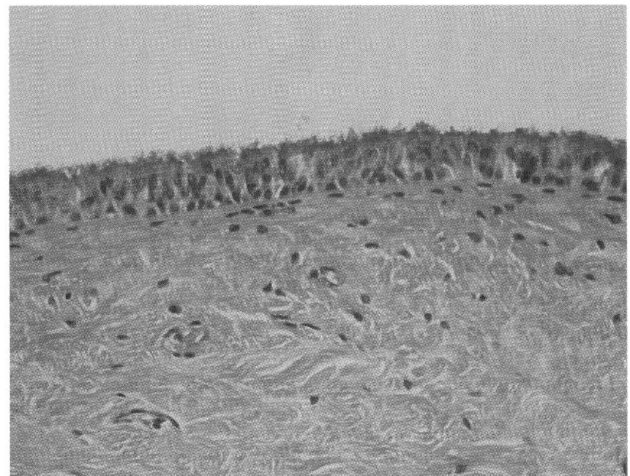

Figure 19.27 Mucocele. This consists of a fibrous walled cyst lined by ciliated, respiratory type epithelium. H&E.

Dermoid cyst

Dermoid cysts are the result of entrapped ectoderm at a site of embryological bony fusion. As such they are usually located in the superior temporal orbit under the eyebrow but may occur superonasally or deep within the orbit. Grossly, the cyst may contain sebaceous material and hair shafts. On histopathological examination the cyst is lined by keratinizing squamous epithelium and there are associated adnexal structures, including pilosebaceous units within the cyst wall (Fig. 19.28). If there has been previous cyst rupture there may be a florid foreign body giant cell reaction to released keratin or hair shafts.

Enterogenous cyst

Enterogenous cysts are rare congenital tumors of the orbit consisting of a fibrocystic mass containing spaces lined by a single layer of mucin-secreting epithelial cells resembling gastrointestinal epithelium. They are considered to be equivalent to those located in the central nervous system usually in the lower cervical and thoracic spine.

Orbital varix

Orbital varix consists of dilated and enlarged orbital veins. This condition may present with intermittent proptosis, which is made worse by performing the Valsalva maneuver. These lesions tend to bleed heavily during surgery and intervention should be avoided. Histological examination of the excised tissue reveals ectactic venous channels often complicated by intraluminal thrombosis that may calcify forming phleboliths.

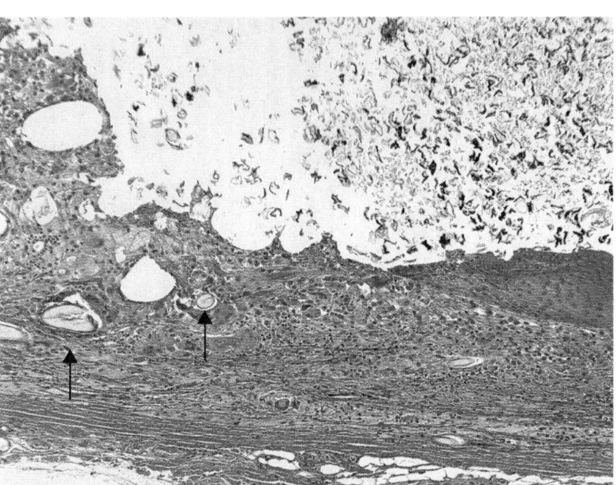

Figure 19.28 Dermoid cyst. On the right the cyst is lined by keratinizing, stratified, squamous epithelium. On the left the cyst wall is broken down in one part with a foreign body giant cell reaction to released keratin and hair shafts (arrows). H&E.

TUMORS OF THE OPTIC NERVE

Glioma

These astrocytic neoplasms usually occur between the ages of 2 and 6 years and may be associated with NF-1. The majority of cases become clinically apparent in the first two decades of life. Malignant astrocytomas of the optic nerve may rarely be seen in older patients. Around 50% of tumors involve the orbital portion of the nerve but the intracranial or chiasmal portions may also be involved. In the orbital portion the tumor may cause proptosis in addition to optic disc swelling and visual loss. CT scan or MRI may be helpful in delineating the location, configuration and extent of the tumor. In over 50% of patients the tumor does not grow but in the remaining cases the tumor does grow and may require surgical intervention. The affected

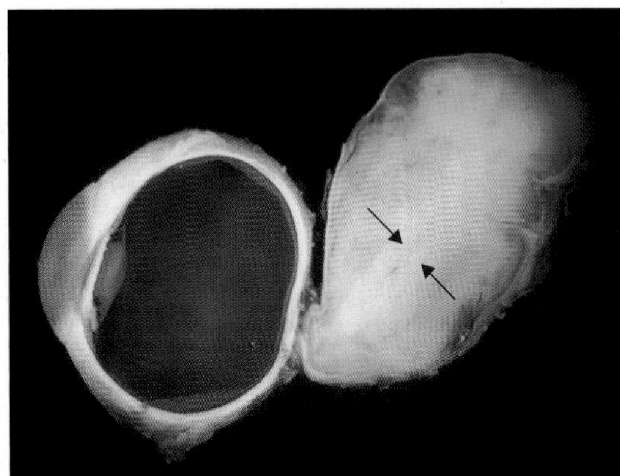

Figure 19.29 Optic nerve glioma. Macroscopic appearance of optic nerve glioma. There is fusiform swelling of the nerve and the outline of the residual optic nerve is barely visible (arrows). (Courtesy of Emeritus Professor W.R. Lee, University of Glasgow.)

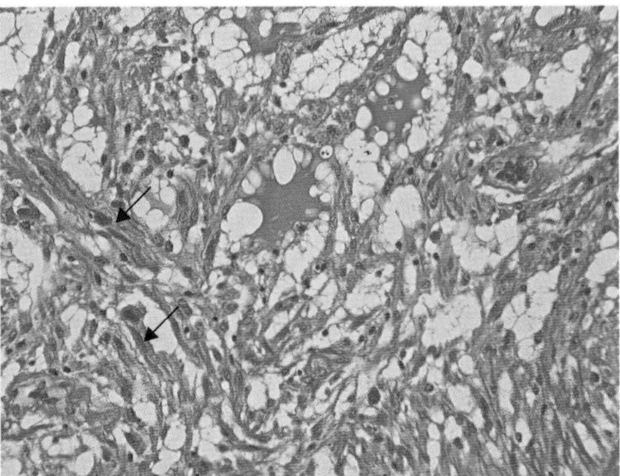

Figure 19.30 Optic nerve glioma. This shows the features of a pilocytic astrocytoma. Areas of cystic degeneration and Rosenthal fibers (arrows) are common in these slow-growing tumors. H&E.

region of the nerve may be excised or if there is extensive tumor with secondary complications such as exposure keratitis then the eye may be removed along with the affected segment of the nerve.

On gross examination there is characteristically a fusiform swelling of the nerve and the residual nerve may be barely visible within the tumor mass (Fig. 19.29). On histological examination the majority of these tumors are identical to intracranial pilocytic astrocytomas (Chapter 15). In older lesions degenerative changes such as myxoid areas and Rosenthal fibers are common (Fig. 19.30). The tumor may induce proliferation of the overlying arachnoid and this hyperplastic tissue may be misdiagnosed as meningioma if the biopsy contains only perineural tissue. Optic nerve gliomas have an excellent prognosis following complete surgical excision although vision is usually sacrificed.

Meningioma

Meningioma of the optic nerve may be primary, arising from the meninges of the optic nerve, or secondary due to extension of an intracranial meningioma. Optic nerve meningioma usually presents with visual loss and proptosis with inferolateral displacement of the globe. Gross optic nerve meningiomas will ensheath the optic nerve, which becomes atrophic due to compression. Meningiomas of the optic nerve characteristically show indolent growth and treatment should therefore be conservative. *En bloc* surgical excision is the treatment of choice. For large tumors this may require removal of the involved section of the optic nerve with the globe attached. Radiotherapy may slow tumor growth but is not curative and radiation retinopathy is a potential complication. On histological examination the appearance is similar to intracranial meningioma with a transitional pattern, sometimes with psammoma bodies is predominating.

SECONDARY TUMORS

Tumors originating from the eye, conjunctiva, eyelid, paranasal sinuses, nasopharynx or intracranial cavity may invade orbital tissue. Intraocular tumors include advanced retinoblastoma and uveal melanoma. Melanoma of the conjunctiva may infiltrate the orbit. The main eyelid tumors that can secondarily involve the orbit include basal cell carcinoma, sebaceous gland carcinoma and squamous cell carcinoma. This is well recognized for sclerosing basal cell carcinomas particularly those situated at the medial canthus which may extend down the medial wall of the orbit (Fig. 19.31). Squamous cell carcinoma, sinonasal carcinoma and

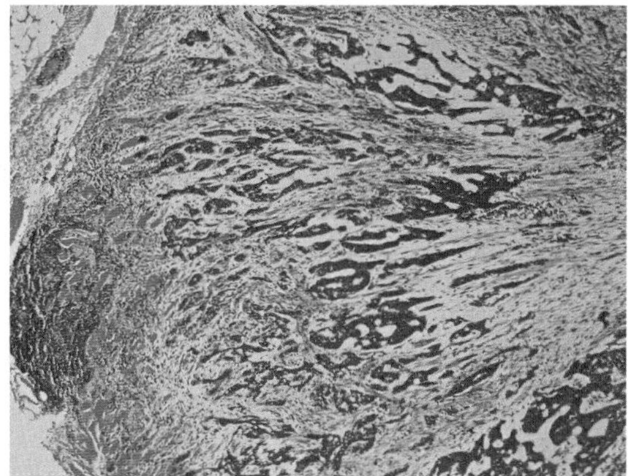

Figure 19.31 Secondary basal cell carcinoma. This basal cell carcinoma has a sclerosing pattern and has invaded into orbital fat and extraocular muscle. H&E.

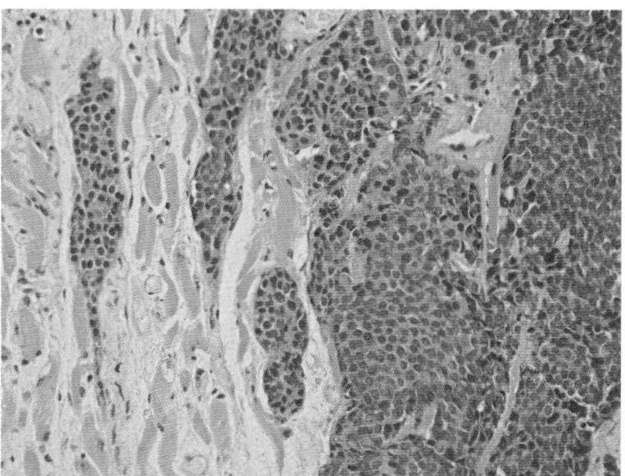

Figure 19.32 Metastatic carcinoid tumor. The tumor is composed of relatively uniform cells with granular, eosinophilic cytoplasm and is infiltrating an extraocular muscle. H&E.

olfactory neuroblastoma may extend into the orbit from the nasopharynx or sinuses. Intracranial meningiomas and rarely glioblastoma may extend to involve the orbit.

METASTASES

In adults most tumors metastatic to the orbit are carcinomas and orbital involvement occurs about one tenth as often spread to the uveal tract occurs. In contrast to children metastatic sarcoma is exceptionally rare. Patients are typically in their sixth and seventh decades, both orbits are equally affected and on occasion bilateral metastases can occur. In general, metastatic tumors to the orbit produce disproportionately severe complaints in comparison with primary orbital tumors. Pain, periorbital swelling, extraocular motility disturbances and decrease in vision may be more frequent, and symptoms develop over a shorter period than with other orbital tumors. Metastatic carcinoma may present a diagnostic challenge as it may occur long after a primary tumor has been treated or as the first sign of an undetected primary neoplasm. In these circumstances immunohistochemistry may be helpful in elucidating a primary site. The most common primary sites are usually the breast, prostate, lung or gastrointestinal tract but metastases from a wide range of primary carcinomas has been described. Metastatic carcinoid tumor in the orbit is also well recognized (Fig. 19.32). Survival following a diagnosis of orbital metastases is generally poor with a median survival for all tumors of between 10.4 and 15.6 months.

In children metastatic disease is usually orbital and uveal involvement is rare. Orbital involvement by neuroblastoma, Ewing's sarcoma, Wilm's tumor and rhabdomyosarcoma may occur.

THE LACRIMAL SYSTEM

Anatomy

Lacrimal gland

The lacrimal gland is pale brown, ovoid in shape (15 mm long) and is located in the shallow lacrimal fossa in the anterosuperior region of the orbit. It is composed of two main lobes, orbital and palpebral, by the levator aponeurosis. Its ducts drain into the superolateral conjunctival fornix. Accessory lacrimal glands (Wolfring and Krause) are located in the tarsal plate and the stroma of the fornix, respectively. The secretory component of the lacrimal gland is formed by lobules containing acini and draining tubules. The acini are formed by cuboidal cells, which secrete glycosaminoglycans and the

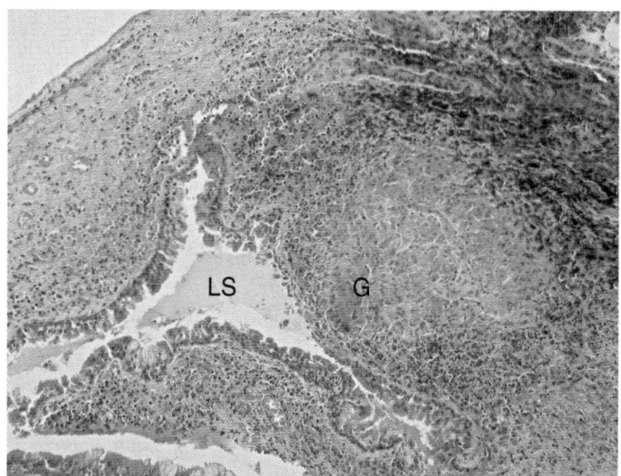

Figure 19.33 Lacrimal sac sarcoidosis. There is a well-formed epithelioid granuloma (G) surrounded by a cuff of lymphocytes situated in the wall of the lacrimal sac (LS). The lacrimal sac is lined by ciliated columnar epithelium with goblet cells. H&E. (Courtesy of Emeritus Professor W.R. Lee, University of Glasgow.)

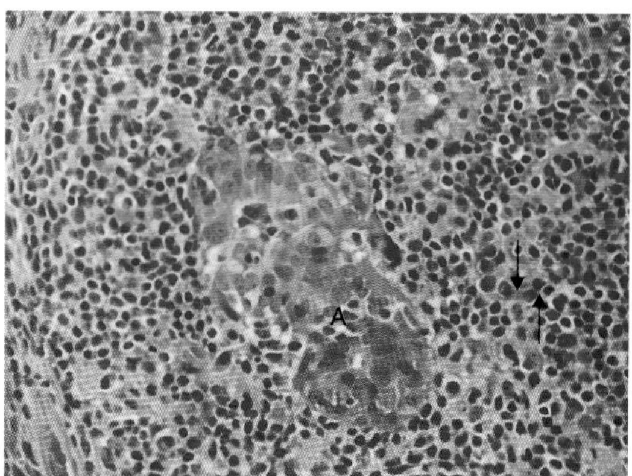

Figure 19.34 Sjögren syndrome. There is a polymorphic lymphoid infiltrate within the lacrimal gland including plasma cells (arrows). Surviving acini (A) are infiltrated by lymphoid cells to form a lymphoepithelial lesion. H&E.

antibacterial substances lysozyme and lactoferrin that are found in the tears. The interstitium contains scattered B cells, T cells and plasma cells, which produce immunoglobulins (IgA and IgM) that are transferred across the epithelium into the ductular system. The secretions from the acini drain into ductules, which are formed by epithelial cells surrounded by myoepithelium. The large drainage ducts (10–12 in number) are accompanied by blood vessels and lymphatics during their course to the superior fornix. The function of the gland is controlled by sympathetic and parasympathetic nerve fibers and the blood supply is via the ophthalmic artery.

Lacrimal drainage system

Tear fluid drains through the punctae at the medial end of the eyelids and through the canaliculi into the lacrimal sac. The sac is located in the lacrimal fossa in the inferomedial part of the orbit, and the duct leads into the nasal cavity. The canaliculi are lined by stratified squamous epithelium and the lacrimal sacs by a stratified columnar epithelium.

Inflammatory and lymphoid lesions of the lacrimal system

The lacrimal gland normally contains a significant population of lymphoid cells. Infections of the lacrimal gland are exceedingly rare but idiopathic inflammation, as previously described, may occur.

Sarcoidosis

Sarcoidosis is a cause of subacute and chronic lacrimal gland enlargement and sarcoid granulomas preferentially localize within the lacrimal gland rather than in other orbital soft tissues. The lacrimal gland is rarely biopsied as there are usually more accessible sites, e.g. conjunctiva, where the diagnosis can be confirmed. On gross examination the gland may be firm. Histological examination will confirm the presence of non-caseating granulomas often surrounded by fibrosis and with a variable accompanying lymphocytic infiltrate. Sarcoidosis may also be a cause of chronic dacryocystitis and is occasionally an incidental finding in a specimen removed at dacryocystectomy (Fig. 19.33).

Sjögren syndrome

In Sjögren syndrome xerostomia and keratoconjunctivitis sicca are associated with a connective tissue disorder. The lacrimal gland contains a diffuse infiltrate of lymphocytes and plasma cells and benign lymphoepithelial lesions may be seen accompanied by acinar atrophy (Fig. 19.34). This condition is considered to predispose to the development of lymphoma.

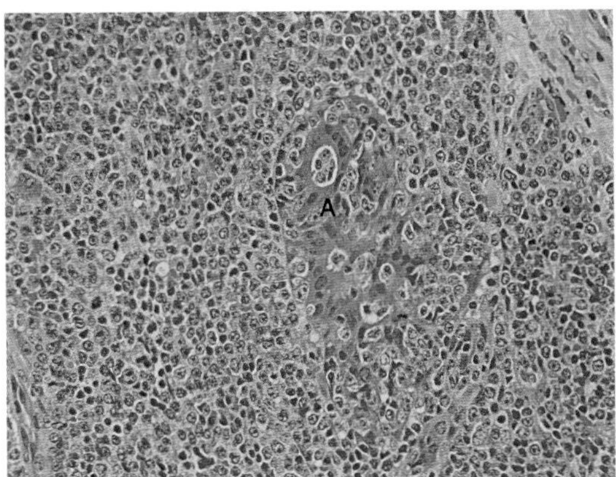

Figure 19.35 Extranodal zone lymphoma of the lacrimal gland. The tumor is composed of a relatively monomorphic population of small to medium-sized lymphoid cells with irregular nuclei. The lymphoid cells infiltrate and destroy the acini (A) of the lacrimal gland. H&E.

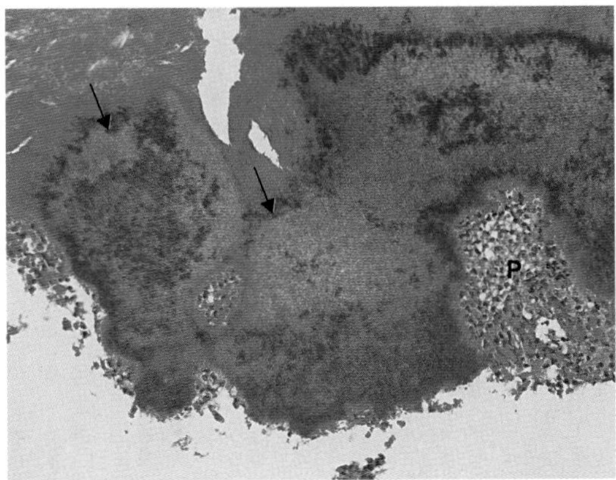

Figure 19.36 *Actinomyces* infection. Histology of characteristic sulfur granule composed of colonies of filamentous bacteria (arrows) associated with a polymorph exudates (P). H&E.

Lymphoma

The lacrimal gland may also by the site of lymphomas. Similar to lymphomas elsewhere in the orbit these are classified according to the WHO classification. Extranodal marginal zone lymphoma (EMZL) (so-called MALT-type) is the most common type (Fig. 19.35) and may arise *de novo* or in a patient with a long history of Sjögren syndrome. EMZL of the lacrimal gland may be treated with radiotherapy but patients should be followed-up as subsequent extraorbital lymphoma is more frequent with lacrimal gland disease compared with EMZL arising in other orbital tissues.

Acute dacryocystitis

Acute dacryocystitis is a common condition manifested clinically by swelling of the lacrimal sac, irritation and epiphora. Infection usually starts primarily in the lacrimal passages but in some cases it is caused by secondary spread of infections from the nose and paranasal sinuses or specific systemic infections. In acute cases an abscess may develop and this may drain through the skin resulting in a permanent external fistula. In chronic cases the excessive production of mucus may lead to a mucocele. Histological examination of chronic dacryocystitis reveals chronic inflammation and fibrosis with ulceration of the lining epithelium. If the contents of a mucocele become inspissated and a foreign body such as an eyelash acts as a nidus, a dacryolith may form. Histology of these frequently shows a mixed bacterial and fungal infection with layers of mucus. In *Actinomyces* infection characteristic 'sulfur granules' may also be expressed from the sac. These sulfur granules consist of colonies of Gram-positive filamentous bacteria (Fig. 19.36).

TUMORS OF THE LACRIMAL SYSTEM

Lacrimal gland tumors

Pleomorphic adenoma (benign mixed tumor)

Pleomorphic adenoma is the most common epithelial tumor of the lacrimal gland, representing 12% of lacrimal fossa lesions. It typically presents in middle age but has been described in virtually every age group. Most tumors arise from the deep orbital lobe and less commonly the palpebral lobe is the site of origin. This tumor is slow growing and painless and presents with proptosis and frequently downward and inward displacement of the globe. The tumor may flatten the sclera and indent bone but frank bone destruction is usually not evident.

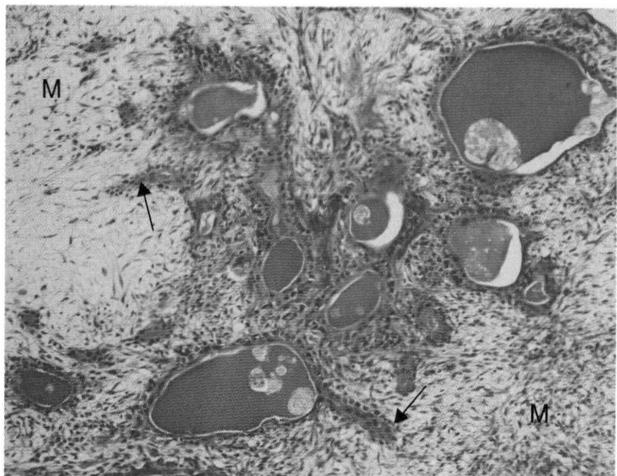

Figure 19.37 Pleomorphic adenoma. The epithelial component consists of a cluster of glands lined by cuboidal epithelium. An outer layer of myoepithelial cells is visible in some areas (arrows). The glands lie in a myxoid stroma (M) containing spindle-shaped myoepithelial cells. H&E.

These tumors are pseudoencapsulated and the excised specimen typically shows surface bosselations. It is therefore important to extensively sample the periphery of the tumor to assess excision. The cut surface often reveals cystic spaces and mucinous areas alternating with fibrous areas.

Histological examination reveals a mixture of epithelial and mesenchymal-like elements (Fig. 19.37). The epithelial component usually consists of acini with an inner layer of uniform cuboidal cells and an outer layer of spindle-shaped myoepithelial cells. In some tumors myoepithelial cells may predominate with sheets of spindle-shaped cells and minimal ductal differentiation. These myoepithelial cells may undergo a range of metaplasias including myxoid tissue, cartilage and rarely bone and fat. Focal squamous metaplasia may also be observed in the epithelial units. Immunohistochemical staining may be useful in defining the two cell populations as the myoepithelial cells are strongly positive for S-100 and smooth muscle actin and weakly positive for cytokeratins. The epithelial cells are strongly positive for cytokeratins and negative for S-100 and smooth muscle actin.

These tumors should be completely excised with an intact pseudocapsule, via a lateral orbitotomy. Incompletely excised tumors recur in about one third of cases and there is a small but significant risk of malignant transformation.

Pleomorphic carcinoma (malignant mixed tumor)

Pleomorphic carcinoma is considered the third most common epithelial tumor of the lacrimal gland and is defined as a pleomorphic adenoma that has undergone malignant transformation. It usually occurs in older patients presumably because malignant transformation occurs relatively late in the history of pleomorphic adenoma. It may present several years after incomplete excision of a benign tumor or with rapid enlargement of a previously asymptomatic or well-tolerated lacrimal gland swelling. Erosion of bone may occur.

Histopathological examination usually reveals a poorly differentiated adenocarcinoma in which a pre-existing pleomorphic carcinoma can be identified. Adenoid cystic carcinoma, squamous cell carcinoma, undifferentiated carcinoma or sebaceous carcinomas have also been described. Radical surgery (exenteration) is the treatment of choice but the prognosis is generally poor.

Adenoid cystic carcinoma

This is the second most common epithelial neoplasm of the lacrimal gland after pleomorphic adenoma. Although it is usually diagnosed in middle-aged or older patients, it frequently occurs in younger patients as well. The history is shorter than for pleomorphic adenoma and patients may present with proptosis, numbness, pain and diplopia because invasion of nerves and extraocular muscles may occur early in tumor development.

The tumors may appear well circumscribed but there is often invasion beyond the pseudocapsule. On histopathological examination these tumors can assume a range of patterns including a cribriform or 'Swiss-cheese' pattern and a sclerosing pattern (Fig. 19.38). An undifferentiated or basaloid pattern is considered to carry a worse prognosis.

Immunohistochemical staining usually shows positivity of cytokeratins and CEA in recognizable duct structures and may show the presence of an S-100 or smooth muscle actin positive myoepithelial cell layer.

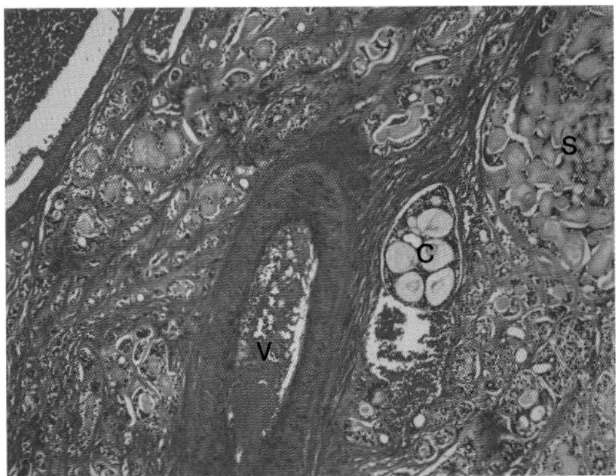

Figure 19.38 Adenoid cystic carcinoma. The tumor is composed of small basaloid cells with some areas displaying a cribriform pattern (C) and other areas with a sclerosing pattern (S). The tumor is infiltrating around a large blood vessel (V). H&E.

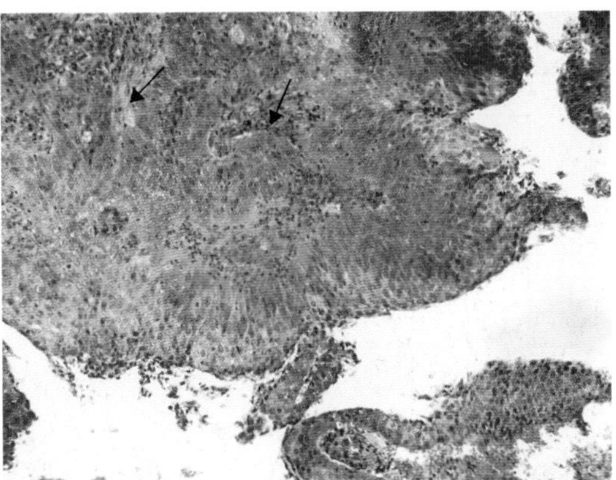

Figure 19.39 Lacrimal sac carcinoma. Transitional cell carcinoma showing a surface papillary architecture with invasion of the underlying stroma (arrows). H&E.

The tumor may be treated by surgery with supplemental radiotherapy or chemotherapy if required. More recently it has been shown that many adenoid cystic carcinomas display positivity for the KIT oncoprotein suggesting that imatinib mesylate may have therapeutic potential in some cases. Positivity for the KIT oncoprotein can be detected with immunohistochemistry.

Other malignant epithelial tumors

A small number of epithelial tumors of the lacrimal gland are adenocarcinomas arising *de novo* with no evidence of a pre-existing benign mixed tumor. Mucoepidermoid carcinoma is another rare form of carcinoma that may arise in the lacrimal gland. They are generally low-grade tumors that show a mixture of squamous and glandular differentiation.

Lacrimal sac tumors

Tumors of the lacrimal sac are uncommon and are usually of epithelial origin. Papillomas may show an exophytic, inverted or mixed growth pattern and the epithelium may be of squamous or transitional cell type. Carcinoma of the lacrimal sac may develop within a papilloma or arise *de novo* (Fig. 19.39). These are locally aggressive tumors and if neglected can invade surrounding structures. Both papillomas and carcinomas are associated with human papilloma virus type 11 and type 18, respectively. Lymphomas of the lacrimal sac are rare and are usually diffuse large B-cell lymphomas.

ORBITAL IMPLANTS

Spherical moulds may be used to reconstruct the orbit following enucleation to give better cosmetic results. These may be composed of a variety of materials with older implants consisting of polyethylene and more modern implants composed of coralline hydroxyapatite. Regardless of composition all implants are constructed with an interconnecting open-pore structure to allow ingrowth of fibrovascular tissue. These orbital implants may fail either because of extrusion or chronic pain, and may be submitted for histopathological examination. Polyethylene implants can be cut and processed directly as the plastic dissolves during processing leaving the fibrovascular tissue that has grown into the mould. Hydroxyapatite implants will require initial decalcification. Histological examination may reveal a chronic inflammatory infiltrate and often a deep-seated area of suppuration (Fig. 19.40). Gram stain may reveal bacteria, which are most commonly Gram-positive cocci.

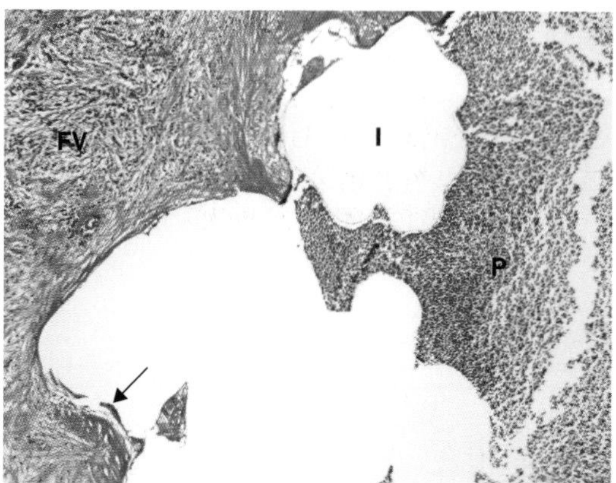

Figure 19.40 Infected orbital implant. The plastic of this implant (I) acts as a scaffold for the ingrowth of fibrovascular tissue (FV). Foreign body giant cells (arrow) surround the implant. This implant has become infected and there are inflammatory cells in the fibrovascular tissue as well as pus (P) surrounding the implant.

THE ORBITAL BIOPSY

With advances in imaging techniques and ancillary clinical studies many orbital masses do not require surgical biopsy. On the other hand many suspected malignant tumors will require a firm diagnosis prior to treatment and other lesions may require excision biopsy to relieve the patient's symptoms. Furthermore, imaging may not be able resolve the difference between certain benign and malignant lesions, for example, idiopathic orbital inflammation and lymphoma, such that biopsy should be considered in all patients without a firm diagnosis. For well-circumscribed orbital tumors, cystic lesions and lacrimal gland tumors excisional biopsy is the treatment of choice. Incisional biopsy may be more appropriate for diffuse orbital lesions, suspected lymphoid lesions or rapidly growing tumors of childhood. Fine-needle aspiration may be helpful for some tumors. Surgical access to lesions in the orbit may be difficult and insufficient or non-representative biopsies may be a problem particular for lesions in both anterior and posterior locations. Anteriorly placed lesions may be approached through the conjunctiva where a tentative biopsy may result in only subconjunctival connective tissue. Due to access insufficient tissue may be obtained from posteriorly situated lesions.

THE EXENTERATION SPECIMEN

An exenteration procedure entails surgical removal of the eyelids, the globe, the optic nerve and the extraocular muscles, the orbital fat and the periosteum. Advanced tumors of the eyelid such as sebaceous gland carcinoma may require exenteration. Neglected basal cell carcinomas can extend down the medial orbital wall and may necessitate inclusion of the ethmoid bones with the specimen. Similarly, malignant tumors of the lacrimal gland may require excision of the superolateral bony wall of the orbit. Occasionally advanced intraocular melanomas with extension into the orbit may require exenteration. In addition to ophthalmic pathology radical resection of the maxilla may be extended to incorporate the orbit. In this case the orbital component is usually separated from the main bulk of the tumor, which is submitted separately for examination by an appropriate specialist pathologist.

The first step is to orientate the specimen, noting that the lashes on the upper eyelid are longer than those on the lower. The medial canthus can be identified by the caruncle and the punctae. The optic nerve should be identified posteriorly and if necessary removal of the fat and superior rectus muscle will allow identification of the tendinous insertion of the superior oblique muscle and the muscular insertion of the inferior oblique muscle. Following orientation any attached bony tissues should be removed for decalcification. The specimen should then be sectioned with the aim to get one block that passes just off the center of the principal lesion and just off the edge of the optic nerve and pupil. The specimen should then be fixed for a further 24 h to ensure adequate penetration of orbital fat. In centers where it is not possible to process large blocks photographic documentation of the gross specimen may help the interpretation of histology. A prolonged processing cycle, such as that used for breast specimens, should be used to improve wax impregnation of orbital fat.

In addition to the main central block further blocks should be taken from lesional tissue and appropriate resection margins. For eyelid tumors radial blocks should be taken from the eyelid skin, and the site of these may be recorded as 'clock hours' on a suitable diagram. For orbital tumors the orbital periosteum should be assessed and the site of blocks may be recorded as medial, lateral, superior or inferior on an appropriate diagram.

CHAPTER 20

DISORDERS OF THE BONY COVERINGS OF THE BRAIN AND SPINE

Robin Reid

INTRODUCTION

The bones surrounding and supporting the brain and spinal cord and the joints which interconnect them are subject to the vast range of pathologies which affect the skeleton. In this brief chapter an effort has been made to discuss those disorders which are seen in the interface between orthopedic and neurosurgical pathology practice, essentially tumors and their radiological and clinical mimics, but also to describe briefly those clinically common disorders which are generally only seen in the laboratory practice in those countries which still have a frequent autopsy practice (Table 20.1).

Table 20.1 Common biopsies in orthopedic/neuropathological practice

	Clinical indication	Major pathologies
Spinal biopsy	Back pain Cord or nerve compression Vertebral collapse Incidental finding of abnormal bone texture/imaging signal	Metastatic carcinoma, myeloma, infection, primary bone tumor (rare) Osteoporosis as diagnosis of exclusion, Paget's disease
Lesions of calvaria	Lump Lytic defect on X-ray	Osteoma, hemangioma, Langerhans cell histiocytosis, myeloma, metastatic carcinoma
Lesions of craniofacial skeleton	Mass, deformity	Fibro-osseous lesions, giant cell reparative granuloma, aneurysmal bone cyst
Lesions of skull base	Mass, cranial nerve palsies	Metastases, myeloma, chordoma, chondrosarcoma
Lesions of sacrum	Cauda equina compression Pelvic mass	Metastases, myeloma, chordoma, teratoma, ependymoma, other rare bone tumors

HANDLING OF SMALL BIOPSIES

Increasingly, many lesions are diagnosed on the basis of percutaneous biopsies guided by imaging such as computed tomography (CT). Ideally, these should be submitted fresh to the pathology department to allow maximum information to be derived from what may be a small amount of tissue. Often, touch preparations allow an initial assessment to be made and help select additional investigations; seeing a small round blue cell tumor, for example, would suggest that a core or part of a core should be sent for cytogenetic analysis, unfixed in tissue transport medium. The increasing availability of molecular biological methods capable of using paraffin-embedded sections may in time supplant classic karyotyping.

The mainstay of diagnosis is, of course, conventional histology supplemented by the now extremely wide range of immunocytochemistry. The latter has diminished the importance of electron microscopy, but if this is considered likely to be of value a small piece should be fixed in glutaraldehyde for subsequent processing. If required, decalcification may be achieved with a range of agents, varying from rapid decalcification by strong acids such as nitric acid, which requires close monitoring to avoid over-decalcification with loss of nuclear staining and which may compromise nucleic acid techniques, through formic acid which is slower but rather more gentle, to EDTA which is the least damaging to the nucleic acids and, although slower, does not usually significantly delay the processing of small biopsies.

TUMORS OF THE SKULL AND SPINE

A similar range of primary and secondary bone tumors affect the skull and spine, and to avoid duplication these will be discussed together with mention of the sites of predilection. A subset of tumors and tumor-like lesions so specifically affect a given area that these are discussed separately.

Certain broad principles can be applied. Most benign spinal tumors tend to affect the posterior vertebral elements: pedicle, lamina, lateral and spinous processes. In contrast most malignant tumors tend to affect the anterior elements, principally the vertebral body. There are, of course, exceptions: both hemangiomas and giant-cell tumors tend to involve the vertebral bodies.

Secondary tumors

Metastatic carcinoma in the spine and myeloma greatly outnumber primary bone tumors. This reflects the relatively high incidence in the general population together with the high frequency with which carcinomas involve the spine, attributable to spread through Batson's prevertebral venous plexus and also by the arterial route.

The commonest primary sites, accounting for over 80% of cases are carcinomas of lung, breast and prostate. All malignancies may metastasize to bone, classically including renal and thyroid. Most metastatic deposits are osteolytic: osteoclastic bone destruction is driven by a vicious cycle mediated by tumor- and bone-derived cytokines and growth factors. Production of parathyroid hormone related protein (PTHrP) by tumor cells is increased by transforming growth factor beta (TGF-β) derived from bone; in turn PTHrP increases osteoblast expression of RANK (receptor activator of NFκB ligand) which activates osteoclasts. Anti-osteoclast drugs such as bisphosphonates are widely used to inhibit this process and treat the associated hypercalcemia.

Bone loss results in mechanical failure of bone with pathological fracture and vertebral collapse (Fig. 20.1). Both this and soft tissue extension may result in nerve root or spinal cord compression. Less often, notably in carcinomas of breast and prostate, the tumor cells stimulate intense reactive new bone formation resulting in osteosclerotic metastases.

Determination of the primary origin of metastatic carcinoma is made on the basis of classic histological features when present, e.g. clear-cell carcinoma of kidney, or in combination with immunocytochemistry with a panel of antibodies. The spine also may be affected by metastatic melanoma, sarcomas of bone or soft tissue origin and neuroblastoma.

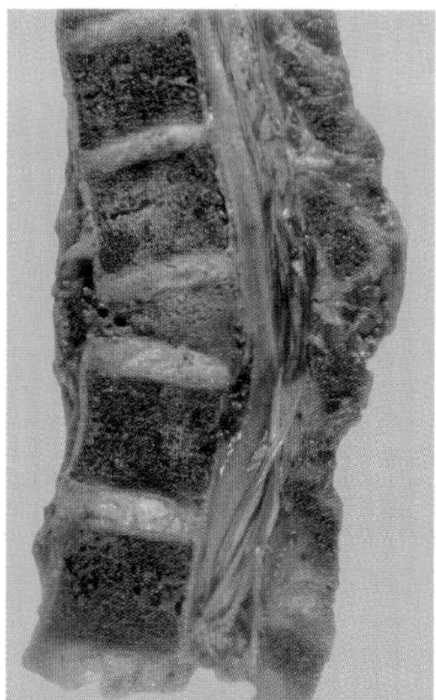

Figure 20.1 Secondary carcinoma in the spine. There is a wedge-shaped collapse of a vertebral body, with good preservation of the adjacent intervertebral discs. The tumor is bulging a little posteriorly towards the spinal canal.

Metastatic carcinomas less commonly involve the skull.

Myeloma

Classically, myeloma presents as a solitary lesion (plasmacytoma) or multiple punched out areas of bone lysis within the vault of the skull (Fig. 20.2a) or vertebral body, the latter often associated with vertebral collapse. It is important to remember that myelomatosis can also cause diffuse osteopenia, which on conventional radiographs cannot reliably be distinguished from simple osteoporosis. Clinical assessment including blood and urine analysis for immunoglobulins, Bence Jones proteins and erythrocyte sedimentation rate (ESR) and bone marrow aspirate are helpful. Biopsy shows sheets of plasma cells (Fig. 20.2b) varying from normal looking to frankly atypical. When well differentiated, detection of light chain restriction, by *in situ* hybridization (preferable to immunocytochemistry), confirms monoclonality.

Myeloma-induced bone destruction is also due to osteoclasts, again activated by RANK, and not accompanied by a comparable increase in osteoblast function as this is inhibited by a number of proteins.

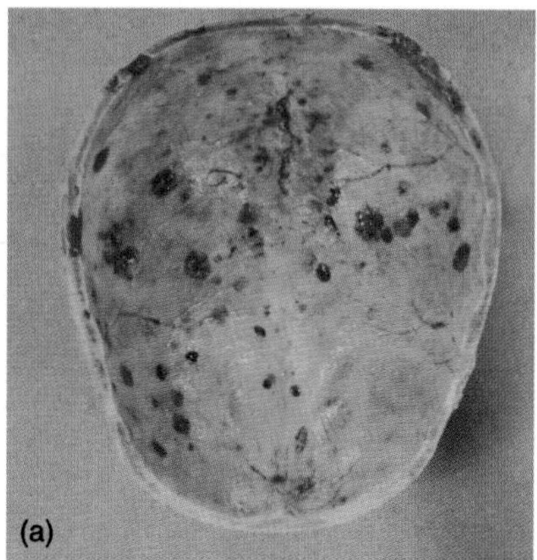

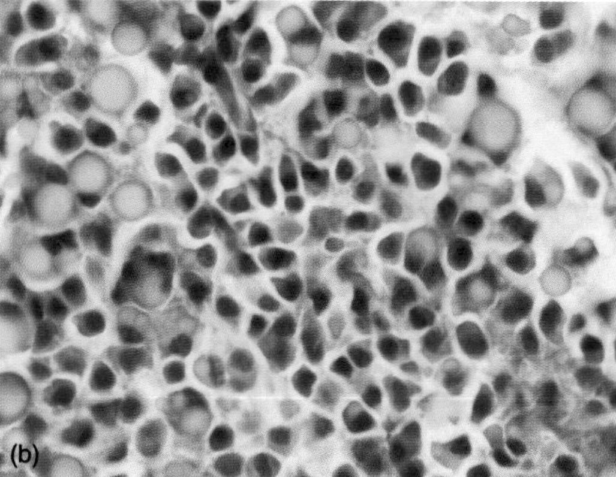

Figure 20.2 Myeloma. (a) This post mortem specimen of skull shows multiple red punched-out lytic lesions. (b) On histology, there are sheets of plasma cells. Numerous eosinophilic globules of immunoglobulin are present in this example. H&E.

Lymphoma

The spine may be involved by primary or secondary lymphomas, both Hodgkin's disease and non-Hodgkin's lymphomas, the latter overwhelmingly predominating in clinical practice.

Primary bone lymphoma is defined as a lymphoma confined to bone both at diagnosis and after 6 months follow-up although more than one bone may be involved. It accounts for around 5% of extranodal lymphomas and around 5% of primary bone tumors. The vast majority of primary bone lymphomas are high grade B-cell non-Hodgkin's lymphomas, expressing leukocyte common antigen (CD45) and B lineage markers such as CD20. CD30 is not uncommonly expressed and some of these tumors express CD10 indicating an origin from follicle center cells. Primary Hodgkin's disease of bone is extremely uncommon.

The full range of lymphomas can secondarily involve bone marrow and bone; a detailed description of the current classification and immunocytochemical findings is beyond the scope of this chapter.

Primary bone tumors

Bone-forming tumors

Osteoma

This is a benign lesion that typically affects the skull vault, presenting as a protuberance on the outer table, or from the paranasal sinuses. Histologically, those arising from the calvarium consist of compact bone with Haversian systems, while those affecting the sinuses tend to more active consisting of woven bone, often with active osteoblasts and osteoclasts. Osteomas are found as part of Gardner syndrome, with polyposis coli and desmoid tumors. Osteomas seldom affect the spine.

Osteoid osteoma

This tumor can affect any bone at any age, but not uncommonly it affects the vertebral column of adolescents and young adults, who complain of back pain, typically relieved by aspirin, and scoliosis.

Histologically, these have a central well-defined nidus which consists of trabeculae of woven bone formed by active osteoblasts and separated by fibrovascular stroma (Fig. 20.3). Numerous active osteoclasts may be seen, representing active bone turnover. The degree of reactive bone sclerosis seen around intracortical osteoid osteomas of long bones is seldom apparent within the spine. By definition osteoid osteomas are small, with a diameter of 1, 1.5 or 2 cm depending on arbitrary criteria. These are benign lesions with limited growth potential which seldom recur after removal. Percutaneous treatment by radiofrequency ablation is widely used, even within the spine.

Osteoblastoma

This is a benign bone tumor histologically very similar to osteoid osteoma from which it is distinguished largely on the basis of size (>2 cm diameter). Clinically, it is less painful than osteoid osteoma; it does have the potential to continue to grow (Fig. 20.4). Osteoblastoma has a significant risk of local recurrence following curettage; this a special problem in the spine and base of skull due to anatomical factors constraining surgical extirpation.

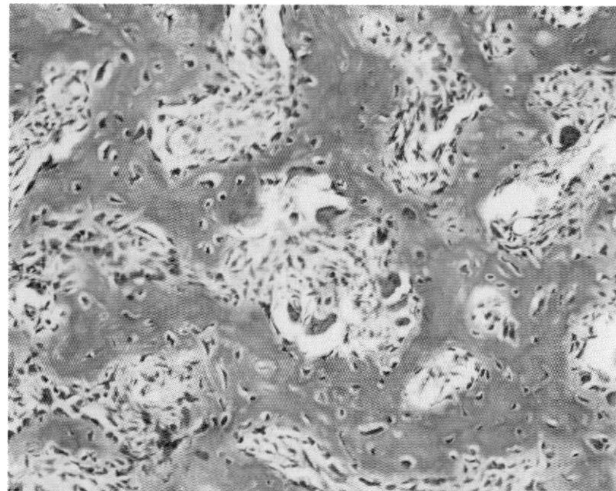

Figure 20.3 Osteoid osteoma. Interconnecting trabeculae of woven bone are separated by a fibrovascular stroma. The bone surfaces are lined by uniform osteoblasts and osteoclasts are also prominent.

Osteosarcoma

Osteosarcoma of the spine and skull is rare: indeed, metastatic osteosarcoma of long bones is more common than primary spinal osteosarcoma. Previous irradiation and Paget's disease predispose to the development of osteosarcoma, usually in older patients. Most spinal osteosarcomas are of high grade with early blood-borne metastases. Rare examples of parosteal osteosarcoma, with characteristic appearances of parallel trabeculae of woven or even lamellar bone separated by a fibroblastic 'stroma' of low histological grade, arise from the bone surface of the skull.

Occasionally, a bone-forming tumor falls into the borderline between an osteoblastoma and an osteosarcoma. These tumors often show more nuclear enlargement, mitotic activity and a more primitive matrix. The term 'aggressive osteoblastoma' formerly applied to these tumors has fallen into disuse. It is likely that these tumors are osteoblastoma-like osteosarcomas, although this diagnosis can only be made with certainty when a

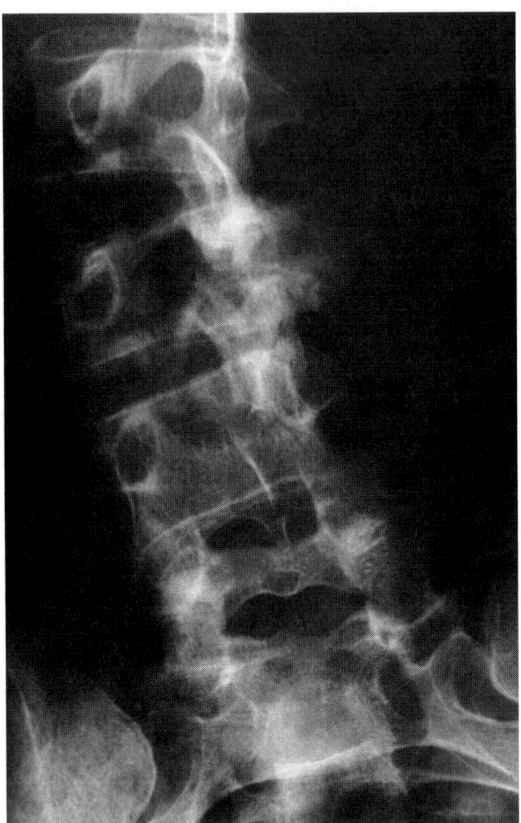

Figure 20.4 Osteoblastoma. This 14-year-old male presented with dull backache. This radiograph shows a sclerotic lesion in the pedicle of the 5th lumbar vertebra.

permeative growth pattern is detected. The practical implication is that these tumors tend to recur and extend locally but metastasize less often. Their anatomical location often leads to the death of the patient.

Cartilage tumors

Cartilage tumors of the spine are uncommon. *Osteocartilaginous exostoses* are seldom seen, other than in patients with multiple exostoses (diaphyseal aclasis) or who have received cranio-spinal irradiation for childhood leukaemia. Symptomatic *enchondromas* are rare indeed. *Chondroblastoma* and *chondromyxoid fibroma*, rare benign bone tumors of cartilaginous type, occasionally affect the base of skull, especially the petrous temporal bone.

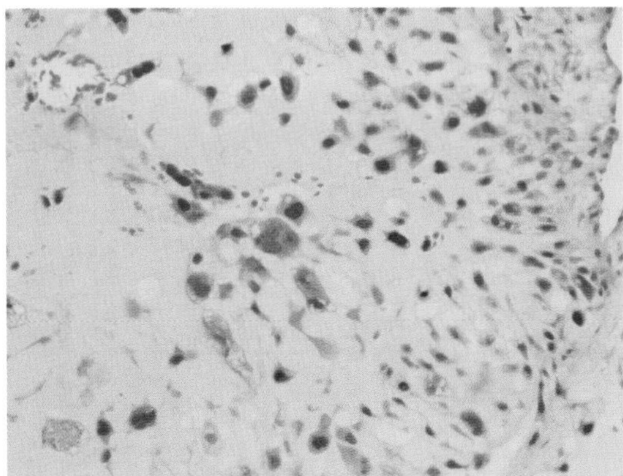

Figure 20.5 Chondrosarcoma. This high-grade tumor consists of tumor cells lying in a pale-staining chondroid matrix. There is considerable variation in cell and nuclear size and shape, a large multinucleated cell is present centrally and a mitotic figure lies to the bottom of the field. H&E.

Chondrosarcomas

Chondrosarcomas of the spine and skull are uncommon. Central chondrosarcomas tend to arise within the vertebral bodies and cause spinal cord compression due to mass effect. Peripheral chondrosarcomas usually arise from pre-existing exostoses and are therefore very uncommon. The vault of the skull is formed by intramembranous rather than endochondral ossification, and therefore cartilage tumors are very uncommon indeed. In contrast, the base of skull is formed by enchondral ossification and chondrosarcomas do arise at this site, often in relation to the petrous temporal bone and clivus. Most chondrosarcomas are slowly growing tumors; even the minority of high-grade tumors tend to metastasize late. Grading is carried out on cytological criteria (Fig. 20.5).

Chordoma

This tumor arises from notochord remnants and therefore can arise at any point along the neuroaxis, but especially at its ends. Thus the sacrum and base of skull – especially the clivus – far exceed in inci-

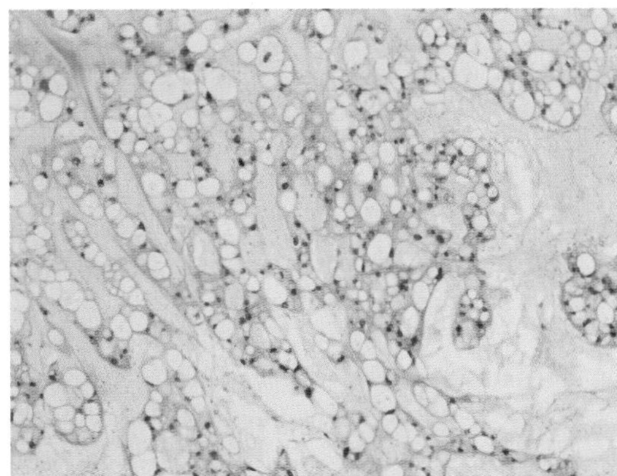

Figure 20.6 Chordoma. Large (physaliphorous) cells with abundant clear cytoplasm lie in packets and cords in a myxoid background. The nuclei are small and darkly stained. H&E.

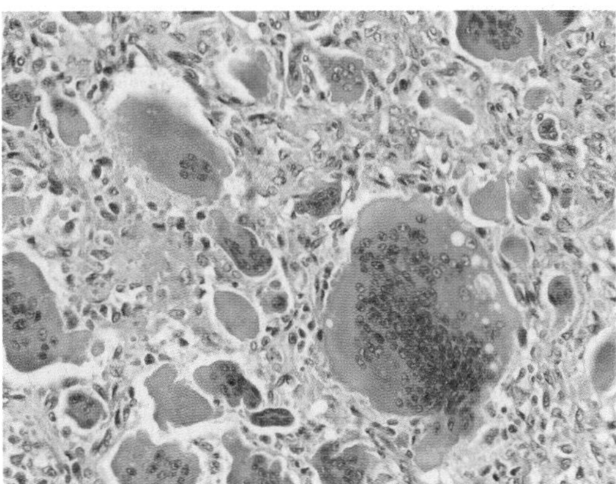

Figure 20.7 Giant cell tumor. Very large multinucleate osteoclasts dominate the field and between them lie ovoid mononuclear cells, whose nuclei resemble those of the giant cells. H&E.

dence the vertebrae, the cervical, thoracic and lumbar being affected in descending order of frequency.

Grossly, these tend to be bulky gelatinous tumors which destroy bone and form large soft-tissue extensions. Within the sacrum they typically bulge anteriorly and can be palpated per rectum (although they should not be biopsied from this approach due to seeding of tumor into the rectal wall). Lateral extension is also seen, particularly noteworthy with lesions in the cervical spine which may present as lateral neck masses which in turn may simulate lymphadenopathy.

Chordomas have a characteristic histological appearance with large 'physaliphorous' (bubble-bearing) cells with cytoplasmic vacuolation, these lying in a myxoid background (Fig. 20.6). There is often much intracellular glycogen, and the diagnosis is supported by the demonstration of cytokeratin, S-100 and epithelial membrane antigen in most cases. The major differential diagnoses are from metastatic carcinoma, particularly renal when the tumor is highly cellular, and chondrosarcoma when the myxoid stroma predominates. A minority of chordomas metastasize, and the rare association of chordoma with a high grade sarcoma (dedifferentiated chordoma) is associated with an especially poor prognosis.

It is increasingly recognized that benign notochordal tumors or hamartomas which are asymptomatic or associated with mild back pain may be found on modern imaging within the vertebral bodies and are important as benign mimics of chordoma, although they may occasionally represent precursors of frank chordomas.

Giant cell tumor

This tumor affects the sacrum and vertebral bodies and very seldom the skull. Before a diagnosis of giant cell tumor is accepted in the craniofacial skeleton, the possibilities of the histologically similar giant cell granuloma and brown tumor of hyperparathyroidism must be excluded, the latter applying also to lesions in the spine and sacrum. The microscopic appearance is distinctive with numerous large osteoclasts evenly spread through the tumor (Fig. 20.7). Interspersed are regular ovoid mononuclear cells, whose nuclei resemble those of the osteoclasts. It is now clear that the mononuclear cells are the tumor cells and the osteoclasts are reactive cells whose recruitment and maturation are driven by cytokines produced by the tumor cells.

Mitotic figures can be numerous, but significant nuclear pleomorphism and abnormal mitotic figures should indicate that this tumor is a sarcoma rich in osteoclasts. True giant cell tumor is locally aggressive and often occurs following curettage, but metastases occur in fewer than 5% of cases. Sometimes true giant cell tumors metastasize, while more commonly this follows sarcomatous

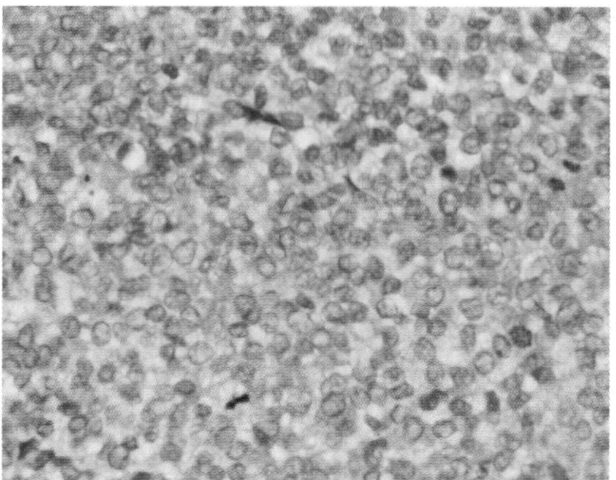

Figure 20.8 Ewing's sarcoma. This 'malignant round cell tumor' consists of sheets of uniform small cells whose nuclei have open chromatin. Mitotic figures are present, but the uniformity of the tumor belies its very aggressive nature. H&E.

transformation, often following previous radiotherapy, especially in the spine where surgical removal is difficult. These tumors therefore represent post-irradiation sarcomas.

Ewing's tumor

This tumor may arise in bone or in soft tissue. Paravertebral soft tissue tumors are not uncommon and large sacral or vertebral tumors are occasionally seen. The tumor is a malignant round cell tumor (Fig. 20.8), now known to be of primitive neuroectodermal type, whose cells often contain glycogen and express CD99. A series of pathognomonic chromosomal translocations are seen, the most common of which, t(11;22)(q24;q12) fuses parts of the *EWS* and *FLI1* genes to form a chimeric protein which acts as a transcriptional activator. These rearrangements can be detected by classic cytogenetic techniques or by molecular pathology.

The differential diagnosis lies in the group of small round blue cell tumors, usually in childhood, of which the main candidates are rhabdomyosarcoma, lymphoma, neuroblastoma and, with increasing frequency, poorly differentiated synovial sarcoma. The main patterns of immuno-staining and the characteristic cytogenetic findings are summarized in Table 20.2.

Aneurysmal bone cyst

This lesion, which usually affects the posterior vertebral elements, consists of a sponge-like mass of tissue with blood-filled spaces. It typically causes an expansile mass, often surrounded by an expanded shell of reactive bone, which may cause spinal cord or nerve root compression. Histologically, there are septae of fibrous tissue with scattered osteoclasts and osteoid matrix and blood-filled spaces which are not lined by endothelial cells (Fig. 20.9). Recurrence is uncommon. Aneurysmal bone cysts have traditionally been regarded as reactive lesions of uncertain etiology, but the presence of translocations within them suggests that they may be neoplastic. The entire specimen should be examined carefully, as aneurysmal bone cyst-like areas may complicate other lesions such as osteoblastomas. The classic differential diagnosis from telangiectatic osteosarcoma is less often seen in the spine than in the appendicular skeleton, but is still worth exclusion by careful examination for frank cytological atypia.

Hemangioma

Hemangiomas of the skull result in a well-defined area of lysis, sometimes with a dramatic spiculated pattern of reactive bone formation (Fig. 20.10). They are usually cavernous in type. Spinal hemangiomas were said to be very common based on extremely thorough autopsy studies but clinically apparent tumors are much less numerous. They have a destructive radiological appearance: thickened vertical bony trabeculae give a striped appearance on plain X-ray and a 'polka-dot' appearance on CT scanning in the horizontal plane. Much less common are frank angiosarcoma and the intermediate group of hemangioendotheliomas, many of which have an epithelioid morphology.

Fibro-osseous lesions of the skull

This term includes a number of lesions in which trabeculae of woven bone form by metaplasia from a fibro-blastic background. The prototype is *fibrous dysplasia*, skull involvement being isolated or as part of generalized polyostotic disease. This process can be affect the facial skeleton, the vault or base of skull, usually with ill-defined margins. Better defined lesions are described as *ossifying fibromas*. A rare subgroup of these, aggressive psammomatous ossifying fibroma, is noteworthy for its tendency to behave in a locally aggressive manner. Its histological appearance, with plump spindle cells and concentric calcified masses (Fig. 20.11), may be confused with a meningioma with psammoma bodies.

Langerhans cell histiocytosis (LCH)

This disorder, which typically presents in childhood and adolescence but which also may affect adults, forms a spectrum from solitary lesions in bone to a disseminated form often seen in infancy. Well-defined lytic defects of the calvaria are commonly seen, classically associated with diabetes insipidus or exophthalmos (Hand–Schuller–Christian syndrome), while vertebral involvement tends to cause vertebral collapse, typically to a flattened 'coin' lesion (vertebra plana). Histologically, LCH is characterized by oval Langerhans cells with abundant pale cytoplasm and cleaved nuclei, often admixed with eosinophils. The Langerhans cells express CD1A and S-100 protein and electron microscopy shows racket-shaped Birbeck granules.

Table 20.2 Malignant round cell tumors in childhood

Tumor	Main positive immunostains	Cytogenetic findings	Molecular basis	Comments
Ewing's sarcoma	CD99 CK, on occasion	t(11;22)(q24;q12) t(21;22)(q22;q12)	*EWS, FLI1* *EWS, ERG*	Other variant translocations found
Alveolar rhabdomyosarcoma	Desmin, MyoD1, myogenin	t(2;13)(q35;q14) T(1;13)(p36;q14)	*PAX3, FKHR* *PAX7, FKHR*	
Desmoplastic small round cell tumor	Cytokeratin, desmin (dot pattern); WT1; NSE (some CD99+ve)	t(11;22)(p13;q12) t(21;22)(q22;q12)	*EWS, WT1* *EWS, ERG*	Almost always intra-abdominal; rare at other sites
Neuroblastoma	NSE, neurofilament, chromogranin, synaptophysin, NB-84	del 1p	*N-myc* amplification	Raised urinary catecholamines
Synovial sarcoma	EMA, CK, calponin (CD99 often +ve)	t(X;18)(p11.23;q11) t(X;18)(p11.21;q11)	*SYT, SSX1* *SYT, SSX2*	
Small-cell osteosarcoma	Alkaline phosphatase by enzyme histochemistry; CD99 rarely positive	No consistent translocations		

NB: In any malignant round cell tumor in childhood it is worth adding terminal deoxynucleotidyl transferase (TdT) to the immunopanel as it is expressed in lymphoblastic lymphoma.

Intradural tumors

Spinal tumors also arise within the intradural space, both from the spinal cord (intramedullary) and from surrounding tissues (extramedullary). Magnetic resonance scanning is the technique of choice to determine the precise location and this largely predicts the histological differential diagnosis. This is summarized in Table 20.3. The major extramedullary intradural tumors are benign nerve sheath tumors especially schwannomas arising from peripheral nerve roots and meningiomas originating from the dura. Each may involve the spinal cord by compression. The major intramedullary tumors are discussed in detail in Chapter 15.

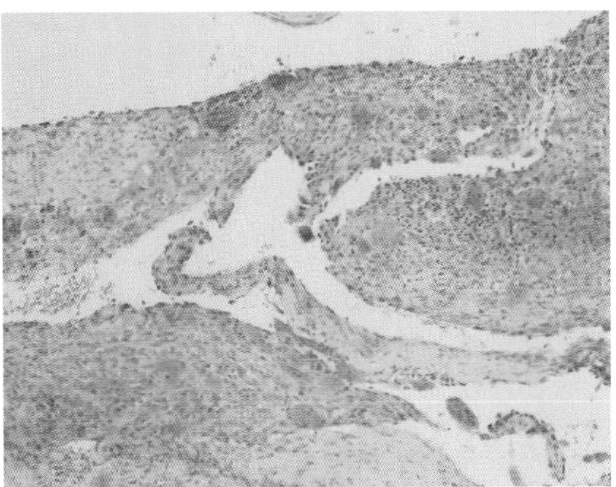

Figure 20.9 Aneurysmal bone cyst. This lesion has a sponge-like architecture, with septa of fibrous tissue containing osteoclasts and delicate osteoid matrix. Blood-filled spaces are not lined by endothelial cells. H&E.

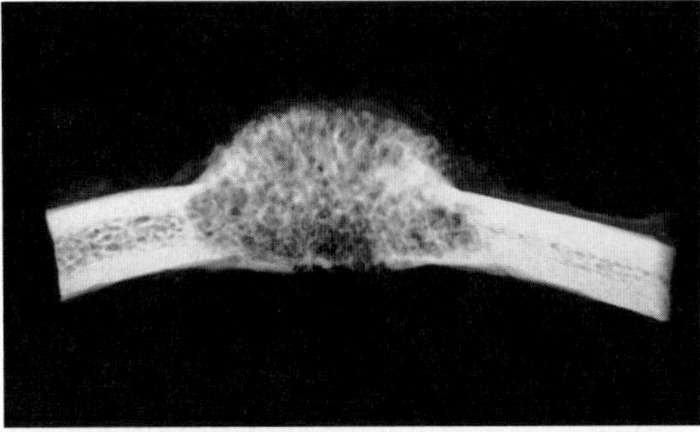

Figure 20.10 Hemangioma of skull. A specimen radiograph shows an expansile lesion with well-defined borders and with a spiculated pattern of bone trabeculae. Histology showed a cavernous hemangioma.

Infection of spine

Tuberculosis and pyogenic osteomyelitis remain important diseases, particularly in developing countries.

Tuberculosis (Pott's disease of the spine)

This is due to blood spread from tuberculosis elsewhere, typically in lung or bowel. In western countries an increase in incidence has followed in the wake of HIV infections. The lower thoracic spine is the commonest site and the infection causes destruction of the intervertebral disc and vertebral body with collapse typically resulting in an angular kyphosis. Spread often occurs along the intervertebral ligaments to adjacent vertebrae. In untreated disease, paraplegia classically follows spread into the extradural space with cord compression aggravated by bone deformity, while there may be associated tuberculous meningitis. Spread from the lumbar spine along the sheath of the psoas muscle may present in the inner aspect of the thigh as a psoas 'cold'

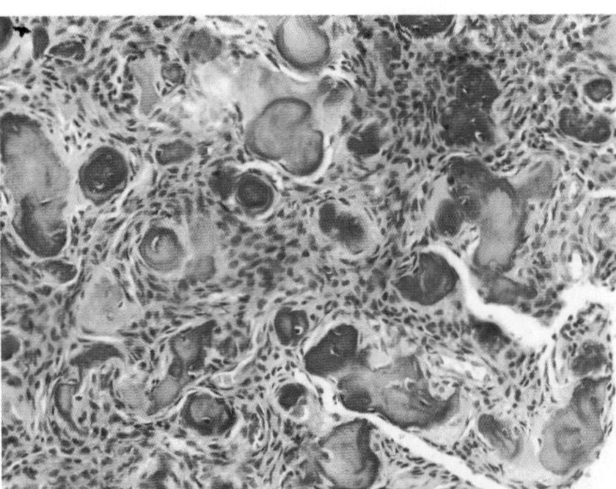

Figure 20.11 Aggressive psammomatous fibro-osseous lesion of skull. This is a cellular lesion composed of plump fibroblastic cells within which large masses of calcified bony matrix, some with concentric lamellations, have formed. H&E.

Table 20.3 Anatomical classification of commoner spinal tumors

Extradural	Intradural extramedullary	Intramedullary
Metastases	Meningioma	Ependymoma
Myeloma	Schwannoma	Astrocytoma
Lymphoma	Metastases	Hemangioblastoma
Chordoma	Epidermoid/dermoid cyst	Lipoma
Osteosarcoma	Lipoma	Epidermoid/dermoid cyst
Chondrosarcoma	Arachnoid cyst	Metastases, e.g. melanoma, carcinoma of breast
Ewing's sarcoma		
Hemangioma		
Osteoid osteoma		
Aneurysmal bone cyst		

abscess. The histological appearances of TB of the spine are of the caseating granulomatous inflammation seen elsewhere.

Pyogenic osteomyelitis

Pyogenic osteomyelitis of the spine occurs especially in the middle aged and elderly and affects the lumbar spine more commonly than the thoracic, the cervical spine being uncommonly involved. Clinically, the disease is often insidious in origin, patients complaining of chronic back pain often worse at night. Infection with Gram-negative bacteria, including *Escherichia coli*, *Proteus*, *Klebsiella* and *Enterobacter* often follows urinary tract infection or instrumentation, while intravenous drug abuse and diabetes mellitus also predispose, particularly to infection by *Staphylococcus aureus*, the commonest responsible agent. The infection initially is localized in bone adjacent to the intervertebral disc or within the disc itself (discitis); in either event, the disc is typically destroyed. Nerve root or cord compression are important complications of advanced disease, usually due to delayed presentation or diagnosis.

Metabolic bone disease

This term includes a variety of generalized skeletal disorders and Paget's disease which may affect one, several or many bones. Only a very brief outline is given and the reader is referred to standard textbooks on metabolic bone diseases.

Paget's disease of bone

This disorder, characterized by excessive and irregular bone turnover and thought to be due primarily to osteoclastic overactivity, can affect any bone but commonly involves the spine and skull. At post mortem around 3% of northern Europeans are affected by the disease, although clearly in many the disorder has been asymptomatic. In the spine, the vertebrae may show an increase in sclerosis or be widened with marginal sclerosis and relative central lucency, the so-called picture frame appearance. In the skull, large areas of lysis (osteoporosis circumscripta) characterize the early predominantly lytic phase of Paget's disease, while in the later phase, in which osteoblastic activity predominates, the skull is thickened with loss of the diploe. In each site the patient may complain of bone pain, deformity and the effects of compression either of nerve (for example the acoustic nerve leading to deafness) or indeed of spinal cord. Histologically, Paget's disease is characterized by exuberant activity of large osteoclasts excavating deep Howship's lacunae filled in by the resulting increase in osteoblastic activity but marked by the basophilic cement lines, which show an irregular mosaic or jigsaw pattern reflecting the resulting irregular bone structure (Fig. 20.12). The marrow is replaced by vascular fibrous tissue.

A small minority of patients develop sarcomas, mainly osteosarcomas or undifferentiated high-grade sarcomas, but the spine is affected less often than its common involvement by Paget's disease might predict.

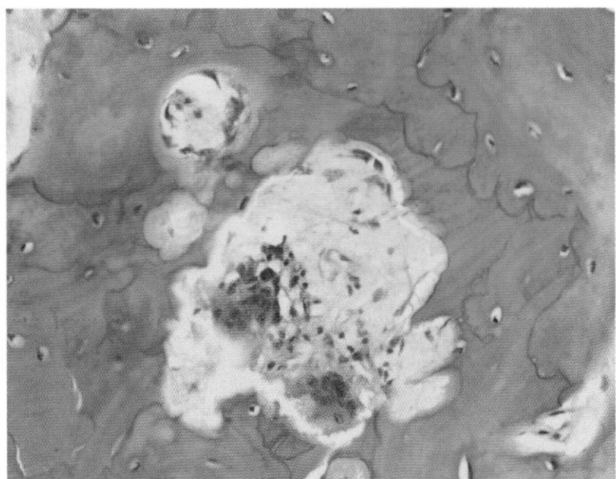

Figure 20.12 Paget's disease. The basophilic cement (reversal) lines in bone are irregular and 'mosaic-like' representing exuberant and irregular activity of large osteoclasts. H&E.

Osteoporosis

Defined as bone mass reduced by 2 standard deviations below the normal, generalized osteoporosis results in microarchitectural deterioration of bone resulting in mechanical failure. This commonly affects the spine, causing compression fractures, often with anterior wedging and bulging of the intervertebral disc through the vertebral end-plate into the vertebral body. With the advent of sophisticated radiological techniques for measuring bone density, only clinically suspicious vertebrae are subject to biopsy.

Hyperparathyroidism

Other than the rare brown tumor of hyperparathyroidism (see giant cell tumor), the typical appearance of increased bone turnover with dissecting resorption of trabeculae, formation of woven bone and marrow fibrosis is seldom seen in surgical practice, but abnormal bone texture may be seen in radiographs in patients with advanced hyperparathyroidism of all forms. The skull shows demineralization with a salt and pepper appearance, while the spine may show erosion of the vertebral end-plates.

Osteomalacia

Osteomalacia, still largely due to dietary deficiency of vitamin D, may cause fractures including vertebral collapse, and rickets may lead to spinal deformity including kyphosis, lordosis and scoliosis. The widened and extensive osteoid seams are only seen on undecalcified sections and are therefore not seen on spinal biopsies. Modern biochemical analysis has largely replaced the need for iliac crest biopsies in this area. Renal osteodystrophy, representing largely the effects of secondary hyperparathyroidism and osteomalacia, is similarly not often the subject of biopsy, but typical radiological appearances include the horizontal striped appearance of the 'rugger jersey spine' with sclerosis adjacent to the vertebral end-plates and central lysis.

Joint disease

The spine contains well over 100 articulations and unsurprisingly is affected by degenerative disease as well as inflammatory arthropathy. Osteoarthritis of the spine (spondylosis) is almost universal in the elderly and is associated with degenerative changes in the intervertebral discs and their narrowing. This leads to involvement of the intervertebral facet joints, characterized pathologically by the usual manifestations of osteoarthritis, namely fibrillation and loss of the articular cartilage with sclerosis and eburnation of the exposed underlying bone, formation of osteophytes and related synovitis. The osteophytes may compromise the intervertebral foramina, leading to nerve root and, in the cervical spine, vertebral artery insufficiency. Spondylosis of the lumbar spine is sometimes associated with degenerative spondylolisthesis where a vertebral body is displaced anteriorly relative to the body below, resulting in narrowing of the spinal canal (spinal stenosis) and nerve root compression.

Rheumatoid arthritis

The clinical features of rheumatoid arthritis are well known and will not be repeated here, other than to indicate that symptoms related to cervical spine involvement are common. These range from pain to severe erosive arthritis, classically causing resorption of the odontoid process. This may result in fracture of the odontoid or atlanto-axial subluxation with basilar invagination.

Seronegative arthropathies

Ankylosing spondylitis is the typical member of this group of diseases, affecting young adult males, over 90% of whom carry the HLA B27 allele. While there may be peripheral arthritis of synovial joints, the brunt of the disease falls on the sacro-iliac and lumbar joints, in severe cases leading to bony fusion (ankylosis) of the apophyseal joints and intervertebral discs. This process advances upwards to involve the thoracic and cervical spine, with fusion of costospinal joints compromising respiratory function. An unrelated condition is ankylosing hyperostosis of the spine, in which ossification of the paravertebral ligaments without disc disease leads to bony union of the spine, especially in the thoracic region.

CHAPTER 21

THE LAW AND FORENSIC NEUROPATHOLOGY

Marjorie Black and Tobias Hatter

INTRODUCTION

Forensic pathologists and neuropathologists should work closely to derive the very best information and evidence for the benefit of the public, the medical profession and the justice system. There have been a number of factors in the United Kingdom in the recent past that have produced change and no doubt working practices in the two specialities will continue to evolve to meet these challenges. These include concerns raised following retention of organs at post mortem examinations at Alder Hey Hospital in Liverpool and in the case of Mr Cyril Isaacs (The Isaac Report) and also:

- In Scotland the Independent Review Group on Organ Retention
- Reviews of the Anatomy Act and the Human Tissue Act
- Coroner's Review and the Shipman Enquiry
- Decline in hospital post mortem examinations

The nature of forensic practice and workload varies throughout the UK (and even more so in mainland Europe and the rest of the world). This is principally due to differing legal systems and employment practice.

LEGAL SYSTEMS IN THE UK

England and Wales

The coroner's system is currently under review following the publication of Dame Janet Smith's reports on the Harold Shipman Inquiry and the Luce Report on Death Certification and Investigation in England, Wales and Northern Ireland, which culminated in the publication of a position paper by the Home Office in March 2004 (www.theshipmaninquiry.org.uk; www.official-documents.co.uk; www.homeoffice.gov.uk/justice).

The exact nature of any changes is not yet known but it appears likely that they will be primarily organizational with the creation of a new medical examiner position to regulate the death certification process. Currently the coroner has jurisdiction under s.8(1) of the Coroners Act 1988 over bodies in his district that have died a violent or unnatural death, have died suddenly and the cause is unknown or have died in prison. A list of reportable deaths is available (see Dorries, 1999, in the Further Reading section). In England and Wales the doctor certifying death must have treated the deceased in life for the final illness and either seen the deceased within

14 days of death or after death. The coroner can instruct a post mortem examination under s.19 of the Act which can either be the basic examination or be one that is deemed to require 'special skills'. A special examination is different and refers to a case where additional investigation is necessary. The coroner must hold an inquest into the death if it falls into any of the categories under s.8(1) above.

Histopathologists, in addition to their primary employment, undertake the majority of coroners' post mortems. These post mortems encompass the full range of non-suspicious deaths and therefore include not only natural disease but also head injuries from accidental falls and vehicular accidents and suicides, for example. Suspicious deaths, however, are referred to Home Office pathologists. To be appointed onto the Home Office list, pathologists require training and experience in forensic pathology.

Scotland

Scotland, in alignment with its separate legal system, has a completely different death investigation process under the auspices of the Crown Office, the branch of the Scottish Executive responsible for the legal system. One of their roles is the investigation of deaths and in the larger offices there will be dedicated 'deaths units' which serve a similar role to that of the coroner.

The fiscal's responsibilities are to investigate certain categories of death with the aim of finding out whether any criminal act has caused or contributed to the death or to discover whether the death has arisen from hazardous circumstances where action may prevent future deaths or injuries.

The types of case that should be referred to the fiscal are specific, regularly revised and are accessible (Independent Review Group on Retention of Organs at Post-mortem – www.show.scot.nhs.uk/scotorgrev). The main groups are unnatural deaths, deaths that have potentially resulted from medical intervention, where there is any concern or allegation of a lack of care or medical mishap and uncertified deaths. In Scotland any doctor can certify the cause of death – they do not need to have known or treated the deceased in life.

The majority of Scotland is covered by full-time forensic pathologists in the cities of Glasgow, Edinburgh, Aberdeen and Dundee who are contracted to the Crown Office to investigate all suspicious and substantial numbers of the non-suspicious deaths. In the more outlying areas the histopathologists are employed in an analogous situation to that in England and Wales.

Under Scots law there is a requirement for evidence to be corroborated. Thus in any death where significant criminal charges may result two pathologists will be instructed and a joint report will be issued.

A fatal accident inquiry (FAI) is the equivalent of the coroner's inquest but has different criteria and outcomes. Mandatory FAIs are required only in deaths in custody and accidental death at work. In other cases the decision as to whether an FAI is held at the discretion of the Lord Advocate, the chief law officer.

RETENTION OF ORGANS AND TISSUES

In a medico-legal post mortem examination consent is not required from the relatives as a legal authority instructs it. The basis for legal retention of organs or tissues is that they are a necessary part of establishing the cause or circumstances of the death. Practice has been modified in recent years in compliance with guidance from the Independent Review Group in Scotland (www.show.scot.nhs.uk/scotorgrev), the Chief Medical Officer and in compliance with the reviews of the Human Tissue Act and the Anatomy Act (www.dh.gov.uk/PublicationsAndStatistics/Publications and www.scotland.gov.uk/Topics/Health). When the pathologist is aware that organ retention is required the coroner/fiscal should be contacted and informed of the reason. They should then inform the relatives. Amendments to the Cremation Regulations now enable separate cremation of organs.

In neuropathology cases best practice is fixation for 2–3 weeks before examination. Alternative practices have been developed to minimize the delay without significantly compromising the examination. Microwave fixation of the brain and sectioning within 24 h has been reported to produce good results. (Barrett *et al.*, 2004) Local practice has evolved such that in many cases only a short period of fixation, of as little as 48 h, is undertaken before sectioning by the neuropathologist. This has resulted in very reasonable results and the brain has been able to be returned to the body without delaying any funeral arrangements. This is dependent on easy access to a neuropathologist. In some cases, particularly where there is diffuse brain damage or epilepsy, it would be possible for the forensic pathologist to sample the brain, after a similar short fixation if possible, and to retain only the relevant slice(s) for subsequent neuropathology (Love, 2004).

It is important, however, that the information, particularly in suspicious deaths, is not compromised and the coroner/fiscal must be willing to accept that in at least some cases there is no acceptable alternative to a significant period of retention.

Full general histology should also be taken in all suspicious deaths in accordance with The Code of Practice for Forensic Pathologists (Royal College of Pathologists) – its use for any purpose other than diagnosis will almost certainly be restricted under the new laws discussed above. In non-suspicious cases the pathologist should comply with best practice guidelines published by the Royal College of Pathologists but must retain tissue only in accordance with the respective legal system (The Coroners (Amendment) Rules 2005 – www.uk-legislation.opsi.gov.uk/si/si2005, www.show.scot.nhs.uk/scotorgrev).

ROLE OF THE EXPERT WITNESS

There are three types of witnesses in law. Ordinary and professional witnesses speak about factual events that have occurred in daily life or during the course of their work, respectively. Expert witnesses speak about factual evidence but are also recognized by the court as having expertise in their subject and can therefore offer opinions. Experts have a duty to provide an independent opinion to the courts and to clearly state evidence and opinion that could be important to either the Crown or the defence. Such opinion should have a scientific foundation and it should be made clear when opinion is based on their experience or on the literature. Experts must be careful not to stray outside their area of expertise.

FORENSIC POST MORTEMS

The aims of a forensic post mortem obviously encompass some of those of a hospital consent examination but there are additional considerations that will vary depending on the nature of the case. These will include:

- Establishing the cause of death
- Determining the circumstances surrounding the death
- Excluding or confirming criminality
- Excluding or confirming whether natural disease has contributed to death
- Investigating the role of any alleged lack of care or misdiagnosis
- Collection of evidence
- Identification

The basic post mortem procedure is no different, but it may require to be modified to the circumstances of the case and there are a number of special techniques that are occasionally required that are little used elsewhere.

The external examination is of more importance than is often the case in hospital cases. Post mortem changes – hypostasis and rigor mortis – should always be assessed and recorded. Careful and thorough documentation of injuries is essential including their nature, size and position – the aim being that the reader can visualize and interpret the injuries without a photograph. Whilst each injury may individually be important, e.g. in determining a weapon, the overall pattern can be equally important in evaluating the circumstances that produced them, e.g. fall versus assault. In suspicious deaths all injuries should be photographed, with a scale where appropriate.

Exclusion of injuries as causal or contributory to death can be at least as important as confirming that death was as a result of violence. External injuries to the scalp and skull fracture (if any) can be vital to the interpretation of the underlying pathology.

GLASGOW DATABASE

In Glasgow, the Department of Forensic Medicine and Science has worked closely with the Department of Neuropathology at the Institute of Neurological Sciences for over 20 years. A recent audit was undertaken to review the number and nature of the cases that were referred by the forensic pathologists to the neuropathologists from 1995 to 2003. This has produced a detailed picture of the nature of the neuropathological deaths that are investigated by forensic pathologists.

Due to the ongoing changes in organ retention practice, the number of whole brains retained for examination after fixation has declined dramatically (Table 21.1). Whole brain retention now occurs in cases in which legal proceedings are likely or the diagnosis is not clear at the initial post mortem stage. Sampling of relevant sections of the brain prior to fixation and referral of the samples to neuropathologists have increased. This technique can give good results but relies on close liaison with a neuropathologist to ensure the correct anatomical regions are sampled adequately depending on the likely diagnosis. Cases in which the diagnosis is relatively straightforward such as extensive disruption of the brain following trauma, bacterial meningitis or brain metastases from a known primary malignancy are usually not referred. The types of cases referred to neuropathology are shown in Table 21.2.

In suspicious deaths and cases of suspected sudden infant death syndrome, negative findings can be as important to document as identifiable pathology, e.g. to exclude significant head trauma in an alleged assault. The contribution of underlying natural disease in trauma cases may also be important to assess. The main reasons for referral of material are outlined below. In cases where survival following injury has been prolonged it may be important to estimate the time period of survival from the initial injury. This can be problematic and at best only a broad timeframe can be estimated. In suspicious cases photographic documentation of pathological lesions may be required.

It is not the intention in this chapter to fully discuss the pathologies that are dealt with elsewhere in the book but rather to address some of the specific forensic issues the pathologist may be presented with. The principal reasons for referring to neuropathology are listed in Table 21.3.

Table 21.1 Changing retention practice

Period	Number of forensic autopsies (yearly average)	Neuropathology retention
1995–1998	2007	240 (12%)
1999–2003	1956	88 (4%)

NATURAL DEATHS

Epilepsy

Epilepsy can cause death from a number of mechanisms and most cases should be referred to the appropriate legal authority, the exception perhaps being status epilepticus, which if clearly documented

Table 21.2 Types of cases referred to neuropathology

Period	Total	Natural	'Stroke'	Trauma	Suspicious	SIDS
1995–1998	240	13 (5.5%)	45 (18.5%)	79 (33%)	78 (32.5%)	25 (10.5%)
1999–2003	88	4 (4.5%)	14 (16%)	16 (18%)	34 (38.5%)	20 (23%)

SIDS, sudden infant death syndrome.

Table 21.3 Principal reasons for referring to neuropathology

Normal or abnormal?
Cause of death?
Diagnose pathology
- Nature
- Distribution
- Severity

Mechanism of damage
- Natural
- Trauma
- Metabolic (e.g. hypoxic–ischemic, hypoglycemia, carbon monoxide)
- Timing of injuries where possible (e.g. subdural hematoma I, diffuse axonal injury)

could be certified as the cause of death without such recourse. Accidental deaths secondary to a seizure, e.g. potential drowning or falls, should be referred as non-natural deaths and the post mortem examination ought to document the findings required to establish such a mechanism of death. It is now recognized that many deaths from epilepsy occur suddenly and unexpectedly, with or without evidence of a seizure, and that asphyxia or inhalation of gastric contents do not need to be postulated to account for these deaths and should not be without clear pathological evidence to support the diagnosis. The definition SUDEP (sudden unexpected death in epilepsy) has been accorded to such cases. It is a diagnosis of exclusion as there are no diagnostic features of such deaths and therefore a full post mortem examination including histology and toxicology is required to rule out other natural disease and intoxication (Black and Graham, 2002).

Neuropathology may identify an anatomical basis for the seizures which may have potential medicolegal implications, e.g. if a head injury occurred as a result of an assault or was sustained in a car accident in which another party was at fault.

Subarachnoid hemorrhage

Naturally occurring subarachnoid hemorrhage (SAH) will present to the forensic pathologist as a sudden unexpected natural death and must be distinguished from that which is secondary to trauma, usually evident from the circumstances of the death and the injuries, if any, identified on external examination.

The majority are secondary to rupture of a saccular aneurysm and the distribution of the blood is appropriate to the site of the aneurysm. The search for the aneurysm should be undertaken at the time of the post mortem examination even if the brain is being retained as the blood clot is adherent after fixation.

There are two specific circumstances where there is substantial medico-legal interest. First, there may be a history of recent headaches which could originate from previous smaller subarachnoid bleeds and there could be litigation if they have been unrecognized by medical personnel. Thus full neuropathology is always recommended in such cases to confirm or eliminate the presence of older hemorrhage with organization and/or hemosiderin staining of meninges.

Second, where the subarachnoid hemorrhage is detected following an episode of trauma the question then arises as to whether the trauma has caused or precipitated the hemorrhage or indeed has the SAH caused the person to fall and subsequently sustain the trauma. If the trauma was part of an assault then there are obvious implications if a causal link is established.

This is a complex problem requiring as much information of the circumstances as is possible. Naturally occurring SAH can have no obvious precipitating event; other causes are associated with an episode that would lead to a catecholamine response and thus rises in blood pressure, heart rate, etc. which could have precipitated the rupture. When the episode is a physical, or even only verbal, altercation then the prosecution may propose that this is the direct cause of the SAH. It is also a possibility that a direct blow to the head could mechanically cause an aneurysm to rupture, particularly if it is thin-walled and friable. The time interval between the incident and collapse/development of the bleed is important; the closer the temporal link the more likely there is a causal connection (Saukko and Knight, 2004).

Intracerebral hemorrhage

Intracerebral hemorrhage (ICH) can also present as a sudden unexpected death and it too can be either natural or secondary to trauma, the latter usually distinguishable by the circumstances and other traumatic injury. Primary spontaneous ICH is most frequently associated with hypertension. This has two medico-legal implications.

First, any event which could result in an episode of raised blood pressure could potentially be linked to the death, e.g. a verbal confrontation or confronting a burglar, much in the same way as for SAH discussed above. Postulating a causal association, if any, between the two events depends on consideration of a number of factors including most importantly the temporal association; the closer in time the two occurred the more likely that there is a link. Caution should always be expressed, however, as most victims are at risk of suffering such an event at any time and it may not be possible to exclude the possibility that the ICH would have happened even without the potential precipitating event.

Second, in a younger or atypical population the possibility that the ICH is secondary to ingestion of illicit drugs should always be considered even if there is no known history of such drug use. Cocaine and amphetamines, including MDMA (ecstasy) are widely abused and are associated with episodes of hypertension and an increased risk of ICH. A full toxicology screen including the suspected drugs must be undertaken in these cases. In some legal systems if the death is considered to be the result of illicit drugs, including the above circumstances, then there is the potential for the supplier of the responsible drugs to be charged with causing the death. (Culpable homicide in Scotland is the equivalent of manslaughter.)

Hypoxic/ischemic brain damage

It is not uncommon for someone to die in hospital with a diagnosis of diffuse hypoxic or ischemic brain damage in circumstances which should result in a medico-legal post mortem examination. Neuropathology can exclude diffuse traumatic injury or other pathology. Whilst retention of the whole brain for the neuropathologist is best practice it is possible to achieve good results in these cases with appropriate sampling for histology. The nature of the insult can then be correlated with the primary event that can often have important medico-legal implications. Examples include:

- Diffuse hypoxic damage following respiratory arrest. This can be a consequence of compression of the neck, either suicidal hanging or ligature/manual strangulation. Whilst often there are external injuries that identify the nature of the trauma, in some instances, e.g. if the ligature is broad and soft and/or removed quickly then it can be very difficult to detect a ligature mark. There may or may not be petechial hemorrhages.
- Such a pattern of damage is also seen secondary to drug overdose. In many hospitals, at best only selective screening of blood or urine is undertaken and at least, in the authors' experience, very few drugs are quantified in the blood. As it is commonly hours or many days before death occurs a blood sample from as soon after admission to hospital as is possible should be retrieved for full toxicological analysis.
- Boundary zone damage secondary to an episode of hypotension. This can be natural, e.g. secondary to myocardial ischemia, or traumatic, e.g. as a consequence of hemorrhage from a stab wound.
- Hypoglycemic damage. It is important that this is distinguished from the above patterns and a cause for it identified if possible.

ACCIDENTAL DEATHS

Road traffic accidents

The cause of death may seem self-evident if there is clear massive head injury but there are often additional injuries identified at post mortem examination that can add valuable information when attempting to reconstruct what happened – even if death is effectively instantaneous. This is even more so when there has been a significant survival period when the nature of the brain injury e.g. DAI/DVI, hypoxia post cardiac arrest can be determined.

There are a number of questions that need to be addressed by the pathologist in road traffic accidents whether the victim is a pedestrian, cyclist or car occupant:

- Do the injuries correspond with the known circumstances of the incident, e.g. a head injury frequently results from secondary impact with the car or ground? Occasionally, the victim may already be lying on the ground and in this instance the pattern of injury could be that of crushing or dragging from being run over.
- Was the accident survivable? If it was did any potential delay in treatment contribute to the death?
- Was there any natural disease, e.g. dementia or effects of alcohol intoxication (acute or chronic), that could have contributed to the accident?

Falls

Falls can be subdivided into two categories in which the pattern of injury is usually quite different.

Simple falls

Death from a head injury occurs frequently after a simple fall (from one's own height or a short height) backwards on to a hard surface. This results in a typical pattern of injury. There is frequently external blunt injury comprising any combination of bruising or abrasion sometimes with a single linear laceration at the site of the impact. In cases where, for example, a thick head of hair is protective and no external injury is present bruising may still be seen on the undersurface of the scalp. A linear skull fracture is often present usually, but not always, at the site of impact and 'contre-coup' fractures of the frontal bones are described. More complex or comminuted fractures are very unusual. A recent review of the files of Forensic Medicine at the University of Glasgow for the years 1994–2004 identifying comminuted fractures found only one case in a simple fall and this fracture involved the roofs of the orbits. The brain may show acute contusional injury opposite the site of impact. The cause of death is usually a subdural hemorrhage which can be of sufficient severity to cause rapid death without identifiable shift and herniation. This pattern of injury is commonly seen associated with alcohol intoxication.

The possibility of an assault resulting in the impact with the ground must always be considered and any injuries suggestive of that, e.g. black eye, bruising to the chin or mouth, should be documented and the possibility raised with the police/legal authorities. Full neuropathology in such cases may identify diffuse traumatic axonal injury of such a severity that it may be considered inconsistent with a simple fall (Geddes *et al.*, 2000).

Falls from a height

These occur in a wide range of circumstances (buildings, mountains, bridges etc.) and can be accidental, suicidal or homicidal – almost always resolved by the circumstantial evidence rather than the pathology. Devastating head injuries including comminuted and compound skull fractures are common, often associated with severe trauma elsewhere. The pattern of injuries can allow determination of how the body landed. A ring fracture of the base of skull indicates primary impact with the ground by the feet/legs and there may be associated fractures of the feet/ankles/lower legs. Alternatively ipsilateral rib and skull fractures indicate impact at these sites. In these circumstances death is rapid and the brain may show lacerations and other evidence of direct trauma. Sometimes there is only minor head injury as the head secondarily impacts with the ground.

Specific injuries from being pushed or deliberately dropped by another person are rarely, if ever, distinguishable within the multiplicity of injuries in such deaths. Occasionally, however, there may be significant injuries that are inconsistent with the fall and indicate a severe assault before the 'fall', e.g. lacerations from a blunt weapon.

In potential falls from lesser heights, e.g. down stairs, death may result from the fall, usually as a result of head or neck injury but may be from natural disease or they may just have collapsed from any variety of causes. You may see scattered blunt injuries, including to the back, from the stair treads but particularly if protected by clothes there may be minimal external injury.

Sporting injuries

Deaths during sporting activities are fortunately uncommon and most frequently cardiac in nature.

Apparently spontaneous intracranial bleeds should be treated with suspicion as they would be rare in the young and the possibility of neck trauma should be considered.

Direct head trauma may occur from contact in high-speed sports, e.g. skiing and other winter sports or motor sports. Neck injury can be found in rugby or diving, for example. The pattern in such deaths is non-specific, reflecting the nature of the impact. There are two sports that are associated with specific neuropathological problems and which may present to the forensic pathologist.

Boxing

Death due to acute injury is now very uncommon but would usually be a consequence of hemorrhage, nearly always subdural, fatal traumatic subarachnoid and extradural hematomas being rare. Long-term sequelae may be identifiable in the brains of ex-boxers who have died from other causes. These include:

- Fenestration of the septum pellucidum
- Neurofibrillary tangles similar to Alzheimer's disease
- Degeneration and depigmentation of the substantia nigra
- Cerebellar and other scarring

Whilst, individually, these abnormalities can be found after isolated head injury, the quartet has been described so frequently and specifically in boxers that there is now little doubt that boxing is responsible (Mason and Purdue, 2000).

Diving

Both the brain and the spinal cord can be affected as part of decompression illness whereby bubbles of inert gas come out of solution as the diver ascends. Death can occur soon after the onset of severe disease following very rapid decompression, during treatment or later. The CNS involvement is most serious and typically includes infarcts of the spinal cord, particularly the lateral and dorsal columns.

HOMICIDE/ASSAULT

A primary role of any medico-legal post mortem examination is to confirm or exclude criminality (if possible). In some cases it may be known that death occurred following an assault, but a full and thorough post mortem is still essential to confirm the causal link between the two events and to determine if there are other factors potentially involved. If there is anything to suggest a significant head injury, either from the nature of the incident or the injuries, then full neuropathology should be carried out in accordance with Royal College of Pathologists' guidelines. Unexpected findings can completely alter the cause of death and the appropriate charges (Black *et al.*, 2003).

A frequent problem is the interpretation of multiple injuries, often including head injuries, as to whether the pattern is that of an assault or an accident. Many people, particularly those with an alcohol problem, can have extremely extensive bruising and internal injury, including rib fractures and intracranial injury. The pattern of the injuries, particularly the distribution and ages of the bruising can be helpful, frequent falls resulting in bruising of varying ages and in appropriate sites. The possibility of repeated assaults would have to be considered and particular attention paid to, for example, the neck where accidental injuries would be less likely.

Sudden death in head injury

In our experience there are not insignificant numbers of cases where death appears to be the result of a head injury, either through circumstance or by exclusion, but in which there is minimal evidence of traumatic brain injury. In many of these deaths there will be a skull fracture, even a basal hinge fracture indicating considerable force has been applied with no apparent brain injury, but in others there may be only minimal meningeal hemorrhage or contusional injury and no skull fracture. Death may be the result of cerebral edema which can be difficult to confirm at post mortem examination. The circumstances are usually of a very sudden death and the failure to demonstrate traumatic brain injury of a severity to account for death probably reflects the limitations of even modern techniques to detect microscopic traumatic brain injury or neurochemical or autonomic dysfunction.

Subdural and extradural hemorrhage

Subdural (SDH) and extradural hemorrhage (EDH) can both cause deaths following an assault, albeit, particularly in the former, accidental causes must be ruled out as discussed above. The occasional ruptured saccular aneurysm presenting as an SDH must also be excluded.

There are a number of additional issues that are important in a medico-legal context:

- The interpretation of injuries to determine the pattern of the assault, e.g. a single blow may result in a charge of culpable homicide or manslaughter being more appropriate.
- Dating of the hemorrhage is difficult but can be important to correlate with an assault. Circumstantial or eye-witness evidence may assist in interpreting the likely time scale but it should always be cautiously expressed. In particular, alternative explanations, e.g. a subsequent fall, should be explored.
- If multiple assailants were involved, is it possible to determine which one inflicted the relevant blow? For example, is the pattern of injury consistent with a propelled blow to the ground causing the SDH rather than kicking whilst on the ground?
- Were the circumstances such that there was the opportunity for medical intervention and if so could it have prevented the death?

Traumatic brain injury

It is now recognized that there is a spectrum of severity of diffuse axonal injury to the brain and that axons can be damaged as a result of mechanisms other than trauma. Extensive studies utilizing both routine H&E stain and β-amyloid precursor protein (β-APP) stains have demonstrated axonal pathology as a consequence of raised intracranial pressure with hypoxic/ischemic damage and hypoglycemia amongst other causes. It is therefore essential that the brain is adequately sampled to allow accurate assessment of the etiology (Geddes *et al.*, 2000; Graham *et al.*, 2004).

Full histology and immunohistochemistry should be undertaken in cases of potential brain injury, for example where there are external injuries on the head, to assess diffuse traumatic axonal injury. This can be useful even when death appears to have occurred relatively quickly (within a few hours) and there is no macroscopic evidence of brain damage. A number of questions may be answerable:

- Was there a significant head injury that may have resulted in e.g. a degree of concussion?
- Was there a significant period of survival after the assault, reflected by β-APP positivity staining?
- Does its presence relate to the nature and degree of the assault, e.g. simple fall/propelled fall/kicking and punching and thus can it help determine which accused was responsible for the death?
- Would the deceased have been able to function after the assault?

Blunt force trauma

Blunt force trauma to the head is a very common type of fatal assault by any combination of foot, fist or blunt weapon. The spectrum of injury is wide and full neuropathological examination is essential. Certain questions arise to which answers should be sought:

- *Can the weapon(s) used be determined?* A patterned injury can indicate the likely nature of the weapon, e.g. a tramline bruise, or imprint bruise, from footwear. The underlying damage can also aid interpretation as in a classic hammer injury comprising a crescentic laceration and/or associated bruising or abrasion with an underlying scalloped skull fracture. Many blunt injuries are individually non-specific but the site and distribution may suggest the nature of the assault.

- *What is the mechanism of death?* There are many possible mechanisms in such cases. These include inhalation of blood, upper airway obstruction (severe facial bone fractures), direct traumatic brain injury, secondary brain damage (ischemic/hypoxic) and intracranial hemorrhage. Assessment of this can have important medicolegal implications, for example when there are multiple accused who may have had different roles in the assault.

Subarachnoid hemorrhage

Traumatic subarachnoid hemorrhage can be a nonspecific part of a head injury but is commonly used to describe a specific entity which is not without controversy. The typical scenario is of a blow to the side of the neck (just below or behind the ear), often in an intoxicated victim, who subsequently collapses, usually but not always, immediately and is found to have a large, basal subtentorial subarachnoid hemorrhage.

In the classical description, the bleeding originating from a tear in the extracranial vertebral artery (caused by sudden abnormal movement at the atlanto-occipital joint) tracks upwards; the mechanism by which the blood breaches the dura is unclear. In other instances no tear can be identified and there remain doubts in some forensic texts as to the existence of such an entity. In some cases, however, a tear can be identified in the vertebral artery in its course at the base of the brain or indeed in the basilar artery, a finding which is most in keeping with the distribution of the blood and for which one does not have to postulate solutions to the above.

In any case when the pathologist is faced with the possibility of such a death the vertebral and basilar arteries should be examined. Many techniques have been described over the years most of which have problems but with which the practising forensic pathologist should be familiar. Angiography either *in situ* or after removal of the brain can be used if the facility is available and may identify a tear but artefactual defects can complicate the picture. The simplest technique is to detach the cerebral hemispheres above the tentorium and then examine the infratentorial structures *in situ*. It is then possible to remove them transecting the cervical spinal cord as low as possible. The Greenfield's technique may be used if a longer segment of cord is desired. If no tear can be identified in the intracranial course then other techniques which involve exposure of the vertebral arteries within the cervical foramina, either at the time of the examination by use of bone-cutting forceps, or after removal of the cervical spine and decalcification can be undertaken (Saukko and Knight, 2004).

Penetrating injury

Penetrating injury of the brain is a not infrequent result of assault with either a knife or a firearm but any projectile and many weapons (including umbrellas and chair legs) can produce such an injury. The nature of the case may not always be immediately recognized particularly if the external injury is small, not obviously penetrating and/or in a slightly distant site, e.g. over the cheek; all circumstances which have been seen within this department in recent years.

In most cases, however, the cause is self-evident and indeed it is not unusual for the weapon to remain stuck within the cranial cavity, the authors having seen such cases involving knives, swords and an axe. Despite this there is still valuable evidence to be gained from the neuropathological examination:

- Documentation of the direction of the wound/track will correlate with the angle of gunshot or how stabbed, bearing in mind the constant imponderables of the relative position, i.e. not everyone is upright and facing the front!
- The length of a stab wound track will approximate to the minimum length of the weapon.
- Reactive changes adjacent to the injury would indicate a period of survival.
- The structures damaged and/or other neuropathology, e.g. subdural hemorrhage, may allow assessment of whether activity was possible subsequent to the assault and whether the injuries would have been amenable to treatment. The former may be particularly relevant in the not too uncommon scenario when stab wounds penetrate the vertebral column and may have damaged the spinal cord.

Pediatric cases

Pediatric forensic neuropathology is increasingly developing into an area where specific expertise is essential. A main recommendation of the Kennedy Report, *Sudden Unexpected Death in Infancy*, is the establishment of a compulsory national protocol for investigation of infant deaths. It also recommends that the post mortem examination should be undertaken by a pediatric pathologist or a forensic pathologist with training in pediatric pathology. If there is suspicion regarding the death the recommendation is that a forensic pathologist should also be involved (www.rcpath.org).

There are two main, difficult and controversial areas where the forensic pathologist may be involved: possible suffocation and head injury.

Possible suffocation

There may be no positive pathological evidence to be found in cases of suffocation. A thorough examination for injuries around the nose and mouth, including dissection of the face, is essential. Full neuropathology should be carried out to look for previous episodes of hypoxic damage in addition to any evidence of trauma. Other findings, e.g. fresh or old hemorrhage in the airways, should be assessed in line with the current scientific literature (Yukawa *et al.*, 1999). Whilst the history may suggest suffocation as a possibility and there may be other supportive findings it should not be stated as a cause of death without clear pathological evidence that could not be accounted for by other explanations.

Head injury

The main problem that will confront the forensic pathologist is subdural hemorrhage with or without skull fracture and retinal hemorrhage. There have been many publications over the years since the entity of shaken baby syndrome was first described by Caffey (Donohoe, 2003). There has been considerable work in this field in recent years, in particular in relation to the mechanism of injury, including shaking and/or impact and the forces required, only some of which are referenced here (Case *et al.*, 2001; Geddes *et al.*, 2001; Geddes and Whitwell, 2004) An alternative explanation to trauma as put forward by Geddes is based on a hypothesis that is considered controversial and has currently been reviewed in the courts. These questions and the time course whereby such injuries cause death is an increasingly complex area. It is our opinion that evidence regarding shaken baby syndrome now requires forensic and paediatric specialists to have regular experience of investigation in baby deaths. In the absence of such a background the role of the forensic pathologist in such a case may now be confirmation of the pathological facts and referral to those with the appropriate expertise.

FURTHER READING

Asa SL.
Tumours of the pituitary gland. Washington DC: Armed Forces Institute of Pathology, 1998.

Aylward GW, Sullivan TJ, Garner A, *et al.*
Orbital involvement in multifocal fibrosclerosis. *Br J Ophthalmol* 1995; **79**:246–9.

Barrett C, Brett F, Grehan D, McDermott MB.
Heat-accelerated fixation and rapid dissection of the pediatric brain at autopsy: a pragmatic approach to the difficulties of organ retention. *Pediatr Dev Pathol* 2004; **7**:595–600.

Bell JE.
Pathogenesis and pathology of neural tube defects. *Obstet Ultrasound* 1994; **2**:28–49.

Bell JE, Becher J-C, Wyatt B, *et al.*
Brain damage and axonal injury in a Scottish cohort of neonatal deaths. *Brain* 2005; **128**:1070–81.

Bell JE, Fryer AA, Collins, *et al.*
Developmental profile of plasma proteins in human fetal cerebrospinal fluid and blood. *Neuropathol App Neurobiol* 1991; **17**:441–56.

Berry M, Butt AM, Wilkin G, Perry VH.
Structure and function of glia in the central nervous system. In: Graham DI, Lantos PL. (Eds) *Greenfield's neuropathology*, 7th edition. London: Arnold, 2002: 75–121.

Bigner DD, McLendon RE, Bruner JM.
Russell and Rubinstein's pathology of tumours of the nervous system, 6th edition. London: Arnold, 1998.

Black M, Fernando R, Graham DI, Kean D.
Unsuspected meningo-encephalitis in a case of assault by blunt force trauma. *Am J Forensic Med Pathol* 2003; **24**:356–60.

Black M, Graham DI.
Sudden death in epilepsy. *Curr Diag Pathol* 2002; **8**:365–72.

Bradley WG (Ed.)
Neurology in clinical practice, 4th edition. Oxford: Butterworth Heinemann, 2004.

Brodal A.
Neurological anatomy in relation to clinical medicine, 3rd edition. Oxford: Oxford University Press, 1981.

Burger PC, Scheithauer BW.
Tumours of the central nervous system. Washington DC: Armed Forces Institute of Pathology, 1994.

Burger PC, Scheithauer BW, Vogel FS.
Surgical pathology of the nervous system and its coverings, 4th edition. New York: Churchill Livingstone, 2002.

Byard RW, Krous HF. (Eds)
Sudden infant death syndrome. London: Arnold, 2001.

Case ME, Graham MA, Handy TC, *et al.* Position paper on fatal abusive head injuries in infants and young children. *Am J Forensic Med Pathol* 2001; 22:112–22.

Cherian S, Whitelaw A, Thoresen M, Love S. The pathogenesis of neonatal post-haemorrhagic hydrocephalus. *Brain Pathol* 2004; **14**:305–11.

Cohen MM, Sulik KK. Perspectives on holosprosencephaly, Part II: central nervous system, craniofacial anatomy, syndrome commentary, diagnostic approach and experimental studies. *J Craniofacial Genet Devel Biol* 1992; 12:196–244.

Cowan F, Rutherford MA, Groenendaal F, *et al.* Origin and timing of brain lesions in term infants with neonatal encephalopathy. *Lancet* 2003; **361**:736.

Coupland SE, Hummel M, Stein H. Ocular adnexal lymphomas: five case presentations and a review of the literature. *Surv Ophthalmol* 2002; **47**:470–90.

Dawson TP, Neal JW, Llewellyn L, Thomas C. *Neuropathology techniques.* London: Arnold, 2003.

Donohoe M. Evidence based medicine and shaken baby syndrome. *Am J Forensic Med Pathol* 2003; **24**:239–42.

Dorries C. *Coroners' courts: a guide to law and practice.* Chichester: John Wiley, 1999.

Duckett S. *Pediatric neuropathology.* Baltimore: Williams & Williams, 1995.

Ellison D, Love S, Chimelli L, Harding BM, Lowe J, Vinters HV. *Neuropathology. A reference text of CNS pathology*, 2nd edition. London: Mosby, 2004.

Esiri MM. *Oppenheimer's diagnostic neuropathology. A practical manual.* Oxford: Blackwell Science, 1996.

Freije WA, Castro-Vargas FE, Fang Z, *et al.* Gene expression profiling of gliomas strongly predicts survival. *Cancer Res* 2004; **64**:6503–10.

Friede RL. *Developmental neuropathology*, 2nd edition. Berlin: Springer Verlag, 1989.

Geddes JF, Hackshaw AK, Vowles GH, *et al.* Neuropathology of inflicted head injury in children. I. Patterns of brain damage. *Brain* 2001; **124**:1290–8.

Geddes JF, Whitwell HL. Inflicted head injury in infants. *Forensic Sci Int* 2004; **146**:83–8.

Geddes JF, Whitwell HL, Graham DI. Traumatic axonal injury: practical issues for diagnosis in medicolegal cases. *Neuropathol Appl Neurobiol* 2000; **26**:105–16.

Geddes JF, Vowles GH, Hackshaw AK, *et al.* Neuropathology of inflicted head injury in children. II. Microscopic brain injury in infants. *Brain* 2001; **124**:1299–306.

Godard S, Getz G, Delorenzi M, *et al.* Classification of human astrocytic gliomas on the basis of gene expression: a correlated group of genes with angiogenic activity emerges as a strong predictor of subtypes. *Cancer Res* 2003; **63**:6613–25.

Golden JA, Harding BN. (Eds) *Pathology and genetics. Developmental neuropathology.* Basel: ISN Neuropath Press, 2004.

Gordon LK. Diagnostic dilemmas in orbital inflammatory disease. *Ocular Immunol Inflamm* 2003; **11**:3–15.

Graeber MB, Blakemore WF, Kreutzberg GW.
Cellular pathology of the central nervous system. In: Graham DI, Lantos PL. (Eds) *Greenfield's neuropathology*, 7th edition. London: Arnold, 2002: 123–91.

Graham D, Montine TJ.
Neurotoxicology. In: Graham DI, Lantos PL. (Eds) *Greenfield's neuropathology*, 7th edition. London: Arnold, 2002: 799–822.

Graham DI, Bell JE, Ironside JW.
Color atlas and text of neuropathology. London: Mosby-Wolfe, 1995.

Graham DI, Lantos PL.
Greenfield's neuropathology, 7th edition. Arnold: London, 2002.

Graham DI, Smith C, Reichard R, *et al.*
Trials and tribulations of using β-amyloid precursor protein immunohistochemistry to evaluate traumatic brain injury in adults. *Forensic Sci Int* 2004; **146**:89–96.

Gray F, de Girolami U, Poirier J.
Escourolle and Poirier. Manual of basic neuropathology, 4th edition. Philadelphia: Butterworth Heinemann, 2004.

Ironside JW, Moss TH, Louis DN, Lowe JS, Weller RO.
Diagnostic pathology of nervous system tumours. London: Churchill-Livingstone, 2002.

Ironside JW, Pickard JD.
Raised intracranial pressure, oedema and hydrocephalus. In: Graham DI, Lantos PL. (Eds) *Greenfield's neuropathology*, 7th edition. London: Arnold, 2002: 193–231.

Iwadate Y, Sakaida T, Hiwasa T, *et al.*
Molecular classification and survival prediction in human gliomas based on proteome analysis. *Cancer Res* 2004; **64**:2496–501.

Jakobiec FA, Bilyk JR, Font RL.
Orbit. In: Spencer WH. (ed.) *Ophthalmic pathology: An atlas and text.* Philadelphia: WB Saunders, 1996.

Jenkins C, Rose GE, Bunce C, *et al.*
Clinical features associated with survival of patients with lymphoma of the ocular adnexa. *Eye* 2003; **17**:809–20.

Kalimo H. (Ed.)
Pathology and genetics: Cerebrovascular diseases. Basel: ISN Neuropath Press, 2005.

Karparti G.
Structural and molecular basis of skeletal muscle diseases. Basel: ISN Neuropath Press, 2002.

Keeling JW. (Ed.)
Fetal and neonatal pathology, 3rd edition. London: Springer, 2001: Chapters 1, 4, 5, 23 and 24.

Kinney HC, Armstrong DD.
Perinatal neuropathology. In: Graham DI, Lantos PL. (Eds) *Greenfield's neuropathology*, 7th edition. London: Arnold, 2002: 519–605.

Kleihues P, Cavenee WK.
Pathology and genetics of tumours of the nervous system. Lyon: IARC Press, 2001.

Krishnakumar S, Subramanian N, Mohan ER, *et al.*
Solitary fibrous tumor of the orbit: a clinicopathologic study of six cases with review of the literature. *Surv Ophthalmol* 2003; **48**:544–54.

Lamont JM, McManamy CS, Pearson AD, *et al.*
Combined histopathological and molecular cytogenetic stratification of medulloblastoma patients. *Clin Cancer Res* 2004; **10**:5482–93.

Lee WR.
Ophthalmic histopathology, 2nd edition. London: Springer Verlag, 2002.

Lindsay KW, Bone I, Callendar R.
Neurology and neurosurgery illustrated, 4th edition. Edinburgh: Churchill Livingstone, 2004.

Love S.
Post mortem sampling of the brain and other tissues in neurodegenerative disease. *Histopathology* 2004; **44**:309–17.

Mason JK, Purdue BN. (Eds)
The pathology of trauma. London: Arnold, 2000.

Midroni G, Bilbao JM.
Biopsy diagnosis of peripheral neuropathy. Butterworth Heinemann, 1995.

Moss TR, Nicoll JAR, Ironside JW.
Intra-operative diagnosis of CNS tumours. London: Arnold, 1997.

Mrak RE, Griffin WST.
Trisomy 21 and the brain. *JNEN* 2004; **63**:670–85.

Norman MG, McGillvray BC, Kalousek DK, *et al.*
Congenital malformations of the brain. New York: Oxford University Press, 1995.

Nutt CL, Mani DR, Betensky RA, *et al.*
Gene expression-based classification of malignant gliomas correlates better with survival than histological classification. *Cancer Res* 2003; **63**:1602–7.

Oldfors A, Tulinius M, Nennesmo I, Harding BN.
Mitochondrial disorders. In: Golden JA, Harding BM. (Eds) *Pathology and genetics. Developmental neuropathology*. Basel: ISN Neuropath Press, 2004: 296–302.

Patten JP.
Neurological differential diagnosis, 2nd edition. London: Springer, 1995.

Perry SR, Rootman J, White VA.
The clinical and pathologic constellation of Wegener's granulomatosis of the orbit. *Ophthalmology* 1997; **104**:683–94.

Pomeroy SL, Tamayo P, Gaasenbeek M, *et al.*
Prediction of central nervous system embryonal tumour outcome based on gene expression. *Nature* 2002; **415**:436–42.

Powers JM.
Peroxisomal disorders. In: Golden JA, Harding BM. (Eds) *Pathology and genetics. Developmental neuropathology*. Basel: ISN Neuropath Press, 2004: 287–96.

Powers JM, De Vivo DC.
Peroxisomal and mitochondrial disorders. In: Graham DI, Lantos PL. (Eds) *Greenfield's neuropathology*, 7th edition. London: Arnold, 2002: 737–788.

Reifenberger G, Louis DN.
Oligodendroglioma: toward molecular definitions in diagnostic neuro-oncology. *J Neuropathol Exp Neurol* 2003; **62**:111–26.

Royal College of Pathologists and the Royal College of Paediatrics and Child Health.
Sudden unexpected death in infancy. London: 2004. (Known as the Kennedy Report.)

Saukko P, Knight B.
Knight's forensic pathology, 3rd edition. London: Arnold, 2004.

Schochet SS, Gray F.
Acquired metabolic disorders. In: Gray F, de Girolami U, Poirier J. (Eds) *Escourolle and Poirier. Manual of basic neuropathology*, 4th edition. Philadelphia: Butterworth Heinemann, 2004: 197–217.

Shields JA, Shields CL, Scartozzi R.
Survey of 1264 patients with orbital tumors and simulating lesions: The 2002 Montgomery Lecture, part 1. *Ophthalmology* 2004; **111**:997–1008.

Simpson JL, Elias S.
Genetics in obstetrics and gynaecology, 3rd edition. Philadelphia: Saunders, 2003.

Smith C, Graham DI.
Extradural and subdural haematomas. In: Kallimo H. (Ed.) *Cerebrovascular diseases.* Basel: ISN Neuropath Press, 2005.

Sotelo C, Triller A.
The central neuron. In: Graham DI, Lantos PL. (Eds) *Greenfield's neuropathology*, 7th edition. London: Arnold, 2002: 1–74.

Squier W. (Ed.)
Acquired damage to the developing brain. Timing and causation. London: Arnold, 2002.

www.cgap.nci.nih.gov

www.dh.gov.uk/PublicationsAndStatistics/Publications/PublicationsAndLegislation

www.dh.gov.uk/PublicationsAndStatistics/Publications/PublicationPolicyAndGuidance

www.genome.gov/

www.homeoffice.gov.uk/justice/

www.neuro.wustl.edu/neuromuscular/ (For information by Alan Pestronk.)

www.official-documents.co.uk/

www.repath.org

www.scotland.gov.uk/Topics/Health

www.show.scot.nhs.uk/scotorgrev

www.theshipmaninquiry.org.uk

www.uk-legislation.opsi.gov.uk/si/si2005

Yukawa N, Carter N, Rutty G, Green M.
Intra-alveolar haemorrhage in sudden infant death syndrome: a cause for concern? *J Clin Pathol* 1999; 52:581–7.

INDEX

Notes: abbreviations used in the index are explained on pp. xv–xvii; page numbers in **bold** refer to tables or figures